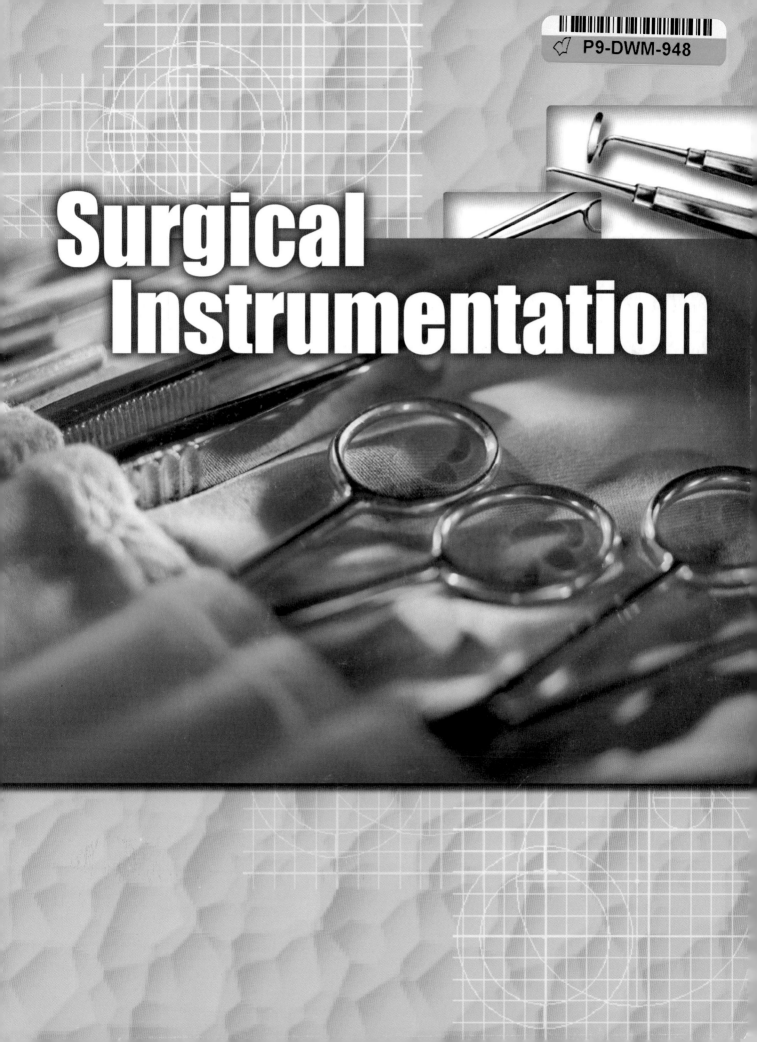

Surgical Instrumentation

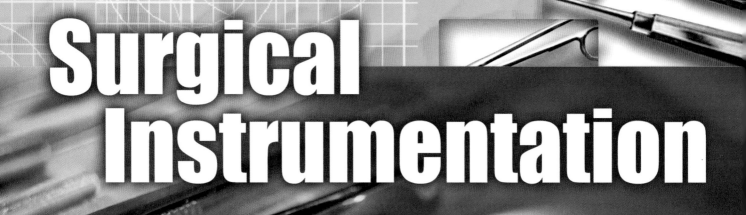

Surgical Instrumentation

Nancymarie Phillips, RN, PhD, RNFA, CNOR

Patricia Kennedy Sedlak, RN, BSN, MEd, RNFA, CST, CNOR

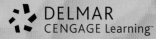

DELMAR
CENGAGE Learning™

Australia • Brazil • Japan • Korea • Mexico • Singapore • Spain • United Kingdom • United States

DEDICATION

This book is dedicated to perioperative students and their educators in all disciplines.

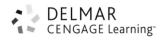

Surgical Instrumentation
Nancymarie Phillips, Patricia Kennedy Sedlak

Vice President, Career and Professional Editorial: Dave Garza

Director of Learning Solutions: Matthew Kane

Executive Editor: Stephen Helba

Senior Acquisitions Editor: Rhonda Dearborn

Managing Editor: Marah Bellegarde

Senior Product Manager: Sarah Prime

Editorial Assistant: Meghan Orvis

Vice President, Career and Professional Marketing: Jennifer Ann Baker

Executive Marketing Manager: Wendy E. Mapstone

Marketing Manager: Nancy Bradshaw

Marketing Coordinator: Erica Ropitzky

Production Director: Carolyn Miller

Content Project Manager: Brooke Greenhouse

Senior Art Director: Jack Pendleton

For product information and technology assistance, contact us at
Cengage Learning Customer & Sales Support, 1-800-354-9706
For permission to use material from this text or product,
submit all requests online at **www.cengage.com/permissions**
Further permissions questions can be emailed to
permissionrequest@cengage.com

Library of Congress Control Number: 2009932218

ISBN-13: 978-1-4018-3297-1

ISBN-10: 1-4018-3297-0

Delmar
Executive Woods
5 Maxwell Drive
Clifton Park, NY 12065
USA

Cengage Learning is a leading provider of customized learning solutions with office locations around the globe, including Singapore, the United Kingdom, Australia, Mexico, Brazil, and Japan. Locate your local office at **www.cengage.com/global**

Cengage Learning products are represented in Canada by Nelson Education, Ltd.

To learn more about Delmar, visit **www.cengage.com/delmar**

Purchase any of our products at your local bookstore or at our preferred online store **www.cengagebrain.com**

Printed in China by China Translation & Printing Services Limited.
2 3 4 5 6 7 15 14 13 12 11

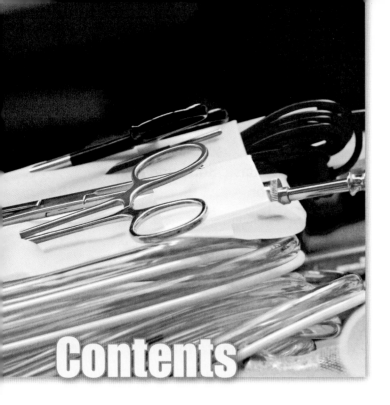

Contents

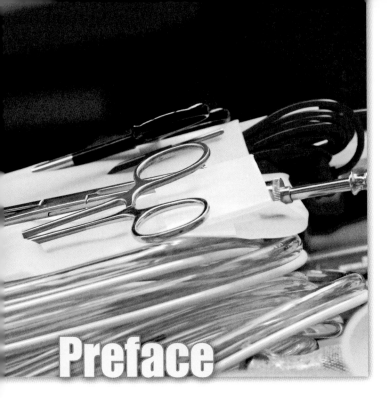

Preface

This text, *Surgical Instrumentation,* is designed for perioperative personnel in all surgical disciplines. Surgeons, nurses, technologists, and technicians will find the design and collections in this book informative and user-friendly. Books about surgical instrumentation have been in print for more than one hundred years. However, none have offered comprehensive collections of instruments used with foundation sets for multiple specialties. They feature individual instruments without providing guidance for establishing or streamlining the set creation process.

THE DEVELOPMENT OF THIS TEXT

The four foundation sets described in this text are designed to be base units for use during procedures that meet the needed instrument weight, length, gage, shape, and material necessary for a safe efficient surgical procedure. The additional instrument groupings, such as those specific to a particular organ or region of the body, can be established as "add-on" sets to be used in combination with the appropriate foundation set.

Every perioperative nurse or surgical technologist who scrubs has encountered sets with instruments that have not been used for many years, yet the items continue to be packed into the tray for no apparent reason. This book may serve as a guide for establishing stan-

dardized instrument sets that will facilitate the count process and ease the burden of inventory control.

ORGANIZATION OF THE TEXT

This text is divided into 15 chapters. Images of the surgical instrumentation are displayed in table form with descriptions and sizes listed.

- *History of Surgical Instrumentation.* The first chapter describes the history of surgical instrumentation and provides background information about the philosophy and contributions of different cultures to the discipline of surgery.

- *Anatomy and Physiology of Surgical Instrumentation.* The materials and characteristics of surgical instruments are explored, as well as the design from handle to tip.

- *Categories of Surgical Instrumentation.* Surgical instruments are designed for specific functions and are grouped into functional categories that define the purpose for each instrument. Specific groupings make it easier to learn the instruments.

- *Considerations for Instrument Set Assembly.* Trays and containers for packaging instruments are described in this chapter. Accountability is a team effort that begins with the construction and assembly of each set.

- *Soft Tissue Foundation Sets.* The foundation sets are designed to meet specific needs for a procedure at a basic level by grouping instruments by category and function.

- *Plastic Surgery Instrumentation.* Instruments specific to the type of plastic surgery procedure are described in combination with foundation sets.

- *General Surgery Instrumentation.* Functional instruments that are added to foundation sets for general surgery are described by organ system and body location.

- *Gynecologic Instrumentation.* Specialty instrumentation specific to the needs for surgery of the female reproductive tract are described.

- *Urologic Instrumentation.* Instrumentation specific to genitourinary procedures of the urethra and kidney are included in this chapter.

- *Basic Bone and Joint Instrumentation.* Many specialties utilize instrumentation to debulk, dissect, or repair bony tissue throughout the body. The bone instruments are used in combination with soft tissue foundation sets according to the location on the body.

- *Head and Neck Procedure Instrumentation.* Upper airway and otorhinolaryngology procedures require specialty instrumentation designed for narrow passages and the soft tissues of the anterior neck and throat.

- *Neurosurgery Instrumentation.* Procedures of the brain and spinal cord use a unique blend of soft tissue sets, compact tissue sets, and microsurgical sets. Instrumentation for procedures of the cranium and spine are described.

- *Cardiovascular and Thoracic Instrumentation.* Instrumentation used for surgical procedures of the lungs, heart, and vascular system is described.

- *Instruments for Microscopic Surgery.* Microsurgery is usually performed on soft tissues. These sets can be used in combination with foundation sets or as stand alone sets.

- *Endoscopic Instrumentation.* The application of endoscopic techniques to multiple specialties is described. Percutaneous and natural orifice endoscopy is described in functional terms.

Surgical Instrumentation has a workbook and online companion web site designed to enhance student learning. Access the online companion web site at www.cengage.com/delmar, by clicking on "Allied Health" on the left navigation menu, and this book's title. Three decks of instrument flash cards, arranged by surgery type, are available as companion products. An instructor's manual is available for faculty.

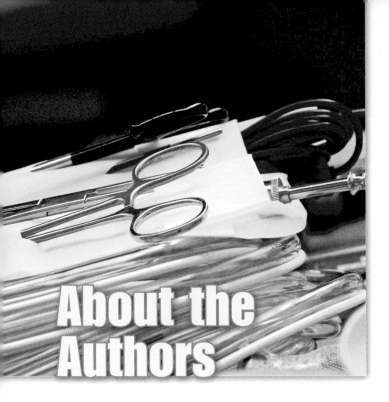

About the Authors

Nancymarie Phillips, RN, PhD, RNFA, CNOR. Dr. Phillips is the Program Director for Perioperative Education at Lakeland Community College in Kirtland, Ohio. Her programs include Perioperative Nursing, Registered Nurse First Assisting, and Surgical Technology. She has authored numerous articles and texts about perioperative patient care. She was the 2006 recipient of the AORN Perioperative Clinical Education Award, the 2006 Lakeland Community College Teaching Excellence Award, and was a nominee for the 2006 *Ohio Magazine* Excellence in Education Award. Dr. Phillips is a member of AORN, AST, and Sigma Theta Tau.

Dr. Phillips has been a perioperative nurse since 1975. In addition, she has worked as a scrub nurse, circulator, first assistant, consultant, author, and educator. She can be reached at nphillips@lakelandcc.edu or nancymphillips@aol.com. Her website is www.nvo.com/delphipro.

Patricia K. Sedlak, RN, BSN, MEd, RNFA, CST, CNOR, is the Director of Surgical Technology and Registered Nurse First Assistant programs at Lorain Community College in Lorain, Ohio, where she produces an award winning Surgical Technology program, which has been the recipient of numerous grants for international work in 2001, 2003, and 2004.

Mrs. Sedlak was the recipient of the 1998 and 2002 Lorain Community College Teaching Excellence Award, the 2002 Ohio Association of Two Year College's (OATYC) Teacher of the Year Award, and the 2003 *Ohio Magazine* Excellence in Education Award.

Mrs. Sedlak has 25 years experience in perioperative nursing and perioperative education and is a member of AORN, AST, and Sigma Theta Tau. She can be reached at patsedlak@comcast.net.

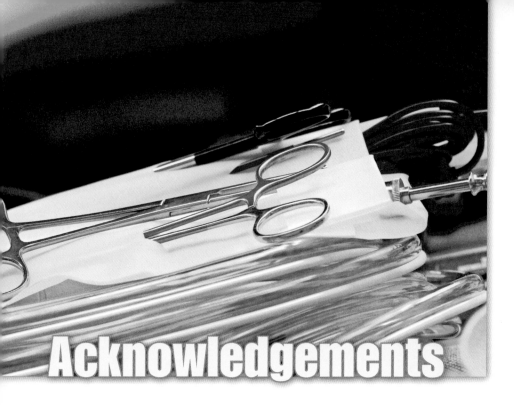

Acknowledgements

The authors wish to thank Rhonda Dearborn, Senior Acquisitions Editor for Delmar, Cengage Learning, and Sarah Prime, Senior Product Manager, for their help and guidance in this project. A special thanks also goes to Regina Elam, CST, Bonnie Venchiarutti, CST, and Denell Lewalk, MLS, Jennifer Gerres, D.P.M. for their assistance in this massive undertaking.

Reviewers

The authors and publisher would like to thank the following reviewers for their feedback during the development process.

Sandra Berch, RN, BSN, CNOR
Surgical Technology Program Director
Indian River Community College
Port St. Lucie, FL

Susan Whaley Boggs, RN, BSN, CNOR
Surgical Technology Program Coordinator
Piedmont Technical College
Greenwood, SC

Gennie Castleberry, BS, CST
Program Director
University of Arkansas for Medical Sciences
Little Rock, AR

Karen L. Chambers, CST-ACLS
Director
Long Island University
Brooklyn, NY

April S. Davis, RN, BSN, CNOR
Faculty for the School of Surgical Technology
Carolinas College of Health Sciences
Charlotte, NC

Alicia Freeman, CST, AAS
Surgical Technology Instructor
Tennessee Technology Center at Paris
Paris, TN

Jane Klick, RN, CNOR
Coordinator Surgical Technology Program
Columbia Public Schools
Columbia, MO

Deborah Pearson, CST, FA, CRCST, CCM
Surgical Technology Program Director/Instructor
D.G. Erwin Technical Center
Tampa, FL

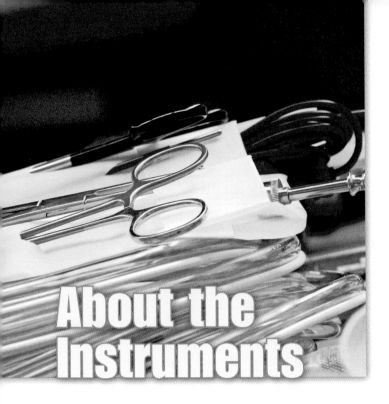

About the Instruments

The instruments appearing in this book have been graciously provided by the following manufacturers:

Accurate Surgical & Scientific Instruments Corporation (ASSI)
www.accuratesurgical.com
300 Shames Drive
Westbury, NY 11590
Phone: 516-333-2570
Toll-free: 800-645-3569
Fax: 516-997-4948
Email: assi@accuratesurgical.com

Cardinal Health
V. Mueller Products and Services
www.cardinal.com
7000 Cardinal Place
Dublin, OH 43017
Phone: 614-757-5000
Toll-free: 800-323-9088

Cook Medical Inc.
www.cookmedical.com
P.O. Box 4195
Bloomington, IN 47402
Phone: 812-339-2235
Toll-free: 800-457-4500
Fax: 800-554-8335
Email: sales.ops@cookmedical.com

Integra LifeSciences Corporation
JARIT Surgical Instruments
Padgett Surgical Instruments
R&B Surgical Instruments
Ruggles Surgical Instruments
www.integra-ls.com
311 Enterprise Drive
Plainsboro, NJ 08536
Phone: 609-275-0500
Fax: 609-275-5363

Karl Storz Endoscopy-America, Inc.
www.karlstorz.com
600 Corporate Pointe 5th Floor
Culver City, CA 90230
Phone: 310-338-8100
Toll-free: 800-421-0837
Fax: 310-410-5527

Miltex, Inc.
www.miltex.com
589 Davies Drive
York, PA 17402
Phone: 717-840-9336
Toll-free: 800-221-1344
Fax: 717-640-9347

Roboz Surgical Instrument Co.
www.roboz.com
P.O. Box 10710
Gaithersburg, MD 20898
Phone: 301-590-0055
Toll-free: 800-424-2974
Fax: 888-424-3121
Email: info@roboz.com

Scanlan International
www.scanlaninternational.com
1 Scanlan Plaza
St. Paul, MN 55107
Phone: 651-298-0997
Toll-free: 800-328-9458
Email: info@scanlangroup.com

Sklar Instruments
www.sklarcorp.com
889 South Matlack Street
West Chester, PA 19382
Phone: 610-430-3200
Toll-free: 800-221-2166
Fax: 610-696-9007
Email: surgi@sklarcorp.com

Sontec Instruments
www.sontecinstruments.com
7248 South Tucson Way
Centennial, CO 80112
Phone: 303-790-9411
Toll-free: 800-821-7496
Fax: 303-792-2606
Email: info@sontecinstruments.com

STERIS Corporation
www.steris.com
5960 Heisley Road
Mentor, OH 44060
Phone: 440-354-2600
Toll-free: 800-548-4873

Surgical Tools, Inc.
www.surgicaltools.com
404A Walnut Ave, SE
Roanoke, VA 24014
Phone: 540-427-0191
Toll-free: 800-774-2040
Fax: 540-427-0193

Teleflex Medical
www.teleflexmedical.com
4024 Stirrup Creek
Research Triangle Park, NC 27703
Phone: 919-544-8000
Toll-free: 866-246-6990
Fax: 919-433-4989

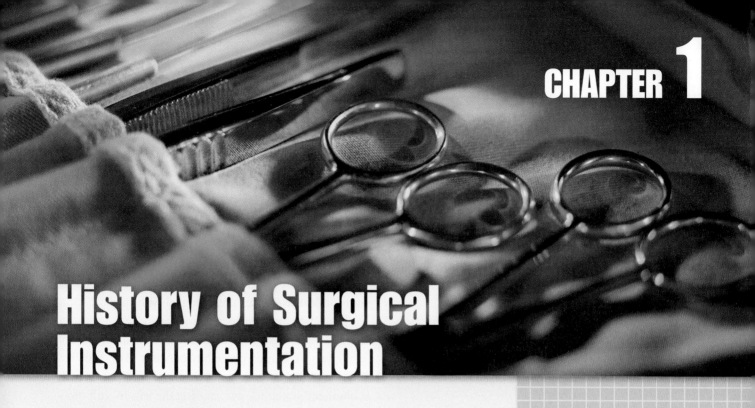

CHAPTER 1

History of Surgical Instrumentation

INTRODUCTION

Since the beginning of time, man has sought to appease the gods and remedy the failings of the human body with the medical and surgical arts. Each culture has historically approached medicine and surgery in a different way and has lent a societal touch to the evolution of surgical practice.

HISTORIC SURGICAL INSTRUMENTATION

Forms of early surgical practice encompassed tending injuries and wounds associated with animal encounters or battles. Some Neolithic tribes were known to have practiced amputation for serious injury, tumors, or infection. Relics of surgical instruments, such as sharpened flints and natural substances like shells, have been found wherever civilizations have been uncovered. Scientists have speculated dates ranging from 10,000 BC for early incisions to 2500 BC for suturing with horsehair or animal tendons.

Hindus developed the earliest known organized practice of surgery (shastrakarma), which is one of the eight branches of Ayurveda (Indian Medicine). Shusruta (circa 800 BC), a medical practitioner from Benares, India, wrote the *Samhita*. In this text he described the need for cleanliness and precision in surgical treatment. His writings were captioned under seven topics: esya (exploration), ahrya (extraction), chedya (excision), lekhya (scarification), vedhya (puncturing), vsraya (evacuation), and sivya (suturing). He based his methods of surgery on his studies of anatomy using dead bodies. Shusruta developed 121 separate surgical instruments of natural materials, such as bone, ivory, mussel shell, and stone. He also advocated the use of hypnosis and wine as anesthetics.

RITUAL AND MAGIC

Prehistoric man performed documented incisional procedures as early as 6000 BC. Scientists speculate that some procedures, such as opening holes into the skull (known as trepanation), were performed for ritualistic or magic reasons. Significant numbers of skulls have been found that indicate the patients lived for many years after the procedure, as new bone growth was identified around the cut edges of the bony holes. Figure 1-1 depicts trepanation instruments used for opening skull bone.

The ancient Egyptians did not feature cutting as a primary medical treatment. Egyptian temple and tomb art indicate that most of the anatomic study involved the embalming of bodies for burial. The religious sects were guardians of physical knowledge and held the internal anatomy sacred. Archeologists discovered papyri that described medical care during this period. American Edwin Smith purchased a 22-page papyrus dating from 1500 BC in 1862 that contained many treatments performed during the ancient times. It was later deciphered by James Henry Breasted. German Egyptologist George Ebers purchased a similar papyrus in 1872 that consisted of 110 pages that dated back to the First Dynasty in 3000 BC. A later papyrus was written as a guide for midwives and those who cared for female patients. These papyri contained medical and surgical references intermingled with magical spells for protection against supernatural forces.

Cataract surgery, known as couching in many ancient lands, was a common procedure between 1345–1200 BC. This surgery was performed by using a rod-like tool with a blunt end to tap the eye, causing the lens to shift away from the pupil. This allowed light to enter. Later methods of performing this procedure included inserting a needle into the eye to dislodge the natural lens (Figure 1-2).

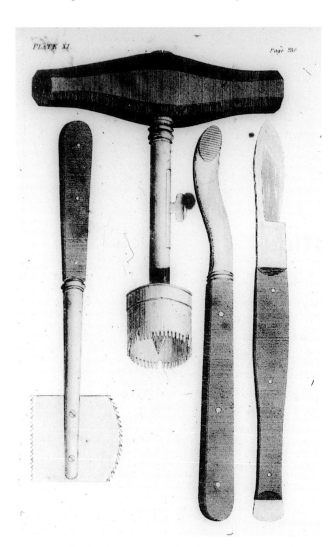

Figure 1-1   Ancient trepanation instruments. *Courtesy of the National Library of Medicine.*

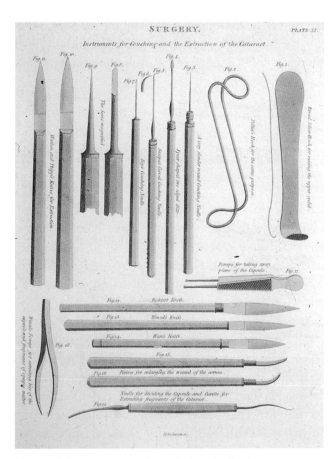

Figure 1-2   Instruments used historically for cataract surgery. *Courtesy of the National Library of Medicine.*

Mesopotamian society (circa 3500 BC) exercised generalized laws and rules governing conduct. They had a concept of comparative worth concerning human life and believed in medical training before commencing practice. The physicians in Mesopotamia identified specific procedures, named each drug used in medical care, and kept records of medical and surgical activities by carving cuneiform figures into clay tablets. Over 20,000 such tablets have been discovered.

Ancient Babylonians (modern-day Iraq) were led by the great King Hammurabi (1795–1750 BC). He established the first known major metropolis and set forth the law that bears his name. The law was clear in regards to medical treatment. A surgeon who successfully treated his nobleman patient would be paid 10 shekels for his labor. If he treated a slave he was paid two shekels, and for treatment of a freeman, he would be paid five shekels. If the nobleman or freeman patient died, the surgeon could lose a hand. If a slave died, the surgeon had to repay the cost of the slave to his master. The law was carved in black diorite stone that stood eight feet tall and was designed like a monument for display in a public location in the city, until it was taken by warring tribes as a trophy. It was discovered in Persia in 1901. The entire code of Hammurabi has been translated into English and is available online at http://www.fordham.edu/halsall, by using the Search button on the left navigation bar and searching for Code of Hammurabi.

Greek civilization gave rise to more organized written texts on medicine and health. The Greeks encouraged a scholarly approach and established formal schools. Most of the surgery performed dealt with war wounds and orthopaedic injury. The Greeks used palm bark and wood bound by moist clay and linen strips to stabilize broken bones like splints. Hippocrates (460–377 BC) used instruments of hardened iron, copper, bronze, and brass. His surgical armamentarium consisted of more than 200 types of surgical instruments. Although physicians were trained in medical and surgical treatments, the main focus of healthcare dealt with diet and exercise.

The early Romans had knowledge of steel. The ancient ruins of Pompeii (circa 310 BC to 79 AD) revealed an instrument manufacturer's place of business with preserved bundles of surgical tools made of several metals wrapped in protective fabric. Homes of physicians revealed beautifully carved boxes for instrument storage. Most of the surgical practice was borrowed from other cultures. Couching was performed as a necessity to displace cataracts. Surgery was considered manual labor and the ancient Roman physicians contributed very little to surgical knowledge. In fact, artists frequently had a greater knowledge of the human body than physicians because they studied corpses during postmortem dissection.

Arabian surgeons established a school for brain surgery in Islam in 800 AD. Other surgical procedures were also performed, such as couching. However, little was known of human anatomy because human dissection was banned by the Koran. During this era, Andalusia (Moorish Spain) was part of the Islamic Empire. A famous skilled Moorish surgeon of the time, El Zahrawi (940–1013 AD), wrote an encyclopedia of 30 volumes referred to as the At-Tasrif to record methods of medical and surgical treatment. He taught his students to treat each patient as an individual and to practice within ethical limits. His writings guided the development of most surgical textbooks in European universities between the 12th and 17th centuries AD. Many of the surgical instruments used during that period were designed by El Zahrawi himself, who personally drew the 200 illustrations for his texts. He is also credited with being the first to use ligatures for hemostasis in surgery. The history and images of El Zahrawi and other Muslim physicians are available online at www.ummah.net/history/scholars.

The Chinese practiced acupuncture and acupressure for at least 2,000 years of recorded history. The central belief of these practices is that there is a mind–body–spirit connection to health and wellness associated with the Ch'i, or life-force. The main focus of health and wellness was not based in surgical procedures, but in a pharmacopoeia of 1,800 medicinal herbs, biologic materials, and chemicals.

The ancient Aztec civilization left little written history, but significant evidence of successful surgery has been unearthed in archeological explorations. They had a strong knowledge of human anatomy because their culture practiced human dissection on their enemies. They felt that they captured the essence of the life-force if they cut the beating heart from the chest of their captives. Blood sacrifice was a daily event. The main feature of their surgical armamentarium was sharp dissection of bone and soft tissues.

SUMMARY

Throughout history, physicians have devised and modified available materials for use in surgical procedures. As scientists contributed new knowledge of metals and eventually synthetics, such as plastics, instrumentation became more functional, incorporating the principles of physics. The increasing knowledge base concerning human anatomy and physiology led physicians to create new tools for exploration and treatment of body regions never surgically treated before. With each successive era, the sophistication of surgical instrumentation has improved significantly.

REFERENCES

Ahmed, M. (2008). Muslim scientists and scholars. Retrieved August 12, 2008, from www.ummah.net/history/scholars.

Haeger, K. (1988). *The illustrated history of surgery.* New York: Bell.

Phillips, N. M. (2007). *Berry and Kohn's operating room technique* (11th ed.). St. Louis: Mosby-Elsevier.

Rutkow, I. M., & Burns, S. B. (1998). *American surgery: An illustrated history.* Philadelphia: Norman Publishing.

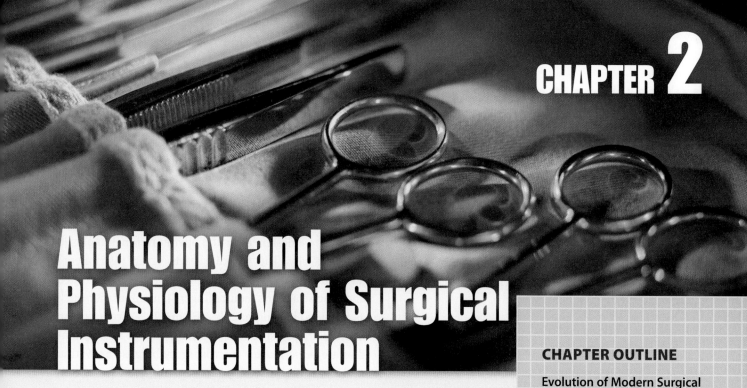

CHAPTER 2

Anatomy and Physiology of Surgical Instrumentation

INTRODUCTION

Surgical instrumentation is the most essential element of an efficient operating room. Surgical procedures require instruments of different sizes, shapes, and chemical composition in order to accomplish specific actions within a patient's body. This chapter describes the importance of the anatomy of surgical instrumentation and why so many types and styles are needed to perform surgical procedures on various types of tissues.

EVOLUTION OF MODERN SURGICAL INSTRUMENTATION

How does a physician improve on a design that has been used since the beginning of recorded medical history? The answer is interesting because many instruments in use today are direct replicas of historic tools. Ambroise Paré (1510–1590) collected surgical instruments for his use in patient care. Most of the surgical tools in the illustration were modeled after instruments used by the ancients. Modern instrumentation is modeled after long-standing styles with modifications to suit contemporary surgical procedures.

ANATOMY OF A SURGICAL INSTRUMENT

Basic design attributes are essentially standardized according to the function of the instrument. Modifications are derived from the baseline instrument. A simple form of instrument anatomy is depicted by the small mosquito hemostat shown in Figure 2-1. It has all the standard design components, such as jaws, box locks, shanks, and handles. The essential standardized design components include the following:

- The working end that contacts the patient's tissues
- The functional mechanism or component that makes the instrument perform its task
- The handle or hand grip held by the operator

With the previous components in mind, the design possibilities are endless. Surgical instruments can be as simple as a single rod or as complex as 15 to 20 moving parts. High tech instrumentation can make contact with the patient through radio frequencies or collimated light waves. Although the contact point is intangible, all of the design elements are present including the functional mechanism and the control used by the operator.

Handle Styles

Handles are designed for the operator's functional grip and dexterity. The working parts of an instrument's jaws commonly dictate the handle style. Controlled and precise actions require fingertip manipulation such as provided by ring handles (Figure 2-2). Compression handles are pressure sensitive for grasping. Spring handles are preferred for microsurgery because activation of the jaws requires only minute motion to effect action on tissues (Figure 2-3). Locking and opposition spring handles are used for secure grasping of heavy or firm tissues such as bone, cartilage, or fascia (Figure 2-4). Pistol grip handles provide additional leverage for several instrument types. Conventional instrumentation for open surgery of the spine, for example, utilizes the pistol grip for cutting and separating bone and tough ligamental fibers (Figure 2-5).

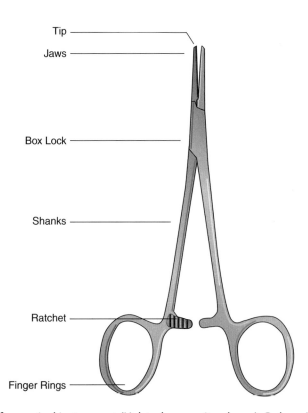

Tip

Jaws

Box Lock

Shanks

Ratchet

Finger Rings

Figure 2-1 Basic anatomy of a surgical instrument (Halsted mosquito clamp). *Delmar/Cengage Learning.*

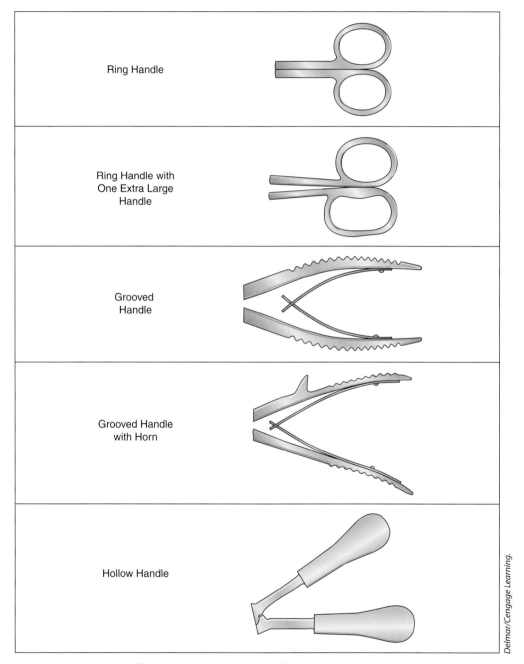

Ring Handle

Ring Handle with
One Extra Large
Handle

Grooved
Handle

Grooved Handle
with Horn

Hollow Handle

Delmar/Cengage Learning.

Figure 2-2   Ring handles and compression handle grips.

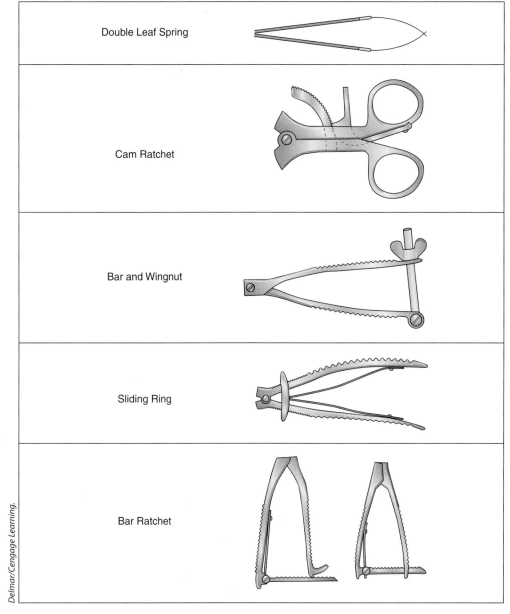

Delmar/Cengage Learning.

Figure 2-3   Spring handles and locking handle grips.

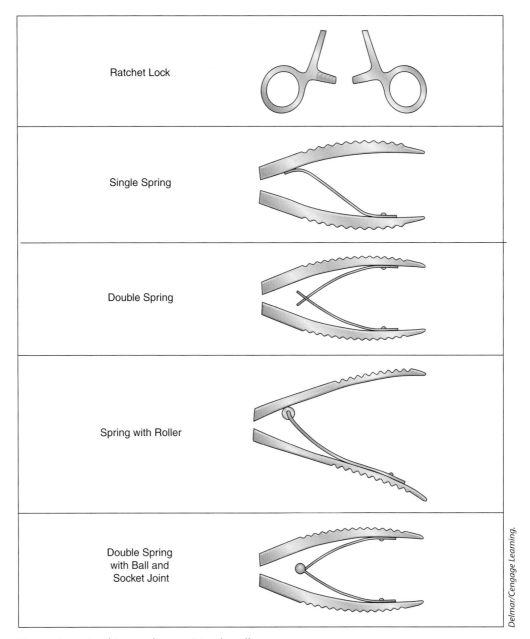

Figure 2-4 Locking and opposition handle system.

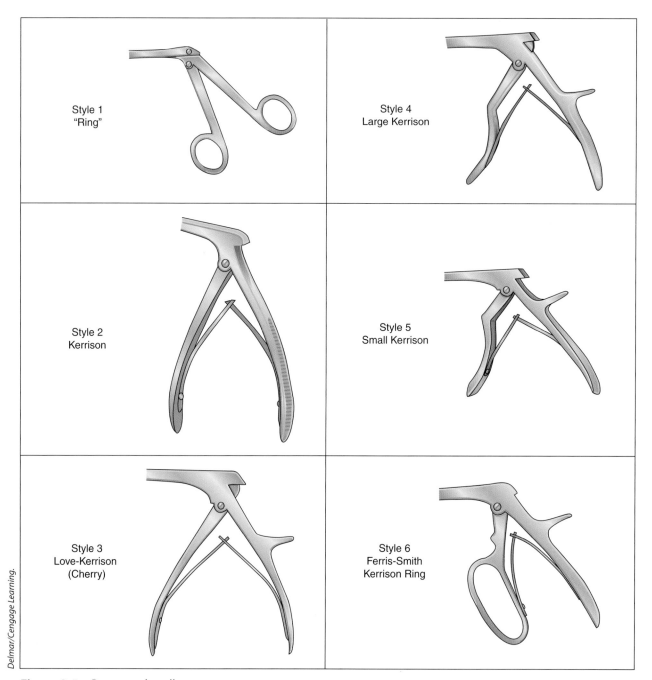

Delmar/Cengage Learning.

Figure 2-5 Rongeurs handles.

Working Mechanism: Joint Styles

The joint style facilitates the precision of the jaws. Three styles are most commonly used (Figure 2-6). Grasping and clamping instruments usually have box lock joints. Overlapping joint styles are common in dissection instruments, such as scissors. Double action joints use the principles of pivots and levers to enable the jaws to grasp, cut, and debulk firm tissues.

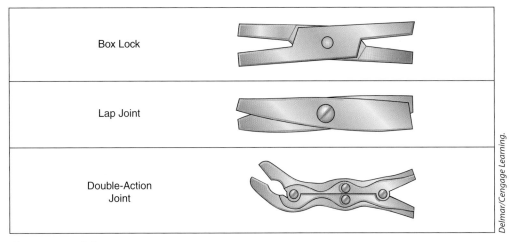

Delmar/Cengage Learning.

Figure 2-6 Joint types.

Tip Styles: Sharp Dissection

Sharp dissection is used to separate tissue planes and divide tissue attachments. The tip styles range from scissors to cutting graspers known as biters, and include knives (Figures 2-7 through 2-13).

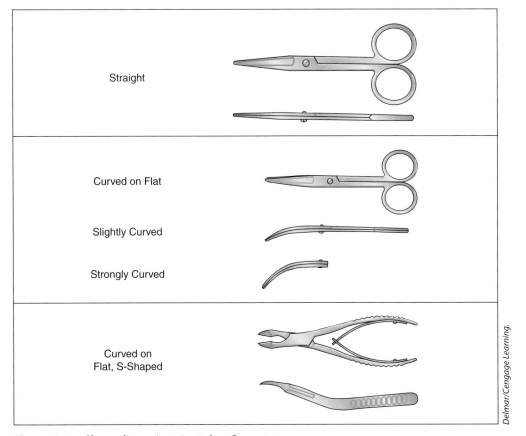

Delmar/Cengage Learning.

Figure 2-7 Sharp dissection tip styles: Curvatures.

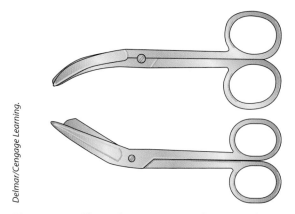

Figure 2-8 Sharp dissection tip styles: Lateral curvatures.

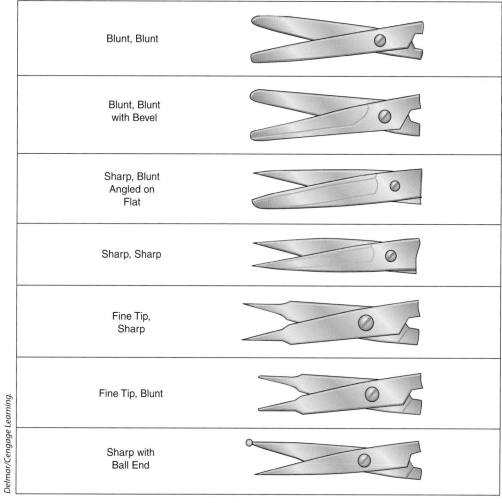

Figure 2-9 Sharp dissection tip styles: Flat.

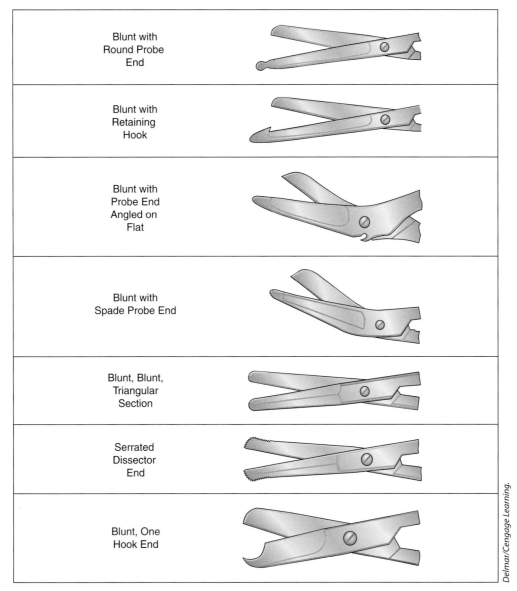

Figure 2-10   Sharp dissection tips: Special configurations.

Blunt with Round Probe End

Blunt with Retaining Hook

Blunt with Probe End Angled on Flat

Blunt with Spade Probe End

Blunt, Blunt, Triangular Section

Serrated Dissector End

Blunt, One Hook End

Delmar/Cengage Learning.

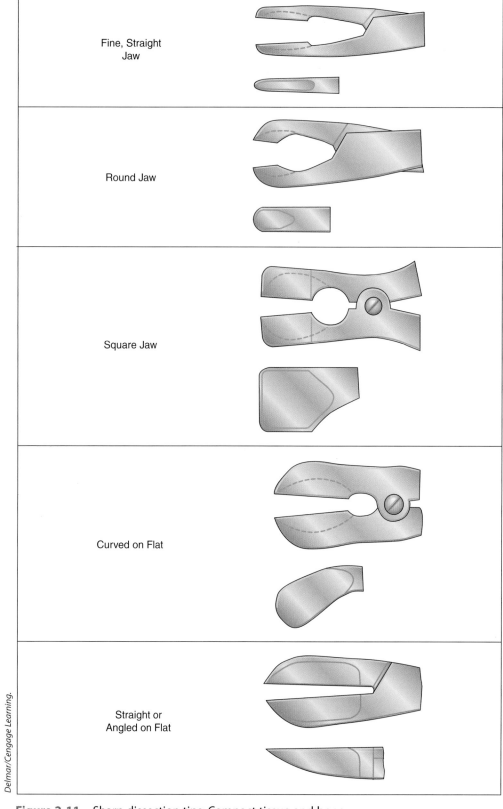

Fine, Straight
Jaw

Round Jaw

Square Jaw

Curved on Flat

Straight or
Angled on Flat

Delmar/Cengage Learning.

Figure 2-11   Sharp dissection tips: Compact tissue and bone.

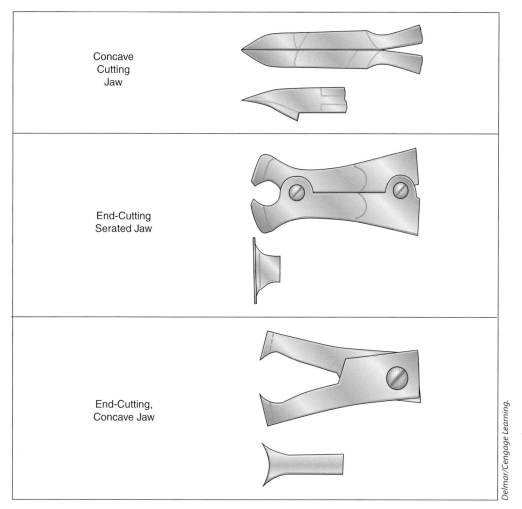

Figure 2-12   Sharp dissection tips: Front cutters.

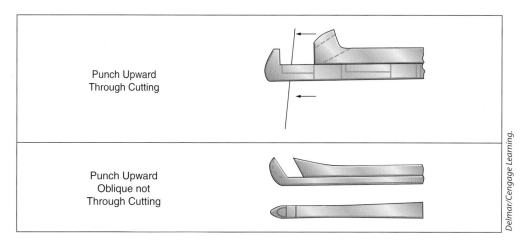

Figure 2-13   Sharp dissection tips: Biters.

Tip Styles: Clamping and Grasping

Clamping and grasping tips are used to hold tissue or items such as sutures or retraction material (e.g., umbilical tapes, silastic vessel loops, Penrose latex drains) (Figure 2-14). Clamping tips are designed to occlude lumens of vessels and other structures as designated by the surgeon. They are primarily used to provide hemostasis, although some noncrushing styles are used to temporarily occlude lumens such as the bowel for surgical repair or incision. Grasping tips are used to hold tissue for manipulation or excision. Some grasping tips have teeth for a more secure attachment to the tissue (Figure 2-15). Most of these

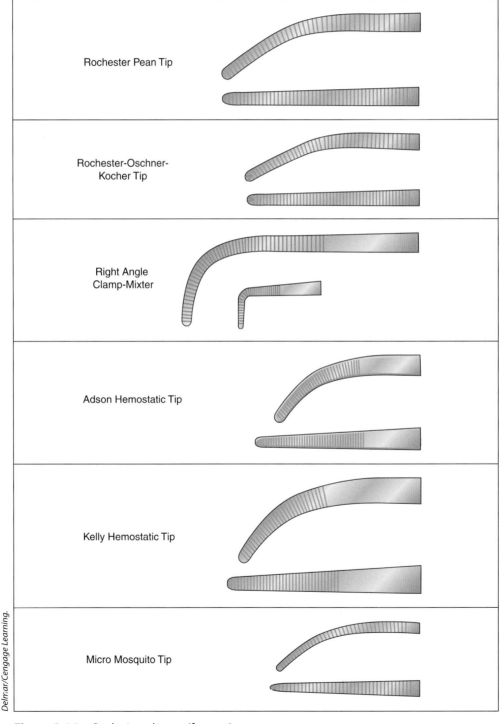

Rochester Pean Tip

Rochester-Oschner-Kocher Tip

Right Angle Clamp-Mixter

Adson Hemostatic Tip

Kelly Hemostatic Tip

Micro Mosquito Tip

Delmar/Cengage Learning.

Figure 2-14   Occlusion clamps (forceps).

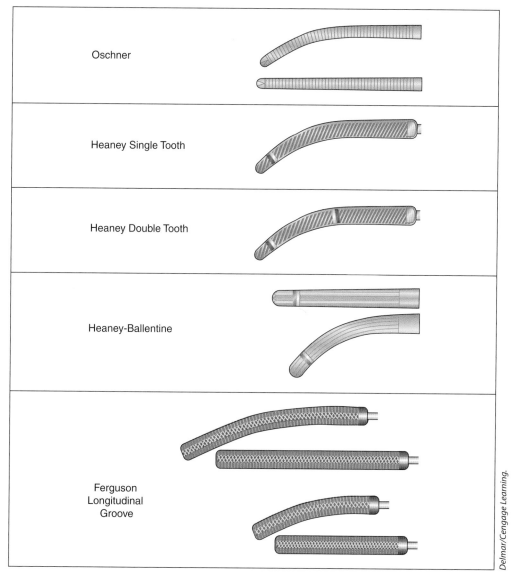

Figure 2-15   Clamps (forceps) with teeth.

Delmar/Cengage Learning.

have serrations over all or part of the instrument's jaws. There are styles for specific use with soft tissue and bone (Figure 2-16).

Tip Styles: Blunt Dissection

Blunt dissection is used to separate tissue planes without causing an incision into tissues (Figure 2-17). Examples include neurosurgery, orthopedics, and plastics for peeling back periosteal layers that cover bone. Other forms of blunt dissection include separating tissue layers such as peritoneal attachments of the bladder flap to the anterior surface of the uterus.

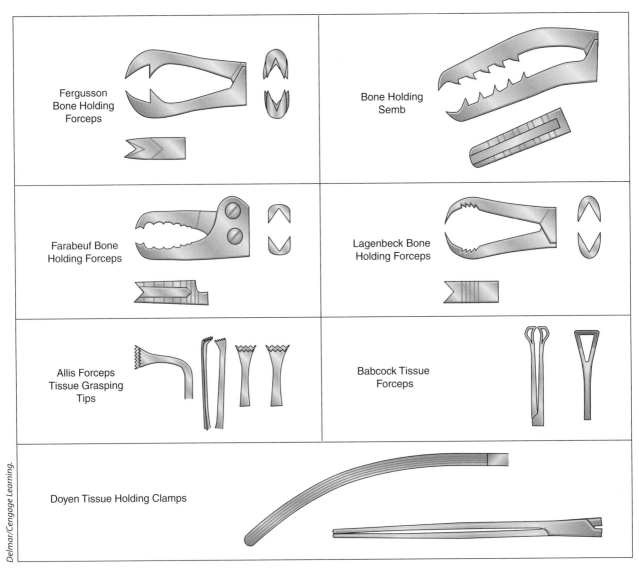

Figure 2-16 Bone and tissue grasping tips.

Fergusson Bone Holding Forceps

Bone Holding Semb

Farabeuf Bone Holding Forceps

Lagenbeck Bone Holding Forceps

Allis Forceps Tissue Grasping Tips

Babcock Tissue Forceps

Doyen Tissue Holding Clamps

Delmar/Cengage Learning.

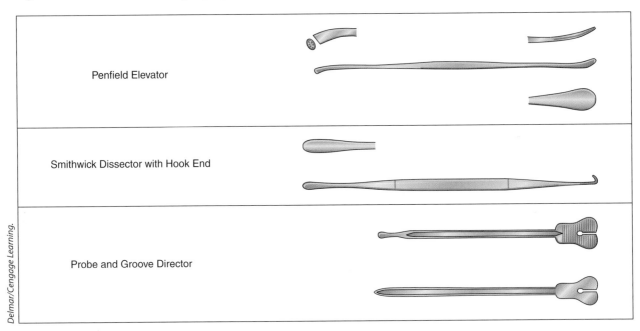

Figure 2-17 Blunt dissection.

Penfield Elevator

Smithwick Dissector with Hook End

Probe and Groove Director

Delmar/Cengage Learning.

CATEGORIES OF SURGICAL INSTRUMENTS

Surgical instrumentation consists of many materials, styles, weights, sizes, and shapes. All categories of instruments can be found in sets for open or endoscopic procedures. The common element is that each instrument has a specific function and should be used only for that purpose. Failure to use the instrument for its intended purpose can cause injury to tissue or damage the instrument's function. All of these styles can be found in standard instrumentation and in endoscopic styles for minimal access surgery. Instrumentation categories as arranged for this text are described as follows:

- *Clamps:* Used for closing circumferentially around an anatomic part either in a crushing or noncrushing manner for hemostasis or occlusion. Standard clamps usually have locking handles, but some forms of microinstrumentation require the operator to maintain grasping pressure to hold tissue. The jaws can be smooth or have serrations (teeth).

- *Grasping and holding forceps:* Used to temporarily secure an anatomic part while it is brought under control, repaired, or connected as appropriate. Graspers are also used to extract foreign bodies. Graspers can have locking or spring compression handles. The jaws can be smooth or finely serrated (toothed).

- *Dissection instrumentation:* Used to separate or incise soft and compact tissues by either sharp or blunt means. Handles can be ring, spring, or pistol style. Scalpels and tissue elevation tools are flat or rounded tips on a rod-like single hand grip. The jaws can be sharp, blunt, serrated, cross-hatched, smooth, or a wire strand.

- *Debulking tools:* Used to intentionally decrease the volume or configuration of soft or compact tissue in a specific target area, debulking can be performed by dissection instrumentation. Handles can be ring, spring, or pistol style. Scraping tools and chisels can be sharp or blunt with a single hand grip. The working end can bite with opposing jaws to cut or pinch off bulky tissue, but not necessarily used for fine separation of defined tissue planes.

- *Probes, cannula, and dilators:* Used to sharply or bluntly expand, tunnel, examine, or create an anatomic passage through which injection, tissue sampling, or decompression can take place.

- *Templates and measuring instrumentation:* Used to mark, calculate, and assess anatomic tissues and landmarks for removal, positioning, implantation, explantation, and/or excision.

- *Retraction and exposure instruments:* Used to provide a clear visual field at the surgical site by displacing and securing tissues and organs.

- *Approximation and closure instrumentation:* Used to align and secure edges of soft and compact tissues for healing. Some approximation devices employ fixation implants such as sutures, staples, clips, wires, screws, and plates.

HOW SURGICAL INSTRUMENTS ARE NAMED

A surgical instrument is commonly named for a person, its appearance, its function, or a nickname.

MATERIALS USED IN THE MANUFACTURE OF SURGICAL INSTRUMENTATION

Materials used in the manufacture of surgical instruments include metals, metal alloys, plastics, silicone, natural latex rubber, and other synthetics. These materials can be used alone or in combination. Care is taken when working with a patient who may be allergic to one or more of these materials. Anaphylaxis can ensue. Currently, there are no rapid standard tests to clinically determine metal allergy or sensitivity. Approximately 10% to 15% of the population has some sensitivity to metals (Hallab, Merritt, & Jacobs, 2001). As metals are degraded by the body, electrochemical processes can cause the immune system to react, manifesting dermatitis, urticaria, and vasculitis. Little is known about the short- or long-term bioavailability of metals as they break down in the system. The metals that most frequently cause sensitivity include the following:

- Nickel
- Beryllium

- Cobalt
- Chromium

And rarely:

- Tantalum
- Titanium
- Vanadium

Nickel is the most common of these metals to cause reaction in a patient.

Metallics

Metals have been in use since copper was hammered into ornaments and tools around 8000 BC. Gold came into use around 6000 BC. Sumerian artifacts dating from 2500 BC demonstrate that copper was made into bronze by adding tin for strength. Other artifacts show that ancient people experimented by adding zinc to create brass. As knowledge of metals increased, ancient Turks found that higher temperatures could cause the iron to separate from ore deposits around 1500 BC. They found that, with repeated heating to 1100°C and hammering the oxygen from the metal, iron became shiny and harder. This type of processed iron was more valuable than gold and became the cornerstone of civilization because of its use in tools and weapons. Cast iron came into popularity in the 14th century AD when the Europeans forged and shaped iron to make cannons.

The most common types of modern metals used in the manufacture of surgical instruments in the 20th and 21st centuries include steel, copper, nickel, titanium, and silver. Combination alloy metals, such as Vitallium (combined cobalt, chromium, tungsten, carbon, manganese, and nickel), have been used in dental and orthopaedic implants since the 1930s. Occasional items such as patient positioning devices are sometimes made of malleable lead or aluminum. With the exception of titanium, all metals have some magnetic properties and cannot be used in the presence of magnetic resonance imaging (MRI).

The chemical elements known to man have been listed together in a chart referred to as the *periodic table of the elements*. Each chemical—whether liquid, gaseous, or solid—is described in terms that reflect its chemical name and symbol, atomic mass weight, and placement in accordance to similar elements. This chart was originally assembled by Russian chemist Dmitri Mendeleev (1834–1907). At the time he created this organized chart, it contained only 63 elements. As of 2008, there are 103 chemicals listed on the periodic table of the elements. Chemical composition descriptions and a downloadable periodic table of the elements are available online at www.webelements.com. The most common types of metals used for surgical instrumentation in surgery are described in the following sections.

Steel

Alloy composition of steel may be iron or carbon based. Most of the instrumentation used in surgery is stainless steel, which is a carbon-based material. Additional components include carbon, silicon, manganese, phosphorus, sulphur, and chromium. Carbon steel was discovered by Tobern Bergman in 1774. This is the forerunner of stainless steel, which was first cast in 1913. Stainless steel was given its name for resisting stains when placed in a vinegar solution. This stainless property is caused by passivation of the chromium that forms the surface layer. It is not really totally stainless, but mostly corrosion and rust resistant. Many industries adopted the term and the alloy for application in aircraft and general use metallic instruments. Stainless steel is sold in bar stock lots referred to as "forgings" graded by its composition. The forgings are exposed to appropriate heat and placed into molds for casting. A large weight is pounded on the mold to cause the metal to take the desired shape and hardness. Several grades are manufactured throughout the world. German-made surgical instruments are commonly preferred in the modern operating room, although many other countries produce forgings suitable for surgical instruments. Steel is hardened into austenite and to martensite by exposure to heat.

400 Series Stainless Steel

Heat-treating and passivation, in combination with a high carbon content, is how instruments requiring a dissection or debulking edge maintain the necessary sharpness to cut both soft and compact or bony tissues. Instruments made of this grade of steel do not readily bend or flex while in use. Other instruments that require this level of hardness are used for secure grasping and holding. Examples of instruments made of 400 series stainless steel include:

- Scissors: Used to dissect soft tissue and suture
- Chisels and osteotomes: Used for debulking and dissecting compact tissue
- Curettes and rasps: Used to debulk soft and compact tissue
- Clamps and hemostats: Crushing and non-crushing for the occlusion of lumens and grasping tissue

- Needle holders: Used for tissue approximation with suture
- Rongeurs: Used to debulk or dissect firm and compact tissue
- Forceps: Used to grasp and hold tissues
- Dilators: Used to sequentially expand a lumen or opening

300 Series Stainless Steel

Instruments that require slight to moderate malleability are composed of 300 series stainless steel. This type of steel is also corrosion resistant. Instruments that are made of 300 series stainless steel include:

- Suction Cannulae: For instillation or removal of fluids and substances
- Probes: For exploration and blunt dissection
- Retractors: Malleable for displacement of tissues to enhance visualization at the surgical site
- Surgical wire
- Surgical steel suture

Copper

Few surgical instruments are made of copper. Those copper instruments in use today are plated with nickel to minimize staining and corrosion. Copper is sometimes preferred for malleable uterine curettes and vascular suction Cannulae. Newer styles of instrumentation are made of malleable 300 grade stainless steel to avoid the use of plated instruments in surgery. The plating wears off with time exposing the bare copper surface.

Titanium

Modern specialty surgical instruments and metallic implants can be made of lightweight, non-magnetic titanium. These instruments are corrosion resistant and very strong. However, repairs to these instruments are costly. Microsurgical instruments, vessel occluding clips, staples, replacement joints, screws, and bone plates are commonly made of titanium because it is inert and lightweight. This metal has been known to science since 1791, but received more scrutiny after 1910 as a specialty metal for surgical application. Titanium is named for the Titans from Greek mythology. They were known for their strength.

Silver

The malleability, stability, and strength of silver make it a good material for metallic tracheotomy tubes and delicate probes, such as those used in the lacrimal ducts of the eye.

SURFACES OF METALLIC SURGICAL INSTRUMENTS

Consideration is given to the surface as a useful or detrimental element of a surgical instrument. The actual surface does not make the instrument more useful, but gives the instrument a preferred appearance. Low reflection or non-reflective surfaces are preferred for use with videoscopic equipment and lasers. The light production of these surgical devices can cause problems with visualization or a reflective injury to the patient's tissues. Basic surface textures are available in surgical instruments. These are as follows:

- Polished: Shiny, high gloss, high reflective like a mirror. Surface is easily marred or damaged by poor instrument care.
- Matte or satin: Low shine, low reflection.
- Ebonized: Blackened, or dull surface. Not reflective.
- Chrome-plating: Chrome over brass or carbon steel; used in floor grade instrumentation, not suitable for surgery. Plating can chip off. Do not place these in an ultrasonic cleaner.
- Ceramic or plastic coating: Provides insulation during electrosurgery.

INSPECTION AND QUALITY CONTROL OF METALLIC SURGICAL INSTRUMENTS

Care of the metallic instrument used in surgery consists of proper handling and usage, cleaning and processing, and packaging and storage. All brand new instrumentation should be cleaned, lubricated, and processed before use in patient care. Stainless steel instrumentation will pit and stain when combined with certain elements. Table 2-1 shows the types of stains and their probable source. Chloride ions found in iodine, blood, and saline cause corrosion and pitting. Use a pencil eraser to determine whether the mark is

TABLE 2-1 Stains on surgical instrumentation

STAIN COLOR	CAUSATIVE AGENT
Rust color or dark orange	Dried blood is autoclaved on the instrument. Discoloration appears like rust. It can also be from soaking in tap water.
Brown	High pH (>7.0: alkaline) detergent or Chlorhexidine solution can cause this type of stain. It can also be from soaking in tap water. Chromium deposits can be a cause. Polyphosphate detergent can cause copper components in the sterilizer to deposit on the instruments in an electrolytic action.
Dark brown	This can be caused by improperly functioning sterilizer. Low pH (<7.0: acidic) detergent or baked on blood can cause this type of stain.
Blue, blackish	Instruments of dissimilar metals cause reverse plating. Chlorides such as blood and saline can be causes.
Gray	This is caused by liquid stain remover used in excess.
Blue-gray	This occurs from chemical disinfectant used in disproportionate concentrations. Use only distilled water for dilutions.
Black	Caused by ammonia exposure. Ammonia is found in many hospital cleansing agents used in surface disinfection. It is not intended for instrumentation.
Multicolor-rainbow	Overheating in the autoclave causes this coloration.
Speckles of light and dark	This is usually caused by water droplets on poorly rinsed and dried instruments.

rust or a surface stain. If the mark rubs off with the eraser, it is a stain. If the discoloration is removed, revealing a different color mark beneath, it is rust. Rusty instruments are unsafe and should be discarded.

Each pit and roughened area represents a weakened area that can harbor microorganisms. Common points of pitting are near the box locks and hinge. Pits can lead to fractures in the joints causing instrument breakage during use. Misuse of instrumentation includes using an instrument for a purpose other than its intended use, such as using a fine needle holder for a heavy needle.

Observe each instrument for stress cracks at the joints, gaps along closed jaws, tight opening and closing action, and generalized appearance.

Inspection of Scissors

Most manufacturers have a recommended test material for use in testing the cutting edge. The scissors should work smoothly, without snagging the cut surface. The cut should be clean and straight. Inspect the tips for burrs and chips. Tips should be completely intact and configured as originally designed, either sharp or blunt. The two halves should not rattle or wobble as they are opened and closed. The screw in the hinge should be

snug. Dissecting forceps are tested in the same manner. The jaw cups of the forceps should cut a clean bite from the test material. There should be no jagged edge.

Inspection of Clamps, Needle Holders, and Graspers

The tips of clamps should meet without slippage when closed over a sheet of paper. The closed jaws should not show any light passage when closed and held in front of a lamp. The box locks should interdigitate smoothly without tightness. The hinge should not wobble or feel loose. The ratchets should click smoothly and hold securely. The instrument should be closed to the first ratchet and lightly tapped on the table. The ratchet should hold and not spring open.

Inspection of Forceps

Forceps should be tested by grasping the forceps between the thumb and forefinger and, using a pinching action, opening and closing them slowly to approximate the tips. The teeth should align without scraping the sides of the opposing side of the forceps. Small items should be picked up without slippage or shifting.

Inspection of Retractors

Handheld retractor blades should hold their shape, yet have slight "give" to protect the patient's organs. Retractors that attach to frames should have secure attaching screws and ratchets (sometimes known as tilts). The retractor should be placed into the holder and given a few tugs to test how well it holds the desired position. The edges of the retractor blades should be smooth and not have any sharp or rough areas.

MAINTENANCE

Basic care of surgical instrumentation involves proper use and cleaning of instruments. Do not leave metallic instruments in chemical sterilant solution for more than 20 minutes, as the instrument surface can be irreparably damaged. Tungsten carbide inserts will dissolve when immersed in benzyl ammonium chloride. Hypochlorite (bleach) should never be used to disinfect instrumentation. It causes pits that can retain bacterial endospores.

Cleaning and Lubrication

Instruments should be cleaned with a neutral pH detergent (7.0) and rinsed thoroughly with distilled water. Blood and body substances should not be allowed to dry on the surfaces. Soaking in tap water or saline is not good for the integrity of the instruments and they should be lubricated with every wash cycle. Water-soluble lubricants should be used because oil-based material does not permit steam or chemical penetration during the sterilization cycle.

Ultrasonic Cleansing

All visible debris and biologic matter should be cleaned from instrumentation before it is placed in the ultrasonic cleaner. Only approved cleaning solutions are used in these machines. Instruments should be completely open and/or disassembled before being placed in the ultrasonic cleaner. Do not overload the unit. Follow the manufacturer's recommendations for loading and processing. Placing dissimilar metals together in the machine can cause an electrolytic reaction that can damage the instrumentation. At the completion of the cycle the instrumentation is removed, rinsed thoroughly, and air dried. The cleaning solution is changed regularly or whenever it becomes visibly soiled.

SUMMARY

Surgical instrumentation has many intricate components that work together for tissue manipulation and alteration. The individual characteristics of the instrumentation are important to the surgeon and the team as they perform the surgical procedure on various tissues within the patient's body. Without the differences in the instrumentation, the procedure would not be as precise and efficient. New styles and materials are developed as new tissue handling needs arise, making the old phrase "necessity is the mother of invention" an instrument manufacturer's favorite mantra.

REFERENCES

Appleby, M. (1998, December). Surgical instrument quality. *Infection Control Today, 2*(12), 20–24.

Burstein, G. T., Hutchings, I. M., & Sasaki, K. (2000, October). Electrochemically induced annealing of stainless steel surfaces. *Nature, 407*(6806), 885–887.

Gardner M. (2002, October). Instrument knowledge: Testing instruments and making the grade. *Infection Control Today, 6*(9), 20.

Hallab, N., Merritt, K., & Jacobs, J. J. (2001, March). Metal sensitivity in patients with orthopaedic implants. *The Journal of Bone and Joint Surgery, 83A*(3), 428–436.

Junge, T. (2002, April). Heavy metals: Metallurgy primer. *Surgical Technologist, 34*(4), 22–29.

Pyrek, K. M. (2002, December). Instrument knowledge: Preventative maintenance extends life of surgical instruments. *Infection Control Today, 6*(12), 20–22.

Ryan, M. P., et al. (February, 2002). Why stainless steel corrodes. *Nature, 415*(6873), 770–774.

Taylor, M., & Campbell, C. (1999, August). Back to basics: Introduction to instruments. *British Journal of Theatre Nursing, 9*(8), 369–371.

Vrancich, A. (2003, March). Instrumental care. *Materials Management in Health Care, 12*(3), 22–25.

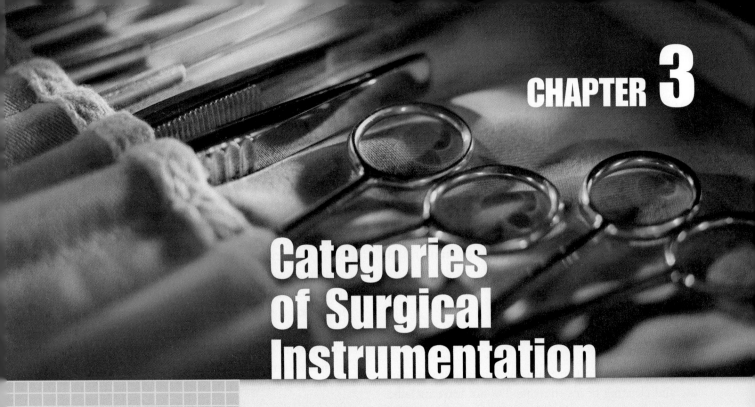

Categories of Surgical Instrumentation

INTRODUCTION

The basic surgical instruments used in the most common procedures are explored here in more depth. In subsequent chapters the instruments will be sorted into functional sets by surgical specialties and additional specialty instruments will be added. The purpose for individualizing the instruments by categories in this chapter is to familiarize the reader with similarities and subtle differences that are commonly confused. Many of the instruments described here are common to multiple types of surgical procedures and not to one specific specialty.

As each specialty chapter develops throughout this text, additional specific instruments will be introduced as appropriate to assist with the creation of functional instrument sets for related procedures. Illustrations and graphics have been obtained from multiple instrument manufacturers in order to utilize the most commonly encountered variations. Some instrument names may vary by company; however, each instrument is described by as many names as known in table format with the accompanying figure number. Special features and characteristics are listed as necessary to augment the learner's knowledge baseline.

CLAMPS

Clamps are used to securely provide hemostasis, hold a segment of tissue or surgical device, or occlude a lumen. Most specialties use similar clamps in varying weights. Most clamps are made from stainless steel for durability and strength; however, some specialties use certain materials; for example, titanium is used in microsurgery for its nonmagnetic property, especially in the presence of magnetic resonance imaging (MRI). The last section in this grouping contains clamps used for tubing that are not intended for use on patient's tissues.

Basic Hemostatic Clamps

Basic hemostatic clamps are designed to stop bleeding by an occlusive motion of the jaws. The basic hemostatic clamps are described and depicted according to size and weight. Other specialty hemostatic clamps will be described in later specialty chapters.

Mosquito Styles

This clamp is known for its fine tip and short jaw style. Although these are common to plastic and vascular procedures, they are commonly found in general sets for use on small structures, such as suture markers and vessel loops. Each set is grouped by a common design.

CLAMP SERRATED THE FULL LENGTH OF JAW TO BOX LOCKS

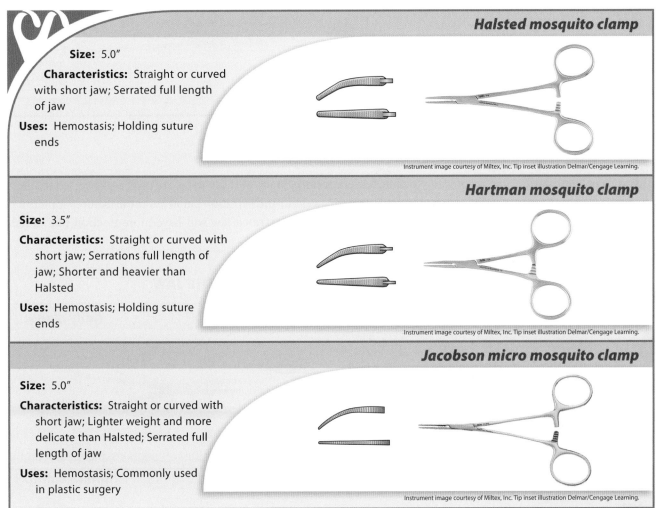

Halsted mosquito clamp

Size: 5.0"

Characteristics: Straight or curved with short jaw; Serrated full length of jaw

Uses: Hemostasis; Holding suture ends

Instrument image courtesy of Miltex, Inc. Tip inset illustration Delmar/Cengage Learning.

FIGURE 3-1

Hartman mosquito clamp

Size: 3.5"

Characteristics: Straight or curved with short jaw; Serrations full length of jaw; Shorter and heavier than Halsted

Uses: Hemostasis; Holding suture ends

Instrument image courtesy of Miltex, Inc. Tip inset illustration Delmar/Cengage Learning.

FIGURE 3-2

Jacobson micro mosquito clamp

Size: 5.0"

Characteristics: Straight or curved with short jaw; Lighter weight and more delicate than Halsted; Serrated full length of jaw

Uses: Hemostasis; Commonly used in plastic surgery

Instrument image courtesy of Miltex, Inc. Tip inset illustration Delmar/Cengage Learning.

FIGURE 3-3

continues

CLAMP SERRATED THE FULL LENGTH OF JAW TO BOX LOCKS *continued*

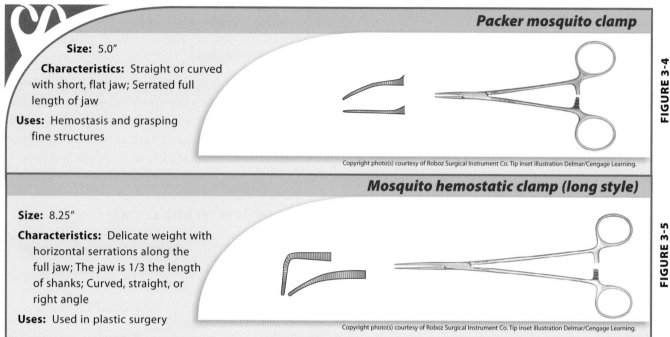

Packer mosquito clamp

Size: 5.0″

Characteristics: Straight or curved with short, flat jaw; Serrated full length of jaw

Uses: Hemostasis and grasping fine structures

Copyright photo(s) courtesy of Roboz Surgical Instrument Co. Tip inset illustration Delmar/Cengage Learning.

Mosquito hemostatic clamp (long style)

Size: 8.25″

Characteristics: Delicate weight with horizontal serrations along the full jaw; The jaw is 1/3 the length of shanks; Curved, straight, or right angle

Uses: Used in plastic surgery

Copyright photo(s) courtesy of Roboz Surgical Instrument Co. Tip inset illustration Delmar/Cengage Learning.

Standard Hemostatic Clamps

This style of hemostatic clamp is common to almost every service. Many of these styles are used and referred to interchangeably. There are distinct differences, particularly in tip, weight, and serration patterns. These features sometimes dictate how the clamp will be used. Consider the fact that a fully serrated jaw will have more traction than a half serrated jaw when applied to a pedicle of tissue.

CLAMP SERRATED HALF THE LENGTH OF THE JAW

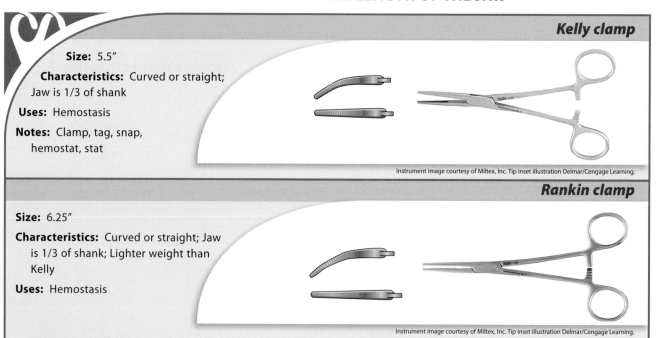

Kelly clamp

Size: 5.5″

Characteristics: Curved or straight; Jaw is 1/3 of shank

Uses: Hemostasis

Notes: Clamp, tag, snap, hemostat, stat

Instrument image courtesy of Miltex, Inc. Tip inset illustration Delmar/Cengage Learning.

Rankin clamp

Size: 6.25″

Characteristics: Curved or straight; Jaw is 1/3 of shank; Lighter weight than Kelly

Uses: Hemostasis

Instrument image courtesy of Miltex, Inc. Tip inset illustration Delmar/Cengage Learning.

CLAMP SERRATIONS THE FULL LENGTH OF THE JAW

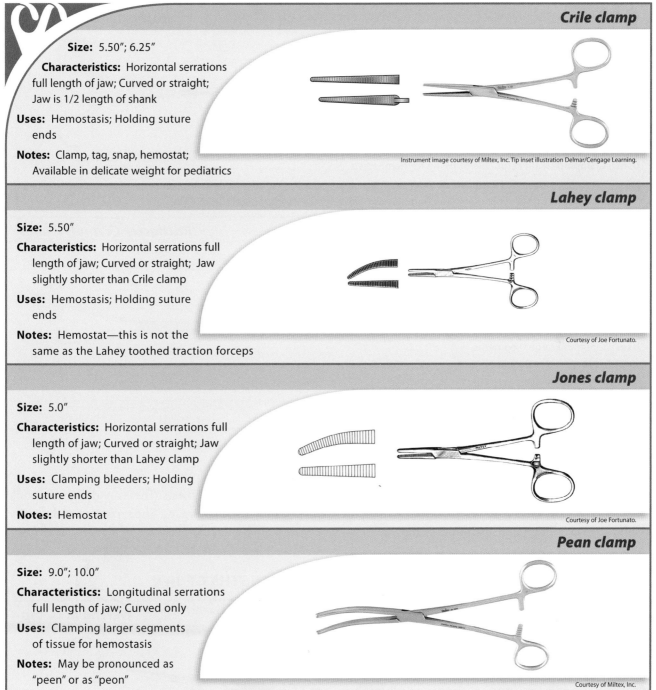

Crile clamp

Size: 5.50"; 6.25"

Characteristics: Horizontal serrations full length of jaw; Curved or straight; Jaw is 1/2 length of shank

Uses: Hemostasis; Holding suture ends

Notes: Clamp, tag, snap, hemostat; Available in delicate weight for pediatrics

Instrument image courtesy of Miltex, Inc. Tip inset illustration Delmar/Cengage Learning.

FIGURE 3-8

Lahey clamp

Size: 5.50"

Characteristics: Horizontal serrations full length of jaw; Curved or straight; Jaw slightly shorter than Crile clamp

Uses: Hemostasis; Holding suture ends

Notes: Hemostat—this is not the same as the Lahey toothed traction forceps

Courtesy of Joe Fortunato.

FIGURE 3-9

Jones clamp

Size: 5.0"

Characteristics: Horizontal serrations full length of jaw; Curved or straight; Jaw slightly shorter than Lahey clamp

Uses: Clamping bleeders; Holding suture ends

Notes: Hemostat

Courtesy of Joe Fortunato.

FIGURE 3-10

Pean clamp

Size: 9.0"; 10.0"

Characteristics: Longitudinal serrations full length of jaw; Curved only

Uses: Clamping larger segments of tissue for hemostasis

Notes: May be pronounced as "peen" or as "peon"

Courtesy of Miltex, Inc.

FIGURE 3-11

continues

CLAMP SERRATIONS THE FULL LENGTH OF THE JAW *continued*

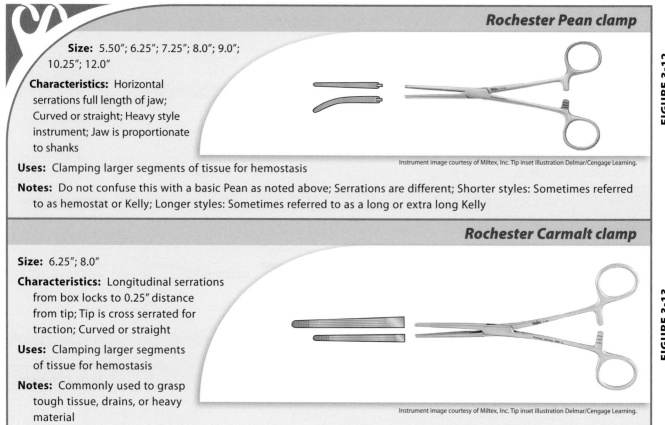

Rochester Pean clamp

Size: 5.50"; 6.25"; 7.25"; 8.0"; 9.0"; 10.25"; 12.0"

Characteristics: Horizontal serrations full length of jaw; Curved or straight; Heavy style instrument; Jaw is proportionate to shanks

Uses: Clamping larger segments of tissue for hemostasis

Notes: Do not confuse this with a basic Pean as noted above; Serrations are different; Shorter styles: Sometimes referred to as hemostat or Kelly; Longer styles: Sometimes referred to as a long or extra long Kelly

Instrument image courtesy of Miltex, Inc. Tip inset illustration Delmar/Cengage Learning.

FIGURE 3-12

Rochester Carmalt clamp

Size: 6.25"; 8.0"

Characteristics: Longitudinal serrations from box locks to 0.25" distance from tip; Tip is cross serrated for traction; Curved or straight

Uses: Clamping larger segments of tissue for hemostasis

Notes: Commonly used to grasp tough tissue, drains, or heavy material

Instrument image courtesy of Miltex, Inc. Tip inset illustration Delmar/Cengage Learning.

FIGURE 3-13

Angled Hemostatic Clamps

These hemostatic clamps are heavier and stronger than most of the standard hemostats. These are designed to hold fuller and tougher bands of tissue, particularly along the edges of highly vascular organs. The serrations and traction ability vary according to the use of the clamp.

SERRATIONS ALONG VARIABLE LENGTHS OF JAW

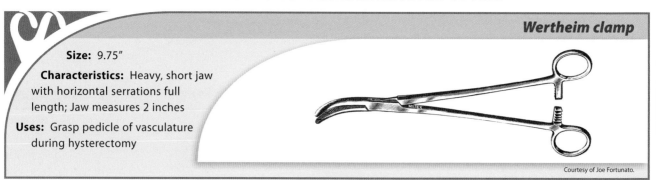

Wertheim clamp

Size: 9.75"

Characteristics: Heavy, short jaw with horizontal serrations full length; Jaw measures 2 inches

Uses: Grasp pedicle of vasculature during hysterectomy

Courtesy of Joe Fortunato.

FIGURE 3-14

SERRATIONS ALONG VARIABLE LENGTHS OF JAW *continued*

Wertheim-Cullen clamp

Size: 8.5″

Characteristics: Heavy, right-angle clamp with longitudinal serrations the distal 1/2 jaw to angle of flexure; Jaw measures 2 inches

Uses: Grasp lower angle of vaginal cuff during abdominal hysterectomy

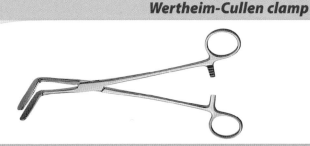

FIGURE 3-15

Moynihan clamp

Size: 8.5″

Characteristics: Intermediate weight with horizontal serrations along the full length of the short right angled jaw

Uses: Grasp tissue along gallbladder attachments and liver bed; Used as a passer for suture around a stalk of tissue

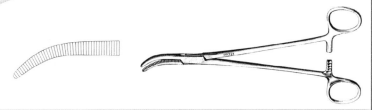

Courtesy of Joe Fortunato.

Notes: Commonly used for circumferential blunt dissection of tubular structures; Can be used for passing suture around or through meticulous vascular beds of tissue such as mesentery

FIGURE 3-16

Baby Mixter clamp

Size: 5.25″

Characteristics: Full right angle with horizontal serrations 1/2 length of jaw; The jaw is 1/3 the length of the shank

Uses: Used for delicate plastic surgery procedures

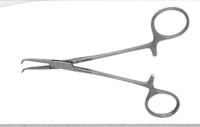

Instruments provided by www.sontecinstruments.com

Notes: Used for circumferential dissection of nerves and vascular structures

FIGURE 3-17

Mixter horizontal clamp

Size: 6.25″; 7.25″

Characteristics: Intermediate weight, long jaw with horizontal serrations the full length of jaw; Curved in a mild right angle or a true right angle

Uses: Grasp tissue along gallbladder attachments and liver bed; Used as a passer for suture around a stalk of tissue

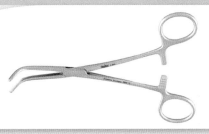

Courtesy of Miltex, Inc.

Notes: Similar function to other Mixter clamps with variations in direction of serrations

FIGURE 3-18

continues

SERRATIONS ALONG VARIABLE LENGTHS OF JAW *continued*

Mixter longitudinal clamp

Size: 9.0"; 11.0"

Characteristics: Intermediate weight, long jaw with longitudinal serrations 3/4 length of jaw; Available in delicate weight

Uses: Grasp tissue along gallbladder attachments and liver bed

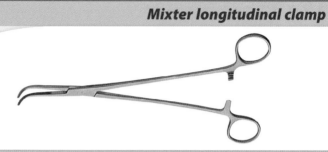

FIGURE 3-19

Mixter horizontal fine clamp

Size: 11.0"

Characteristics: Delicate weight with 45 mm curved jaw

Uses: Grasp tissue along gallbladder attachments and liver bed; Used as a passer for suture around a stalk of tissue

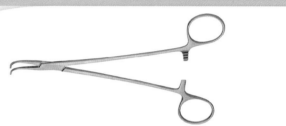

FIGURE 3-20

Gemini Mixter clamp

Size: 5.5"; 7.0"; 8.0"; 9.0"; 11.0"

Characteristics: Delicate weight with horizontal serrations the full length of the jaw; The jaw is 1/3 the length of the shanks

Uses: Grasp tissue along gallbladder attachments and liver bed; Used as a passer for suture around a stalk of tissue

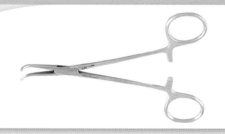

FIGURE 3-21

Schnidt hemostatic forceps, closed rings

Size: 7.50"

Characteristics: Intermediate weight clamp with horizontal serrations 1/2 way along the jaw; The jaw is 1/4 the length of the shanks; Curved

Uses: Commonly used for tonsils; Used for passing suture around or under tissue

Notes: Referred to as tonsil clamp

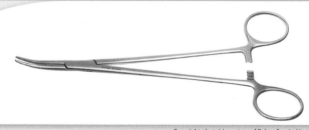

FIGURE 3-22

SERRATIONS ALONG VARIABLE LENGTHS OF JAW *continued*

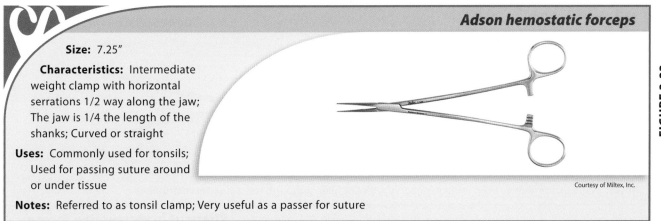

Adson hemostatic forceps

Size: 7.25″

Characteristics: Intermediate weight clamp with horizontal serrations 1/2 way along the jaw; The jaw is 1/4 the length of the shanks; Curved or straight

Uses: Commonly used for tonsils; Used for passing suture around or under tissue

Notes: Referred to as tonsil clamp; Very useful as a passer for suture

Courtesy of Miltex, Inc.

FIGURE 3-23

Hemostatic Clamps with a Tooth or Teeth at Tip (Traumatic)

These clamps are commonly used for higher levels of traction and enclosing the distal aspect of tissue within the confines of the clamp. It clearly delineates the distal tip for dissection.

HEAVY TO INTERMEDIATE WEIGHT CLAMPS (CURVED/STRAIGHT)

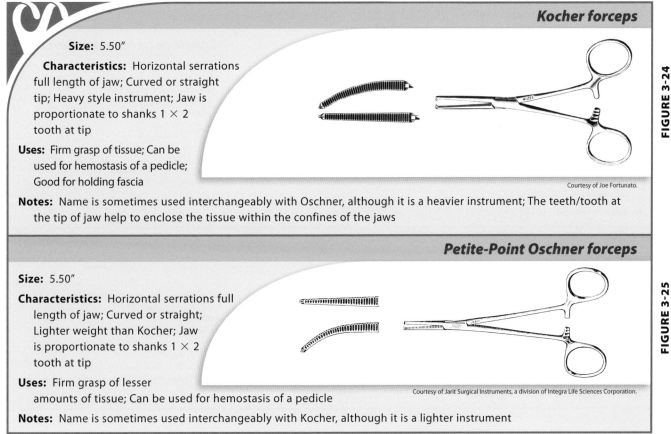

Kocher forceps

Size: 5.50″

Characteristics: Horizontal serrations full length of jaw; Curved or straight tip; Heavy style instrument; Jaw is proportionate to shanks 1 × 2 tooth at tip

Uses: Firm grasp of tissue; Can be used for hemostasis of a pedicle; Good for holding fascia

Courtesy of Joe Fortunato.

Notes: Name is sometimes used interchangeably with Oschner, although it is a heavier instrument; The teeth/tooth at the tip of jaw help to enclose the tissue within the confines of the jaws

FIGURE 3-24

Petite-Point Oschner forceps

Size: 5.50″

Characteristics: Horizontal serrations full length of jaw; Curved or straight; Lighter weight than Kocher; Jaw is proportionate to shanks 1 × 2 tooth at tip

Uses: Firm grasp of lesser amounts of tissue; Can be used for hemostasis of a pedicle

Courtesy of Jarit Surgical Instruments, a division of Integra Life Sciences Corporation.

Notes: Name is sometimes used interchangeably with Kocher, although it is a lighter instrument

FIGURE 3-25

continues

HEAVY TO INTERMEDIATE WEIGHT CLAMPS (CURVED/STRAIGHT) *continued*

Rochester Oschner forceps

Size: 6.25"; 7.25"; 8.0"; 9.0"; 10.0"

Characteristics: Horizontal serrations full length of jaw; Curved or straight tip; Heavy style instrument; Jaw is proportionate to shanks 1 × 2 tooth at tip

Uses: Firm grasp of tissue; Can be used for hemostasis of a pedicle

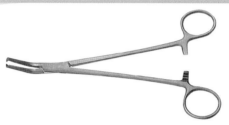

Courtesy of Miltex, Inc.

Notes: Name is sometimes used interchangeably with Oschner, although it is a heavier instrument

FIGURE 3-26

Phaneuf hysterectomy forceps

Size: 8.0"

Characteristics: Longitudinal serrations the full length of the jaw; The jaw is 1/4 the length of the shanks; Straight or angled jaw; Jaw is short; Shanks are longer in proportion 1 × 2 tooth at the tip

Uses: Firm grasp of shorter, thicker pedicles of tissue; Can be used for hemostasis

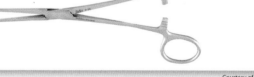

Photo supplied courtesy of Cardinal Health, V. Mueller® Products and Services. All rights reserved.

Notes: Distinguished from other 1 × 2 toothed clamp by shortness of the jaw; Commonly used for the uterine artery

FIGURE 3-27

Lovelace hemostatic forceps

Size: 6.25"

Characteristics: Cross serrations the full length of the jaw; The jaw is 1/2 the length of the shanks; Straight jaw 1 × 2 tooth at the tip

Uses: Firm grasp of shorter, thicker pedicles of tissue; Can be used for hemostasis

Courtesy of Miltex, Inc.

Notes: Intermediate weight of the 1 × 2 toothed clamp styles

FIGURE 3-28

Allen clamp

Size: 8.0"

Characteristics: Intermediate weight; Jaw is straight with longitudinal serrations 1 × 2 teeth at the tip

Uses: Firm grasp of tissue; Can be used for hemostasis of a fine tissue pedicle

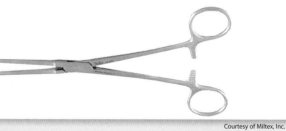

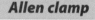

Courtesy of Miltex, Inc.

Notes: Resembles a 1 × 2 toothed Kocher clamp, but lighter weight

FIGURE 3-29

Edge Hemostasis and Grasping Clamps

These clamps have locking ratchets for secure gripping. Traction is commonly placed on these styles of clamps. Most have an open area and serrations along variable aspects of the jaw or tip to provide a non-slip surface. Most of these clamps can be found in many types of basic instrument sets in multiple numbers.

VARIABLE SERRATIONS ALONG LENGTH OR TIP OF JAW

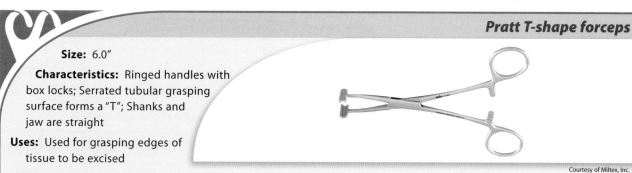

Pratt T-shape forceps

Size: 6.0″

Characteristics: Ringed handles with box locks; Serrated tubular grasping surface forms a "T"; Shanks and jaw are straight

Uses: Used for grasping edges of tissue to be excised

Notes: Commonly used on vaginal rugae during colporrhaphy; Crushing and traumatic to tissues

Courtesy of Miltex, Inc.

FIGURE 3-30

Pennington hemostatic forceps

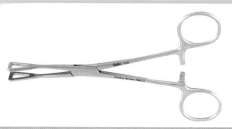

Size: 6.0″; 8.0″

Characteristics: Ringed handles with open triangular serrated grasping edges; Shanks and jaws are straight

Uses: Used for grasping and stabilizing large cut edges of tissue intended for approximation

Courtesy of Miltex, Inc.

Notes: Commonly used in cesarean section to grasp the incised edges of the uterus; Provides hemostasis of the uterine vessels imbedded in the myometrium; Used by body piercing personnel to stabilize cutaneous tissue for perforation

FIGURE 3-31

Lovelace gallbladder forceps

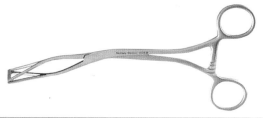

Size: 7.25″

Characteristics: Ringed handles with open triangular serrated grasping edges; Shanks are curved at the box locks and jaws are straight; The jaws measure 1″; Intermediate weight

Uses: Used for grasping and stabilizing mobile structures such as the gallbladder

Courtesy of Miltex, Inc.

Notes: Firmly grasps structures with moderate traction

FIGURE 3-32

Foerster sponge forceps

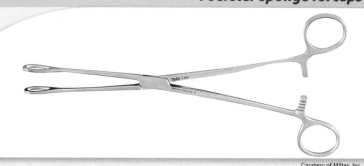

Size: 7.0″; 9.5″

Characteristics: Ringed handles with open oval serrated or smooth grasping edges; Shanks are straight or mildly curved at the box locks; Intermediate weight

Uses: Used for grasping and stabilizing mobile structures; Can be used to grasp cut edges of the uterus for hemostasis

Courtesy of Miltex, Inc.

Notes: Firmly grasps structures with moderate traction; Commonly used for sponge forceps and prepping; Also known as ring forceps; Curved forceps are commonly used in amniotic and placental removal from the endometrial cavity during childbirth

FIGURE 3-33

continues

VARIABLE SERRATIONS ALONG LENGTH OR TIP OF JAW *continued*

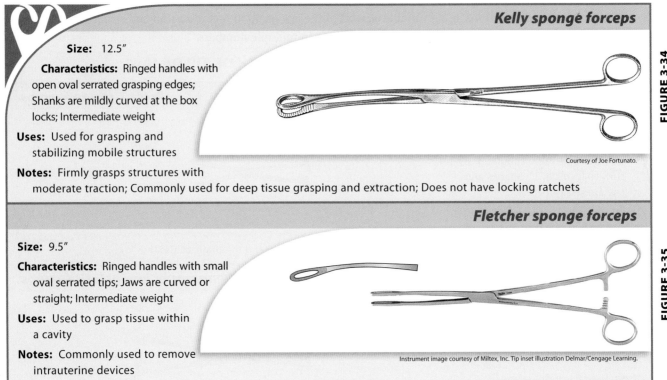

Kelly sponge forceps

Size: 12.5″

Characteristics: Ringed handles with open oval serrated grasping edges; Shanks are mildly curved at the box locks; Intermediate weight

Uses: Used for grasping and stabilizing mobile structures

Notes: Firmly grasps structures with moderate traction; Commonly used for deep tissue grasping and extraction; Does not have locking ratchets

Courtesy of Joe Fortunato.

FIGURE 3-34

Fletcher sponge forceps

Size: 9.5″

Characteristics: Ringed handles with small oval serrated tips; Jaws are curved or straight; Intermediate weight

Uses: Used to grasp tissue within a cavity

Notes: Commonly used to remove intrauterine devices

Instrument image courtesy of Miltex, Inc. Tip inset illustration Delmar/Cengage Learning.

FIGURE 3-35

Hemostatic Clamp with Teeth Along the Inner Jaw

These clamps have unique grasping teeth that maintain the tissue in a stationary position for lateral dissection. The surgeon will commonly use two of each at a time and cut medially or bilaterally along the length of the jaw with either a knife or curved scissors. One clamp will remain on the pedicle and the other will remain attached to the excised organ or tissue specimen.

VARIABLE SERRATIONS ALONG LENGTH OF JAW ON HEAVY TO INTERMEDIATE WEIGHT CLAMP

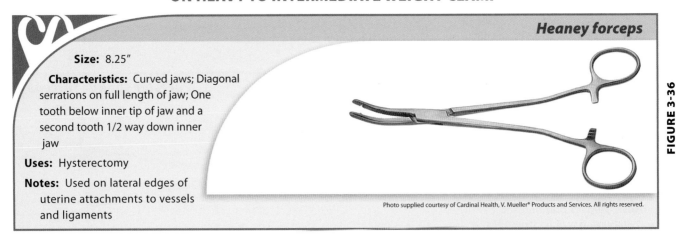

Heaney forceps

Size: 8.25″

Characteristics: Curved jaws; Diagonal serrations on full length of jaw; One tooth below inner tip of jaw and a second tooth 1/2 way down inner jaw

Uses: Hysterectomy

Notes: Used on lateral edges of uterine attachments to vessels and ligaments

Photo supplied courtesy of Cardinal Health, V. Mueller® Products and Services. All rights reserved.

FIGURE 3-36

VARIABLE SERRATIONS ALONG LENGTH OF JAW
ON HEAVY TO INTERMEDIATE WEIGHT CLAMP *continued*

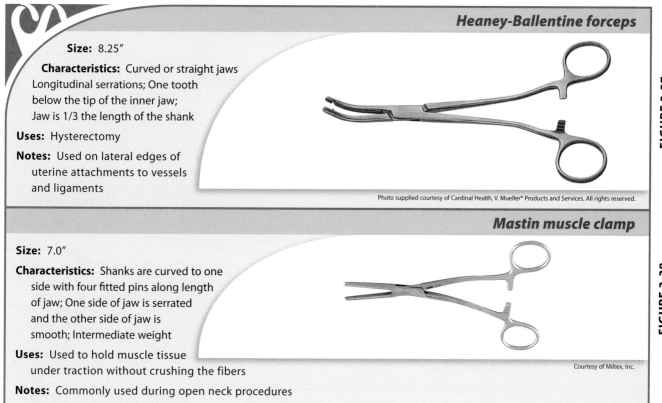

Heaney-Ballentine forceps

Size: 8.25″

Characteristics: Curved or straight jaws
Longitudinal serrations; One tooth
below the tip of the inner jaw;
Jaw is 1/3 the length of the shank

Uses: Hysterectomy

Notes: Used on lateral edges of
uterine attachments to vessels
and ligaments

FIGURE 3-37

Mastin muscle clamp

Size: 7.0″

Characteristics: Shanks are curved to one
side with four fitted pins along length
of jaw; One side of jaw is serrated
and the other side of jaw is
smooth; Intermediate weight

Uses: Used to hold muscle tissue
under traction without crushing the fibers

Notes: Commonly used during open neck procedures

FIGURE 3-38

Non-Crushing Clamps

These clamps have a softer grip and feel. The shanks and jaws have some give to the metal that allow for a firm occlusion of a lumen without crushing the structure. They are commonly used to hold a structure or gently occlude a lumen.

VARIABLE SERRATIONS ON A LIGHTER WEIGHT CLAMP

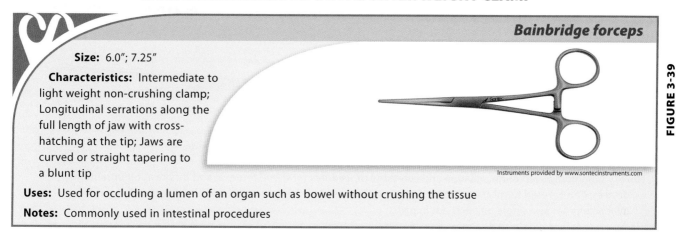

Bainbridge forceps

Size: 6.0″; 7.25″

Characteristics: Intermediate to
light weight non-crushing clamp;
Longitudinal serrations along the
full length of jaw with cross-
hatching at the tip; Jaws are
curved or straight tapering to
a blunt tip

Uses: Used for occluding a lumen of an organ such as bowel without crushing the tissue

Notes: Commonly used in intestinal procedures

FIGURE 3-39

continues

VARIABLE SERRATIONS ON A LIGHTER WEIGHT CLAMP *continued*

Baby Doyen forceps

Size: 6.5″

Characteristics: Jaws are curved or straight and longer than the shanks; The jaws are flexible and diagonally serrated with a flattened appearance

Uses: Grasps the body of an organ without crushing

Notes: Intermediate to light weight

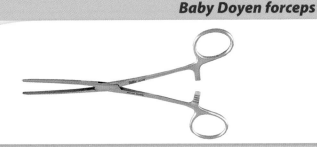

Courtesy of Miltex, Inc.

FIGURE 3-40

Doyen forceps

Size: 9.0″

Characteristics: Jaws are curved or straight and longer than the shanks; The jaws are slightly malleable and longitudinally serrated

Uses: Grasps the body of a larger organ such as a lung without crushing

Notes: Provides mild atraumatic traction

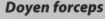

Courtesy of Miltex, Inc.

FIGURE 3-41

Kocher intestinal forceps

Size: 10.5″

Characteristics: Jaws are 2/3 the length of the shanks with longitudinal serrations; The jaws have mild flexibility and can be curved or straight

Uses: Used to grasp pedicles without crushing

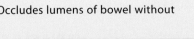

Courtesy of Miltex, Inc.

Notes: Differs from Kocher clamp because it is atraumatic (toothless) and longer; Occludes lumens of bowel without tissue destruction; Closely resembles a Doyen clamp

FIGURE 3-42

Bozeman sponge forceps

Size: 10.5″

Characteristics: Horizontal serrations 1/2 the length of the jaws; The body of the instrument has a slight "S" curve; The jaws can be curved or straight; Intermediate weight; Atraumatic

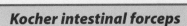

Courtesy of Miltex, Inc.

Uses: Used to probe and grasp tissue within a cavity

Notes: Commonly used during dilation and curettage procedures for tissue retrieval and for grasping intrauterine devices; Can be used for packing the uterine cavity; Not used for hemostasis or pedicles; Frequently found in a gynecology set as a single unit and not in pairs

FIGURES 3-43

Tube Occluding and Securing Clamps

The clamps in this section are named for the facility that requested or suggested a specific design. All of these are smooth, without coarse serrations, so clamped or secured tubing is not damaged in the holding process. These are not used on the patient's tissues.

CLAMPS FOR OCCLUSION OF TUBES

St. Vincent tube occluding clamp

Size: 6.5″

Characteristics: Smooth curved jaws; Intermediate to heavy weight for firm control

Uses: Used to occlude moderate thickness of tubing

Notes: Applies even occlusive pressure without damaging the tubing; Resembles a short curved pean; Not interchangeable with a curved pean because there are no serrations

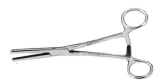

Copyright photo(s) courtesy of Roboz Surgical Instrument Co.

FIGURE 3-44

Presbyterian Hospital tube occluding clamp

Size: 7.0″

Characteristics: Smooth straight jaws; Heavy weight

Uses: Used to occlude moderate to heavy tubing such as chest tubes

Notes: Applies even occlusive pressure without damaging the tubing

Courtesy of Miltex, Inc.

FIGURE 3-45

U.S. pattern tube occluding clamp (with guard)

Size: 5.75″; 7.5″

Characteristics: Lightly serrated straight jaws with guard over the box locks to prevent crimping of the tubing

Uses: Used to occlude thick tubing such as cardiac cannulae

Notes: Applies even occlusive pressure without damaging the tubing; Serrations are shallow and provide minimal traction for secure tube holding action; Not for use on thin to moderate tubes

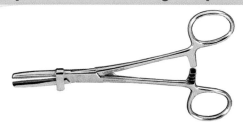

Courtesy of Miltex, Inc.

FIGURE 3-46

Vorse clamp

Size: 6.0″

Characteristics: Intermediate to heavy weight tubing clamp with a straight bluntly serrated jaw

Uses: Occludes tubing without crushing

Notes: Short jaw commonly used for temporary chest tube occlusion; Available with box lock guard

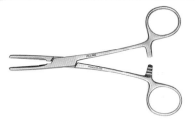

Pilling branded instrumentation courtesy of Teleflex Medical.

FIGURE 3-47

Towel and Drape Clamps

Towel and drape clamps are found on many types of sets. Some surgeons do not use these because they may impair the integrity of the drape. If placed on a drape they should be placed only once to prevent contamination of the sterile field. Care is taken not to grasp the patient's skin through the drape when applying this clamp. Some varieties penetrate and others are non-perforating. The most common types are described here. Some specialty drape clamps will be described in the specialty chapters. Many facilities refer to these clamps as "towel clips."

TOWEL AND DRAPE CLAMPS

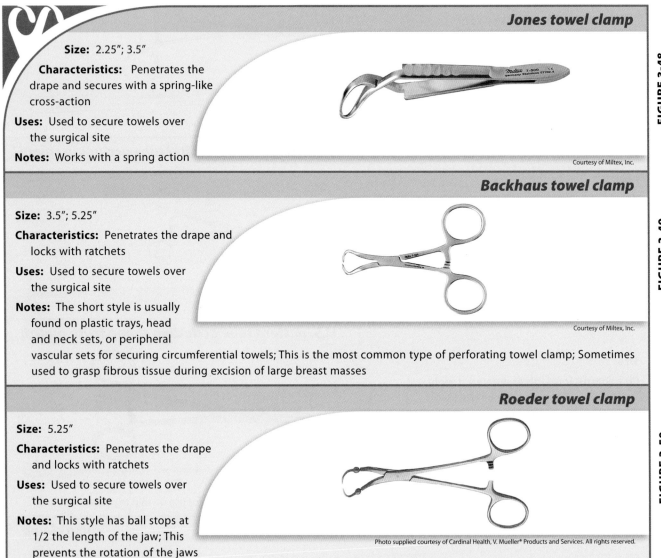

Jones towel clamp

Size: 2.25"; 3.5"

Characteristics: Penetrates the drape and secures with a spring-like cross-action

Uses: Used to secure towels over the surgical site

Notes: Works with a spring action

Courtesy of Miltex, Inc.

FIGURE 3-48

Backhaus towel clamp

Size: 3.5"; 5.25"

Characteristics: Penetrates the drape and locks with ratchets

Uses: Used to secure towels over the surgical site

Notes: The short style is usually found on plastic trays, head and neck sets, or peripheral vascular sets for securing circumferential towels; This is the most common type of perforating towel clamp; Sometimes used to grasp fibrous tissue during excision of large breast masses

Courtesy of Miltex, Inc.

FIGURE 3-49

Roeder towel clamp

Size: 5.25"

Characteristics: Penetrates the drape and locks with ratchets

Uses: Used to secure towels over the surgical site

Notes: This style has ball stops at 1/2 the length of the jaw; This prevents the rotation of the jaws of the clamp from the unsterile undersurface to the sterile surface

Photo supplied courtesy of Cardinal Health, V. Mueller® Products and Services. All rights reserved.

FIGURE 3-50

TOWEL AND DRAPE CLAMPS *continued*

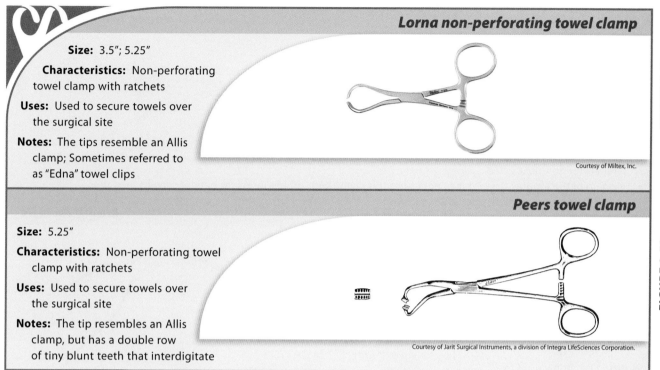

Lorna non-perforating towel clamp

Size: 3.5"; 5.25"

Characteristics: Non-perforating towel clamp with ratchets

Uses: Used to secure towels over the surgical site

Notes: The tips resemble an Allis clamp; Sometimes referred to as "Edna" towel clips

Courtesy of Miltex, Inc.

FIGURE 3-51

Peers towel clamp

Size: 5.25"

Characteristics: Non-perforating towel clamp with ratchets

Uses: Used to secure towels over the surgical site

Notes: The tip resembles an Allis clamp, but has a double row of tiny blunt teeth that interdigitate

Courtesy of Jarit Surgical Instruments, a division of Integra LifeSciences Corporation.

FIGURE 3-52

GRASPING FORCEPS

The purpose of this instrument type is to grasp or hold tissues or structures such as ducts or calculi.

Ring-Handled Grasping Forceps

Non-Crushing Grasping Forceps

JAWS ARE SERRATED AND OPEN OR SEATED WITH RUBBER JAW LINERS

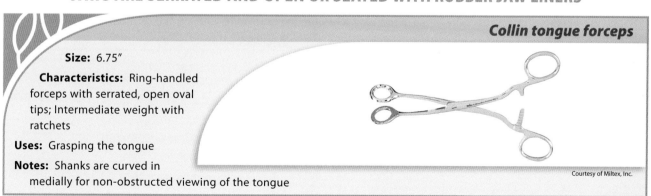

Collin tongue forceps

Size: 6.75"

Characteristics: Ring-handled forceps with serrated, open oval tips; Intermediate weight with ratchets

Uses: Grasping the tongue

Notes: Shanks are curved in medially for non-obstructed viewing of the tongue

Courtesy of Miltex, Inc.

FIGURE 3-53

continues

JAWS ARE SERRATED AND OPEN OR SEATED WITH RUBBER JAW LINERS *continued*

Young tongue forceps

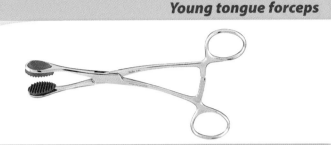

Size: 6.5"

Characteristics: Ring-handled forceps with open oval tips fitted with soft rubber insets for traction; Intermediate weight with ratchets

Notes: Shanks are curved laterally for non-obstructed viewing of the tongue; Care is taken not to use this clamp with rubber insets for patient sensitive to latex

Courtesy of Miltex, Inc.

FIGURE 3-54

Magill forceps

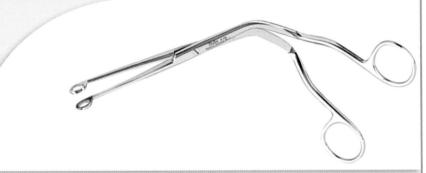

Size: 7.0"; 9.0"

Characteristics: Long-angled forceps without ratchets with serrated small, open oval tips

Uses: Used to grasp tubing as it is passed through the oropharynx

Notes: Commonly used by anesthesia personnel to position nasogastric, nasotracheal, or endotracheal tubes at the back of the patient's throat during anesthesia

Courtesy of Miltex, Inc.

FIGURE 3-55

Blake gallstone forceps

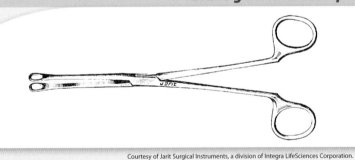

Size: 8.5"

Characteristics: Intermediate weight ring-handled forceps without ratchets; The jaw is open and oval-shaped with surface serrations; Curved or straight

Uses: Used to grasp calculus from the cystic duct

Courtesy of Jarit Surgical Instruments, a division of Integra LifeSciences Corporation.

Notes: Can be used for retrieval of polyps from the endometrial cavity of the uterus or stones from the gallbladder or duct; The soft feel of the instrument allows for some tactile sense when direct vision is not possible

FIGURE 3-56

Perforating Grasping Forceps

These graspers have toothed structures at the tip of the jaw for a firm, piercing grip that uses opposing prongs without crushing the structures.

PERFORATING GRASPING FORCEPS

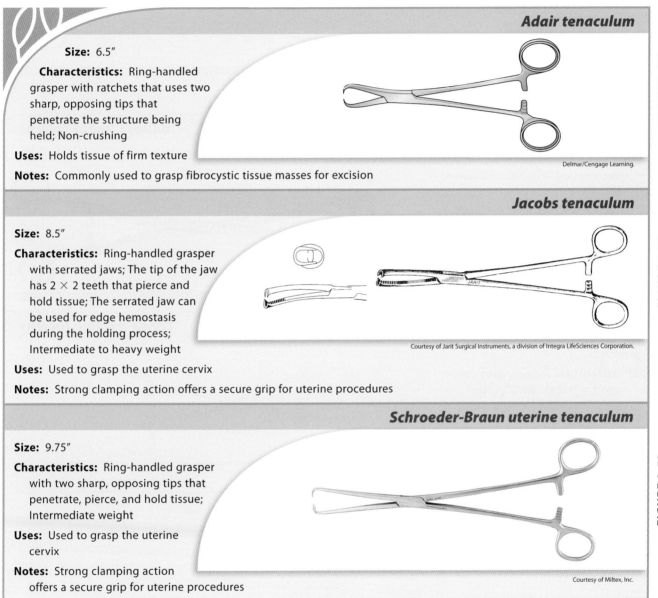

Adair tenaculum

Size: 6.5″

Characteristics: Ring-handled grasper with ratchets that uses two sharp, opposing tips that penetrate the structure being held; Non-crushing

Uses: Holds tissue of firm texture

Notes: Commonly used to grasp fibrocystic tissue masses for excision

Delmar/Cengage Learning.

FIGURE 3-57

Jacobs tenaculum

Size: 8.5″

Characteristics: Ring-handled grasper with serrated jaws; The tip of the jaw has 2 × 2 teeth that pierce and hold tissue; The serrated jaw can be used for edge hemostasis during the holding process; Intermediate to heavy weight

Uses: Used to grasp the uterine cervix

Notes: Strong clamping action offers a secure grip for uterine procedures

Courtesy of Jarit Surgical Instruments, a division of Integra LifeSciences Corporation.

FIGURE 3-58

Schroeder-Braun uterine tenaculum

Size: 9.75″

Characteristics: Ring-handled grasper with two sharp, opposing tips that penetrate, pierce, and hold tissue; Intermediate weight

Uses: Used to grasp the uterine cervix

Notes: Strong clamping action offers a secure grip for uterine procedures

Courtesy of Miltex, Inc.

FIGURE 3-59

continues

PERFORATING GRASPING FORCEPS *continued*

Schroeder uterine vulsellum forceps

Size: 10.0"

Characteristics: Ring-handled grasper with four sharp, opposing tips that penetrate, pierce, and hold tissue; Curved, angled, or straight; Intermediate weight

Uses: Used to grasp the uterine cervix

Notes: Strong clamping action offers a secure grip for uterine procedures

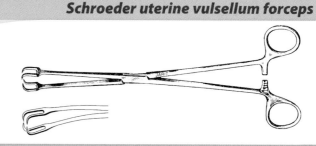

Courtesy of Jarit Surgical Instruments, a division of Integra LifeSciences Corporation.

FIGURE 3-60

Billroth tumor forceps

Size: 11.0"

Characteristics: Ring-handled grasper with 4 × 4 sharp, opposing tips that penetrate, pierce, and hold tissue; Straight; Intermediate to heavy weight

Uses: Used to grasp fibroid tumors

Notes: Strong perforating clamp

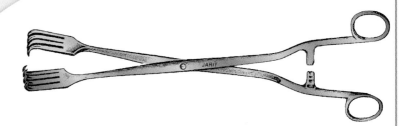

Courtesy of Jarit Surgical Instruments, a division of Integra LifeSciences Corporation.

FIGURE 3-61

Lahey traction forceps

Size: 6.25"

Characteristics: Ring-handled grasper with 3 × 3 sharp teeth in opposing jaws; Intermediate weight with locking ratchets

Uses: Used to grasp fibrous tissue

Notes: Commonly used in general surgery to grasp fibrous breast or thyroid tissue

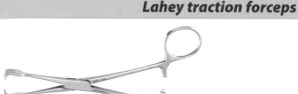

Courtesy of Miltex, Inc.

FIGURE 3-62

Non-Perforating Grasping Forceps

These graspers use serrations at the tip of the jaw or a circumferential design to securely hold tissue causing minimal trauma.

NON-PERFORATING GRASPING FORCEPS

Allis tissue forceps

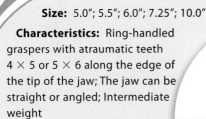

Size: 5.0″; 5.5″; 6.0″; 7.25″; 10.0″

Characteristics: Ring-handled graspers with atraumatic teeth 4 × 5 or 5 × 6 along the edge of the tip of the jaw; The jaw can be straight or angled; Intermediate weight

Uses: Holding tissue edges

Courtesy of Miltex, Inc.

Notes: One of the most commonly used instruments in the surgical setup; Longer Allis forceps are used in general surgery; Angled Allis forceps are used in hemorrhoid ligation for occlusion banding

FIGURE 3-63

Allis Adair tissue forceps

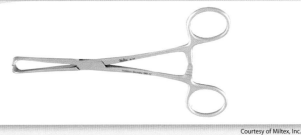

Size: 6.5″

Characteristics: Ring-handled graspers with atraumatic teeth 9 × 10 along the edge of the tip of the jaw; Straight

Uses: Holding wide tissue edges

Courtesy of Miltex, Inc.

Notes: Tip of jaw is very wide; Commonly used in place of Pratt T clamp for grasping edges under traction

FIGURE 3-64

Babcock tissue forceps

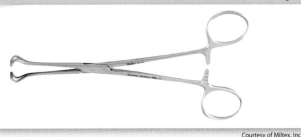

Size: 6.25″; 8.25″; 9.5″

Characteristics: Ring-handled forceps with a circumferential jaw that has longitudinal serrations across the edge of the tip of the jaw; Intermediate weight to light weight; Atraumatic

Uses: Used to hold delicate tissues and tubular structures

Courtesy of Miltex, Inc.

Notes: Has a soft touch and feels mildly malleable

FIGURE 3-65

continues

NON-PERFORATING GRASPING FORCEPS *continued*

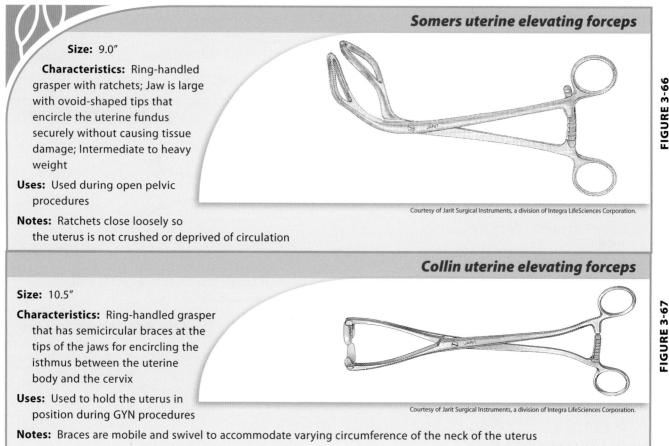

Somers uterine elevating forceps

Size: 9.0″

Characteristics: Ring-handled grasper with ratchets; Jaw is large with ovoid-shaped tips that encircle the uterine fundus securely without causing tissue damage; Intermediate to heavy weight

Uses: Used during open pelvic procedures

Notes: Ratchets close loosely so the uterus is not crushed or deprived of circulation

Courtesy of Jarit Surgical Instruments, a division of Integra LifeSciences Corporation.

FIGURE 3-66

Collin uterine elevating forceps

Size: 10.5″

Characteristics: Ring-handled grasper that has semicircular braces at the tips of the jaws for encircling the isthmus between the uterine body and the cervix

Uses: Used to hold the uterus in position during GYN procedures

Notes: Braces are mobile and swivel to accommodate varying circumference of the neck of the uterus

Courtesy of Jarit Surgical Instruments, a division of Integra LifeSciences Corporation.

FIGURE 3-67

Non-Ring-Handled Grasping Forceps

These forceps are commonly referred to as "pick-ups." They resemble tweezers. This set of forceps is not all-inclusive and is limited to the types most frequently found in basic instrument sets.

Non-Ring-Handled Grasping Forceps Without Teeth

Surgeons will frequently refer to non-toothed varieties as "thumb forceps" or "smooth pick-ups" even though they have fine serrations at the tip. Handle styles will vary according to the location of the tissue and surgeon's preference. The shanks of several of the bayonet styles and intermediate weight forceps have a stop peg to prevent overcompensated grasping of tissue that can cause crushing of the fibers. Additional non-ring-handled grasping forceps without teeth will be described in the appropriate specialty chapters.

NON-RING-HANDLED GRASPING FORCEPS WITHOUT TEETH

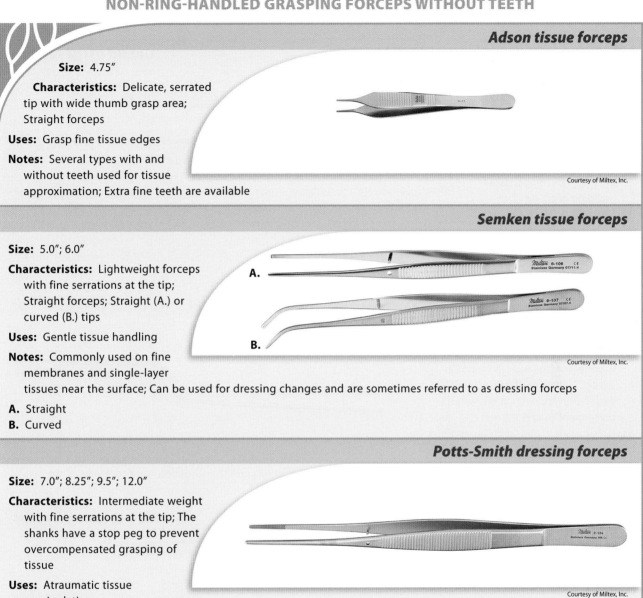

Adson tissue forceps

Size: 4.75"

Characteristics: Delicate, serrated tip with wide thumb grasp area; Straight forceps

Uses: Grasp fine tissue edges

Notes: Several types with and without teeth used for tissue approximation; Extra fine teeth are available

Courtesy of Miltex, Inc.

FIGURE 3-68

Semken tissue forceps

Size: 5.0"; 6.0"

Characteristics: Lightweight forceps with fine serrations at the tip; Straight forceps; Straight (A.) or curved (B.) tips

Uses: Gentle tissue handling

Notes: Commonly used on fine membranes and single-layer tissues near the surface; Can be used for dressing changes and are sometimes referred to as dressing forceps

A. Straight
B. Curved

Courtesy of Miltex, Inc.

FIGURE 3-69

Potts-Smith dressing forceps

Size: 7.0"; 8.25"; 9.5"; 12.0"

Characteristics: Intermediate weight with fine serrations at the tip; The shanks have a stop peg to prevent overcompensated grasping of tissue

Uses: Atraumatic tissue manipulation

Notes: Commonly used on fine membranes and single-layer tissues; Can be used for dressing changes and are sometimes referred to as dressing forceps

Courtesy of Miltex, Inc.

FIGURE 3-70

Cushing forceps

Size: 7.0"; 7.25"

Characteristics: Light to intermediate weight forceps with fine serrations at the tip; The proximal end is beveled for use as a blunt dissector; The handle is longitudinally grooved to fit the bulk of the thumb and pad of the index finger

Uses: Used on very delicate tissue

Notes: Frequently used during dissection; Handles can be straight or bayonet style; The handle grooves can vary

A. Serrated, Gutch handle, scraper end
B. Serrated, bayonet, scraper end

Courtesy of Miltex, Inc.

FIGURE 3-71

continues

NON-RING-HANDLED GRASPING FORCEPS WITHOUT TEETH *continued*

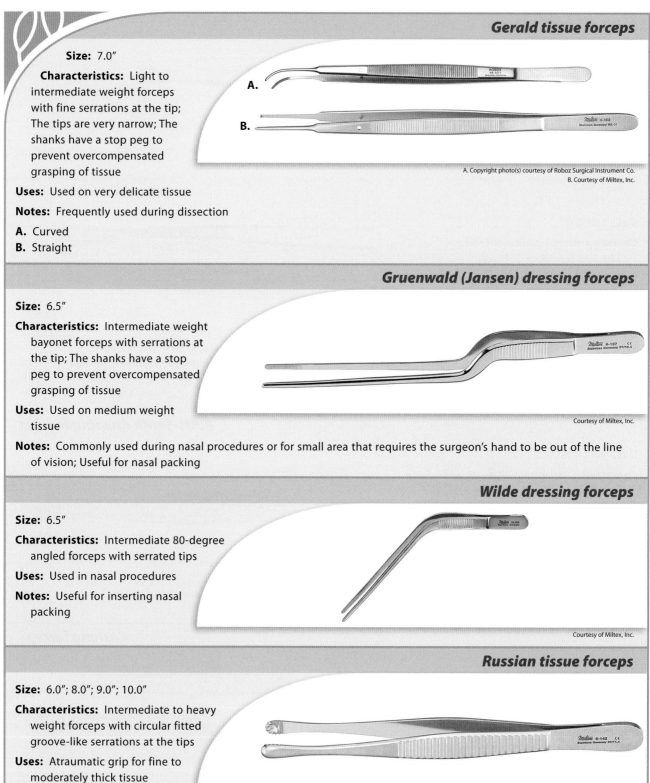

Gerald tissue forceps

Size: 7.0″

Characteristics: Light to intermediate weight forceps with fine serrations at the tip; The tips are very narrow; The shanks have a stop peg to prevent overcompensated grasping of tissue

Uses: Used on very delicate tissue

Notes: Frequently used during dissection

A. Curved

B. Straight

A. Copyright photo(s) courtesy of Roboz Surgical Instrument Co.
B. Courtesy of Miltex, Inc.

FIGURE 3-72

Gruenwald (Jansen) dressing forceps

Size: 6.5″

Characteristics: Intermediate weight bayonet forceps with serrations at the tip; The shanks have a stop peg to prevent overcompensated grasping of tissue

Uses: Used on medium weight tissue

Notes: Commonly used during nasal procedures or for small area that requires the surgeon's hand to be out of the line of vision; Useful for nasal packing

Courtesy of Miltex, Inc.

FIGURE 3-73

Wilde dressing forceps

Size: 6.5″

Characteristics: Intermediate 80-degree angled forceps with serrated tips

Uses: Used in nasal procedures

Notes: Useful for inserting nasal packing

Courtesy of Miltex, Inc.

FIGURE 3-74

Russian tissue forceps

Size: 6.0″; 8.0″; 9.0″; 10.0″

Characteristics: Intermediate to heavy weight forceps with circular fitted groove-like serrations at the tips

Uses: Atraumatic grip for fine to moderately thick tissue

Notes: Sometimes referred to as Mayo Russians

Courtesy of Miltex, Inc.

FIGURE 3-75

NON-RING-HANDLED GRASPING FORCEPS WITHOUT TEETH *continued*

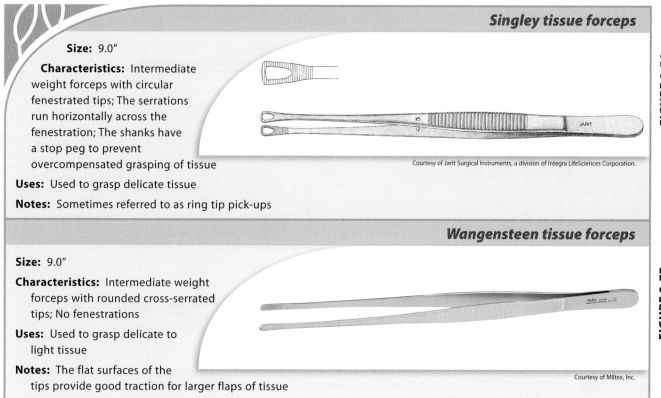

Singley tissue forceps

Size: 9.0″

Characteristics: Intermediate weight forceps with circular fenestrated tips; The serrations run horizontally across the fenestration; The shanks have a stop peg to prevent overcompensated grasping of tissue

Uses: Used to grasp delicate tissue

Notes: Sometimes referred to as ring tip pick-ups

Courtesy of Jarit Surgical Instruments, a division of Integra LifeSciences Corporation.

FIGURE 3-76

Wangensteen tissue forceps

Size: 9.0″

Characteristics: Intermediate weight forceps with rounded cross-serrated tips; No fenestrations

Uses: Used to grasp delicate to light tissue

Notes: The flat surfaces of the tips provide good traction for larger flaps of tissue

Courtesy of Miltex, Inc.

FIGURE 3-77

Non-Ring-Handled Forceps with Teeth

These forceps are commonly referred to as "pick-ups." They resemble tweezers. This set of forceps is not all inclusive and is limited to the types most frequently found in basic instrument sets. Handle styles will vary according to the location of the tissue and surgeon's preference. The shanks of several of the bayonet styles and intermediate weight forceps have a stop peg to prevent overcompensated grasping of tissue that can cause crushing of the fibers. Additional non-ring-handled grasping forceps with teeth will be described in the appropriate specialty chapters.

NON-RING-HANDLED GRASPING FORCEPS WITH TEETH

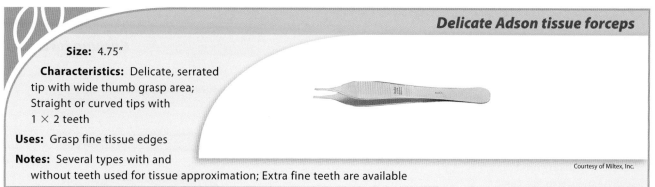

Delicate Adson tissue forceps

Size: 4.75″

Characteristics: Delicate, serrated tip with wide thumb grasp area; Straight or curved tips with 1 × 2 teeth

Uses: Grasp fine tissue edges

Notes: Several types with and without teeth used for tissue approximation; Extra fine teeth are available

Courtesy of Miltex, Inc.

FIGURE 3-78

continues

NON-RING-HANDLED GRASPING FORCEPS WITH TEETH *continued*

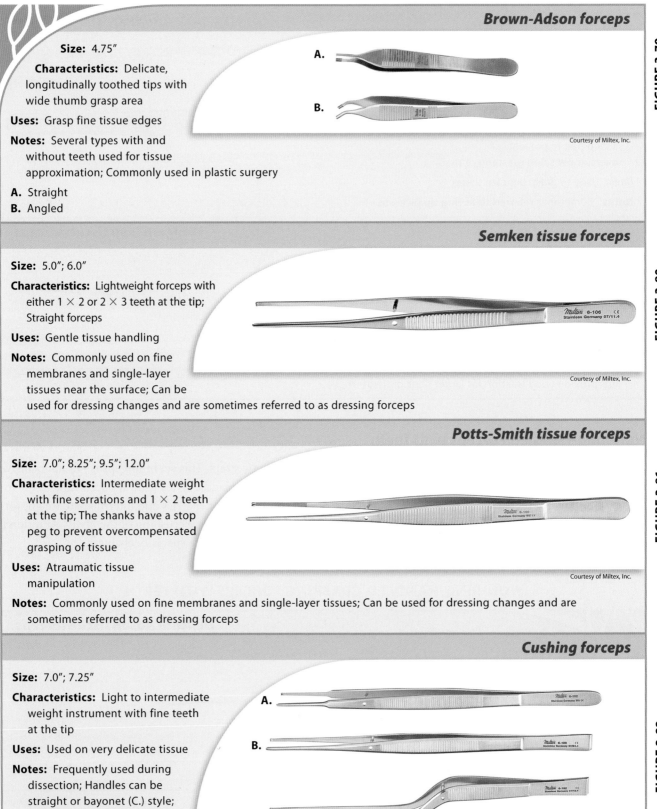

Brown-Adson forceps

Size: 4.75"

Characteristics: Delicate, longitudinally toothed tips with wide thumb grasp area

Uses: Grasp fine tissue edges

Notes: Several types with and without teeth used for tissue approximation; Commonly used in plastic surgery

A. Straight
B. Angled

A.
B.

Courtesy of Miltex, Inc.

FIGURE 3-79

Semken tissue forceps

Size: 5.0"; 6.0"

Characteristics: Lightweight forceps with either 1 × 2 or 2 × 3 teeth at the tip; Straight forceps

Uses: Gentle tissue handling

Notes: Commonly used on fine membranes and single-layer tissues near the surface; Can be used for dressing changes and are sometimes referred to as dressing forceps

Courtesy of Miltex, Inc.

FIGURE 3-80

Potts-Smith tissue forceps

Size: 7.0"; 8.25"; 9.5"; 12.0"

Characteristics: Intermediate weight with fine serrations and 1 × 2 teeth at the tip; The shanks have a stop peg to prevent overcompensated grasping of tissue

Uses: Atraumatic tissue manipulation

Notes: Commonly used on fine membranes and single-layer tissues; Can be used for dressing changes and are sometimes referred to as dressing forceps

Courtesy of Miltex, Inc.

FIGURE 3-81

Cushing forceps

Size: 7.0"; 7.25"

Characteristics: Light to intermediate weight instrument with fine teeth at the tip

Uses: Used on very delicate tissue

Notes: Frequently used during dissection; Handles can be straight or bayonet (C.) style; The handle grooves can vary from Gutch (A.) to standard (B.)

A. 1 × 2 teeth, Gutch handle, scraper end
B. 1 × 2 teeth, scraper end
C. 1 × 2 teeth, bayonet, scraper end

A.
B.
C.

Courtesy of Miltex, Inc.

FIGURE 3-82

NON-RING-HANDLED GRASPING FORCEPS WITH TEETH *continued*

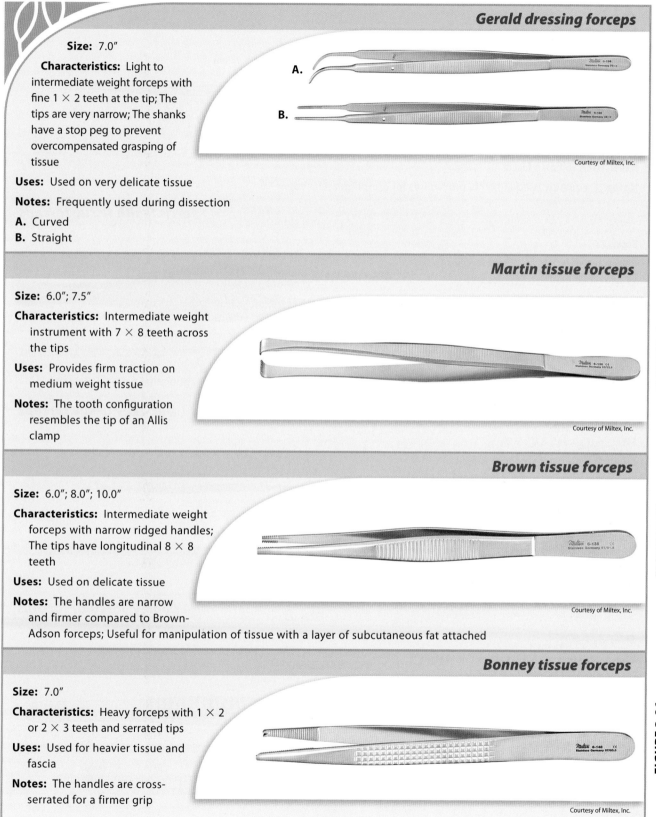

Gerald dressing forceps

Size: 7.0″

Characteristics: Light to intermediate weight forceps with fine 1 × 2 teeth at the tip; The tips are very narrow; The shanks have a stop peg to prevent overcompensated grasping of tissue

Uses: Used on very delicate tissue

Notes: Frequently used during dissection

A. Curved
B. Straight

Courtesy of Miltex, Inc.

FIGURE 3-83

Martin tissue forceps

Size: 6.0″; 7.5″

Characteristics: Intermediate weight instrument with 7 × 8 teeth across the tips

Uses: Provides firm traction on medium weight tissue

Notes: The tooth configuration resembles the tip of an Allis clamp

Courtesy of Miltex, Inc.

FIGURE 3-84

Brown tissue forceps

Size: 6.0″; 8.0″; 10.0″

Characteristics: Intermediate weight forceps with narrow ridged handles; The tips have longitudinal 8 × 8 teeth

Uses: Used on delicate tissue

Notes: The handles are narrow and firmer compared to Brown-Adson forceps; Useful for manipulation of tissue with a layer of subcutaneous fat attached

Courtesy of Miltex, Inc.

FIGURE 3-85

Bonney tissue forceps

Size: 7.0″

Characteristics: Heavy forceps with 1 × 2 or 2 × 3 teeth and serrated tips

Uses: Used for heavier tissue and fascia

Notes: The handles are cross-serrated for a firmer grip

Courtesy of Miltex, Inc.

FIGURE 3-86

continues

NON-RING-HANDLED GRASPING FORCEPS WITH TEETH *continued*

Kelly tissue forceps

Size: 9.0"

Characteristics: Intermediate weight forceps with 1 × 2, 2 × 3, or 3 × 4 teeth; The shanks have a stop peg to prevent overcompensated grasping of tissue; The handle style is Gutch

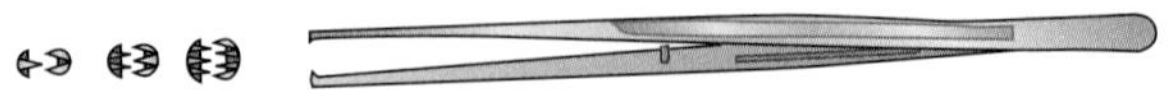

Uses: Used to grasp fascia

Notes: Frequently used in hernia procedures for grasping fascial edges

Delmar/Cengage Learning.

FIGURE 3-87

Ferris Smith tissue forceps

Size: 7.0"

Characteristics: Heavyweight forceps with wide platform handles with cross-hatched grooves for a firm grip; The teeth are 1 × 2 or 2 × 3 over serrated tips

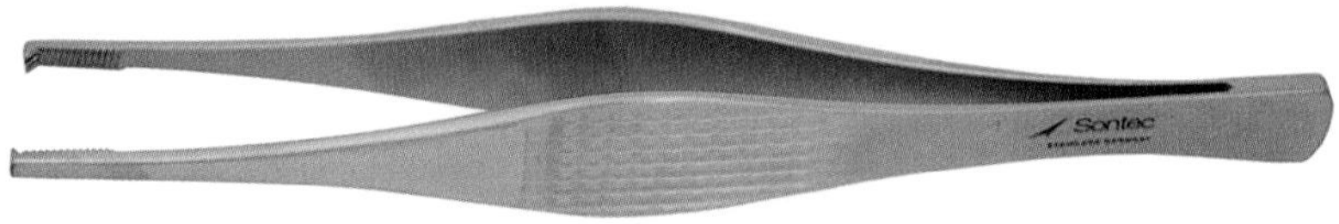

Uses: Used for firm or fibrous tissue

Instruments provided by www.sontecinstruments.com

Notes: Commonly used in colon-rectal surgery for grasping the perineal fascia during abdominal perineal resection

FIGURE 3-88

DeBakey tissue forceps

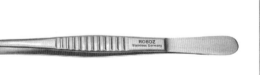

Size: 6.0"; 7.75"; 8.0"; 9.0"

Characteristics: Intermediate weight forceps with longitudinal fine teeth and matching grooves

Uses: Used for most vascular and general surgery procedures

Notes: Atraumatic forceps; The favorite tool of many surgeons; The straight tips narrow toward the distal end and interdigitate

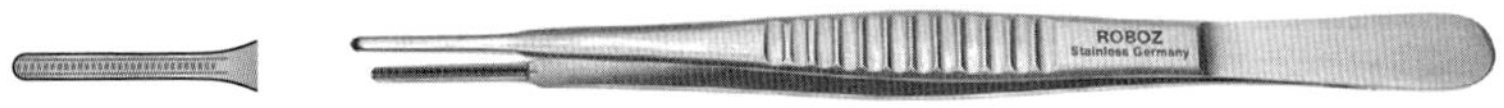

Copyright photo(s) courtesy of Roboz Surgical Instrument Co. Tip inset illustration Delmar/Cengage Learning.

FIGURE 3-89

Cooley vascular forceps

Size: 6.0"; 8.0"

Characteristics: Intermediate to fine weight forceps with longitudinal teeth and matching grooves; The straight tips narrow toward the distal grooved end and interdigitate

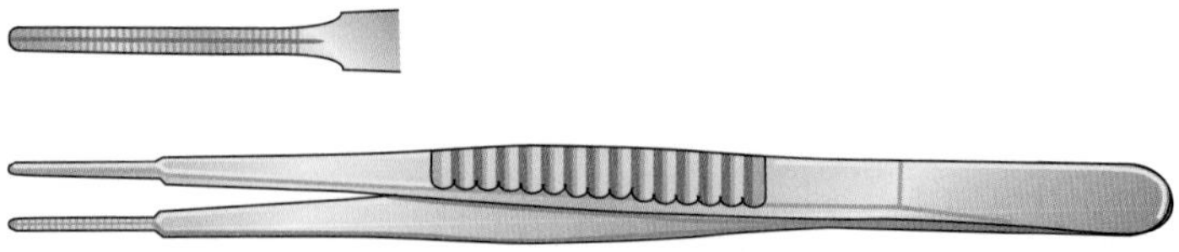

Uses: Used for most vascular and general surgery procedures

Delmar/Cengage Learning.

Notes: Atraumatic forceps with 2 mm wide tips Similar to DeBakey forceps, but with a reverse jaw configuration

FIGURE 3-90

Comparison Between DeBakey and Cooley jaw types

Characteristics: Approximation versus interdigitation

Uses: Found on clamps, forceps, and many styles of graspers

Notes: Cross-section of DeBakey and Cooley jaw types

A. DeBakey jaw
B. Cooley jaw

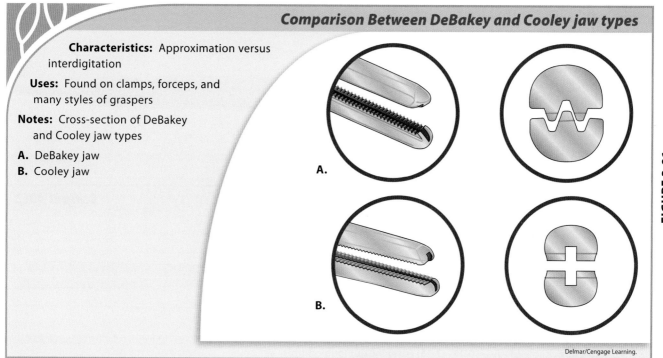

FIGURE 3-91

Delmar/Cengage Learning.

DISSECTION INSTRUMENTATION

Instrumentation used in dissection can be sharp or blunt. Sharp dissection is performed by incising anatomic planes, non-anatomic planes, or scars from former surgery, or by transecting specific tissue layers. Blunt dissection is performed by placing an instrument between the anatomic planes or tissue layers to cause separation of the fibers. In many instances, the best blunt dissection tool is the surgeon's forefinger wrapped in a single layer of Raytec or a Foerster sponge forceps clamped around a rolled sponge. Regardless of the method employed, the end result is a division of layers. In some cases portions of the tissue are intentionally removed to create space or prepared as a specimen and sent for pathologic examination.

Considerations for dissection include provision for hemostasis and prevention of peripheral damage of adjacent structures. In certain disease states such as tumors or necrosis, identification of anatomic layers is extremely difficult. This can be complicated by the use of poor quality instrumentation. Damaged or broken instruments can cause serious injury during the dissection process.

Sharp Dissection Instrumentation

Sharp dissection instruments commonly have a bladed edge. This means that the working component is machined or honed to a fine edge without chips or burrs to slice through tissue without interruption. Primary sharp dissection instruments include single blade knives. Secondary sharp dissection instruments commonly have two blades that work in opposition to cut tissue, such as scissors or ring-handled punches.

Scalpels and Knives

Scalpels and knives are single-handled instruments that are designed to attach to a disposable blade. Through history scalpels and the knife edge were permanently attached and required frequent sharpening. Disposable blades are more efficient and provide a fresh sharp edge for an individual patient.

SCALPELS AND KNIVES

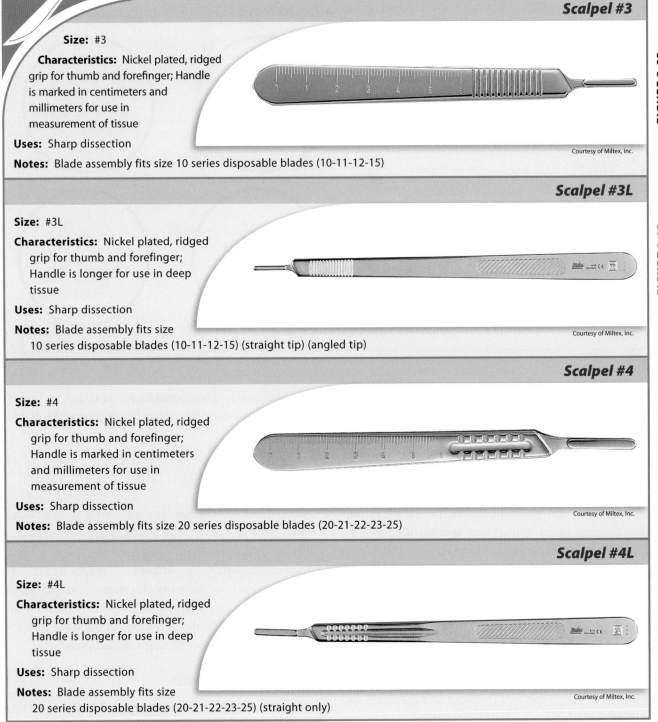

Scalpel #3

Size: #3

Characteristics: Nickel plated, ridged grip for thumb and forefinger; Handle is marked in centimeters and millimeters for use in measurement of tissue

Uses: Sharp dissection

Notes: Blade assembly fits size 10 series disposable blades (10-11-12-15)

Courtesy of Miltex, Inc.

FIGURE 3-92

Scalpel #3L

Size: #3L

Characteristics: Nickel plated, ridged grip for thumb and forefinger; Handle is longer for use in deep tissue

Uses: Sharp dissection

Notes: Blade assembly fits size 10 series disposable blades (10-11-12-15) (straight tip) (angled tip)

Courtesy of Miltex, Inc.

FIGURE 3-93

Scalpel #4

Size: #4

Characteristics: Nickel plated, ridged grip for thumb and forefinger; Handle is marked in centimeters and millimeters for use in measurement of tissue

Uses: Sharp dissection

Notes: Blade assembly fits size 20 series disposable blades (20-21-22-23-25)

Courtesy of Miltex, Inc.

FIGURE 3-94

Scalpel #4L

Size: #4L

Characteristics: Nickel plated, ridged grip for thumb and forefinger; Handle is longer for use in deep tissue

Uses: Sharp dissection

Notes: Blade assembly fits size 20 series disposable blades (20-21-22-23-25) (straight only)

Courtesy of Miltex, Inc.

FIGURE 3-95

SCALPELS AND KNIVES *continued*

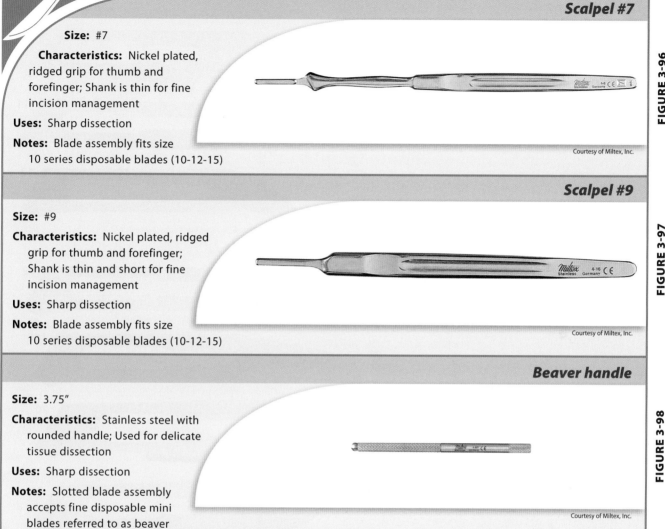

Scalpel #7

FIGURE 3-96

Size: #7

Characteristics: Nickel plated, ridged grip for thumb and forefinger; Shank is thin for fine incision management

Uses: Sharp dissection

Notes: Blade assembly fits size 10 series disposable blades (10-12-15)

Courtesy of Miltex, Inc.

Scalpel #9

FIGURE 3-97

Size: #9

Characteristics: Nickel plated, ridged grip for thumb and forefinger; Shank is thin and short for fine incision management

Uses: Sharp dissection

Notes: Blade assembly fits size 10 series disposable blades (10-12-15)

Courtesy of Miltex, Inc.

Beaver handle

FIGURE 3-98

Size: 3.75"

Characteristics: Stainless steel with rounded handle; Used for delicate tissue dissection

Uses: Sharp dissection

Notes: Slotted blade assembly accepts fine disposable mini blades referred to as beaver blades; Flat end of blade fits into slot and handle chuck is turned like a screw motion until blade is held secure; Also called miniature blade handle

Courtesy of Miltex, Inc.

continues

SCALPELS AND KNIVES *continued*

Scalpel blades

Characteristics: Standard blade assortment for scalpel handles

Uses: Sharp dissection

Notes: Each blade is individually wrapped in perforation resistant foil; Blades are disposable (see handle description for size matching with blade)

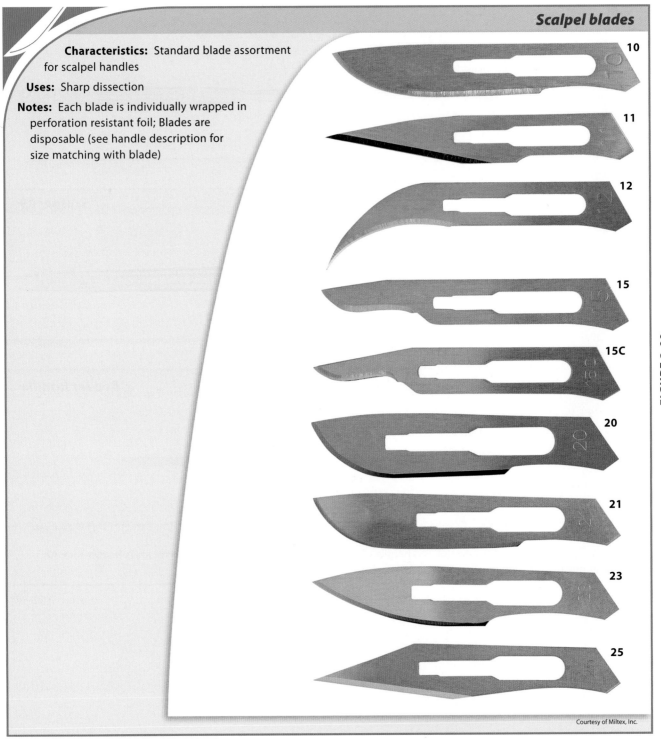

10

11

12

15

15C

20

21

23

25

Courtesy of Miltex, Inc.

FIGURE 3-99

Scissors

Scissors use opposing blades for sharp dissection. Scissors can also be used for blunt dissection by inserting the closed tips into a tissue plane, then gently opening the blades widely to spread the fibers. This procedure is referred to as Hilton's maneuver and is commonly used in areas densely packed with vessels and nerves. This procedure is also useful for opening abscess sacs for incision and drainage. Some surgeons use this blunt-method maneuver with round-tipped scissors. In deep tissues, this maneuver serves as a method for blind palpation during dissection as an extension of the surgeon's fingers.

Most standard scissors are primarily intended for right-handed use; however, many manufacturers offer left-handed styles of scissors and other ring-handled instruments by special order. Left-handed scissors may be packaged into specialty sets labeled with a particular surgeon's name for easy identification.

This section covers the most basic styles of scissors that are commonly found in basic instrument sets for general, neurologic, minor soft tissue, and vascular surgery. Additional specialty scissors will be added within each specialty chapter.

Many combinations of handle and blade styles and tip configurations are available. Some manufacturers offer an option of electrosurgical current as a mode of function. Scissors with electrosurgical capabilities cannot be sharpened and must be used with all the safeguards associated with protecting the patient and team from stray current and accumulation of energy.

SCISSORS

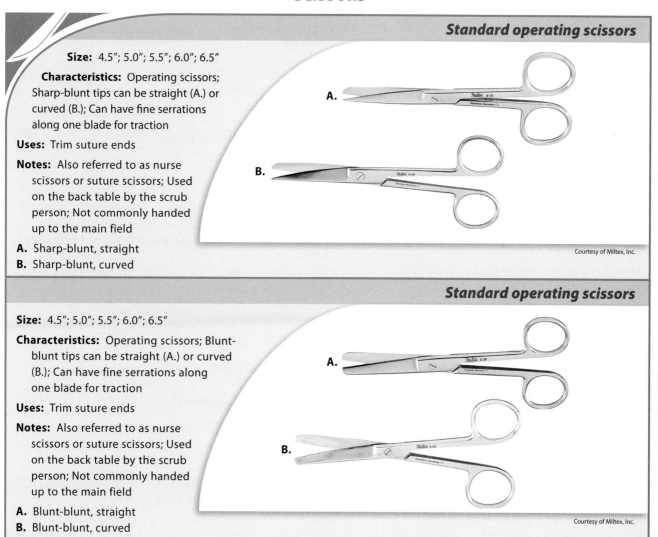

Standard operating scissors

Size: 4.5"; 5.0"; 5.5"; 6.0"; 6.5"

Characteristics: Operating scissors; Sharp-blunt tips can be straight (A.) or curved (B.); Can have fine serrations along one blade for traction

Uses: Trim suture ends

Notes: Also referred to as nurse scissors or suture scissors; Used on the back table by the scrub person; Not commonly handed up to the main field

A. Sharp-blunt, straight
B. Sharp-blunt, curved

Courtesy of Miltex, Inc.

FIGURE 3-100

Standard operating scissors

Size: 4.5"; 5.0"; 5.5"; 6.0"; 6.5"

Characteristics: Operating scissors; Blunt-blunt tips can be straight (A.) or curved (B.); Can have fine serrations along one blade for traction

Uses: Trim suture ends

Notes: Also referred to as nurse scissors or suture scissors; Used on the back table by the scrub person; Not commonly handed up to the main field

A. Blunt-blunt, straight
B. Blunt-blunt, curved

Courtesy of Miltex, Inc.

FIGURE 3-101

continues

SCISSORS *continued*

Standard operating scissors

Size: 4.5″; 5.0″; 5.5″; 6.0″; 6.5″

Characteristics: Operating scissors; Sharp-sharp tips can be straight (A.) or curved (B.); Can have fine serrations along one blade for traction

Uses: Trim suture ends

Notes: Also referred to as nurse scissors or suture scissors; Used on the back table by the scrub person; Not commonly handed up to the main field

A. Sharp-sharp, straight
B. Sharp-sharp, curved

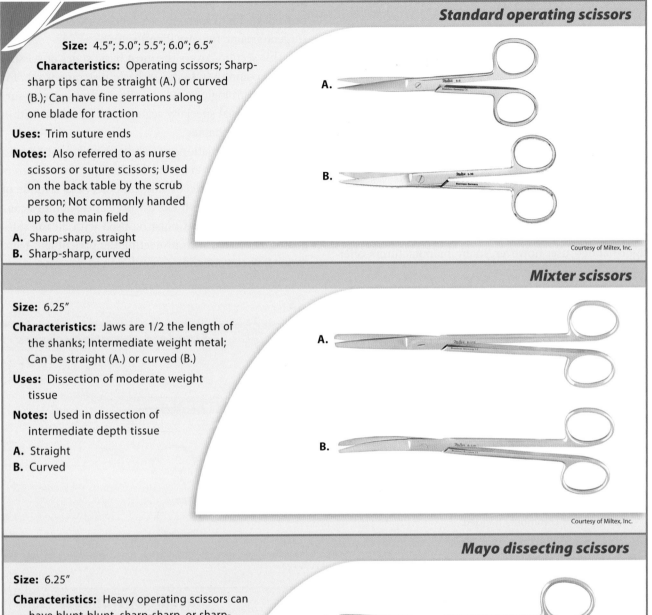

Courtesy of Miltex, Inc.

FIGURE 3-102

Mixter scissors

Size: 6.25″

Characteristics: Jaws are 1/2 the length of the shanks; Intermediate weight metal; Can be straight (A.) or curved (B.)

Uses: Dissection of moderate weight tissue

Notes: Used in dissection of intermediate depth tissue

A. Straight
B. Curved

Courtesy of Miltex, Inc.

FIGURE 3-103

Mayo dissecting scissors

Size: 6.25″

Characteristics: Heavy operating scissors can have blunt-blunt, sharp-sharp, or sharp-blunt tips; Can be straight (A.) or curved (B.)

Notes: Found in most instrument sets in both curved and straight styles; Curved are used on patient tissue; Straight are used to cut suture

A. Straight
B. Curved

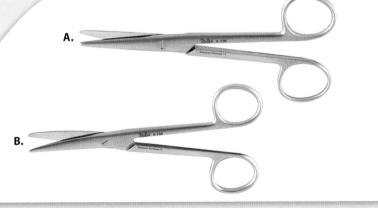

Courtesy of Miltex, Inc.

FIGURE 3-104

SCISSORS *continued*

Mayo operating scissors

Size: 5.5″; 6.75″; 9.0″

Characteristics: Heavy operating scissors can have sharp-sharp (A.), blunt-blunt (B.), or heavy-blunt (C.) tips; Can be curved or straight

Uses: Dissection of heavy to thick tissue

Notes: Found in most instrument sets in both curved and straight configurations with assorted tip styles

A. Sharp-sharp, straight
B. Blunt-blunt, curved
C. Heavy-blunt, straight

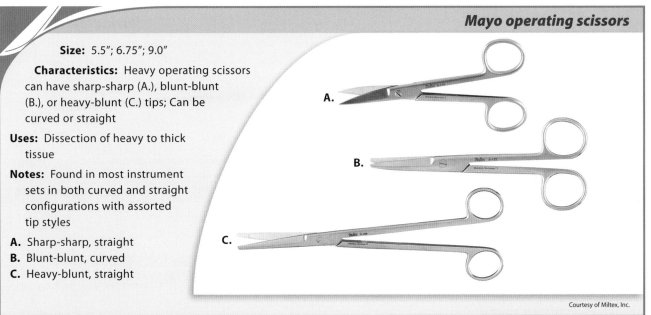

Courtesy of Miltex, Inc.

FIGURE 3-105

Metzenbaum scissors

Size: 5.5″; 7.0″; 8.0″; 9.0″; 11.0″; 14.5″

Characteristics: Fine, lightweight scissors with blunt-blunt tips; Jaws are 1/2 the length of the shanks; Available in curved and straight styles

Uses: Dissection of fine tissue

Notes: Found on most instrument sets; The most commonly used style is curved

A. Standard curved
B. Long curved
C. Delicate curved
D. Long delicate curved

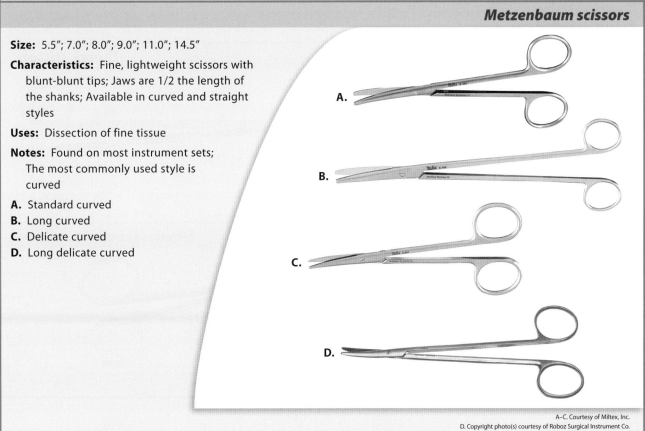

A–C. Courtesy of Miltex, Inc.
D. Copyright photo(s) courtesy of Roboz Surgical Instrument Co.

FIGURE 3-106

continues

SCISSORS *continued*

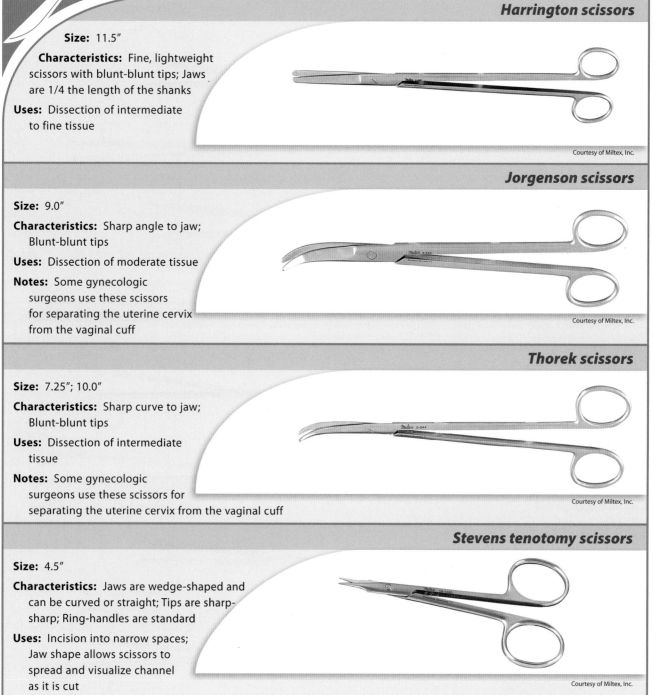

Harrington scissors

Size: 11.5"

Characteristics: Fine, lightweight scissors with blunt-blunt tips; Jaws are 1/4 the length of the shanks

Uses: Dissection of intermediate to fine tissue

Courtesy of Miltex, Inc.

FIGURE 3-107

Jorgenson scissors

Size: 9.0"

Characteristics: Sharp angle to jaw; Blunt-blunt tips

Uses: Dissection of moderate tissue

Notes: Some gynecologic surgeons use these scissors for separating the uterine cervix from the vaginal cuff

Courtesy of Miltex, Inc.

FIGURE 3-108

Thorek scissors

Size: 7.25"; 10.0"

Characteristics: Sharp curve to jaw; Blunt-blunt tips

Uses: Dissection of intermediate tissue

Notes: Some gynecologic surgeons use these scissors for separating the uterine cervix from the vaginal cuff

Courtesy of Miltex, Inc.

FIGURE 3-109

Stevens tenotomy scissors

Size: 4.5"

Characteristics: Jaws are wedge-shaped and can be curved or straight; Tips are sharp-sharp; Ring-handles are standard

Uses: Incision into narrow spaces; Jaw shape allows scissors to spread and visualize channel as it is cut

Courtesy of Miltex, Inc.

FIGURE 3-110

SCISSORS *continued*

Stevens tenotomy scissors ribbon type handle

Size: 4.5″

Characteristics: Jaws are wedge-shaped and can be curved or straight; Tips are sharp-sharp; Handles are flattened into a ribbon-style for a wider stabilizing grip

Uses: Incision into narrow spaces

Notes: Ribbon handles

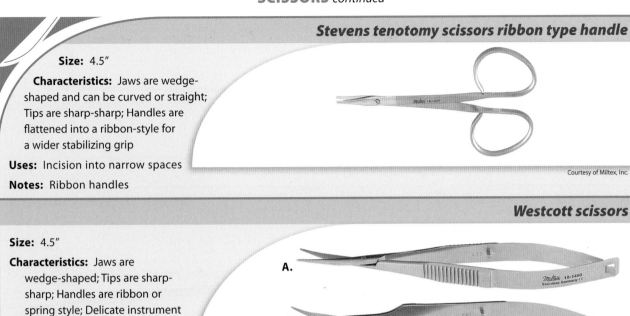

Courtesy of Miltex, Inc.

FIGURE 3-111

Westcott scissors

Size: 4.5″

Characteristics: Jaws are wedge-shaped; Tips are sharp-sharp; Handles are ribbon or spring style; Delicate instrument

Uses: Incision into narrow spaces

Notes: Similar to Stevens tenotomy; Ribbon handle; Spring style

A. Utility scissors

B. Tenotomy scissors

A.

B.

Courtesy of Miltex, Inc.

FIGURE 3-112

Martin cartilage scissors

Size: 8.0″

Characteristics: Tip is wedge-shaped; The curved blades have fine serrations for traction

Uses: Used for cutting cartilage

Notes: The wedge-shaped tip is used for blunt entry into a cartilaginous area; The serrations provide a secure cutting surface after dissection of the planes

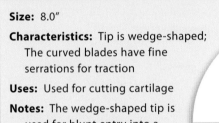

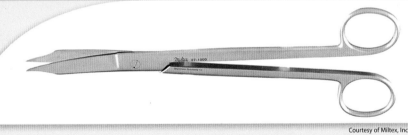

Courtesy of Miltex, Inc.

FIGURE 3-113

Potts-Smith scissors

Size: 7.0″; 7.5″

Characteristics: Jaw is 1/4 the length of the shanks and right-angled to specified degree; Sharp-sharp tips; 25, 45, or 60 degrees

Uses: Used to open and trim blood vessel edges

Notes: Available in two blade lengths:

• 20 mm intermediate weight (A.)
• 13 mm delicate weight (B.)

A. Intermediate weight

B. Delicate weight

A.

B.

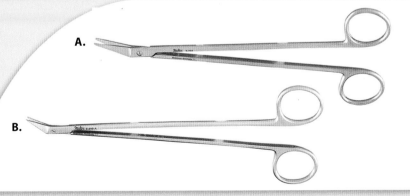

Courtesy of Miltex, Inc.

FIGURE 3-114

continues

SCISSORS *continued*

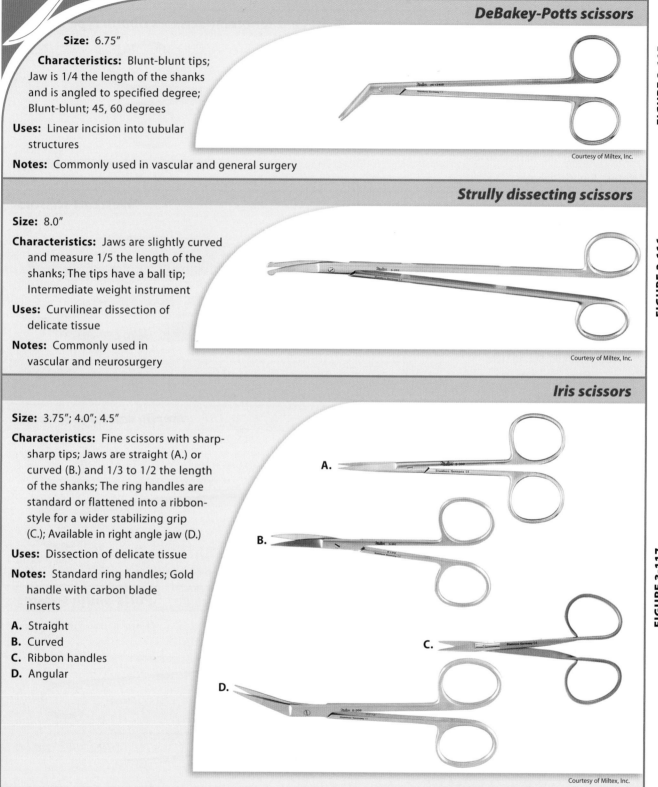

DeBakey-Potts scissors

Size: 6.75″

Characteristics: Blunt-blunt tips; Jaw is 1/4 the length of the shanks and is angled to specified degree; Blunt-blunt; 45, 60 degrees

Uses: Linear incision into tubular structures

Notes: Commonly used in vascular and general surgery

Courtesy of Miltex, Inc.

FIGURE 3-115

Strully dissecting scissors

Size: 8.0″

Characteristics: Jaws are slightly curved and measure 1/5 the length of the shanks; The tips have a ball tip; Intermediate weight instrument

Uses: Curvilinear dissection of delicate tissue

Notes: Commonly used in vascular and neurosurgery

Courtesy of Miltex, Inc.

FIGURE 3-116

Iris scissors

Size: 3.75″; 4.0″; 4.5″

Characteristics: Fine scissors with sharp-sharp tips; Jaws are straight (A.) or curved (B.) and 1/3 to 1/2 the length of the shanks; The ring handles are standard or flattened into a ribbon-style for a wider stabilizing grip (C.); Available in right angle jaw (D.)

Uses: Dissection of delicate tissue

Notes: Standard ring handles; Gold handle with carbon blade inserts

A. Straight
B. Curved
C. Ribbon handles
D. Angular

Courtesy of Miltex, Inc.

FIGURE 3-117

SCISSORS *continued*

Lister bandage scissors

Size: 3.5″; 4.5″; 5.5″; 7.25″; 8.0″

Characteristics: The jaws are right angles; The upper blade is blunt; The lower blade is slightly longer with a wedge-probe tip; Ring handles can be equal in size (A.) or have a larger thumb handle for wide stabilization (B.)

Uses: Used to cut thick tissue or dressing material; Some obstetricians use them for cutting the umbilical cord

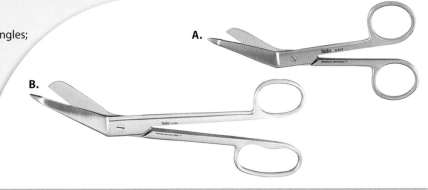

Courtesy of Miltex, Inc.

Notes: The lower probe-wedge tip acts as a protector for unseen tissue during cutting action; Can be used to cut circumferential bandages without unwrapping them from a patient's limb

A. Ring handles equal in size
B. With one large finger ring

FIGURE 3-118

Bandage and utility scissors

Size: 6.5″; 7.5″

Characteristics: Durable lightweight metal; The jaws are right angles; The upper blade is blunt; the lower serrated blade is slightly longer with a wedge-probe tip; Ring handles are heat-stable plastic and have a larger thumb handle for wide stabilization

Uses: Used to cut thick dressing material

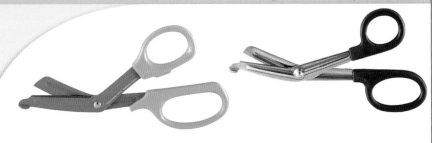

Courtesy of Miltex, Inc.

Notes: Not used for patient tissue; Some manufacturers coat the blades with fluoride to prevent adhesive tape build up; Handles can be color coded

FIGURE 3-119

Wire-Cutting scissors

Size: 4.25″; 4.75″

Characteristics: Blades are 1/4 the length of the shanks and jaws have one serrated blade at a 45-degree angle; Available in straight (A.) and angled (B.) styles; Tips are blunt-blunt

Uses: Used only for cutting wire suture or intermediate pins

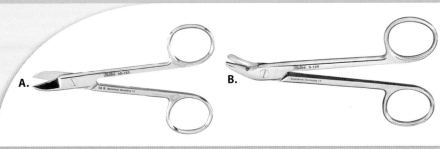

Courtesy of Miltex, Inc.

Notes: Angled style is most frequently used

A. Straight
B. Angled

FIGURE 3-120

continues

SCISSORS *continued*

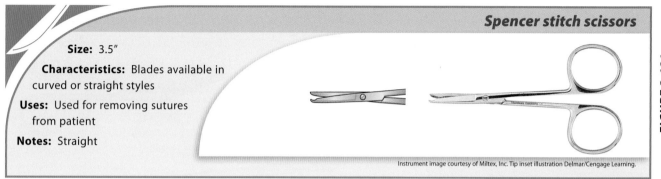

Spencer stitch scissors

Size: 3.5"

Characteristics: Blades available in curved or straight styles

Uses: Used for removing sutures from patient

Notes: Straight

Instrument image courtesy of Miltex, Inc. Tip inset illustration Delmar/Cengage Learning.

FIGURE 3-121

Biopsy Forceps

Biopsy forceps sharply dissect tissue for pathologic examination and are not commonly found on standard instrument sets. They are added as needed. The sharpness of the cutting edges outlines the margins to be studied by the pathologist. Use of dull instruments causes tissue distortion and crushing that can cause the diagnostic process to be delayed or inaccurate. Incisional biopsies are performed with biopsy forceps by biting into the tissue that is being studied. The sample is not all inclusive of the entire diseased segment. Many of these biopsy forceps were designed for use on the uterus, but can be used for other tissues as needed. Keep in mind that after the biopsy is taken, there is a need for appropriate hemostasis.

BIOPSY FORCEPS

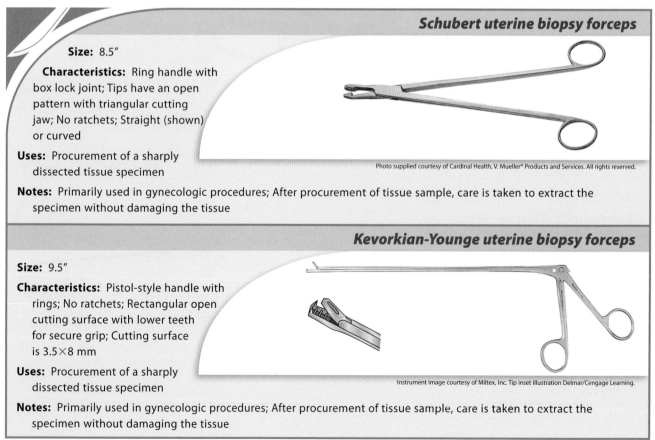

Schubert uterine biopsy forceps

Size: 8.5"

Characteristics: Ring handle with box lock joint; Tips have an open pattern with triangular cutting jaw; No ratchets; Straight (shown) or curved

Uses: Procurement of a sharply dissected tissue specimen

Photo supplied courtesy of Cardinal Health, V. Mueller® Products and Services. All rights reserved.

Notes: Primarily used in gynecologic procedures; After procurement of tissue sample, care is taken to extract the specimen without damaging the tissue

FIGURE 3-122

Kevorkian-Younge uterine biopsy forceps

Size: 9.5"

Characteristics: Pistol-style handle with rings; No ratchets; Rectangular open cutting surface with lower teeth for secure grip; Cutting surface is 3.5×8 mm

Uses: Procurement of a sharply dissected tissue specimen

Instrument image courtesy of Miltex, Inc. Tip inset illustration Delmar/Cengage Learning.

Notes: Primarily used in gynecologic procedures; After procurement of tissue sample, care is taken to extract the specimen without damaging the tissue

FIGURE 3-123

BIOPSY FORCEPS *continued*

Eppendorfer uterine biopsy forceps

Size: 8.5"

Characteristics: Pistol-style handle with rings; No ratchets; Oval open cutting surface; No teeth; No ratchets

Uses: Procurement of a sharply dissected tissue specimen

Notes: Primarily used in gynecologic procedures; After procurement of tissue sample, care is taken to extract the specimen without damaging the tissue

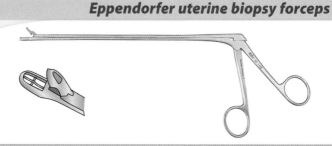

Instrument image courtesy of Miltex, Inc. Tip inset illustration Delmar/Cengage Learning.

FIGURE 3-124

Tischler cervical punch biopsy forceps

Size: 9.75"

Characteristics: Oval cutting surface with a cup style jaw; Cup interdigitates with lower jaw for cleaner cut on tougher tissue; Pistol-style handle with one large ring grip for fingers and spring action closure; No ratchets 6 × 3 × 1.5 mm specimen

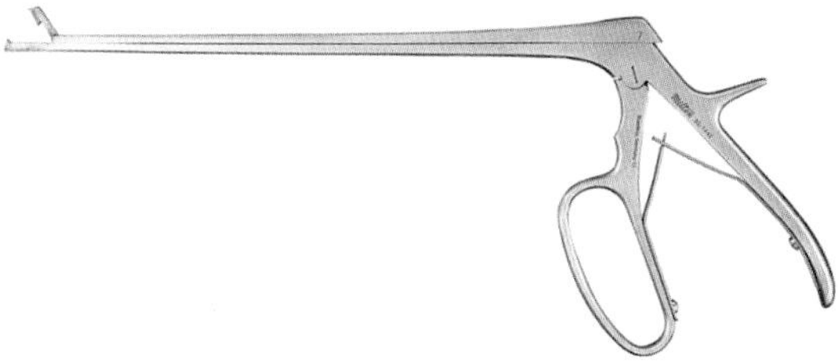

Uses: Procurement of a sharply dissected tissue specimen

Notes: Primarily used in gynecologic procedures; After procurement of tissue sample, care is taken to extract the specimen without damaging the tissue

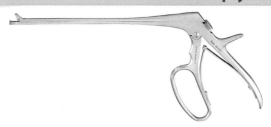

Courtesy of Miltex, Inc.

FIGURE 3-125

Townsend "mini bite" cervical biopsy forceps

Size: 7.5"

Characteristics: Pistol-style handle with one large ring for fingers; No ratchets; Slide lock at joint; Oval cup cutting surface with interdigitating cutting surfaces; No ratchets 4.2 × 2.3 × 1 mm specimen

Uses: Procurement of a sharply dissected tissue specimen

Notes: Primarily used in gynecologic procedures; After procurement of tissue sample, care is taken to extract the specimen without damaging the tissue

Courtesy of Miltex, Inc.

FIGURE 3-126

Braasch (Buie) bladder biopsy forceps

Size: 13.0"

Characteristics: Narrow shaft for passage through urethra into the bladder; Modified pistol-style handle with single finger lever action; Oval approximating cup cutting surface 3.5 mm specimen

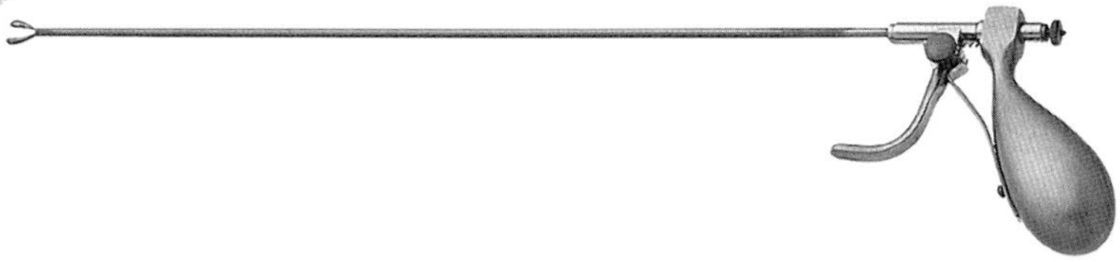

Uses: Procurement of a sharply dissected soft-tissue specimen

Notes: Can be used with most genitourinary instrumentation; Shaft is very delicate and can be inadvertently bent or damaged if mishandled

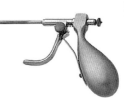

Photo supplied courtesy of Cardinal Health, V. Mueller® Products and Services. All rights reserved.

FIGURE 3-127

continues

BIOPSY FORCEPS *continued*

Interchangeable handles with rotating shafts

Size: 10.0"; 14.0"; 16.0"

Characteristics: Handles for rotating shafts can be purchased separately and fitted interchangeably with several types of rotating shafts and cutting surfaces for a 4 × 8 specimen; Pistol-style handles in two configurations

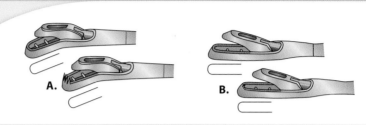

A.

B.

Delmar/Cengage Learning.

FIGURE 3-128

Uses: Procurement of a sharply dissected tissue specimen

Notes: Pistol-style handles Yeoman handle with rings; Turrell handle with spring-action grip; The style of interchangeable shafts with cutting surfaces:

- Straight-smooth cut
- Straight with teeth
- Angled jaw smooth cut
- Angled jaw with teeth

A. Turrell biopsy forceps
B. Yeoman biopsy forceps

Yeoman biopsy forceps

Size: 9.0"; 13.0"; 15.0"

Characteristics: Pistol-style handle with rings; Oval cutting surfaces for 3.5 × 10 mm specimen; No teeth; No ratchets

Uses: Procurement of a sharply dissected tissue specimen

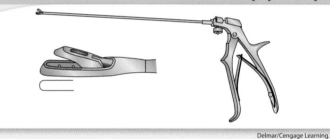

Delmar/Cengage Learning.

FIGURE 3-129

MANUAL COMPACT TISSUE DISSECTION: BONE KNIVES AND SAWS

Langenbeck metacarpal saw

Size: 9.25"

Characteristics: The serrated blade is 4.5" long; Handle is smooth

Uses: Cuts through compact tissue

Notes: Size is appropriate for use on small wrist bones; Can be used for pediatric amputations

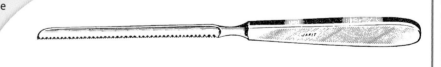

Courtesy of Jarit Surgical Instruments, a division of Integra LifeSciences Corporation.

FIGURE 3-130

MANUAL COMPACT TISSUE DISSECTION: BONE KNIVES AND SAWS *continued*

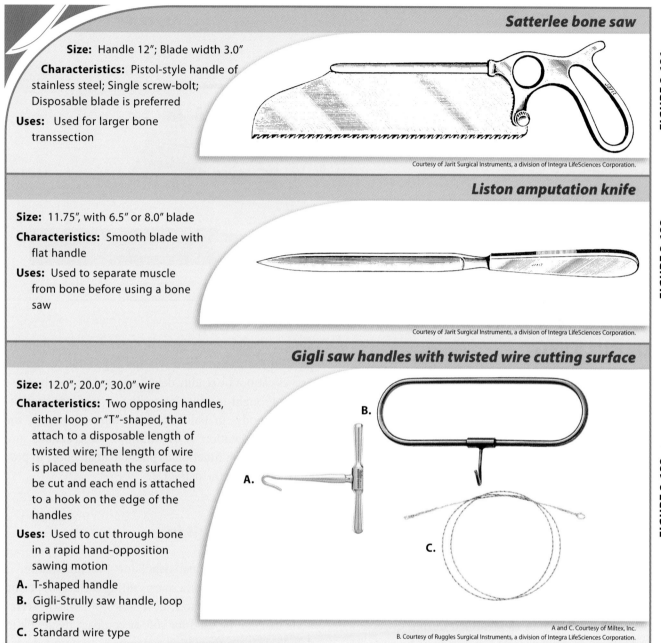

Satterlee bone saw

Size: Handle 12"; Blade width 3.0"

Characteristics: Pistol-style handle of stainless steel; Single screw-bolt; Disposable blade is preferred

Uses: Used for larger bone transsection

FIGURE 3-131

Courtesy of Jarit Surgical Instruments, a division of Integra LifeSciences Corporation.

Liston amputation knife

Size: 11.75", with 6.5" or 8.0" blade

Characteristics: Smooth blade with flat handle

Uses: Used to separate muscle from bone before using a bone saw

FIGURE 3-132

Courtesy of Jarit Surgical Instruments, a division of Integra LifeSciences Corporation.

Gigli saw handles with twisted wire cutting surface

Size: 12.0"; 20.0"; 30.0" wire

Characteristics: Two opposing handles, either loop or "T"-shaped, that attach to a disposable length of twisted wire; The length of wire is placed beneath the surface to be cut and each end is attached to a hook on the edge of the handles

Uses: Used to cut through bone in a rapid hand-opposition sawing motion

A. T-shaped handle

B. Gigli-Strully saw handle, loop gripwire

C. Standard wire type

FIGURE 3-133

A and C. Courtesy of Miltex, Inc.
B. Courtesy of Ruggles Surgical Instruments, a division of Integra LifeSciences Corporation.

Punches

Biopsies and sharp dissection performed with tissue punches are commonly core, or cylindrical in shape. The most common configuration of the cutting blade of a punch is round. Punches can be used for soft or compact tissue. The margins of the tissue specimen taken as a biopsy should be clear of the neoplasm. This is accomplished by using a punch that is a few millimeters wider in diameter than the excisional focus. An excisional biopsy is all inclusive of the area to be studied up to and including clear margins of healthy tissue. Disposable punches are preferred because a sharp edge is assured for each patient. Reusable styles are difficult to sharpen and become dull easily. Punches are not found on most instrument sets; however, they are available as separately wrapped instruments.

PUNCHES

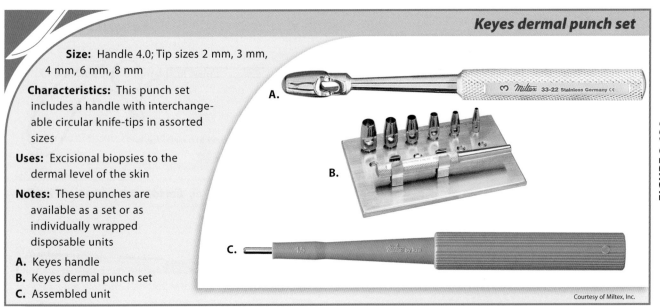

Keyes dermal punch set

Size: Handle 4.0; Tip sizes 2 mm, 3 mm, 4 mm, 6 mm, 8 mm

Characteristics: This punch set includes a handle with interchange-able circular knife-tips in assorted sizes

Uses: Excisional biopsies to the dermal level of the skin

Notes: These punches are available as a set or as individually wrapped disposable units

A. Keyes handle
B. Keyes dermal punch set
C. Assembled unit

A.

B.

C.

Courtesy of Miltex, Inc.

FIGURE 3-134

DEBULKING

The process of debulking is performed to reduce hypertrophic (enlarged) areas of abnormal tissue or to decrease the bulk of necrotic material for the promotion of healing by reepithilialization. Hypertrophic overgrowth of tissue or neoplasm can happen to any type of cell—ranging from soft tissue to compact bone. Debulking as a form of dissection does not include the careful separation of tissue layers by cutting linear incisions through defined planes. Debulking involves scraping or tearing away tissue from the surface to an underlying level demonstrated to be as clear of disease as possible. It is not always a precise measurement and does not clearly delineate tissue planes as identified during dissection. Debulking can be performed manually or by a mechanized device. Common manual debulking instruments will be described in this section. Specialized mechanical debulking devices will be described in the appropriate specialty chapters.

Some hypertrophy is benign and some is the result of malignancy. Each type of overgrowth has the potential to cause impairment or even death. Benign hypertrophy is potentially serious if the process causes obstruction or interference with the normal body processes. Benign tissues can be carefully dissected as hemostasis is maintained. Malignancy has the potential

for spreading to other areas of the body, causing multiple disturbances to organ systems in general. Malignant tissues cannot be readily debulked, or cut away, because this is thought to cause spreading or seeding throughout the body. In palliative procedures, however, the main consideration is to minimize obstructions and restore as much function as possible in an effort to provide comfort to the patient.

Manual Debulking

Sharp to blunt manual debulking instrumentation is characterized by either a sharp cutting surface, opposing cutting/grasping surfaces, or a series of abrasive serrations that can be used for soft or compact tissue. Blunt debulking instrumentation generally has a rounded edge or a grooved configuration that permits the surgeon to peel away layers of soft tissue and muscle. These are commonly wrapped separately to prevent dulled edges caused by repeated processing by steam sterilization.

NOTE: Curettes and debulking instruments have working surfaces that are measured either numerically or in millimeters. Measurement methods differ between manufacturers and are represented here as appropriate. Smaller measurement numbers on the handle indicate a smaller, more delicate working surface. Sizes listed in the chart are the way they will be seen on the handle.

SHARP TO BLUNT MANUAL DEBULKING CURETTES

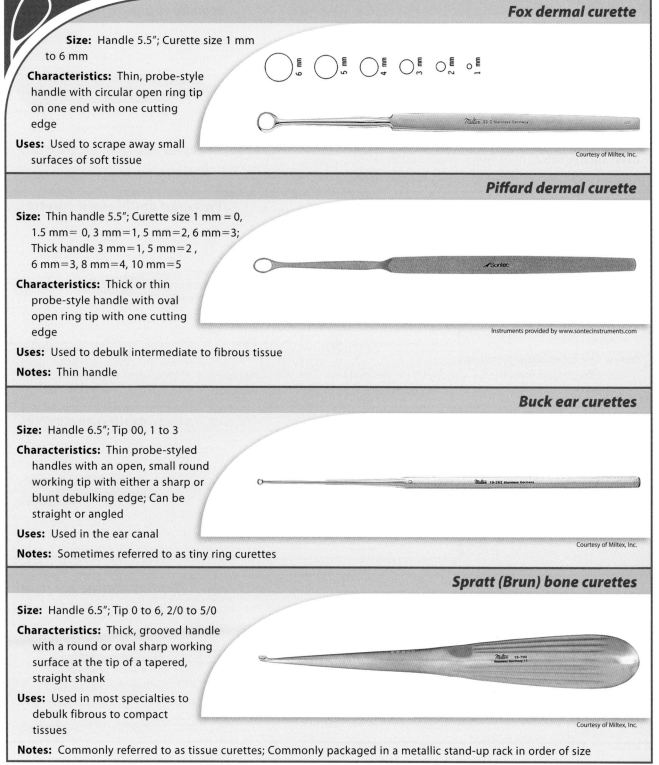

Fox dermal curette

Size: Handle 5.5"; Curette size 1 mm to 6 mm

Characteristics: Thin, probe-style handle with circular open ring tip on one end with one cutting edge

Uses: Used to scrape away small surfaces of soft tissue

6 mm · 5 mm · 4 mm · 3 mm · 2 mm · 1 mm

Courtesy of Miltex, Inc.

FIGURE 3-135

Piffard dermal curette

Size: Thin handle 5.5"; Curette size 1 mm = 0, 1.5 mm= 0, 3 mm=1, 5 mm=2, 6 mm=3; Thick handle 3 mm=1, 5 mm=2 , 6 mm=3, 8 mm=4, 10 mm=5

Characteristics: Thick or thin probe-style handle with oval open ring tip with one cutting edge

Uses: Used to debulk intermediate to fibrous tissue

Notes: Thin handle

Instruments provided by www.sontecinstruments.com

FIGURE 3-136

Buck ear curettes

Size: Handle 6.5"; Tip 00, 1 to 3

Characteristics: Thin probe-styled handles with an open, small round working tip with either a sharp or blunt debulking edge; Can be straight or angled

Uses: Used in the ear canal

Notes: Sometimes referred to as tiny ring curettes

Courtesy of Miltex, Inc.

FIGURE 3-137

Spratt (Brun) bone curettes

Size: Handle 6.5"; Tip 0 to 6, 2/0 to 5/0

Characteristics: Thick, grooved handle with a round or oval sharp working surface at the tip of a tapered, straight shank

Uses: Used in most specialties to debulk fibrous to compact tissues

Courtesy of Miltex, Inc.

Notes: Commonly referred to as tissue curettes; Commonly packaged in a metallic stand-up rack in order of size

FIGURE 3-138

continues

SHARP TO BLUNT MANUAL DEBULKING CURETTES *continued*

Scoville ruptured disc curettes

Size: Handle 10.0"

Characteristics: Thick, grooved handle with a sharp, scoop-shaped oval working surface at the tip of a long, tapered, straight shank; The cutting end is angled up or down measuring 4 × 10 mm

Uses: Used to debulk deep fibrous or compact tissue

Notes: Commonly used in spinal surgery for disc debulking

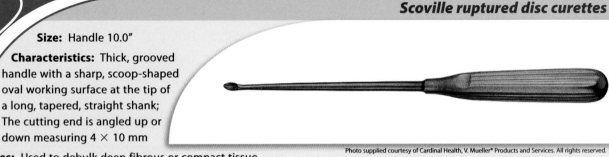

FIGURE 3-139

Volkman double-end curettes

Size: 5.0"; 5.5"; 6.5"; 8.0"

Characteristics: Double-ended handle with a sharp, scoop-shaped oval and round working surfaces of two sizes; Straight shank

Uses: Used to debulk fibrous or compact tissue

Notes: The scoop-shaped ends face two different directions; The 5.5" size curette has two oval ends (Tips 5 × 10 mm and 6 × 20 mm); Other sizes have one oval and one round end; 6 × 10 mm and 7 mm diameter; 8 × 14 mm and 10 mm diameter; 9 × 18 mm and 11 mm diameter

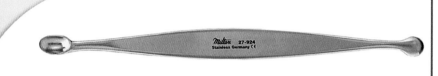

FIGURE 3-140

Sims uterine curettes

Size: Handle 11.0"; Tip size 00 to 01 to 6

Characteristics: Hoop-shaped oval sharp debulking surface on a long malleable shank; Sharp on one side, blunt on the other

Uses: Used inside the uterus

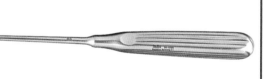

FIGURE 3-141

Thomas uterine curettes

Size: Handle 11.0"; Tip size 1 to 6

Characteristics: Hoop-shaped oval blunt debulking surface on a long malleable shank; Blunt

Uses: Used inside the uterus

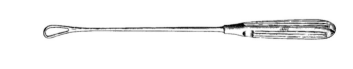

FIGURE 3-142

ELEVATORS AND STRIPPERS: BLUNT DEBULKING INSTRUMENTS

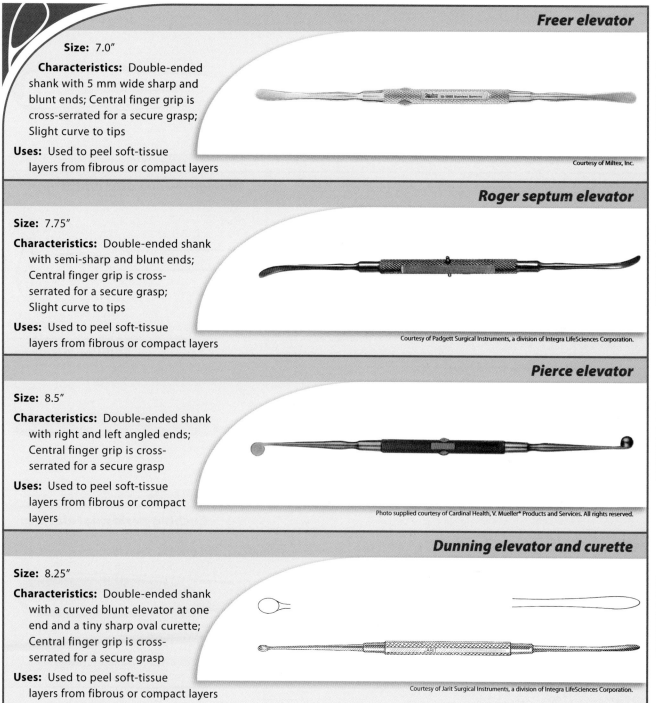

Freer elevator

Size: 7.0"

Characteristics: Double-ended shank with 5 mm wide sharp and blunt ends; Central finger grip is cross-serrated for a secure grasp; Slight curve to tips

Uses: Used to peel soft-tissue layers from fibrous or compact layers

Courtesy of Miltex, Inc.

FIGURE 3-143

Roger septum elevator

Size: 7.75"

Characteristics: Double-ended shank with semi-sharp and blunt ends; Central finger grip is cross-serrated for a secure grasp; Slight curve to tips

Uses: Used to peel soft-tissue layers from fibrous or compact layers

Courtesy of Padgett Surgical Instruments, a division of Integra LifeSciences Corporation.

FIGURE 3-144

Pierce elevator

Size: 8.5"

Characteristics: Double-ended shank with right and left angled ends; Central finger grip is cross-serrated for a secure grasp

Uses: Used to peel soft-tissue layers from fibrous or compact layers

Photo supplied courtesy of Cardinal Health, V. Mueller® Products and Services. All rights reserved.

FIGURE 3-145

Dunning elevator and curette

Size: 8.25"

Characteristics: Double-ended shank with a curved blunt elevator at one end and a tiny sharp oval curette; Central finger grip is cross-serrated for a secure grasp

Uses: Used to peel soft-tissue layers from fibrous or compact layers

Courtesy of Jarit Surgical Instruments, a division of Integra LifeSciences Corporation.

FIGURE 3-146

continues

ELEVATORS AND STRIPPERS: BLUNT DEBULKING INSTRUMENTS *continued*

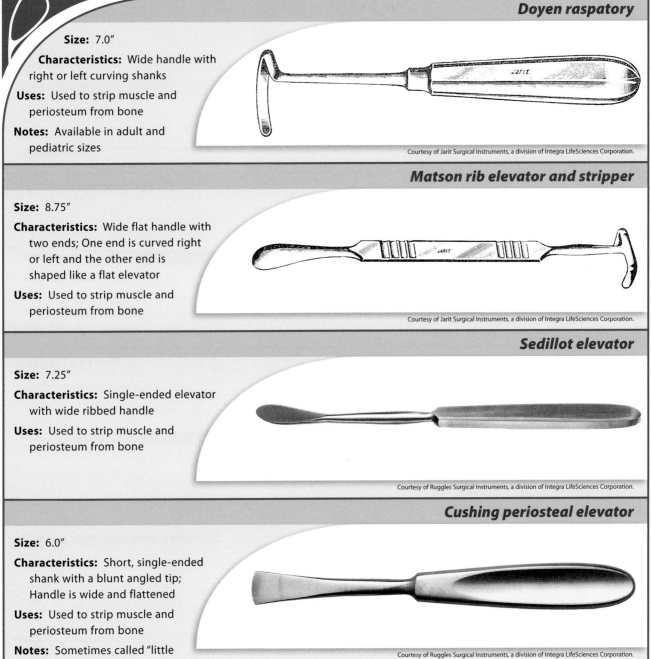

Doyen raspatory

Size: 7.0"

Characteristics: Wide handle with right or left curving shanks

Uses: Used to strip muscle and periosteum from bone

Notes: Available in adult and pediatric sizes

Courtesy of Jarit Surgical Instruments, a division of Integra LifeSciences Corporation.

FIGURE 3-147

Matson rib elevator and stripper

Size: 8.75"

Characteristics: Wide flat handle with two ends; One end is curved right or left and the other end is shaped like a flat elevator

Uses: Used to strip muscle and periosteum from bone

Courtesy of Jarit Surgical Instruments, a division of Integra LifeSciences Corporation.

FIGURE 3-148

Sedillot elevator

Size: 7.25"

Characteristics: Single-ended elevator with wide ribbed handle

Uses: Used to strip muscle and periosteum from bone

Courtesy of Ruggles Surgical Instruments, a division of Integra LifeSciences Corporation.

FIGURE 3-149

Cushing periosteal elevator

Size: 6.0"

Characteristics: Short, single-ended shank with a blunt angled tip; Handle is wide and flattened

Uses: Used to strip muscle and periosteum from bone

Notes: Sometimes called "little joker"

Courtesy of Ruggles Surgical Instruments, a division of Integra LifeSciences Corporation.

FIGURE 3-150

ELEVATORS AND STRIPPERS: BLUNT DEBULKING INSTRUMENTS *continued*

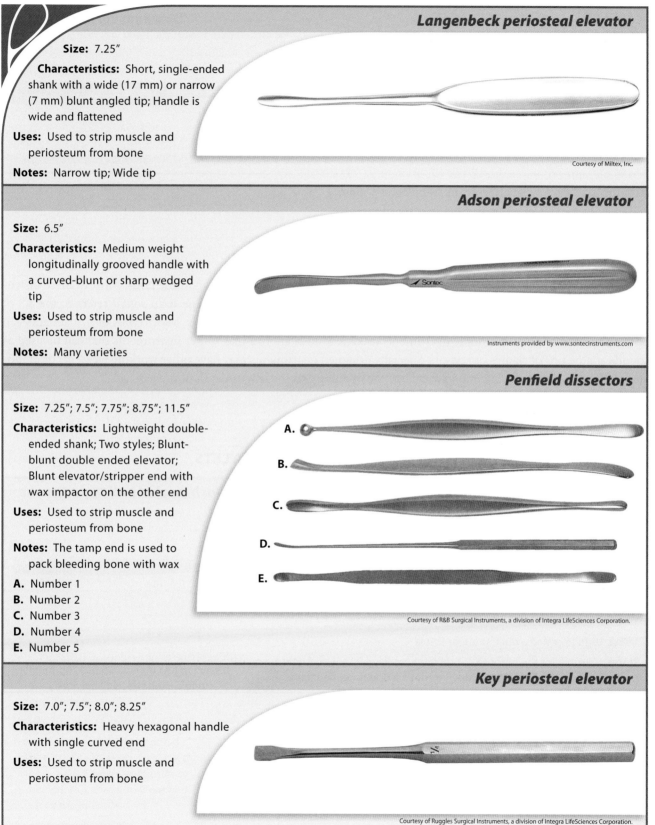

Langenbeck periosteal elevator

Size: 7.25″

Characteristics: Short, single-ended shank with a wide (17 mm) or narrow (7 mm) blunt angled tip; Handle is wide and flattened

Uses: Used to strip muscle and periosteum from bone

Notes: Narrow tip; Wide tip

Courtesy of Miltex, Inc.

FIGURE 3-151

Adson periosteal elevator

Size: 6.5″

Characteristics: Medium weight longitudinally grooved handle with a curved-blunt or sharp wedged tip

Uses: Used to strip muscle and periosteum from bone

Notes: Many varieties

Instruments provided by www.sontecinstruments.com

FIGURE 3-152

Penfield dissectors

Size: 7.25″; 7.5″; 7.75″; 8.75″; 11.5″

Characteristics: Lightweight double-ended shank; Two styles; Blunt-blunt double ended elevator; Blunt elevator/stripper end with wax impactor on the other end

Uses: Used to strip muscle and periosteum from bone

Notes: The tamp end is used to pack bleeding bone with wax

A. Number 1
B. Number 2
C. Number 3
D. Number 4
E. Number 5

A.
B.
C.
D.
E.

Courtesy of R&B Surgical Instruments, a division of Integra LifeSciences Corporation.

FIGURE 3-153

Key periosteal elevator

Size: 7.0″; 7.5″; 8.0″; 8.25″

Characteristics: Heavy hexagonal handle with single curved end

Uses: Used to strip muscle and periosteum from bone

Courtesy of Ruggles Surgical Instruments, a division of Integra LifeSciences Corporation.

FIGURE 3-154

continues

ELEVATORS AND STRIPPERS: BLUNT DEBULKING INSTRUMENTS *continued*

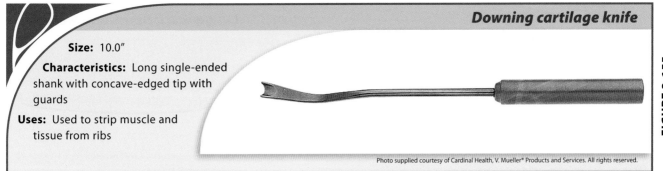

Downing cartilage knife

Size: 10.0"

Characteristics: Long single-ended shank with concave-edged tip with guards

Uses: Used to strip muscle and tissue from ribs

FIGURE 3-155

PROBES AND DILATORS

Dilators and probes are used to expand and explore a natural or created opening in the body. Most of these instruments are blunt; however, some have knives that are incorporated in the tips. The term *sound* refers to the act of blindly, but gently, inserting an instrument into an opening to feel how deep it is. Many types of instruments can be used to "sound" a wound. Some instruments used as sounds are rod-like. Other instruments that can be used as sounds are the tips of clamps or scissors. Specially designed instruments may have other working elements or graduated surfaces that serve to intentionally enlarge the opening and the length/depth of the passage.

Measurement and Expansion

SOUNDS, TUNNELERS, AND STYLETS

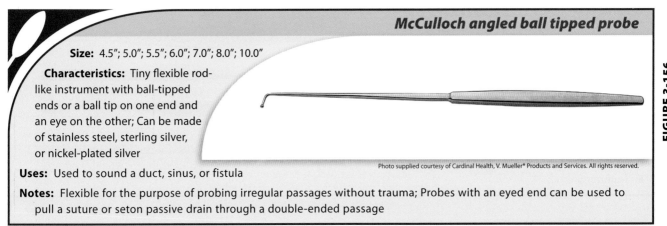

McCulloch angled ball tipped probe

Size: 4.5"; 5.0"; 5.5"; 6.0"; 7.0"; 8.0"; 10.0"

Characteristics: Tiny flexible rod-like instrument with ball-tipped ends or a ball tip on one end and an eye on the other; Can be made of stainless steel, sterling silver, or nickel-plated silver

Uses: Used to sound a duct, sinus, or fistula

Notes: Flexible for the purpose of probing irregular passages without trauma; Probes with an eyed end can be used to pull a suture or seton passive drain through a double-ended passage

FIGURE 3-156

SOUNDS, TUNNELERS, AND STYLETS *continued*

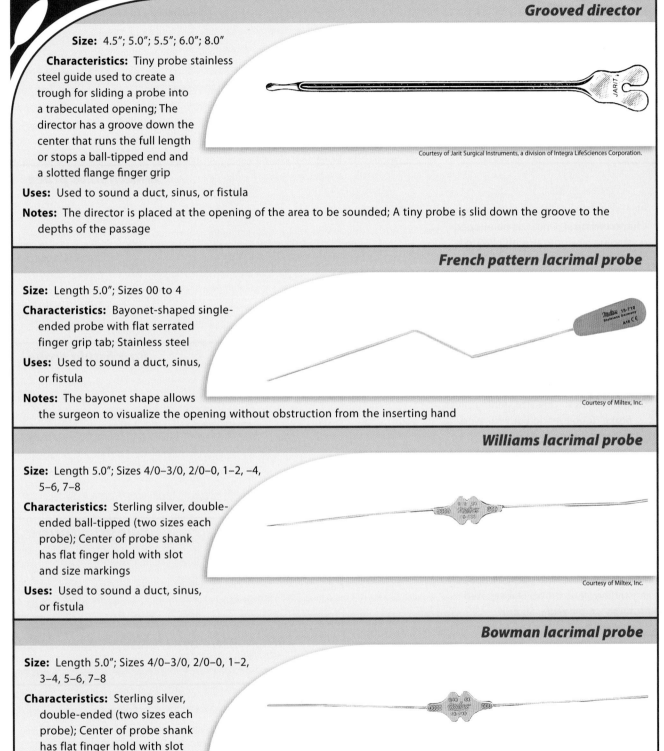

Grooved director

Size: 4.5"; 5.0"; 5.5"; 6.0"; 8.0"

Characteristics: Tiny probe stainless steel guide used to create a trough for sliding a probe into a trabeculated opening; The director has a groove down the center that runs the full length or stops a ball-tipped end and a slotted flange finger grip

Uses: Used to sound a duct, sinus, or fistula

Notes: The director is placed at the opening of the area to be sounded; A tiny probe is slid down the groove to the depths of the passage

Courtesy of Jarit Surgical Instruments, a division of Integra LifeSciences Corporation.

FIGURE 3-157

French pattern lacrimal probe

Size: Length 5.0"; Sizes 00 to 4

Characteristics: Bayonet-shaped single-ended probe with flat serrated finger grip tab; Stainless steel

Uses: Used to sound a duct, sinus, or fistula

Notes: The bayonet shape allows the surgeon to visualize the opening without obstruction from the inserting hand

Courtesy of Miltex, Inc.

FIGURE 3-158

Williams lacrimal probe

Size: Length 5.0"; Sizes 4/0–3/0, 2/0–0, 1–2, –4, 5–6, 7–8

Characteristics: Sterling silver, double-ended ball-tipped (two sizes each probe); Center of probe shank has flat finger hold with slot and size markings

Uses: Used to sound a duct, sinus, or fistula

Courtesy of Miltex, Inc.

FIGURE 3-159

Bowman lacrimal probe

Size: Length 5.0"; Sizes 4/0–3/0, 2/0–0, 1–2, 3–4, 5–6, 7–8

Characteristics: Sterling silver, double-ended (two sizes each probe); Center of probe shank has flat finger hold with slot and size markings

Uses: Used to sound a duct, sinus, or fistula

Courtesy of Miltex, Inc.

FIGURE 3-160

continues

SOUNDS, TUNNELERS, AND STYLETS *continued*

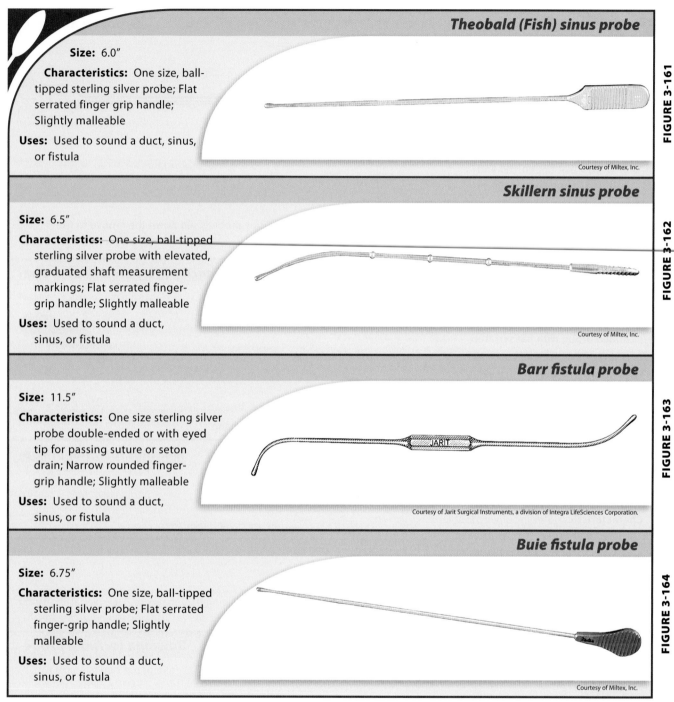

Theobald (Fish) sinus probe

Size: 6.0"

Characteristics: One size, ball-tipped sterling silver probe; Flat serrated finger grip handle; Slightly malleable

Uses: Used to sound a duct, sinus, or fistula

Courtesy of Miltex, Inc.

FIGURE 3-161

Skillern sinus probe

Size: 6.5"

Characteristics: One size, ball-tipped sterling silver probe with elevated, graduated shaft measurement markings; Flat serrated finger-grip handle; Slightly malleable

Uses: Used to sound a duct, sinus, or fistula

Courtesy of Miltex, Inc.

FIGURE 3-162

Barr fistula probe

Size: 11.5"

Characteristics: One size sterling silver probe double-ended or with eyed tip for passing suture or seton drain; Narrow rounded finger-grip handle; Slightly malleable

Uses: Used to sound a duct, sinus, or fistula

Courtesy of Jarit Surgical Instruments, a division of Integra LifeSciences Corporation.

FIGURE 3-163

Buie fistula probe

Size: 6.75"

Characteristics: One size, ball-tipped sterling silver probe; Flat serrated finger-grip handle; Slightly malleable

Uses: Used to sound a duct, sinus, or fistula

Courtesy of Miltex, Inc.

FIGURE 3-164

SOUNDS, TUNNELERS, AND STYLETS *continued*

Pratt rectal probe

Size: 11.0"

Characteristics: One size, ball-tipped sterling silver probe; Rounded finger-grip handle; Slightly malleable

Uses: Used to sound a duct, sinus, or fistula

Notes: Slightly heavier gauge than a Skillern probe

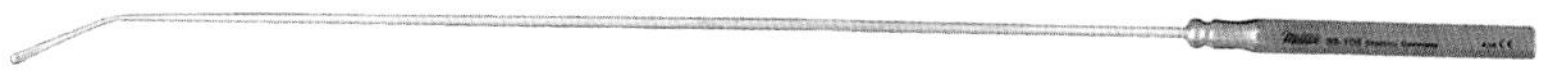

Courtesy of Miltex, Inc.

FIGURE 3-165

Mayo common duct probe

Size: 10.0"; Sizes 15 fr, 18 fr

Characteristics: Single-ended olive-tipped probe with flat grooved handle; Shaft is malleable

Uses: Used to sound a duct or tubular structure

Notes: The tip resembles a small solid olive-shaped knob on the end of the shaft

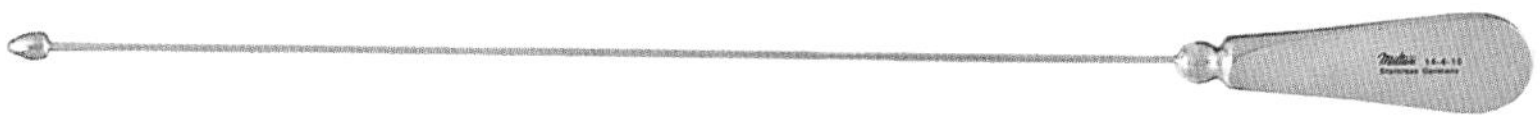

Courtesy of Miltex, Inc.

FIGURE 3-166

Bakes common duct dilator

Size: 8.75"

Characteristics: Single-ended bullet-tipped probe with short cylindrical handle; Shaft is malleable

Uses: Used to sound a duct or tubular structure

Notes: The tip resembles a bullet shape on the end of a slender shaft

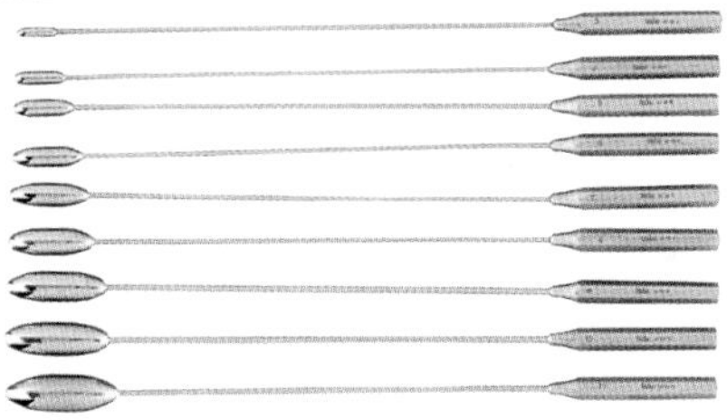

Courtesy of Miltex, Inc.

FIGURE 3-167

Stewart crypt hook

Size: 8.5"

Characteristics: Crook-shaped probe with a ball tip; Single-ended; Stainless steel; Open-looped handle

Uses: Used to probe an anal crypt

Notes: Probe is inserted in anus and used to separate the wall of the crypt from the dentate line; The roof is incised and permitted to drain

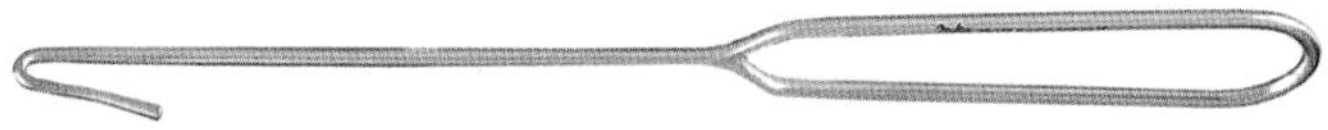

Courtesy of Miltex, Inc.

FIGURE 3-168

continues

SOUNDS, TUNNELERS, AND STYLETS *continued*

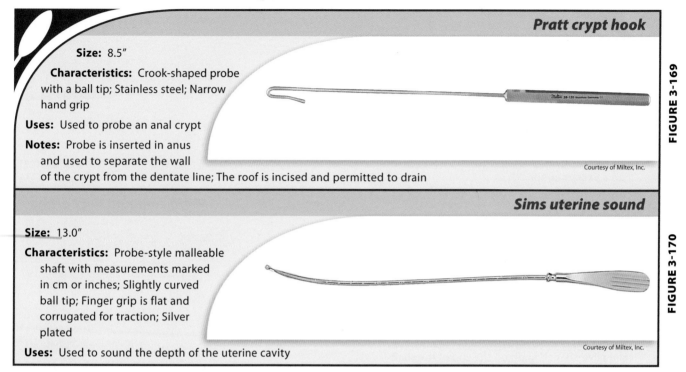

Pratt crypt hook

FIGURE 3-169

Size: 8.5"

Characteristics: Crook-shaped probe with a ball tip; Stainless steel; Narrow hand grip

Uses: Used to probe an anal crypt

Notes: Probe is inserted in anus and used to separate the wall of the crypt from the dentate line; The roof is incised and permitted to drain

Courtesy of Miltex, Inc.

Sims uterine sound

FIGURE 3-170

Size: 13.0"

Characteristics: Probe-style malleable shaft with measurements marked in cm or inches; Slightly curved ball tip; Finger grip is flat and corrugated for traction; Silver plated

Uses: Used to sound the depth of the uterine cavity

Courtesy of Miltex, Inc.

MANUAL GRADUATED DILATORS

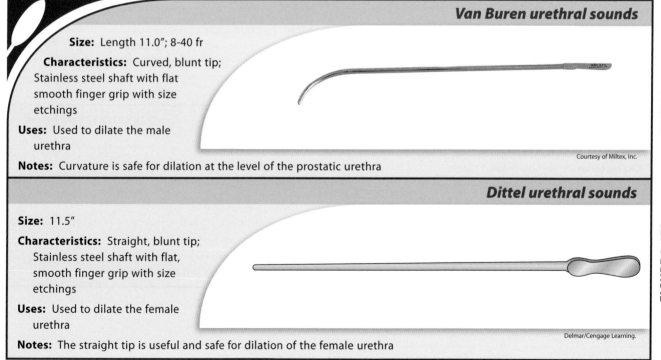

Van Buren urethral sounds

FIGURE 3-171

Size: Length 11.0"; 8–40 fr

Characteristics: Curved, blunt tip; Stainless steel shaft with flat smooth finger grip with size etchings

Uses: Used to dilate the male urethra

Notes: Curvature is safe for dilation at the level of the prostatic urethra

Courtesy of Miltex, Inc.

Dittel urethral sounds

FIGURE 3-172

Size: 11.5"

Characteristics: Straight, blunt tip; Stainless steel shaft with flat, smooth finger grip with size etchings

Uses: Used to dilate the female urethra

Notes: The straight tip is useful and safe for dilation of the female urethra

Delmar/Cengage Learning.

MANUAL GRADUATED DILATORS *continued*

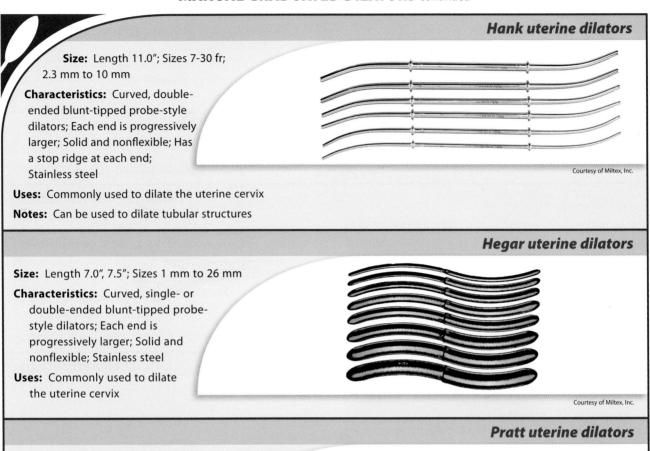

Hank uterine dilators

Size: Length 11.0"; Sizes 7-30 fr; 2.3 mm to 10 mm

Characteristics: Curved, double-ended blunt-tipped probe-style dilators; Each end is progressively larger; Solid and nonflexible; Has a stop ridge at each end; Stainless steel

Uses: Commonly used to dilate the uterine cervix

Notes: Can be used to dilate tubular structures

Courtesy of Miltex, Inc.

FIGURE 3-173

Hegar uterine dilators

Size: Length 7.0", 7.5"; Sizes 1 mm to 26 mm

Characteristics: Curved, single- or double-ended blunt-tipped probe-style dilators; Each end is progressively larger; Solid and nonflexible; Stainless steel

Uses: Commonly used to dilate the uterine cervix

Courtesy of Miltex, Inc.

FIGURE 3-174

Pratt uterine dilators

Size: Length 11.5"; Sizes 13 to 15 fr

Characteristics: Curved, double-ended blunt-tipped probe-style dilators; Each end is progressively larger; Solid and nonflexible; Stainless steel

Uses: Commonly used to dilate the uterine cervix

Courtesy of Jarit Surgical Instruments, a division of Integra LifeSciences Corporation.

FIGURE 3-175

MECHANIZED DILATORS

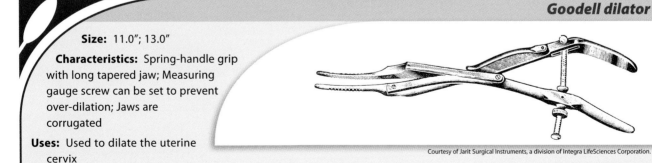

Goodell dilator

Size: 11.0"; 13.0"

Characteristics: Spring-handle grip with long tapered jaw; Measuring gauge screw can be set to prevent over-dilation; Jaws are corrugated

Uses: Used to dilate the uterine cervix

Notes: Mechanical cervical dilators with smooth jaws and without the measuring screw are commonly called Wilie's or Starlinger's dilators

Courtesy of Jarit Surgical Instruments, a division of Integra LifeSciences Corporation.

FIGURE 3-176

continues

MECHANIZED DILATORS *continued*

Trousseau tracheal dilator

Size: 4.25"; 5.25"

Characteristics: Ring handles with spring mechanism in handles; Two blunt-tipped, right-angled jaws for tracheal space dilation

Uses: Used to open the incision for tracheostomy

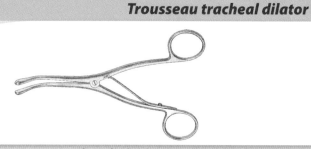

Courtesy of Jarit Surgical Instruments, a division of Integra LifeSciences Corporation.

FIGURE 3-177

LaBorde tracheal dilator

Size: 5.5"

Characteristics: Ring handles with spring mechanism in handles; Three blunt-tipped, right-angled jaws for tracheal space dilation

Uses: Used to open the incision for tracheostomy

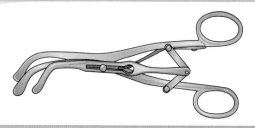

Delmar/Cengage Learning.

FIGURE 3-178

Otis urethrotome

Size: 11.0"

Characteristics: Straight dilation assembly with two cutting blade surfaces to release strictured urethral tissues

Uses: Used to enlarge the urethral passage

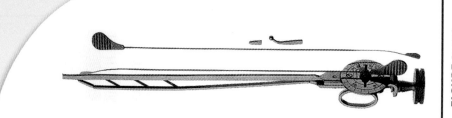

Courtesy of Jarit Surgical Instruments, a division of Integra LifeSciences Corporation.

FIGURE 3-179

MEASURING DEVICES

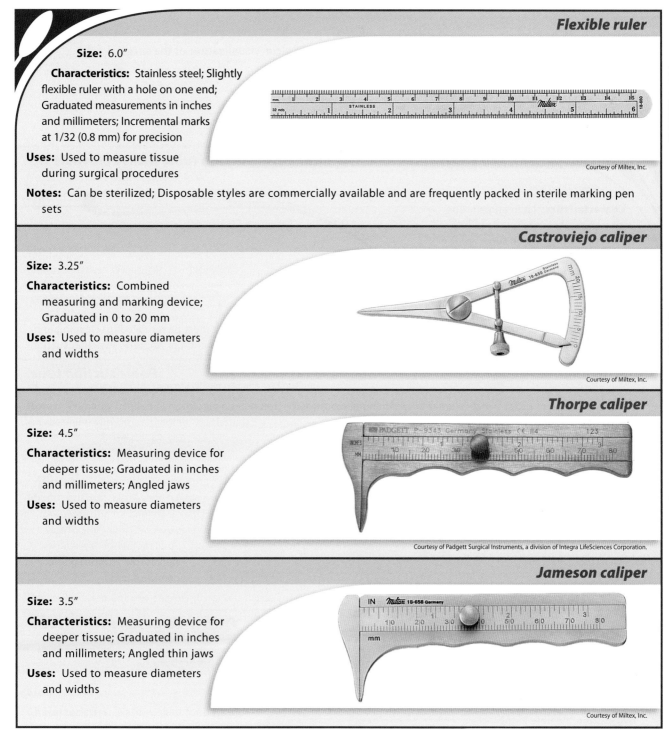

FIGURE 3-180

Flexible ruler

Size: 6.0″

Characteristics: Stainless steel; Slightly flexible ruler with a hole on one end; Graduated measurements in inches and millimeters; Incremental marks at 1/32 (0.8 mm) for precision

Uses: Used to measure tissue during surgical procedures

Notes: Can be sterilized; Disposable styles are commercially available and are frequently packed in sterile marking pen sets

Courtesy of Miltex, Inc.

FIGURE 3-181

Castroviejo caliper

Size: 3.25″

Characteristics: Combined measuring and marking device; Graduated in 0 to 20 mm

Uses: Used to measure diameters and widths

Courtesy of Miltex, Inc.

FIGURE 3-182

Thorpe caliper

Size: 4.5″

Characteristics: Measuring device for deeper tissue; Graduated in inches and millimeters; Angled jaws

Uses: Used to measure diameters and widths

Courtesy of Padgett Surgical Instruments, a division of Integra LifeSciences Corporation.

FIGURE 3-183

Jameson caliper

Size: 3.5″

Characteristics: Measuring device for deeper tissue; Graduated in inches and millimeters; Angled thin jaws

Uses: Used to measure diameters and widths

Courtesy of Miltex, Inc.

EVACUATION AND INSTALLATION INSTRUMENTATION

Removal of blood and body fluids from the surgical site promotes clear visualization of the surgical field.

Evacuation Instrumentation

SUCTION TIPS

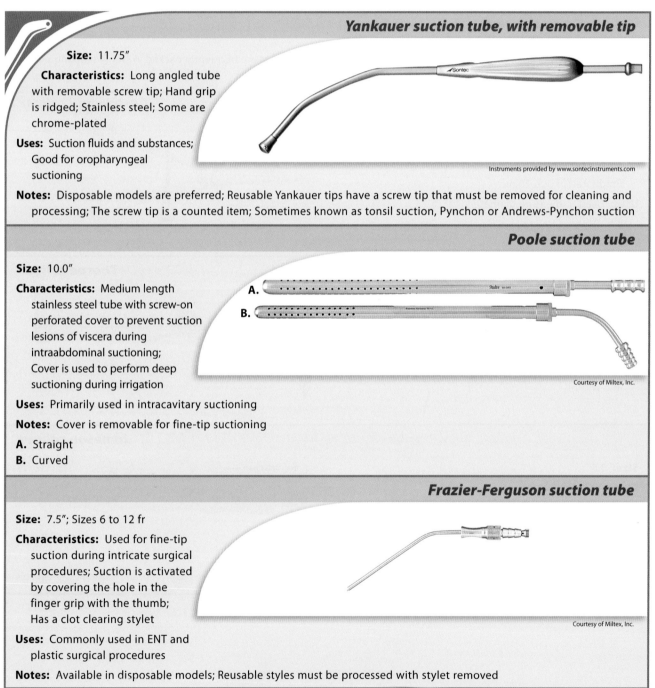

Yankauer suction tube, with removable tip

Size: 11.75"

Characteristics: Long angled tube with removable screw tip; Hand grip is ridged; Stainless steel; Some are chrome-plated

Uses: Suction fluids and substances; Good for oropharyngeal suctioning

Instruments provided by www.sontecinstruments.com

Notes: Disposable models are preferred; Reusable Yankauer tips have a screw tip that must be removed for cleaning and processing; The screw tip is a counted item; Sometimes known as tonsil suction, Pynchon or Andrews-Pynchon suction

FIGURE 3-184

Poole suction tube

Size: 10.0"

Characteristics: Medium length stainless steel tube with screw-on perforated cover to prevent suction lesions of viscera during intraabdominal suctioning; Cover is used to perform deep suctioning during irrigation

A.

B.

Courtesy of Miltex, Inc.

Uses: Primarily used in intracavitary suctioning

Notes: Cover is removable for fine-tip suctioning

A. Straight
B. Curved

FIGURE 3-185

Frazier-Ferguson suction tube

Size: 7.5"; Sizes 6 to 12 fr

Characteristics: Used for fine-tip suction during intricate surgical procedures; Suction is activated by covering the hole in the finger grip with the thumb; Has a clot clearing stylet

Courtesy of Miltex, Inc.

Uses: Commonly used in ENT and plastic surgical procedures

Notes: Available in disposable models; Reusable styles must be processed with stylet removed

FIGURE 3-186

SUCTION TIPS *continued*

Baron suction tube

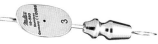

Size: 3.0"; Sizes 3, 5, 7 fr

Characteristics: Used for fine-tip suction during intricate surgical procedures; Suction is activated by covering the hole in the finger grip with the thumb; Smaller than Frazier-Ferguson suction tips; Has a clot-clearing stylet

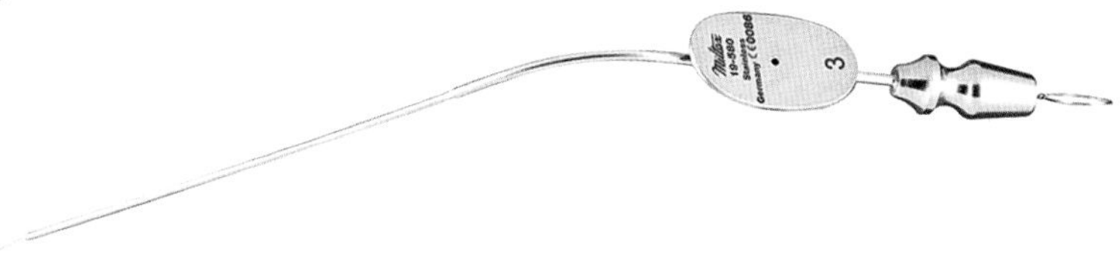

Uses: Commonly used in small surgical areas

Notes: Reusable styles must be processed with stylet removed

Courtesy of Miltex, Inc.

FIGURE 3-187

Adson suction tube

Size: 6.0"; 8.0"; Sizes 11 or 15 fr

Characteristics: Used for fine-tip suction during intricate surgical procedures; Suction is activated by covering the hole in the finger grip with the thumb; Smaller than Frazier-Ferguson suction tips; Has a clot-clearing stylet

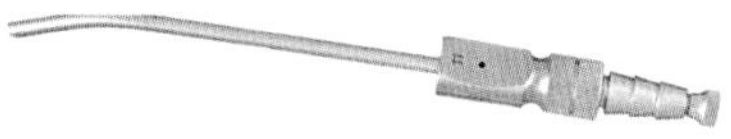

Uses: Commonly used in small surgical areas

Notes: Reusable stylets must be processed with stylet removed

Courtesy of Miltex, Inc.

FIGURE 3-188

Buie suction tube

Size: 16.0"

Characteristics: No stylet; Stainless steel suction tip; Suction is activated by covering the hole in the finger grip with the thumb

Uses: Commonly used in rigid endoscopic procedures of the upper and the lower gastrointestinal tract

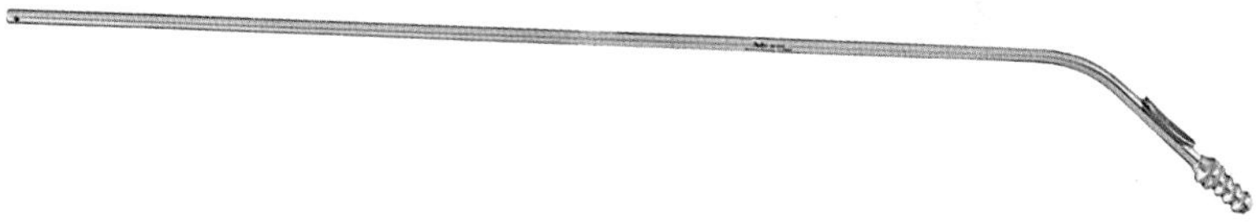

Courtesy of Miltex, Inc.

FIGURE 3-189

Injection and Irrigation Devices

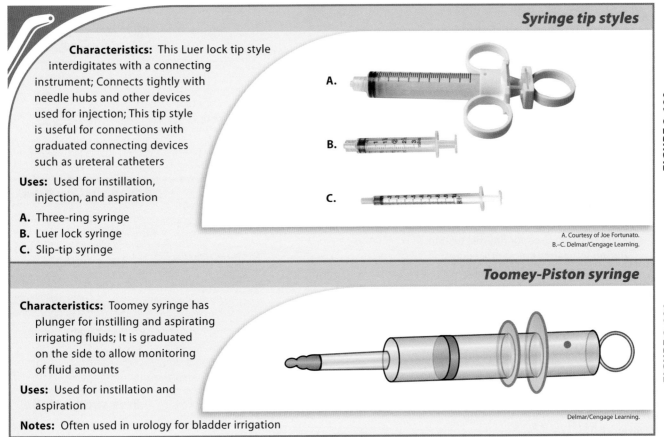

SYRINGES

Syringe tip styles

Characteristics: This Luer lock tip style interdigitates with a connecting instrument; Connects tightly with needle hubs and other devices used for injection; This tip style is useful for connections with graduated connecting devices such as ureteral catheters

Uses: Used for instillation, injection, and aspiration

A. Three-ring syringe
B. Luer lock syringe
C. Slip-tip syringe

A. Courtesy of Joe Fortunato.
B.–C. Delmar/Cengage Learning.

FIGURE 3-190

Toomey-Piston syringe

Characteristics: Toomey syringe has plunger for instilling and aspirating irrigating fluids; It is graduated on the side to allow monitoring of fluid amounts

Uses: Used for instillation and aspiration

Notes: Often used in urology for bladder irrigation

Delmar/Cengage Learning.

FIGURE 3-191

RETRACTION AND EXPOSURE

Retractors are used to stabilize and displace anatomic structures in a surgical field in order to provide visual exposure. There are two basic styles of retractors commonly used in surgery—(1) manual, handheld and (2) self-retaining, free-mounted or bed-mounted. Handheld retractors are held by the first assistant. Self-retaining retractors work on the principle of counter-traction secured with a locking mechanism. Use of any retractor requires knowledge and skill associated with anatomic structures and should only be placed and held by adequately trained personnel.

Retractors

Handheld Retractors

Handheld retractors do not require the application of over-tight pulling to provide a clear visual field. They are dynamically designed to be held comfortably with one hand in a natural position. Some larger manual retractors, when repeatedly held in a prolonged pose, can contribute to repetitive stress injury with resultant carpal tunnel syndrome.

HANDHELD RETRACTORS

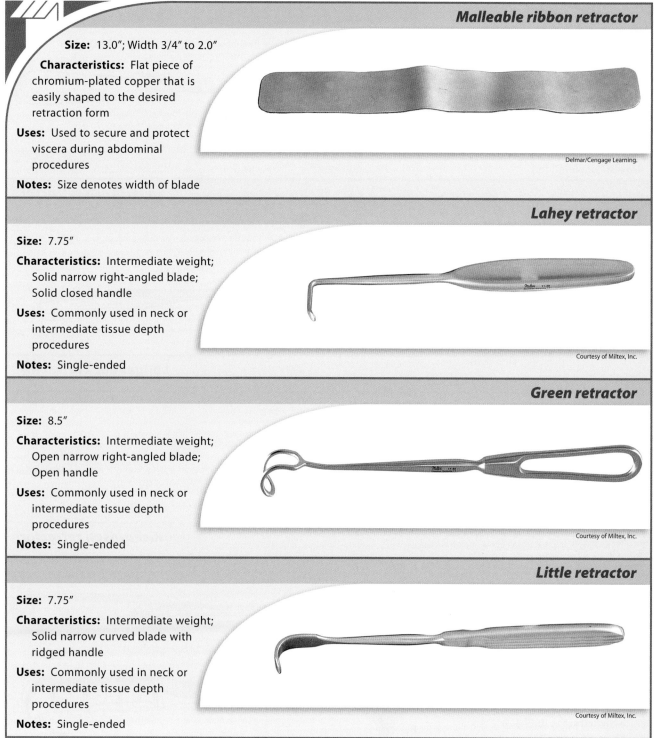

Malleable ribbon retractor

Size: 13.0"; Width 3/4" to 2.0"

Characteristics: Flat piece of chromium-plated copper that is easily shaped to the desired retraction form

Uses: Used to secure and protect viscera during abdominal procedures

Notes: Size denotes width of blade

Delmar/Cengage Learning.

FIGURE 3-192

Lahey retractor

Size: 7.75"

Characteristics: Intermediate weight; Solid narrow right-angled blade; Solid closed handle

Uses: Commonly used in neck or intermediate tissue depth procedures

Notes: Single-ended

Courtesy of Miltex, Inc.

FIGURE 3-193

Green retractor

Size: 8.5"

Characteristics: Intermediate weight; Open narrow right-angled blade; Open handle

Uses: Commonly used in neck or intermediate tissue depth procedures

Notes: Single-ended

Courtesy of Miltex, Inc.

FIGURE 3-194

Little retractor

Size: 7.75"

Characteristics: Intermediate weight; Solid narrow curved blade with ridged handle

Uses: Commonly used in neck or intermediate tissue depth procedures

Notes: Single-ended

Courtesy of Miltex, Inc.

FIGURE 3-195

continues

HANDHELD RETRACTORS *continued*

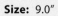

Cushing vein retractor

Size: 9.0"

Characteristics: Intermediate weight; Closed narrow right-angled blade with curved lip; Open handle

Uses: Commonly used in neck or intermediate tissue depth procedures

Notes: Single-ended

Courtesy of Miltex, Inc.

FIGURE 3-196

Sauerbruch retractor

Size: 9.0"

Characteristics: Intermediate weight; Closed narrow right-angled blade with curved lip; Ridged cylindrical handle

Uses: Commonly used in neck or intermediate tissue depth procedures

Courtesy of Miltex, Inc.

FIGURE 3-197

Langenbeck retractor

Size: 8.0"

Characteristics: Right-angle retractor; Flat solid hand grip; Blade length can vary

Uses: Used for layers closer to the surface

Notes: Single-ended

Courtesy of Miltex, Inc.

FIGURE 3-198

Richardson retractor

Size: 9.5"

Characteristics: Right-angle retractor; Blade width can vary; Handle can be open loop style (A.) or hollow closed (B.); Both have finger ridges for a secure grip

Uses: Used for several layers including deep body wall

Notes: Single-ended; Similar to Kelly retractor, but has a shorter blade; Common blade size 2.0" × 3/4" is used frequently for open appendectomy (appendicele)

A. Loop handle
B. Hollow grip handle

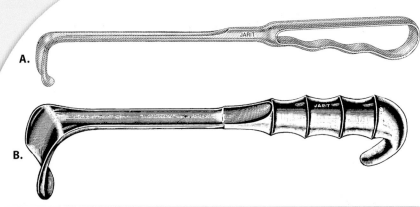

Courtesy of Jarit Surgical Instruments, a division of Integra LifeSciences Corporation.

FIGURE 3-199

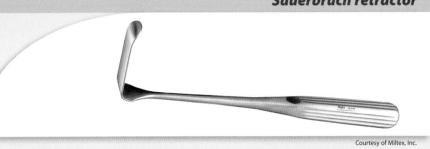
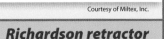

HANDHELD RETRACTORS *continued*

Kelly retractor

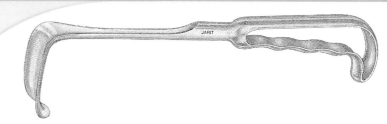

Size: 9.50"; 9.75"; 10.0"

Characteristics: Right-angle retractor; Blade length can vary; Handle can be open loop style (shown) or hollow closed; Both have finger ridges for a secure grip

Uses: Used for several layers including deep body wall

Notes: Single-ended; Similar to Richardson retractor, but has a longer blade

Courtesy of Jarit Surgical Instruments, a division of Integra LifeSciences Corporation.

FIGURE 3-200

Deaver retractor

Size: 12.0"; Sizes 1.0", 1.5", 2.0", 3.0", 4.0"

Characteristics: Flat semi-firm large curved blade with "S" curve at hand grip for traction; Size is denoted for width of blade; Slightly flexible; Hollow grip handle available

Uses: Used for several layers including deep body wall

Notes: Pediatric Deaver blade is measured in increments of 1/8" up to 7/8"; When used to retract an organ, a moist laparotomy sponge should be placed between the retractor blade and the structure

A. Flat handle
B. Hollow grip handle

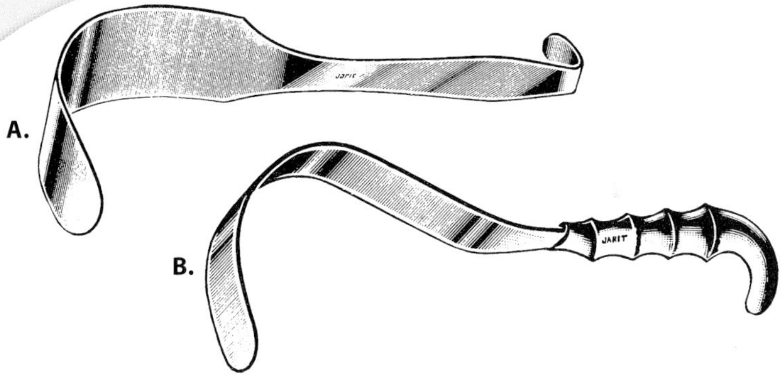

Courtesy of Jarit Surgical Instruments, a division of Integra LifeSciences Corporation.

FIGURE 3-201

Harrington retractor

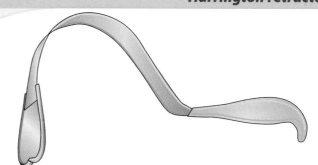

Size: 9.0"; 12.0"

Characteristics: Flat, large curved blade with hollow hand grip for traction; Size is denoted for width of blade; Slightly flexible; Heart-shaped viscera protector at the tip to prevent perforation

Uses: Used to retract the liver

Notes: Commonly called "sweetheart" or "valentine" retractor

Delmar/Cengage Learning.

FIGURE 3-202

Heaney-Simon retractor

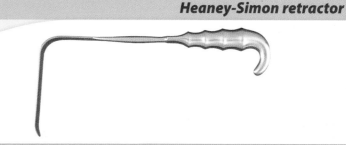

Size: 11.0"; Size 4.5"

Characteristics: Right-angle retractor with elongated 1.0" wide blade; Hollow hand grip with ridges

Uses: Used for several layers including deep body wall

Notes: Single-ended

Courtesy of Miltex, Inc.

FIGURE 3-203

continues

HANDHELD RETRACTORS *continued*

De Lee universal retractor

Size: 9.5″

Characteristics: Right-angled retractor with 2.75″ × 2.0″ blade; Scooped out blade surface provides additional lateral wall retraction; Hollow grip handle

Uses: Used for several layers including narrow incisions into body wall

Notes: Used often in obstetrics to retract bladder during Cesarean section

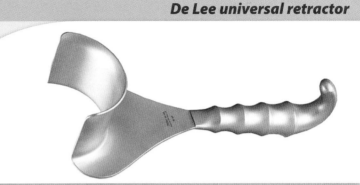

Courtesy of Miltex, Inc.

FIGURE 3-204

Doyen retractor

Size: 9.0″; Sizes 1.75″, 2.0″, 2.25″

Characteristics: Right-angled retractor with solid posterior thumb hook hand grip; Blade is long and squared with blunt edges

Uses: Used for several layers including deep body wall

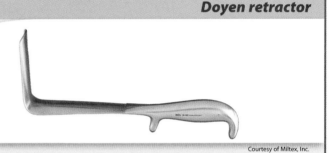

Courtesy of Miltex, Inc.

FIGURE 3-205

Mayo abdominal retractor

Size: 10.0″

Characteristics: Right-angled retractor with solid anterior thumb hook hand grip; Blade is wide and curved under with blunt edges

Uses: Used for body wall

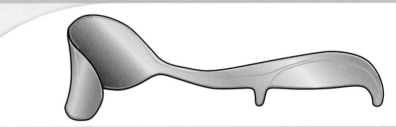

Delmar/Cengage Learning.

FIGURE 3-206

Allison retractor

Size: 12.75″

Characteristics: Flexible layered wire hoop that is atraumatic to friable tissue; Solid handle

Uses: Used to retract lung tissue

Notes: Looks like a flattened wire baking whisk; Relatively large sections of tissue can be retracted without injury

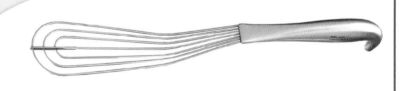

Courtesy of Miltex, Inc.

FIGURE 3-207

HANDHELD RETRACTORS *continued*

Davidson scapula retractor

Size: Blade 3.5″ × 3.25″

Characteristics: Acutely angled wide bladed retractor; Solid ridged handle

Uses: Used to retract the scapula

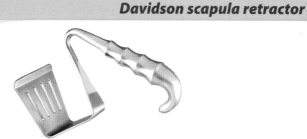

Courtesy of Miltex, Inc.

FIGURE 3-208

Rake retractor

Size: 5.0″; 6.0″

Characteristics: Single-ended prong-tipped; Stainless steel; Spring-flex retraction end available with one to three prongs; Sharp and blunt prong styles

Uses: Used for layers closer to the surface

Notes: Prongs on rake grasp tissue securely; Cannot use rake retractors near areas in risk for perforation such as vessels, nerves, or viscera

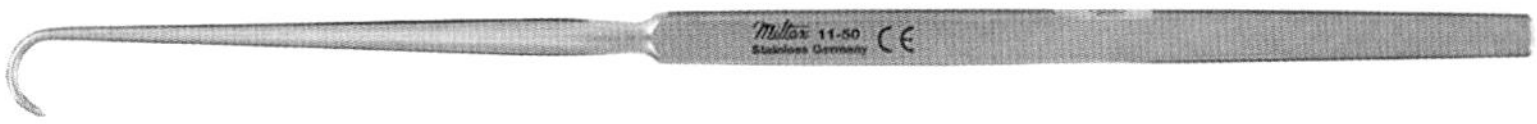

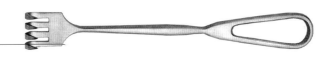

Courtesy of Miltex, Inc.

FIGURE 3-209

Volkman retractor

Size: 4.5″; 8.0″; 8.5″; 9.0″

Characteristics: Single-ended prong-tipped; Stainless steel; One to six prongs; Sharp and blunt prong styles

Uses: Used for layers closer to the surface

Notes: Open or closed handle styles

Courtesy of Ruggles Surgical Instruments, a division of Integra LifeSciences Corporation.

FIGURE 3-210

Murphy retractor

Size: 7.5″

Characteristics: Single-ended prong-tipped; Stainless steel; Two to six prongs; Sharp and blunt prong styles; Egyptian; Ankh–shaped handle with thumb hooks and finger ring for secure grasp

Uses: Used for layers closer to the surface

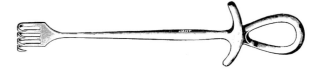

Courtesy of Jarit Surgical Instruments, a division of Integra LifeSciences Corporation.

FIGURE 3-211

continues

HANDHELD RETRACTORS *continued*

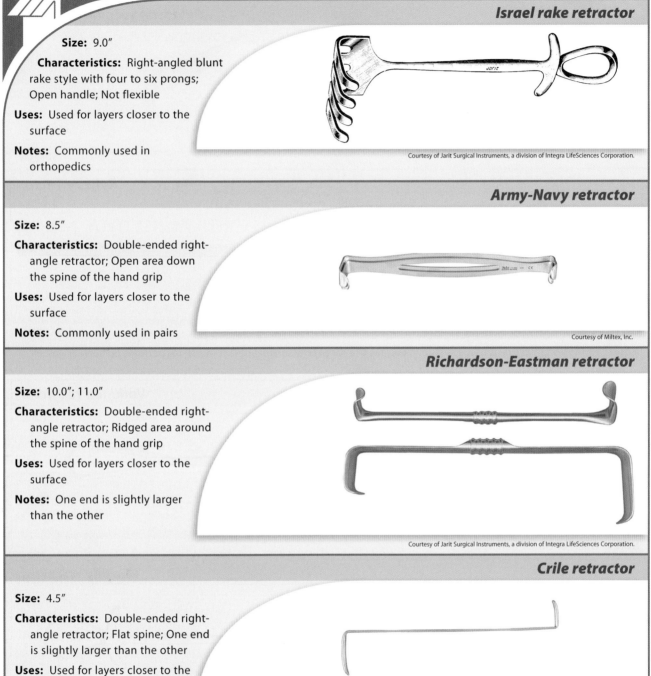

Israel rake retractor

Size: 9.0"

Characteristics: Right-angled blunt rake style with four to six prongs; Open handle; Not flexible

Uses: Used for layers closer to the surface

Notes: Commonly used in orthopedics

Courtesy of Jarit Surgical Instruments, a division of Integra LifeSciences Corporation.

FIGURE 3-212

Army-Navy retractor

Size: 8.5"

Characteristics: Double-ended right-angle retractor; Open area down the spine of the hand grip

Uses: Used for layers closer to the surface

Notes: Commonly used in pairs

Courtesy of Miltex, Inc.

FIGURE 3-213

Richardson-Eastman retractor

Size: 10.0"; 11.0"

Characteristics: Double-ended right-angle retractor; Ridged area around the spine of the hand grip

Uses: Used for layers closer to the surface

Notes: One end is slightly larger than the other

Courtesy of Jarit Surgical Instruments, a division of Integra LifeSciences Corporation.

FIGURE 3-214

Crile retractor

Size: 4.5"

Characteristics: Double-ended right-angle retractor; Flat spine; One end is slightly larger than the other

Uses: Used for layers closer to the surface

Notes: The ends point in opposite directions; When the working end is in the tissue, the opposite end serves as the finger grip

Courtesy of Miltex, Inc.

FIGURE 3-215

HANDHELD RETRACTORS *continued*

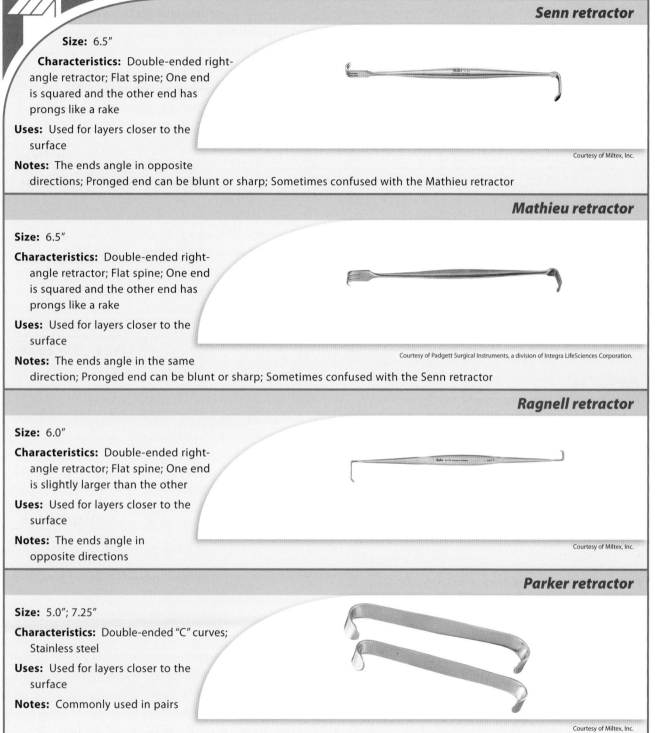

Senn retractor

Size: 6.5"

Characteristics: Double-ended right-angle retractor; Flat spine; One end is squared and the other end has prongs like a rake

Uses: Used for layers closer to the surface

Notes: The ends angle in opposite directions; Pronged end can be blunt or sharp; Sometimes confused with the Mathieu retractor

Courtesy of Miltex, Inc.

FIGURE 3-216

Mathieu retractor

Size: 6.5"

Characteristics: Double-ended right-angle retractor; Flat spine; One end is squared and the other end has prongs like a rake

Uses: Used for layers closer to the surface

Notes: The ends angle in the same direction; Pronged end can be blunt or sharp; Sometimes confused with the Senn retractor

Courtesy of Padgett Surgical Instruments, a division of Integra LifeSciences Corporation.

FIGURE 3-217

Ragnell retractor

Size: 6.0"

Characteristics: Double-ended right-angle retractor; Flat spine; One end is slightly larger than the other

Uses: Used for layers closer to the surface

Notes: The ends angle in opposite directions

Courtesy of Miltex, Inc.

FIGURE 3-218

Parker retractor

Size: 5.0"; 7.25"

Characteristics: Double-ended "C" curves; Stainless steel

Uses: Used for layers closer to the surface

Notes: Commonly used in pairs

Courtesy of Miltex, Inc.

FIGURE 3-219

continues

HANDHELD RETRACTORS *continued*

Kleinert-Kutz hook retractor

Size: 5.0"; Sizes 3 mm, 5 mm, 7 mm

Characteristics: Extremely sharp single hook on a narrow shaft; Slightly flexible

Uses: Used for layers closer to the surface

Courtesy of Miltex, Inc.

FIGURE 3-220

Gillies (Converse) retractor

Size: 7.0"

Characteristics: Extremely sharp single hook on a narrow shaft; Smaller hook than Kleinert-Kutz

Uses: Used for layers closer to the surface

Courtesy of Miltex, Inc.

FIGURE 3-221

Freer skin hook

Size: 6.0"

Characteristics: Tiny double hook on a narrow shaft; Hooks can be blunt or sharp; Distance between prongs is 2.5 mm

Uses: Used for layers closer to the surface

Courtesy of Miltex, Inc.

FIGURE 3-222

Joseph hook

Size: 6.25"

Characteristics: Sharp single hook (A.) or double hook (B.) on a narrow shaft; Double prongs can be 2 mm-10 mm apart

Uses: Used for layers closer to the surface

A. Single prong
B. Double prong

A.

B.

Courtesy of Miltex, Inc.

FIGURE 3-223

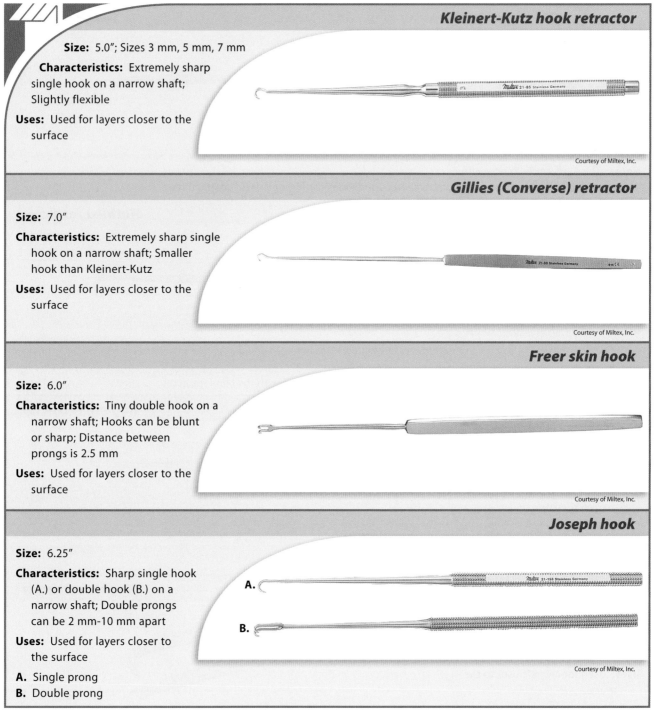

Self-Retaining Retractors

Self-retaining retractors provide exposure without causing physical strain on the surgical team. Care is taken when placing the components of the retractor because inadvertent structures could become entrapped and damaged. A locking or stabilizing mechanism is built in to each style. Some use screws and some use a ratchet system. Each self-retaining retractor has a primary frame that locks to hold tissues in position. Some styles have detachable blades, hooks, rakes, or traction.

SELF-RETAINING RETRACTORS

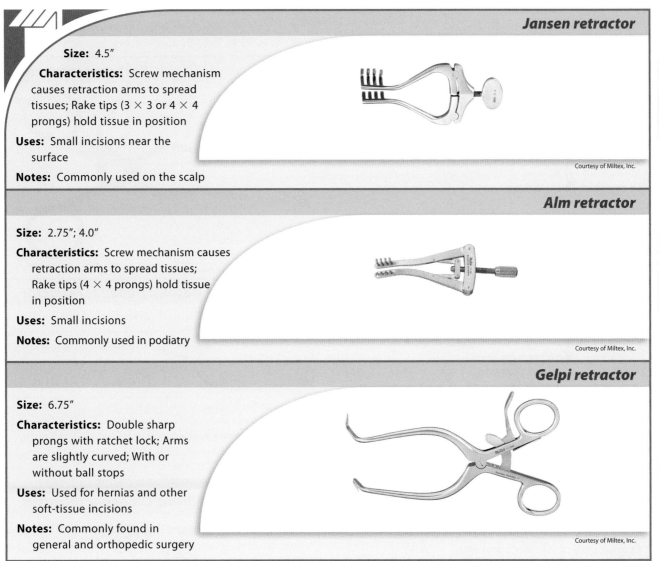

Jansen retractor

Size: 4.5″

Characteristics: Screw mechanism causes retraction arms to spread tissues; Rake tips (3 × 3 or 4 × 4 prongs) hold tissue in position

Uses: Small incisions near the surface

Notes: Commonly used on the scalp

Courtesy of Miltex, Inc.

FIGURE 3-224

Alm retractor

Size: 2.75″; 4.0″

Characteristics: Screw mechanism causes retraction arms to spread tissues; Rake tips (4 × 4 prongs) hold tissue in position

Uses: Small incisions

Notes: Commonly used in podiatry

Courtesy of Miltex, Inc.

FIGURE 3-225

Gelpi retractor

Size: 6.75″

Characteristics: Double sharp prongs with ratchet lock; Arms are slightly curved; With or without ball stops

Uses: Used for hernias and other soft-tissue incisions

Notes: Commonly found in general and orthopedic surgery

Courtesy of Miltex, Inc.

FIGURE 3-226

continues

SELF-RETAINING RETRACTORS *continued*

Weitlaner retractor

Size: 4.0"; 5.5"; 6.5"; 8.0"; 9.5"

Characteristics: Double-armed blades with ratchet lock; Tips have sharp or blunt rake prongs that interdigitate when closed

Uses: Used for small deep incisions

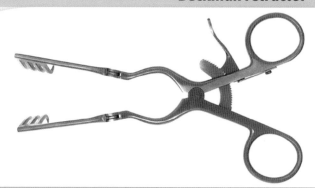

Notes: Straight arms separate and secure the tissue; More than one can be used at opposing ends of the incision; Used by almost every surgical service

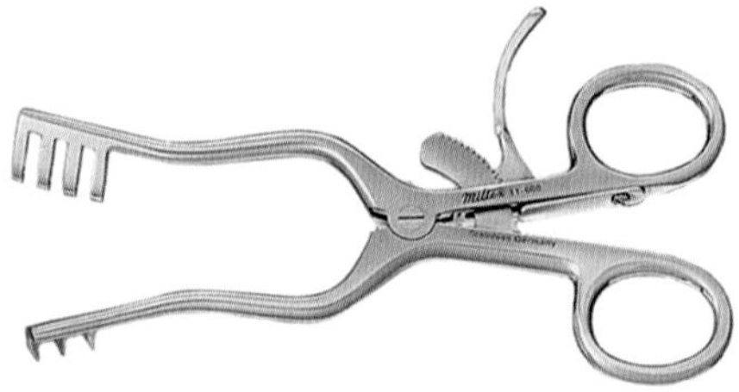

FIGURE 3-227

Beckman retractor

Size: 12.5"

Characteristics: Double-armed blades with ratchet lock; Tips are mounted on hinged arms and have sharp 4 × 4 rake prongs

Uses: Used for small deep incisions

FIGURE 3-228

Adson cerebellar retractor

Size: 7.5"

Characteristics: Double-armed blades with ratchet lock; Arms are curved to overlie the body part; Tips have sharp 4 × 4 rake prongs that match up evenly when closed; The prongs do not interdigitate; Straight and curved arms are available

Uses: Used for brain surgery

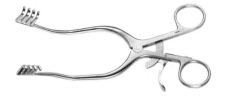

FIGURE 3-229

O'Sullivan-O'Connor retractor

Size: 3" Blades

Characteristics: Circular frame with side wall retractors; Three interchangeable right-angle blades that attach with a bolt and wing nut assembly to retract the viscera; Small style available for vaginal use

Uses: Used for pelvic incisions

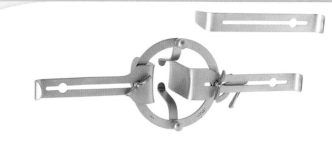

Notes: Specially designed for gynecological procedures using Pfannenstiel incision; Observe for wing nut during the counting procedure; Main circular frame is hinged and does not disassemble for cleaning and processing

FIGURE 3-230

SELF-RETAINING RETRACTORS *continued*

Balfour retractor

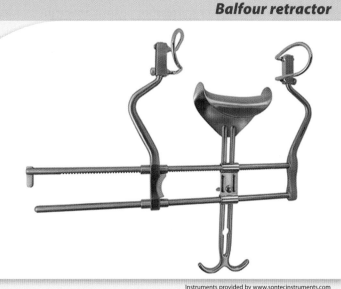

Size: 7.0"; 10.0"

Characteristics: Adjustable lateral side wall solid or open retractor blades that traverse a stainless steel bar into a locking position; A curved Mayo-style bladder blade attaches with a wing nut; Incision and body wall are supported on three sides

Uses: Used for abdominal incisions

Notes: Bladder blade can be used alone as a retractor during cesarean sections; Observe for wing nut during the counting procedure; This retractor disassembles for cleaning and processing

Instruments provided by www.sontecinstruments.com

FIGURE 3-231

Finochietto retractor

Size: Spread 85 mm or 6.0" to 12.0"

Characteristics: Bilateral side wall retractor that spreads across ratchets by turning a crank; Heavy duty instrument for holding firm tissue; Infant and pediatric sizes available; Straight or curved arms can be used; A lever is depressed to release the traction

Uses: Used for thoracic incisions

Notes: Can be aluminum or stainless steel; Fixed blades (curved arms) or interchangeable blades (Burford; straight arms)

Courtesy of Jarit Surgical Instruments, a division of Integra LifeSciences Corporation.

FIGURE 3-232

Denis Browne adult retractor set

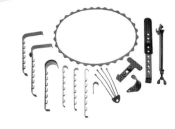

Characteristics: Designed for upper abdominal procedures or biliary procedures on the obese patient; Allows patient arms to be out, rather than along body

Uses: Gastric, spleen, hepatic surgery

Photo supplied courtesy of Cardinal Health, V. Mueller® Products and Services. All rights reserved.

FIGURE 3-233

Bed-Mounted Self-Retaining Retractors

Bed-mounted retractors are attached to the side rail of the operating bed frame at the level of the mattress. A long side-mount supporting post with a securing bolt is aligned with the railing and tightened. The post is part of the sterile apparatus and remains sterile above the level of the patient's body. The screw mechanism and the securing bolt are manipulated by the circulator as the supporting post is attached to the operating bed rail. This lower segment is considered unsterile after the attaching procedure. The upper end of the post remains sterile for assembly of the primary retractor system. Care is taken not to permit the supporting post to rest against the patient's tissues. Pressure against the arm, for example, could cause a permanent brachial palsy.

Once the supporting post is mounted a large frame is attached that encircles the incision. Retractor blades are slid onto the frame with the blade inserted into the incision. As the blades are tightened onto the frame and directed laterally, exposure of the surgical site is provided without causing strain on the team.

Bed-mounted retractors are commonly packaged in two or more processing trays because of excessive weight and number of components.

BED-MOUNTED SELF-RETAINING RETRACTORS

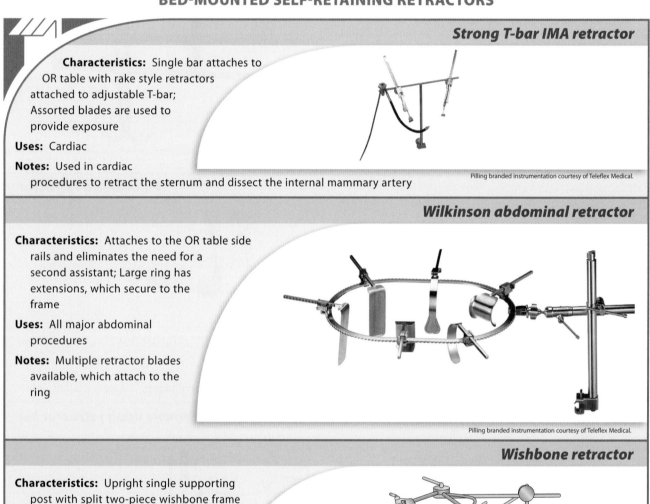

Strong T-bar IMA retractor

Characteristics: Single bar attaches to OR table with rake style retractors attached to adjustable T-bar; Assorted blades are used to provide exposure

Uses: Cardiac

Notes: Used in cardiac procedures to retract the sternum and dissect the internal mammary artery

Pilling branded instrumentation courtesy of Teleflex Medical.

FIGURE 3-234

Wilkinson abdominal retractor

Characteristics: Attaches to the OR table side rails and eliminates the need for a second assistant; Large ring has extensions, which secure to the frame

Uses: All major abdominal procedures

Notes: Multiple retractor blades available, which attach to the ring

Pilling branded instrumentation courtesy of Teleflex Medical.

FIGURE 3-235

Wishbone retractor

Characteristics: Upright single supporting post with split two-piece wishbone frame from which retractor blades are secured

Uses: All major abdominal procedures

Notes: Multiple retractor blades available including Deavers, fence blades, hoes, Kellys, malleable, Mayo blades, and Richardsons

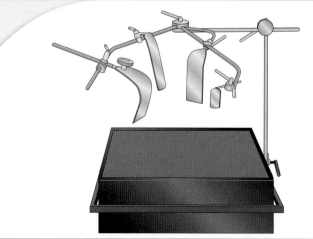

Delmar/Cengage Learning.

FIGURE 3-236

BED-MOUNTED SELF-RETAINING RETRACTORS *continued*

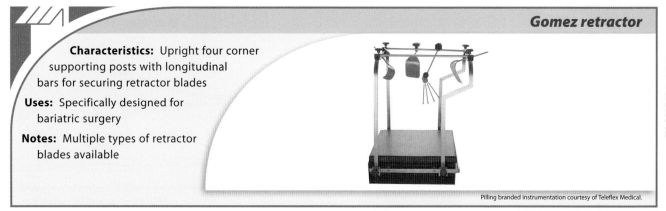

Gomez retractor

Characteristics: Upright four corner supporting posts with longitudinal bars for securing retractor blades

Uses: Specifically designed for bariatric surgery

Notes: Multiple types of retractor blades available

Pilling branded instrumentation courtesy of Teleflex Medical.

FIGURE 3-237

APPROXIMATION AND CLOSURE INSTRUMENTATION

Suturing Instrumentation

The superficial closure of the surgical site is the outermost manifestation of the surgical procedure the patient can visualize. Use of the correct suture in the correct needle holder promotes a satisfactory appearance. Proper care of the instrument assures that it will remain serviceable for many uses. Using a needle holder to load a scalpel blade onto a handle can cause the jaws to misalign and should be avoided particularly if the jaws are lined with diamond dust or special metal. Replacement can be costly. Needle holders are not designed for torque. A damaged needle holder may fail to hold a needle in position at a critical time during the surgical procedure harming the patient and creating ire in the surgeon. A Kelly or short Pean is more suited to this task and is less costly to repair.

Needle holders are sometimes referred to as needle drivers. The majority of the needles used with a needle holder have a curve. Straight needles, with the exception of some ocular and endoscopic styles, are used without a driver.

Handle styles range from ring to spring configurations. The jaws are short and can be smooth, finely cross-serrated, notched, or inset with diamond dust or carbide.

NEEDLE HOLDERS

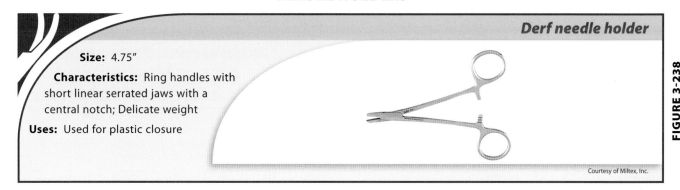

Derf needle holder

Size: 4.75″

Characteristics: Ring handles with short linear serrated jaws with a central notch; Delicate weight

Uses: Used for plastic closure

Courtesy of Miltex, Inc.

FIGURE 3-238

continues

NEEDLE HOLDERS *continued*

Webster needle holder

Size: 4.75"; 5.0"

Characteristics: Ring handles with a variety of jaws: cross-serrated, smooth, or diamond dust inset; Delicate weight

Uses: Used for plastic closure

Notes: Similar to Halsey needle holder

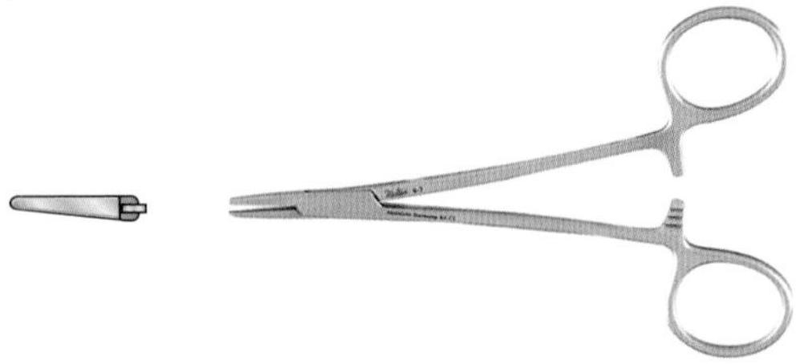

Instrument image courtesy of Miltex, Inc. Tip inset illustration Delmar/Cengage Learning.

FIGURE 3-239

Halsey needle holder

Size: 5.0"

Characteristics: Ring handles with cross-serrated (B.) or smooth (A.) jaws; Light weight

Uses: Used for plastic closure

A. Smooth jaws
B. Serrated jaws

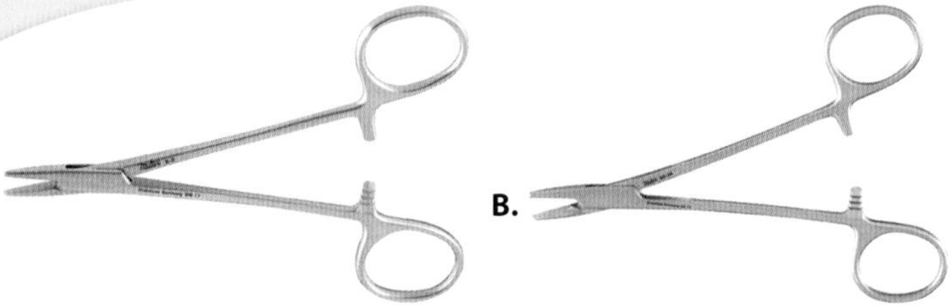

Courtesy of Miltex, Inc.

FIGURE 3-240

Olsen-Hegar needle holder

Size: 4.75"; 5.5"; 6.5"; 7.25"

Characteristics: Ring handles with serrated jaws; Scissors built in at the box locks

Uses: Used for intermediate weight suture

Notes: Commonly used by plastic surgeons when placing multiple stitches

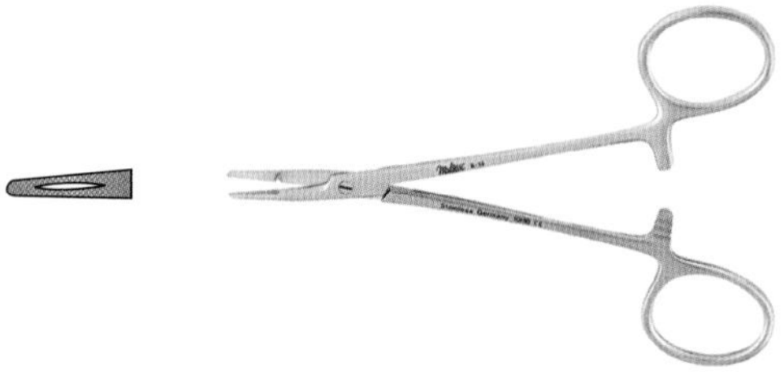

Instrument image courtesy of Miltex, Inc. Tip inset illustration Delmar/Cengage Learning.

FIGURE 3-241

Converse needle holder

Size: 4.25"

Characteristics: Larger ring handles with short jaw; Longitudinal serrations

Uses: Used for plastic closure

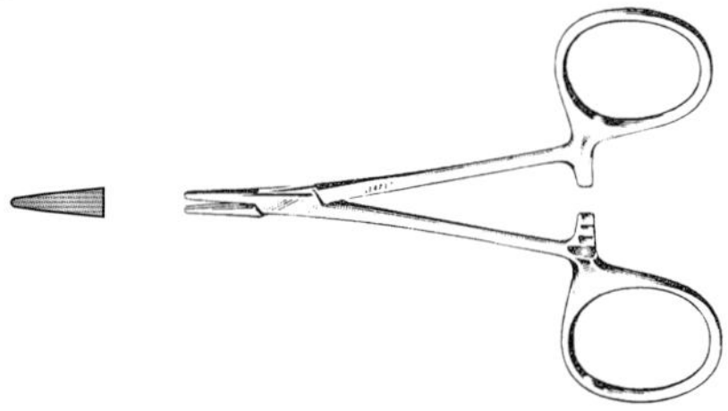

Courtesy of Jarit Surgical Instruments, a division of Integra LifeSciences Corporation. Tip inset illustration Delmar/Cengage Learning.

FIGURE 3-242

NEEDLE HOLDERS *continued*

Mayo-Hegar needle holder

Size: 5.0"; 6.0"; 7.0"; 8.0"; 10.5"

Characteristics: Ring handles with heavy jaws; Cross-serrated with central notch

Uses: Used for intermediate to heavy weight suture

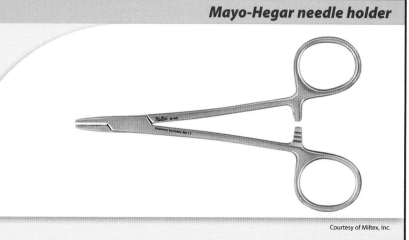

Courtesy of Miltex, Inc.

FIGURE 3-243

Crile-Wood needle holder

Size: 6.0"; 7.0"; 8.0"; 9.0"

Characteristics: Ring handles with intermediate weight jaws; Cross-serrated with narrow central notch

Uses: Used for light to intermediate weight suture

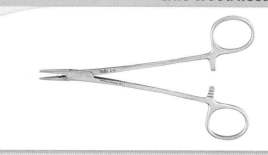

Courtesy of Miltex, Inc.

FIGURE 3-244

Gillies-Sheehan needle holder

Size: 6.5"

Characteristics: One jaw is fenestrated to carry a suture; Both jaws are cross-serrated; Curved or straight with built-in scissors; Ring handles with one off-set finger ring

Uses: Used for light to intermediate weight suture

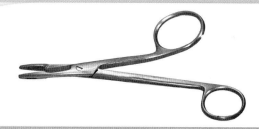

Courtesy of Padgett Surgical Instruments, a division of Integra LifeSciences Corporation.

FIGURE 3-245

Sarot needle holder

Size: 7.0"; 10.5"

Characteristics: Ring handles with medially curved shanks; Fine jaws with cross-serrations; Central notch

Uses: Used for light to intermediate weight suture

Notes: Commonly used in vascular surgery

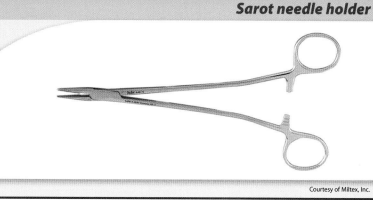

Courtesy of Miltex, Inc.

FIGURE 3-246

continues

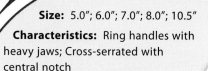

NEEDLE HOLDERS *continued*

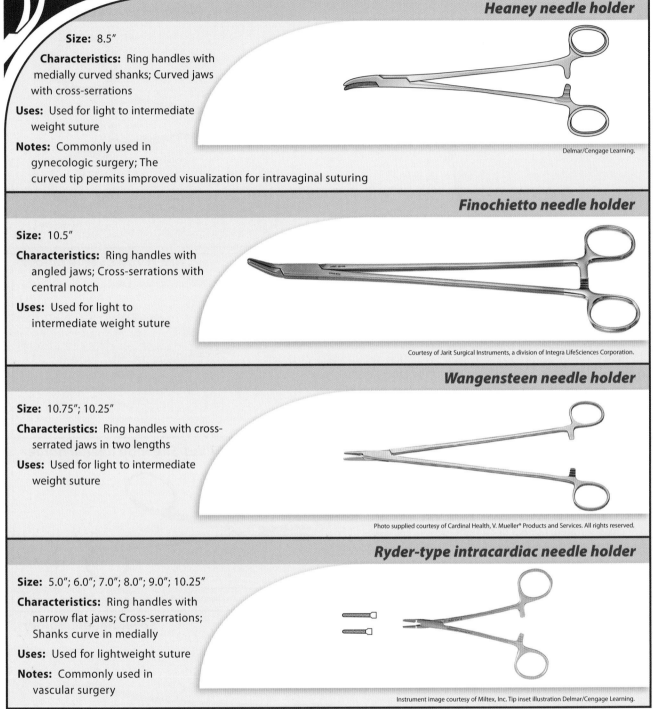

Heaney needle holder

Size: 8.5″

Characteristics: Ring handles with medially curved shanks; Curved jaws with cross-serrations

Uses: Used for light to intermediate weight suture

Notes: Commonly used in gynecologic surgery; The curved tip permits improved visualization for intravaginal suturing

Delmar/Cengage Learning.

FIGURE 3-247

Finochietto needle holder

Size: 10.5″

Characteristics: Ring handles with angled jaws; Cross-serrations with central notch

Uses: Used for light to intermediate weight suture

Courtesy of Jarit Surgical Instruments, a division of Integra LifeSciences Corporation.

FIGURE 3-248

Wangensteen needle holder

Size: 10.75″; 10.25″

Characteristics: Ring handles with cross-serrated jaws in two lengths

Uses: Used for light to intermediate weight suture

Photo supplied courtesy of Cardinal Health, V. Mueller® Products and Services. All rights reserved.

FIGURE 3-249

Ryder-type intracardiac needle holder

Size: 5.0″; 6.0″; 7.0″; 8.0″; 9.0″; 10.25″

Characteristics: Ring handles with narrow flat jaws; Cross-serrations; Shanks curve in medially

Uses: Used for lightweight suture

Notes: Commonly used in vascular surgery

Instrument image courtesy of Miltex, Inc. Tip inset illustration Delmar/Cengage Learning.

FIGURE 3-250

SUTURE AND LIGATURE CARRIERS

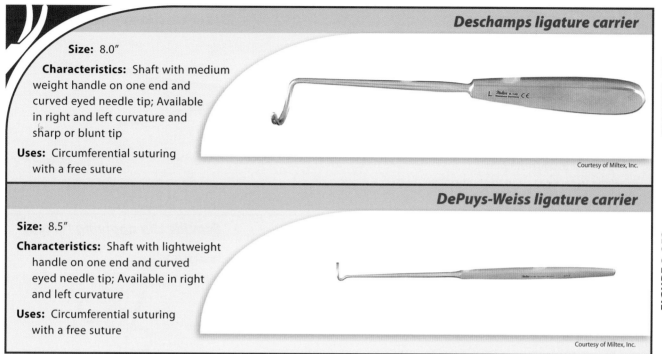

Deschamps ligature carrier

Size: 8.0"

Characteristics: Shaft with medium weight handle on one end and curved eyed needle tip; Available in right and left curvature and sharp or blunt tip

Uses: Circumferential suturing with a free suture

Courtesy of Miltex, Inc.

FIGURE 3-251

DePuys-Weiss ligature carrier

Size: 8.5"

Characteristics: Shaft with lightweight handle on one end and curved eyed needle tip; Available in right and left curvature

Uses: Circumferential suturing with a free suture

Courtesy of Miltex, Inc.

FIGURE 3-252

Single Clip Appliers

Single metallic or absorbable clips can be secured with an applicator forceps. Disposable models are commercially available with preloaded clips.

SINGLE CLIP APPLIERS

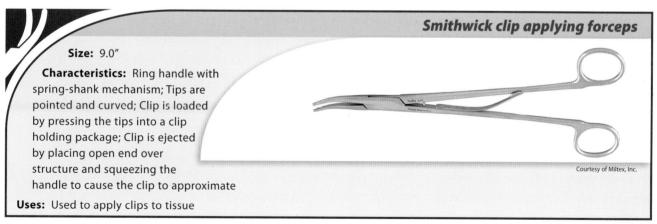

Smithwick clip applying forceps

Size: 9.0"

Characteristics: Ring handle with spring-shank mechanism; Tips are pointed and curved; Clip is loaded by pressing the tips into a clip holding package; Clip is ejected by placing open end over structure and squeezing the handle to cause the clip to approximate

Uses: Used to apply clips to tissue

Courtesy of Miltex, Inc.

FIGURE 3-253

continues

SINGLE CLIP APPLIERS *continued*

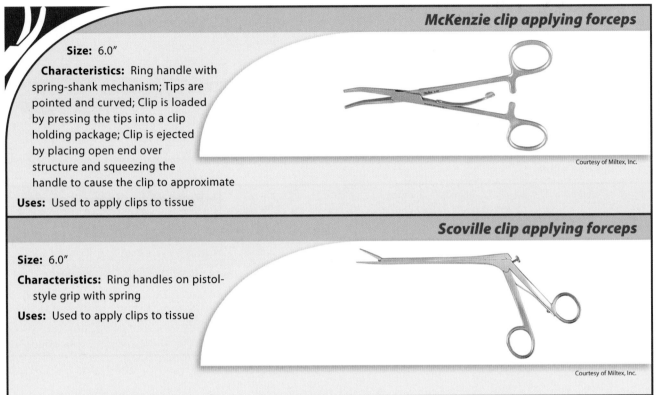

McKenzie clip applying forceps

Size: 6.0"

Characteristics: Ring handle with spring-shank mechanism; Tips are pointed and curved; Clip is loaded by pressing the tips into a clip holding package; Clip is ejected by placing open end over structure and squeezing the handle to cause the clip to approximate

Uses: Used to apply clips to tissue

Courtesy of Miltex, Inc.

FIGURE 3-254

Scoville clip applying forceps

Size: 6.0"

Characteristics: Ring handles on pistol-style grip with spring

Uses: Used to apply clips to tissue

Courtesy of Miltex, Inc.

FIGURE 3-255

SUMMARY

Surgical instrumentation takes many forms and has many functions. Assembling sets of the appropriate instrumentation for the planned surgical procedure requires knowledge of the case and the preferences of the surgeon. Most facilities have standardized sets that can be used for many different services. In the subsequent chapters of this text, more specialized instruments will be introduced and assembled into functional sets that meet the needs associated with the performance of particular surgeries.

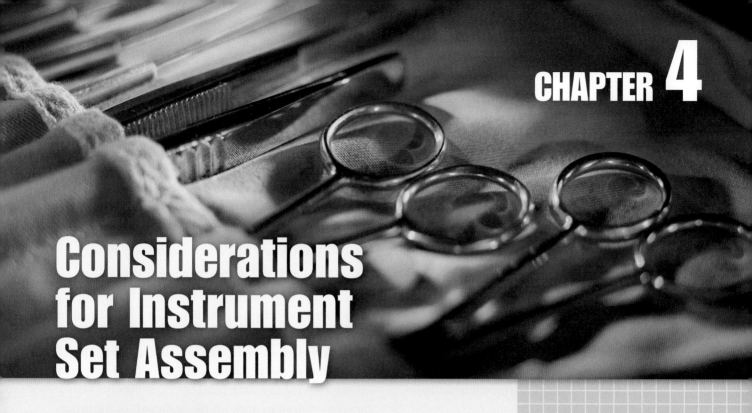

CHAPTER 4

Considerations for Instrument Set Assembly

INTRODUCTION

Each surgical procedure requires a collection of instruments for the safe, efficient, and effective performance of the intended operation. Sets are constructed based on logical assumptions premised in a practical hierarchical order. Advance planning in set construction can permit the set to be used for many types of procedures with the addition of a few individually wrapped instruments. Selection of the proper set of instruments is based on several factors; these include, but are not limited to, the following:

1. The resources available to the facility.
2. The nature of the planned procedure.
3. The potential for a secondary procedure.
4. The positioning of the patient.
5. The preferences of the primary surgeon.
6. Patient-specific indicators (e.g., size of body habitus, concurrent comorbidity).
7. The type of anesthesia employed for the procedure.

The following nine universal characteristics govern instrument set selection regardless of the procedure being performed. The essentials of procedural instrument planning include, but are not limited to, the following:

1. A method for entering the patient's body
   a. Sharp dissection—incision through the skin
   b. Blunt dissection and/or dilation—separation of layers between planes
   c. Natural orifice—oral, aural, nasal, anal, urethral, or vaginal entrance
   d. Tissue transcendence with nonionizing radiation or other non-tangible element—laser, ultrasound, x-ray, or electricity

2. Provision of exposure

   a. Manual retractor—Richardson, Senn, or other manual retractor

   b. Self-retaining retractor—Balfour, O'Sullivan-O'Connor, Scott retractor and stays

3. Creation of a clear working area

   a. Organ displacement with instruments or sponges—packing bowel and structures out of the surgical field with silastic sheeting and laparotomy sponges

   b. Containment and protection of adjacent structures—sterile plastic bowel bag

4. A method of hemostasis

   a. Clamping—use of a hemostat to occlude bleeding

   b. Establishing tamponade—deployment of embolization coils or sclerosing agent

5. Manipulation of adjacent structures

   a. Anastomosis—connection of tubular structures

   b. Repair—closure of deep layers as in hernia

6. Capture of target tissue

   a. Biopsy—a piece of tissue is procured for testing

   b. Removal

      1) Excisional removal—target tissue is removed

      2) Incisional removal—sample of target tissue is removed

7. Evacuation of blood, fluid, and other body substances

   a. Suctioning—material is removed from the surgical site by negative pressure

   b. Irrigation and aspiration—therapeutic solution is instilled, then removed, by negative pressure

   c. Ultrasonic fragmentation and aspiration—high frequency sound is used to break cells apart and the material is removed by negative pressure

   d. Debridement—debulking of necrotic or hypertrophic tissue or tumor

8. Retrieval of foreign material for accountability

   a. Sponges—packing is removed after use

   b. Instruments—all items used during the procedure are accounted for

9. Approximation of entry point(s)

   a. Suturing edges—closure, or approximation of incised tissues

   b. Closure of a cavity within a cavity—primary or secondary approximation of incised edges

A majority of surgical procedures are performed by entering the patient's body through the skin and require the use of the same or similar instruments, regardless of the procedural intent below the surface. After entering the superficial layers, additional instruments are used to perform the main part of the procedure according to the tissue type and techniques used to effect the end result. Standardization of instrument sets is an efficient and cost effective way to plan for needed resources. This includes selecting instruments from each category as appropriate for each surgical procedure in a consistent manner.

In planning for the construction of a functional set of instruments, consideration is given to assembling the set in a way that permits processing for sterile use and packaging in a way that allows for individual instrument retrieval in a systematic and organized manner. The packaging must permit all of the instrumentation surfaces to remain in contact with the sterilization process for the appropriate period of time. The arrangement and stabilization of the instruments involves sorting and stringing the instruments in an open position on specialized racks to accomplish thorough processing. The racks, sometimes referred to as "stringers," are designed to slip through the ring handles and hold the instruments open (Figure 4-1). The process for placing the instruments on the racks is referred to as "stringing the instruments on the stringers." Any instrument that passes through the sterilization process in a closed position is considered unsterile because the sterilant is unable to contact all surfaces. If one instrument is unsterile it renders the remainder of the instruments unsterile by cross-contamination. Although the outer wrapper or container bears a date of processing, there is no expiration date unless the package contains medications or other unstable chemical agents.

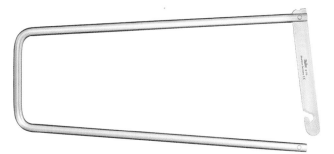

Figure 4-1 Instrument rack, also referred to as a stringer. *Courtesy of Miltex, Inc.*

INSTRUMENT CONTAINERS AND TRAYS

After the individual instruments are strung on stringers, the loaded stringers are placed in a tray with other loose instruments, such as scalpel handles and retractors. Several types of trays are commercially available and are described in the following sections.

Perforated Trays

The most common type of tray is the perforated tray. It can be made of stainless steel, aluminum, or high impact plastic. The entire tray has small one-eighth inch evenly spaced openings or holes over the entire surface of the bottom and the sides or can be made of an interwoven metallic mesh. The tray must be durable and stable for the type of sterilization method available. The perforations permit the sterilant to penetrate throughout the inner basket to all surfaces.

The standard stainless steel perforated tray is a stand-alone, open top pan fashioned into a sturdy square or rectangle configuration for ease of stacking and storage (Figure 4-2). The racks of instruments fit evenly within the confines of the tray. Other types of stand-alone trays have perforated hinged lids and a series of pegs to hold instruments apart and do not require the instruments to be on racks (Figure 4-3). Stand-alone trays are wrapped in double thickness woven or nonwoven fabric wrappers. Most facilities have standardized to nonwoven fabric wrappers because they are disposable and more durable than woven varieties that must be laundered and patched regularly. Some manufacturers have recycling programs that re-

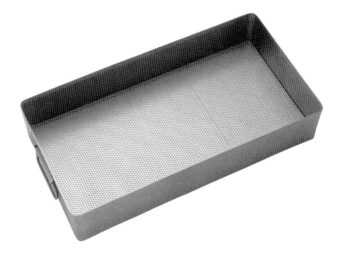

Figure 4-2 Stainless steel sterilization tray, without lid. *Photo supplied courtesy of Cardinal Health, V. Mueller® Products and Services. All rights reserved.*

process used nonwoven wrappers. Woven wrappers have a limited number of uses and each use must be tracked by stamper marks that denote serviceability. Any fabric- or paper-wrapped item will be sealed with chemical indicator tape that changes color in the presence of steam or certain gases. The tape should always be peeled off the woven fabric wrappers and broken without peeling from the nonwoven wrappers. Peeling

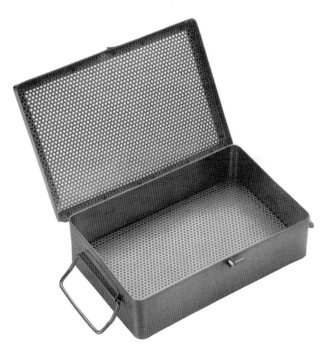

Figure 4-3 Sterilization tray, with lid. *Photo supplied courtesy of Cardinal Health, V. Mueller® Products and Services. All rights reserved.*

tape from nonwoven wrappers disturbs the integrity of the package, permitting contamination during the unwrapping process. Failing to remove all the tape from woven fabric wrappers causes problems with the laundering process.

Closed Rigid Containers

Mesh baskets and high impact plastic trays are not stand-alone trays. They are nested into an aluminum or composite plastic box-like structure with a locking lid referred to as a closed container (Figure 4-4). The lid has a gasket seal that permits the tight closure necessary to maintain sterility after processing and locks with a tamper evident device. In some closed containers with nested baskets, the lid and bottom of the closed container have one-way filtered vents for the escape of steam or other sterilants. A wrapper is not used. If the internal surface is damp upon opening, the contents of the closed container are considered contaminated because the filter has become saturated. This process causes capillary action that permits passive diffusion of microorganisms. Some types of closed containers are not vented. Occasionally some condensation will build up and pool in the non-vented containers. This is considered to be sterile condensate and does not indicate contamination of the set.

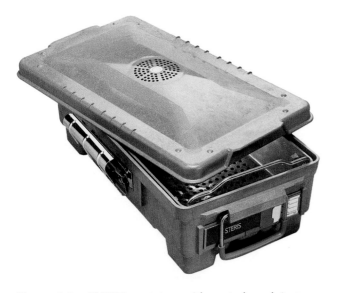

Figure 4-4 AMSCO container with nested mesh instrument basket. *Courtesy of the STERIS Corporation. Reprinted with permission.*

ASSEMBLY OF INSTRUMENT SETS

Standardized instrument sets are a collection of instruments that are used for related surgical procedures. Each time a particular set is assembled it is required to have specific numbers of each needed instrument. Instrument sets are assembled in the central processing department and sterilized for use in surgical procedures.

Determining Instrument Set Contents

Knowledge of the procedure to be performed and the anatomy of the organ system involved is important when determining what should be included in an instrument set. The best way to be sure all instrumentation needs are met is to follow an organized system of categorization. Categories to consider when creating a useful set of instruments are listed in Table 4-1.

Key elements to include in every set will depend on its intended use. Most sets will have several types of dissection instruments, clamps, graspers, retractors, and closure tools. Not all sets will have probes, dilators, or debulking equipment unless they are necessary for the intended procedure.

TABLE 4-1	Categories of instruments to consider when creating an instrument set
Clamping instruments
Grasping forceps
Dissection instruments
Debulking instruments
Probing and dilation instruments
Evacuation and instillation instruments
Retraction and exposure instruments
Approximation and closure instruments
Specialty devices

Counts and Accountability

Each set will have standardized quantities of specific instruments. Counting the instruments is made easier when the items are packed in even numbers. The team, particularly the scrub person and the circulating nurse, are responsible for performing a baseline instrument count and a closing instrument count. Additional counts are required if a cavity within a cavity is closed. This accountability is important for patient and team safety, inventory control, and infection control. Safety considerations involve prevention of puncture wounds for the team and retained objects for the patient. Inventory control is addressed by not inadvertently tossing an instrument into the trash or sending it out with the laundry. Infection control involves containment of contamination. If an instrument leaves the field during use, it could carry blood and body fluids to an unsuspecting person who could accidentally handle the contaminated item without the protection of gloves. Not all contamination is visible to the naked eye.

Accountability can be accomplished in several ways. The most common method employs an inventory sheet provided with each sterile set that validates the items packaged in the processing department by name and number. The processing personnel count the instruments and document the total numbers on a count sheet when wrapping and processing the set for use in the operating room. The packing counts are recorded on an inventory count sheet that is then used by the scrub person and circulating nurse to set a baseline when the set is opened for a procedure. The same count sheet is used at the end of the case for the closing counts performed by the scrub person and the circulating nurse. The totals are reconciled and documented on the patient's chart as correct or incorrect according to facility policy. Any incorrect count requires a repeat count until the totals are correct. If no resolution is made concerning the incorrectness of a count then the surgeon is notified, the search of the environment is continued, and an x-ray of the surgical site may need to be taken. A resolved count is documented as correct if the missing item is located. If the missing item is not found then the count is documented as incorrect and all steps in the search process are recorded on the appropriate forms designated by the facility.

Accountability during a surgical procedure can be managed by developing a few simple habits when functioning in the scrub role. Some suggestions include, but are not limited to, the following:

1. One-for-one: Every time an armed needle holder is passed, retrieve the used needle back on the instrument before passing the next suture.

2. Be consistent: Establish the set-up by always setting up the same way, in the same order. If an instrument is not in its place, it will likely be obvious to the eye.

3. Be tidy: Do not permit instruments to accumulate and clutter the sterile field. It is difficult to locate instruments when they are randomly placed.

4. Be organized: Place every instrument in the same place on the sterile instrument table after each use. This helps to keep an ongoing count and accountability.

Maintaining an organized and tidy sterile field creates a sense of efficiency and safety that facilitates the performance of the procedure without adverse event.

OVERVIEW OF PROCESSING OPTIONS

The surgical processing department has several methods of processing the instrument sets and rendering them sterile. The most common sterilization methods are steam under pressure, chemicals in gas, and chemicals in solution. The characteristics of the instrument set are the determining factors as to which method of sterilization is appropriate. Most metallic instruments made of stainless steel, titanium, silver, and copper can be sterilized by steam because they can tolerate heat and moisture. Heat and moisture-sensitive instruments made of plastic or synthetics are commonly sterilized by chemicals in gas. Items commercially packaged and processed by the manufacturer are usually sterilized by radiation or microwaves. These methods are not available in hospitals. Each item processed in the surgical processing department has a specific method for safe processing that is described in writing by the manufacturer.

SUMMARY

Instrument sets are assembled according to the types of procedures for which they will be used. The sets are packaged in trays or containers and processed to render them sterile according to manufacturer's recommendations. The contents of the individual sets are determined according to the standardized inventory lists that are packed within the tray and used as count sheets during the surgical procedure.

REFERENCES

Barrett, A. (1999, March). Instrument standardization. *Infection Control Today*, 3(3), 60–63.

Marvin, E. (1999, February). Instrument inventory systems: Or what it takes to never lose another towel clip. *Infection Control Today*, 3(2), 60–62.

Phillips, N. M. (2007). *Berry and Kohn's operating room technique* (11th ed.). St. Louis: Mosby-Elsevier.

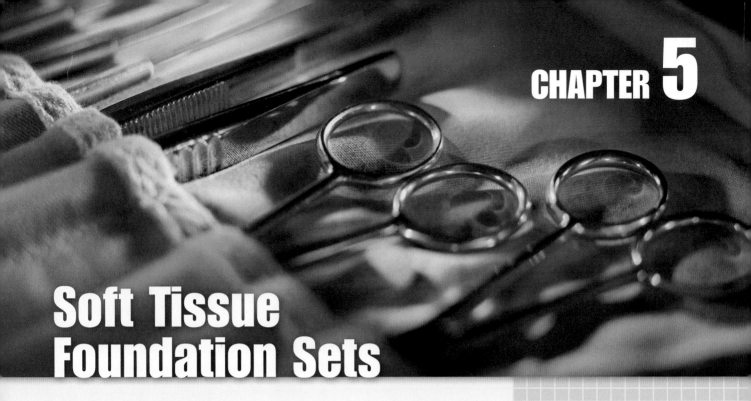

CHAPTER 5

Soft Tissue Foundation Sets

INTRODUCTION

Soft tissue sets are groups of instruments used to work with tissue layers such as the epidermis, dermis, adipose, subcutaneous, muscle, fascia, and fibrous tissues. The length of the instruments in a soft tissue set will vary according to the procedure to be performed. For example, procedures performed near the surface of the body use short (approximately 4.0″ to 6.0″), intermediate weight instrumentation. Mid-depth procedures commonly use medium instruments (approximately 6.5″ to 8.0″), and deep procedures, such as laparotomy, require long instruments (approximately 8.5″ to 12.0″). In contrast, when planning the instrumentation for a deeper procedure, take into consideration that the surface layers must first be entered. This process uses shorter instruments first followed by medium length instruments for dissection. The long instruments are used to perform the intended procedure. Facilities that designate short and long sets will require one of each set for most abdominal procedures. This chapter describes three foundation or baseline sets from which procedures can be performed through soft tissue at three tissue depths. An optional extra long foundation add-on set is included as external to the three primary sets. They are as follows:

1. Short foundation set: Excisional soft tissue set
2. Medium foundation set: Soft tissue dissection set
3. Long foundation set: Laparotomy set
4. (Optional) Extra-long foundation add-ons

This chapter will describe and discuss the soft tissue aspect of short to medium length instrument set planning by category. The last foundation set—the laparotomy set—contains the longest instruments that are logically contained within a set. It is not cost effective to include all possible instruments that could conceivably be used in all circumstances in every set. Logical sequencing of instrumentation needs for the tissue layers will help the scrub person decide which foundation set is the most useful for the intended procedure. Specialty trays can be added to complete the set-up. The soft tissue sets in this chapter will form the foundation for the creation of specialty sets in subsequent chapters.

SHORT FOUNDATION SET

Short foundation sets can be used for superficial procedures, excisions, and biopsies. Most procedures performed near the surface of the body can utilize this collection of instruments as a foundation. Surgeon-specific requests and preferences can be added as standard or as "add-ons" when the set is opened for use.

Excisional Set

Excisional sets are commonly used to dissect tissue above the fascial layers, although they can be used for patients of small stature or a child. The instrumentation need not be longer than 6.0″ unless the patient is significantly obese. Many excisional procedures are performed to obtain biopsies, realign tissues as in scar revision, or procure tissue for autografting.

Excisional Set – CLAMPS

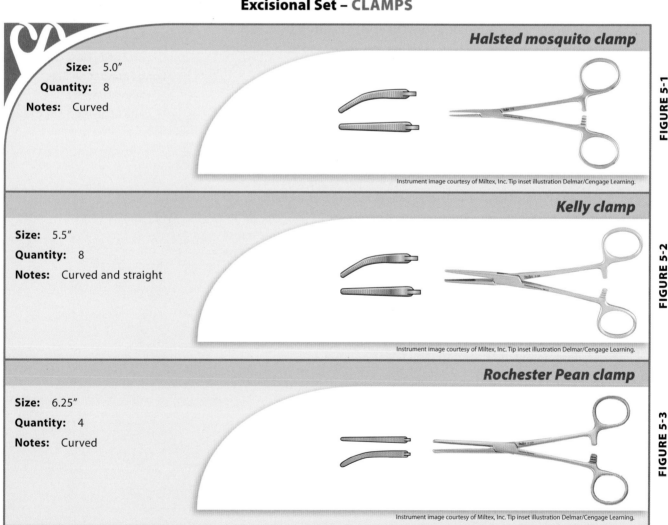

Halsted mosquito clamp

Size: 5.0″
Quantity: 8
Notes: Curved

Instrument image courtesy of Miltex, Inc. Tip inset illustration Delmar/Cengage Learning.

FIGURE 5-1

Kelly clamp

Size: 5.5″
Quantity: 8
Notes: Curved and straight

Instrument image courtesy of Miltex, Inc. Tip inset illustration Delmar/Cengage Learning.

FIGURE 5-2

Rochester Pean clamp

Size: 6.25″
Quantity: 4
Notes: Curved

Instrument image courtesy of Miltex, Inc. Tip inset illustration Delmar/Cengage Learning.

FIGURE 5-3

Excisional Set – CLAMPS *continued*

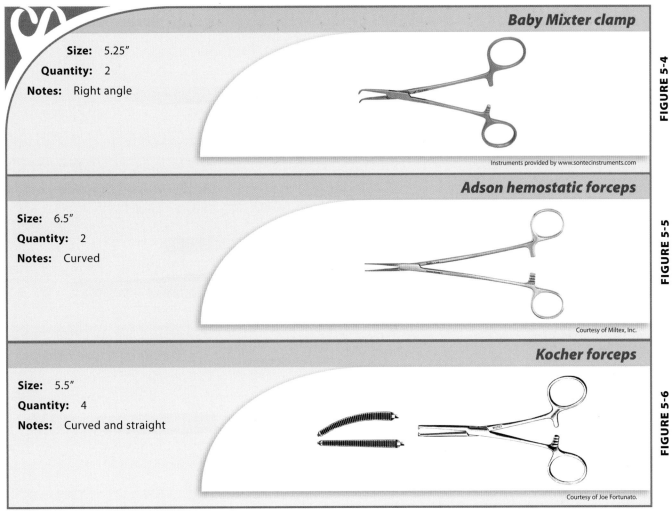

Baby Mixter clamp

Size: 5.25″
Quantity: 2
Notes: Right angle

Instruments provided by www.sontecinstruments.com

FIGURE 5-4

Adson hemostatic forceps

Size: 6.5″
Quantity: 2
Notes: Curved

Courtesy of Miltex, Inc.

FIGURE 5-5

Kocher forceps

Size: 5.5″
Quantity: 4
Notes: Curved and straight

Courtesy of Joe Fortunato.

FIGURE 5-6

Excisional Set – GRASPING FORCEPS

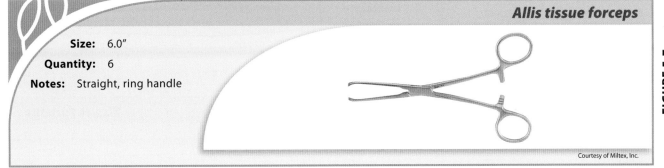

Allis tissue forceps

Size: 6.0″
Quantity: 6
Notes: Straight, ring handle

Courtesy of Miltex, Inc.

FIGURE 5-7

continues

Excisional Set – GRASPING FORCEPS *continued*

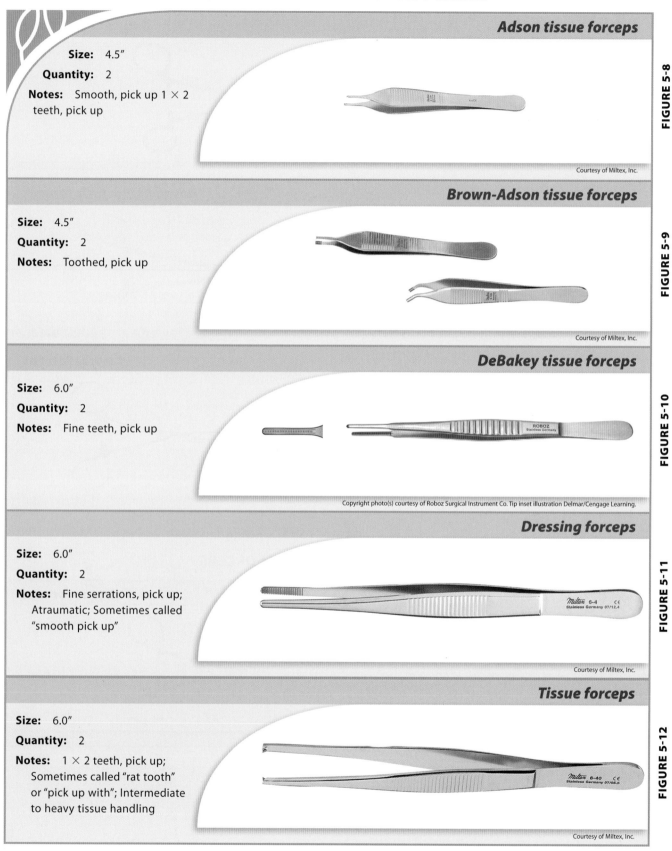

Adson tissue forceps

Size: 4.5"

Quantity: 2

Notes: Smooth, pick up 1 × 2 teeth, pick up

Courtesy of Miltex, Inc.

FIGURE 5-8

Brown-Adson tissue forceps

Size: 4.5"

Quantity: 2

Notes: Toothed, pick up

Courtesy of Miltex, Inc.

FIGURE 5-9

DeBakey tissue forceps

Size: 6.0"

Quantity: 2

Notes: Fine teeth, pick up

Copyright photo(s) courtesy of Roboz Surgical Instrument Co. Tip inset illustration Delmar/Cengage Learning.

FIGURE 5-10

Dressing forceps

Size: 6.0"

Quantity: 2

Notes: Fine serrations, pick up; Atraumatic; Sometimes called "smooth pick up"

Courtesy of Miltex, Inc.

FIGURE 5-11

Tissue forceps

Size: 6.0"

Quantity: 2

Notes: 1 × 2 teeth, pick up; Sometimes called "rat tooth" or "pick up with"; Intermediate to heavy tissue handling

Courtesy of Miltex, Inc.

FIGURE 5-12

Excisional Set – DISSECTION INSTRUMENTS

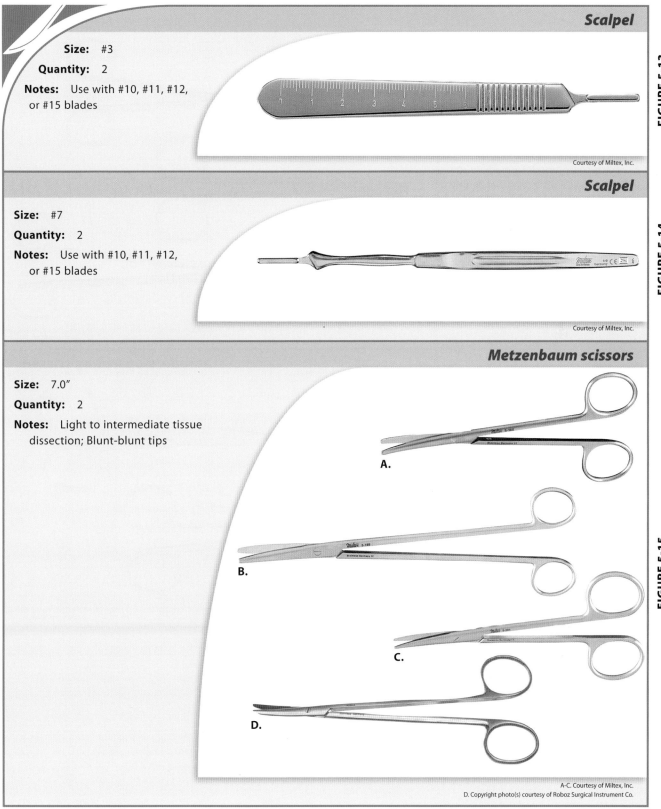

Scalpel

FIGURE 5-13

Size: #3

Quantity: 2

Notes: Use with #10, #11, #12, or #15 blades

Courtesy of Miltex, Inc.

Scalpel

FIGURE 5-14

Size: #7

Quantity: 2

Notes: Use with #10, #11, #12, or #15 blades

Courtesy of Miltex, Inc.

Metzenbaum scissors

FIGURE 5-15

Size: 7.0″

Quantity: 2

Notes: Light to intermediate tissue dissection; Blunt-blunt tips

A.

B.

C.

D.

A-C. Courtesy of Miltex, Inc.
D. Copyright photo(s) courtesy of Roboz Surgical Instrument Co.

continues

Excisional Set – DISSECTION INSTRUMENTS *continued*

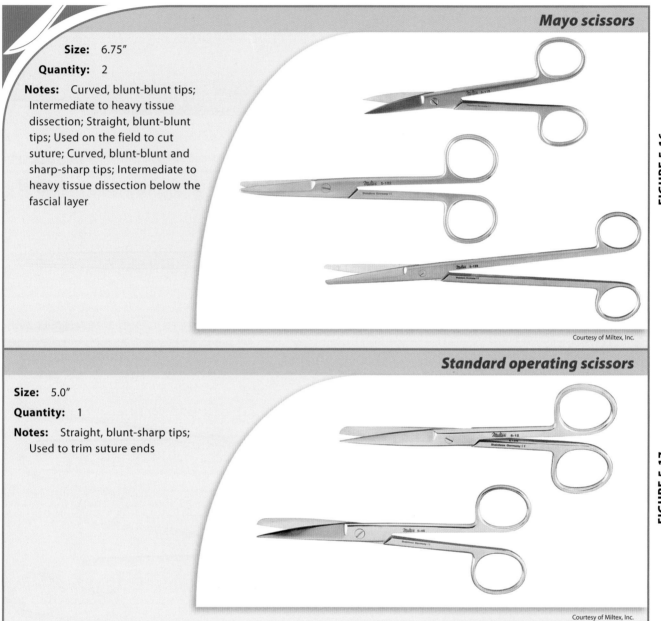

Mayo scissors

Size: 6.75"

Quantity: 2

Notes: Curved, blunt-blunt tips; Intermediate to heavy tissue dissection; Straight, blunt-blunt tips; Used on the field to cut suture; Curved, blunt-blunt and sharp-sharp tips; Intermediate to heavy tissue dissection below the fascial layer

Courtesy of Miltex, Inc.

FIGURE 5-16

Standard operating scissors

Size: 5.0"

Quantity: 1

Notes: Straight, blunt-sharp tips; Used to trim suture ends

Courtesy of Miltex, Inc.

FIGURE 5-17

Excisional Set – DISSECTION INSTRUMENTS *continued*

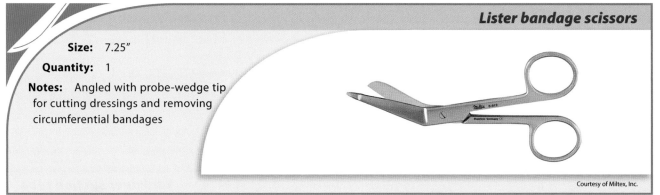

Lister bandage scissors

Size: 7.25"

Quantity: 1

Notes: Angled with probe-wedge tip for cutting dressings and removing circumferential bandages

Courtesy of Miltex, Inc.

FIGURE 5-18

Excisional Set – DEBULKING INSTRUMENTS

None: Can be added if wound debridement is required

Excisional Set – PROBES AND DILATORS

None: Can be added if sinus tract or fistula is present

Excisional Set – EVACUATION AND INSTILLATION INSTRUMENTS

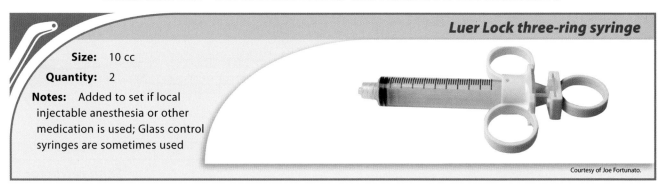

Luer Lock three-ring syringe

Size: 10 cc

Quantity: 2

Notes: Added to set if local injectable anesthesia or other medication is used; Glass control syringes are sometimes used

Courtesy of Joe Fortunato.

FIGURE 5-19

continues

Excisional Set – EVACUATION AND INSTILLATION INSTRUMENTS *continued*

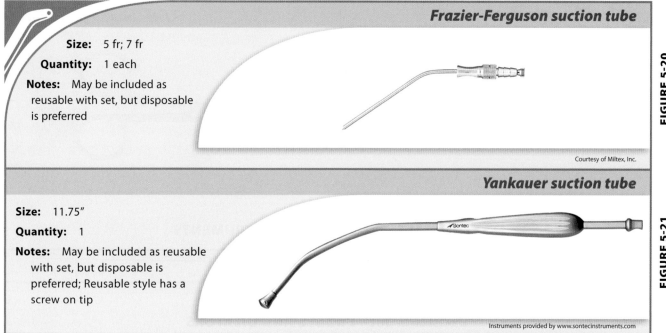

Frazier-Ferguson suction tube

Size: 5 fr; 7 fr

Quantity: 1 each

Notes: May be included as reusable with set, but disposable is preferred

Courtesy of Miltex, Inc.

FIGURE 5-20

Yankauer suction tube

Size: 11.75″

Quantity: 1

Notes: May be included as reusable with set, but disposable is preferred; Reusable style has a screw on tip

Instruments provided by www.sontecinstruments.com

FIGURE 5-21

Excisional Set – RETRACTION AND EXPOSURE INSTRUMENTS

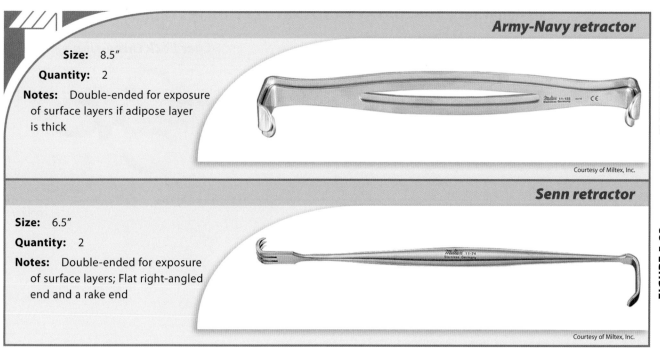

Army-Navy retractor

Size: 8.5″

Quantity: 2

Notes: Double-ended for exposure of surface layers if adipose layer is thick

Courtesy of Miltex, Inc.

FIGURE 5-22

Senn retractor

Size: 6.5″

Quantity: 2

Notes: Double-ended for exposure of surface layers; Flat right-angled end and a rake end

Courtesy of Miltex, Inc.

FIGURE 5-23

Excisional Set – RETRACTION AND EXPOSURE INSTRUMENTS *continued*

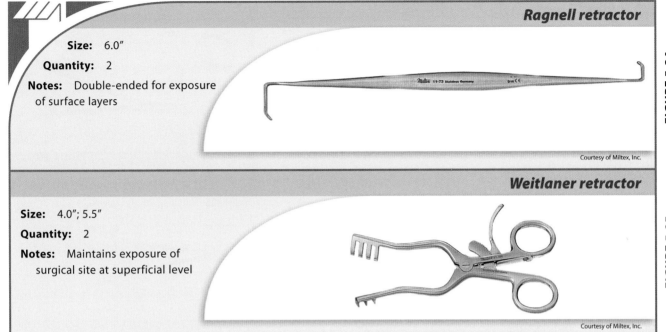

Ragnell retractor

Size: 6.0"

Quantity: 2

Notes: Double-ended for exposure of surface layers

FIGURE 5-24

Courtesy of Miltex, Inc.

Weitlaner retractor

Size: 4.0"; 5.5"

Quantity: 2

Notes: Maintains exposure of surgical site at superficial level

FIGURE 5-25

Courtesy of Miltex, Inc.

Excisional Set – APPROXIMATION AND CLOSURE INSTRUMENTS

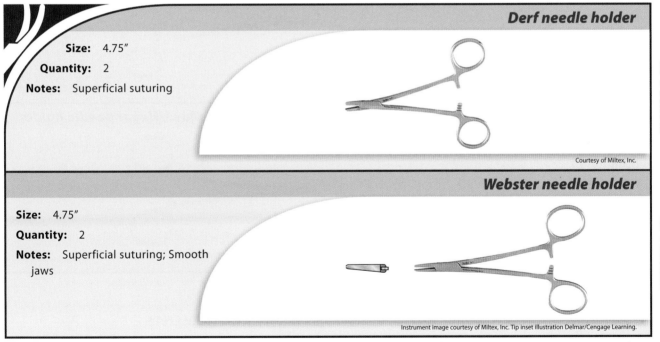

Derf needle holder

Size: 4.75"

Quantity: 2

Notes: Superficial suturing

FIGURE 5-26

Courtesy of Miltex, Inc.

Webster needle holder

Size: 4.75"

Quantity: 2

Notes: Superficial suturing; Smooth jaws

FIGURE 5-27

Instrument image courtesy of Miltex, Inc. Tip inset illustration Delmar/Cengage Learning.

continues

Excisional Set – APPROXIMATION AND CLOSURE INSTRUMENTS *continued*

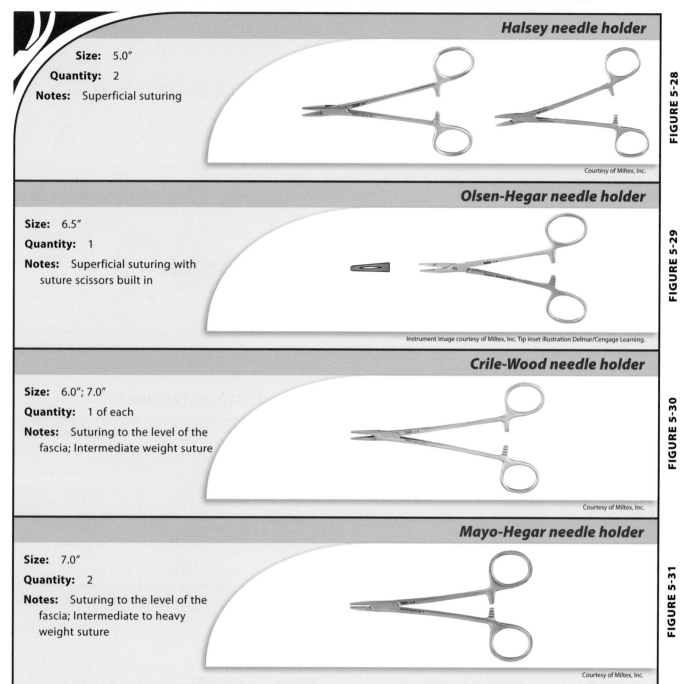

Halsey needle holder

Size: 5.0"

Quantity: 2

Notes: Superficial suturing

Courtesy of Miltex, Inc.

FIGURE 5-28

Olsen-Hegar needle holder

Size: 6.5"

Quantity: 1

Notes: Superficial suturing with suture scissors built in

Instrument image courtesy of Miltex, Inc. Tip inset illustration Delmar/Cengage Learning.

FIGURE 5-29

Crile-Wood needle holder

Size: 6.0"; 7.0"

Quantity: 1 of each

Notes: Suturing to the level of the fascia; Intermediate weight suture

Courtesy of Miltex, Inc.

FIGURE 5-30

Mayo-Hegar needle holder

Size: 7.0"

Quantity: 2

Notes: Suturing to the level of the fascia; Intermediate to heavy weight suture

Courtesy of Miltex, Inc.

FIGURE 5-31

Excisional Set – SPECIALTY SPECIFIC INSTRUMENTS

None: Add specialty instruments as appropriate

MEDIUM FOUNDATION SETS

Soft Tissue Dissection

Soft tissue dissection sets can be used for most areas of the body that do not surpass a tissue depth of 6 to 8 inches. Procedures in this grouping include hernias, excisional breast biopsy, excision of a lipoma, placement of percutaneous tubes, ostomy take-down, and incision and drainage of superficial abscess and other tissue layers within the reach of the instruments on the set. Longer instruments can be added as needed.

Soft Tissue Dissection – CLAMPS

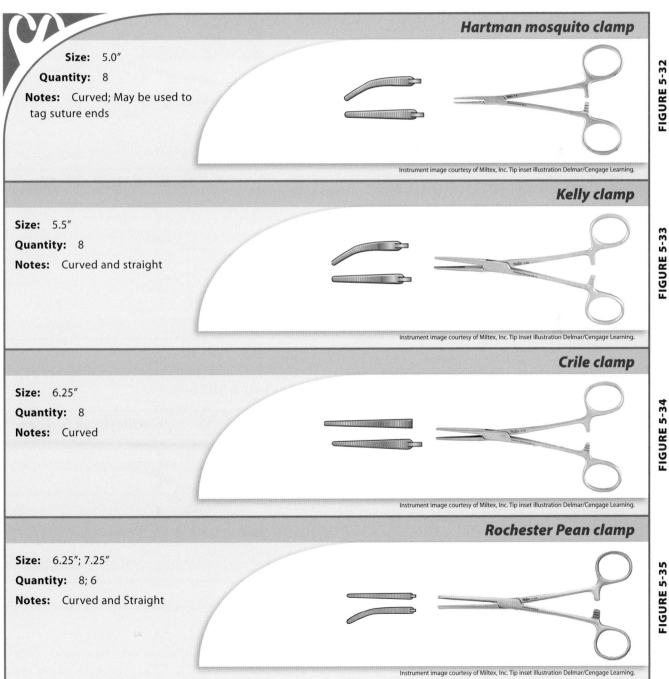

Hartman mosquito clamp

Size: 5.0"
Quantity: 8
Notes: Curved; May be used to tag suture ends

Instrument image courtesy of Miltex, Inc. Tip inset illustration Delmar/Cengage Learning.

FIGURE 5-32

Kelly clamp

Size: 5.5"
Quantity: 8
Notes: Curved and straight

Instrument image courtesy of Miltex, Inc. Tip inset illustration Delmar/Cengage Learning.

FIGURE 5-33

Crile clamp

Size: 6.25"
Quantity: 8
Notes: Curved

Instrument image courtesy of Miltex, Inc. Tip inset illustration Delmar/Cengage Learning.

FIGURE 5-34

Rochester Pean clamp

Size: 6.25"; 7.25"
Quantity: 8; 6
Notes: Curved and Straight

Instrument image courtesy of Miltex, Inc. Tip inset illustration Delmar/Cengage Learning.

FIGURE 5-35

continues

Soft Tissue Dissection – CLAMPS *continued*

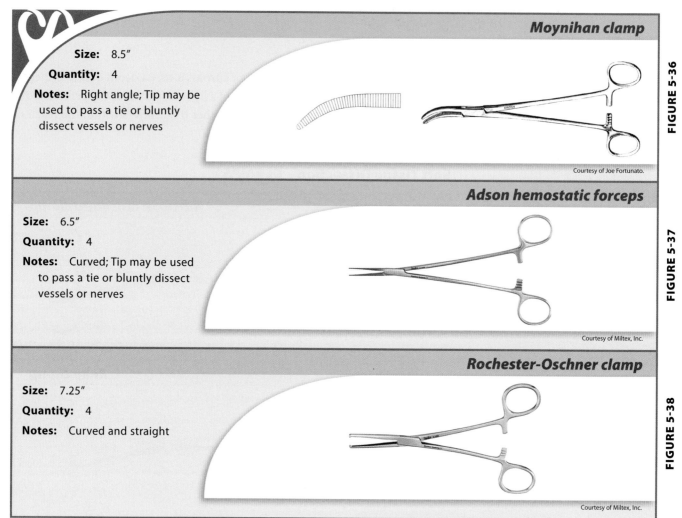

Moynihan clamp

Size: 8.5″

Quantity: 4

Notes: Right angle; Tip may be used to pass a tie or bluntly dissect vessels or nerves

Courtesy of Joe Fortunato.

FIGURE 5-36

Adson hemostatic forceps

Size: 6.5″

Quantity: 4

Notes: Curved; Tip may be used to pass a tie or bluntly dissect vessels or nerves

Courtesy of Miltex, Inc.

FIGURE 5-37

Rochester-Oschner clamp

Size: 7.25″

Quantity: 4

Notes: Curved and straight

Courtesy of Miltex, Inc.

FIGURE 5-38

Soft Tissue Dissection – GRASPING FORCEPS

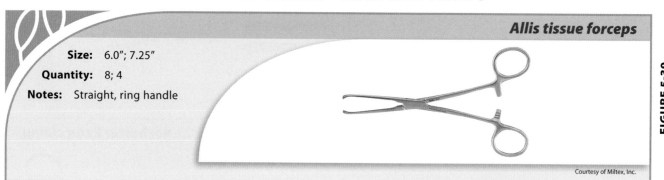

Allis tissue forceps

Size: 6.0″; 7.25″

Quantity: 8; 4

Notes: Straight, ring handle

Courtesy of Miltex, Inc.

FIGURE 5-39

Soft Tissue Dissection – GRASPING FORCEPS *continued*

Babcock tissue forceps

Size: 6.25"; 8.25"

Quantity: 2 of each

Notes: Use to grasp delicate tissues at the level of the peritoneum or bowel

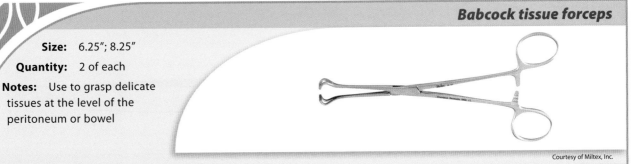

Courtesy of Miltex, Inc.

FIGURE 5-40

Adson tissue forceps

Size: 4.5"

Quantity: 2

Notes: Smooth, pick up; 1 × 2 teeth, pick up

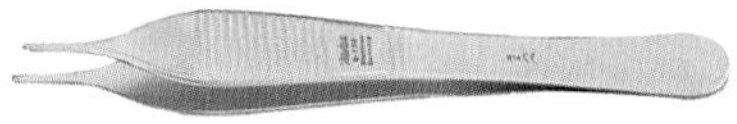

Courtesy of Miltex, Inc.

FIGURE 5-41

Brown-Adson tissue forceps

Size: 4.5"

Quantity: 2

Notes: Multi-toothed, pick up

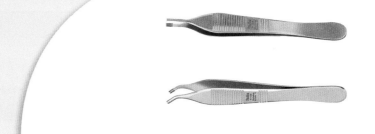

Courtesy of Miltex, Inc.

FIGURE 5-42

DeBakey tissue forceps

Size: 6.0"; 8.0"

Quantity: 2 of each

Notes: Fine teeth, pick up

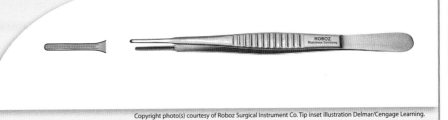

Copyright photo(s) courtesy of Roboz Surgical Instrument Co. Tip inset illustration Delmar/Cengage Learning.

FIGURE 5-43

continues

Soft Tissue Dissection – GRASPING FORCEPS *continued*

Dressing forceps

Size: 6.0"; 7.0"; 10.0"

Quantity: 2 of each

Notes: Fine serrations, pick up; Atraumatic; Can be used to place deep packing at the end of the case

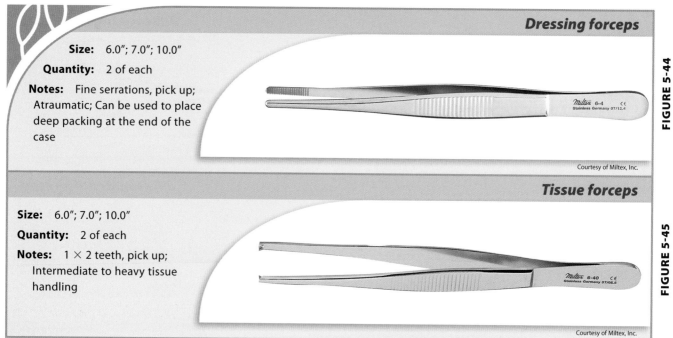

Courtesy of Miltex, Inc.

FIGURE 5-44

Tissue forceps

Size: 6.0"; 7.0"; 10.0"

Quantity: 2 of each

Notes: 1 × 2 teeth, pick up; Intermediate to heavy tissue handling

Courtesy of Miltex, Inc.

FIGURE 5-45

Soft Tissue Dissection – DISSECTION INSTRUMENTS

Scalpel

Size: #3

Quantity: 2

Notes: Use with #10, #11, #12, or #15 blades

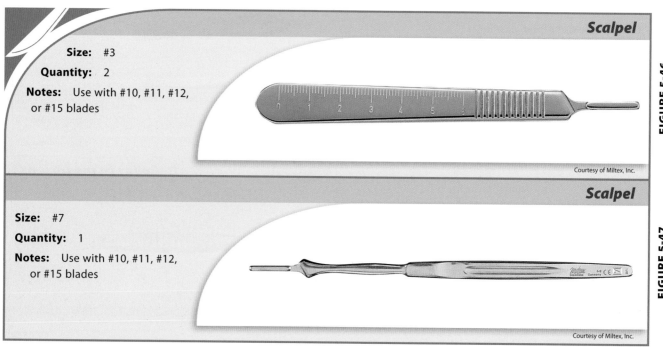

Courtesy of Miltex, Inc.

FIGURE 5-46

Scalpel

Size: #7

Quantity: 1

Notes: Use with #10, #11, #12, or #15 blades

Courtesy of Miltex, Inc.

FIGURE 5-47

Soft Tissue Dissection – DISSECTION INSTRUMENTS *continued*

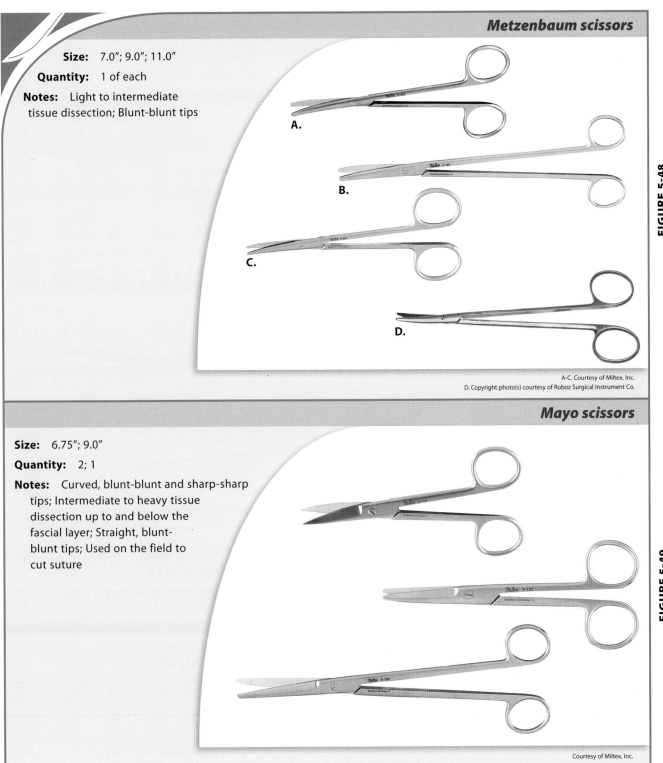

Metzenbaum scissors

Size: 7.0"; 9.0"; 11.0"

Quantity: 1 of each

Notes: Light to intermediate tissue dissection; Blunt-blunt tips

A.

B.

C.

D.

A-C. Courtesy of Miltex, Inc.
D. Copyright photo(s) courtesy of Roboz Surgical Instrument Co.

FIGURE 5-48

Mayo scissors

Size: 6.75"; 9.0"

Quantity: 2; 1

Notes: Curved, blunt-blunt and sharp-sharp tips; Intermediate to heavy tissue dissection up to and below the fascial layer; Straight, blunt-blunt tips; Used on the field to cut suture

Courtesy of Miltex, Inc.

FIGURE 5-49

continues

Soft Tissue Dissection – DISSECTION INSTRUMENTS *continued*

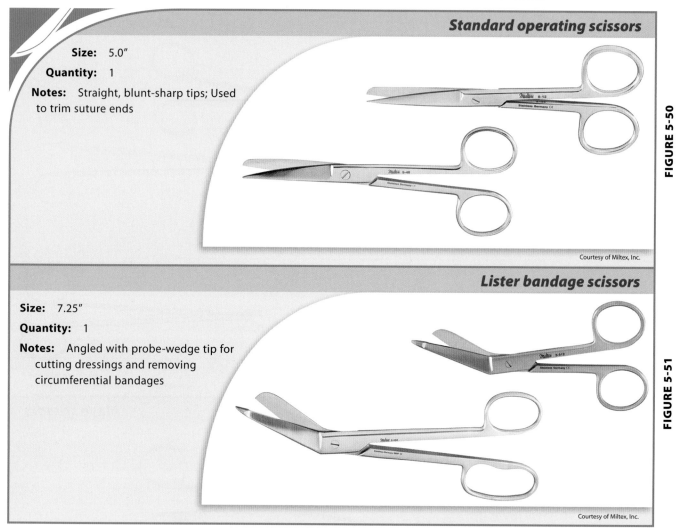

Standard operating scissors

Size: 5.0″

Quantity: 1

Notes: Straight, blunt-sharp tips; Used to trim suture ends

Courtesy of Miltex, Inc.

Lister bandage scissors

Size: 7.25″

Quantity: 1

Notes: Angled with probe-wedge tip for cutting dressings and removing circumferential bandages

Courtesy of Miltex, Inc.

FIGURE 5-50

FIGURE 5-51

Soft Tissue Dissection – DEBULKING INSTRUMENTS

None: Can be added if wound debridement is required

Soft Tissue Dissection – PROBES AND DILATORS

None: Can be added if sinus tract or fistula is present

Soft Tissue Dissection – EVACUATION AND INSTILLATION INSTRUMENTS

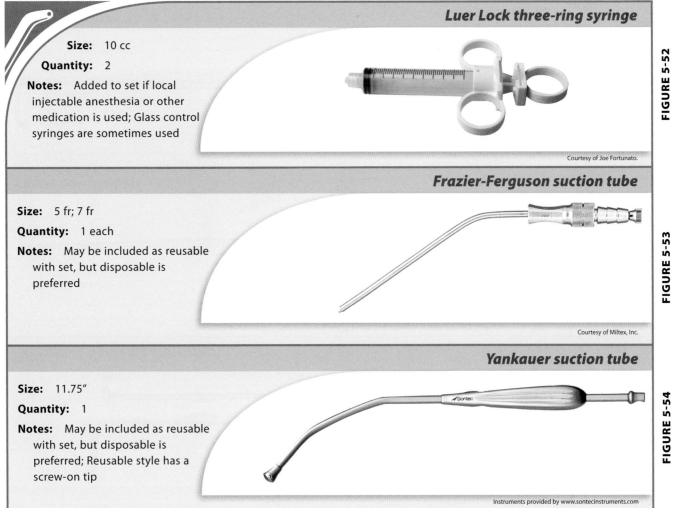

Luer Lock three-ring syringe

Size: 10 cc

Quantity: 2

Notes: Added to set if local injectable anesthesia or other medication is used; Glass control syringes are sometimes used

Courtesy of Joe Fortunato.

FIGURE 5-52

Frazier-Ferguson suction tube

Size: 5 fr; 7 fr

Quantity: 1 each

Notes: May be included as reusable with set, but disposable is preferred

Courtesy of Miltex, Inc.

FIGURE 5-53

Yankauer suction tube

Size: 11.75"

Quantity: 1

Notes: May be included as reusable with set, but disposable is preferred; Reusable style has a screw-on tip

Instruments provided by www.sontecinstruments.com

FIGURE 5-54

Soft Tissue Dissection – RETRACTION AND EXPOSURE INSTRUMENTS

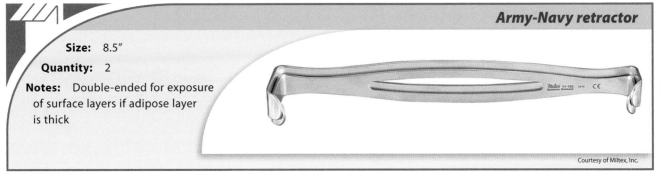

Army-Navy retractor

Size: 8.5"

Quantity: 2

Notes: Double-ended for exposure of surface layers if adipose layer is thick

Courtesy of Miltex, Inc.

FIGURE 5-55

continues

Soft Tissue Dissection – RETRACTION AND EXPOSURE INSTRUMENTS *continued*

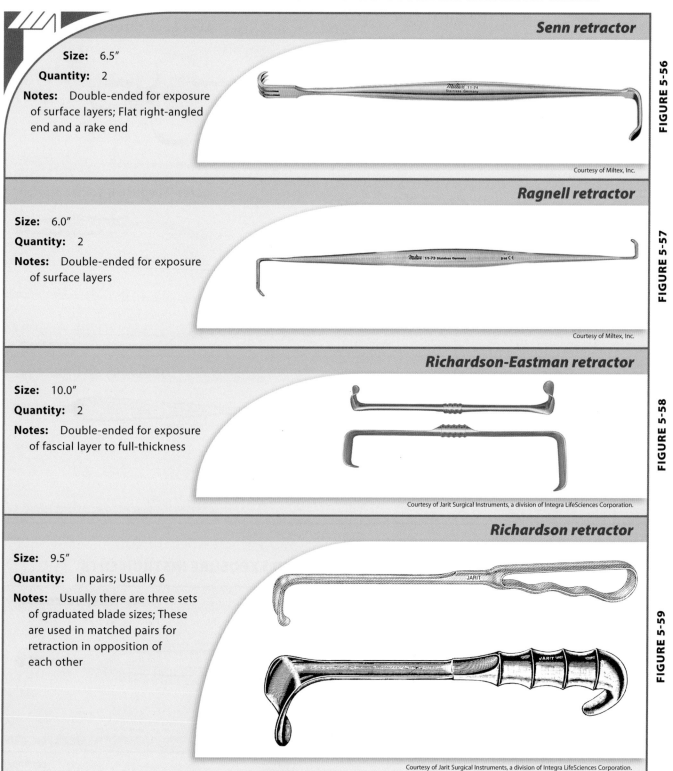

Senn retractor

Size: 6.5"

Quantity: 2

Notes: Double-ended for exposure of surface layers; Flat right-angled end and a rake end

Courtesy of Miltex, Inc.

FIGURE 5-56

Ragnell retractor

Size: 6.0"

Quantity: 2

Notes: Double-ended for exposure of surface layers

Courtesy of Miltex, Inc.

FIGURE 5-57

Richardson-Eastman retractor

Size: 10.0"

Quantity: 2

Notes: Double-ended for exposure of fascial layer to full-thickness

Courtesy of Jarit Surgical Instruments, a division of Integra LifeSciences Corporation.

FIGURE 5-58

Richardson retractor

Size: 9.5"

Quantity: In pairs; Usually 6

Notes: Usually there are three sets of graduated blade sizes; These are used in matched pairs for retraction in opposition of each other

Courtesy of Jarit Surgical Instruments, a division of Integra LifeSciences Corporation.

FIGURE 5-59

Soft Tissue Dissection – RETRACTION AND EXPOSURE INSTRUMENTS *continued*

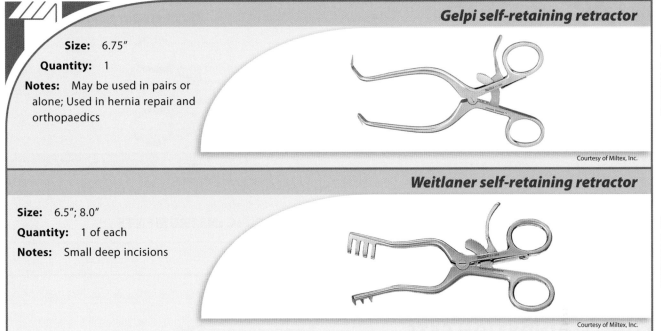

Gelpi self-retaining retractor

Size: 6.75″

Quantity: 1

Notes: May be used in pairs or alone; Used in hernia repair and orthopaedics

Courtesy of Miltex, Inc.

FIGURE 5-60

Weitlaner self-retaining retractor

Size: 6.5″; 8.0″

Quantity: 1 of each

Notes: Small deep incisions

Courtesy of Miltex, Inc.

FIGURE 5-61

Soft Tissue Dissection – APPROXIMATION AND CLOSURE INSTRUMENTS

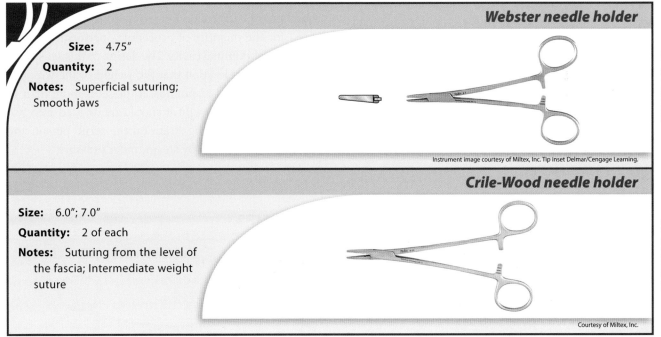

Webster needle holder

Size: 4.75″

Quantity: 2

Notes: Superficial suturing; Smooth jaws

Instrument image courtesy of Miltex, Inc. Tip inset Delmar/Cengage Learning.

FIGURE 5-62

Crile-Wood needle holder

Size: 6.0″; 7.0″

Quantity: 2 of each

Notes: Suturing from the level of the fascia; Intermediate weight suture

Courtesy of Miltex, Inc.

FIGURE 5-63

continues

Soft Tissue Dissection – APPROXIMATION AND CLOSURE INSTRUMENTS *continued*

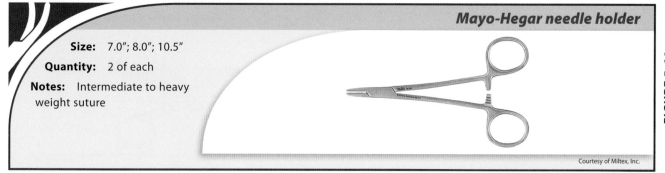

Mayo-Hegar needle holder

Size: 7.0"; 8.0"; 10.5"

Quantity: 2 of each

Notes: Intermediate to heavy weight suture

Courtesy of Miltex, Inc.

FIGURE 5-64

Soft Tissue Dissection – SPECIALTY SPECIFIC INSTRUMENTS

None: Added as needed

LONG FOUNDATION SETS

Instrument sets that are used below the level of the fascia and enter the peritoneal cavity include many of the instruments from the excisional and short sets. The main difference in these sets is instrument length. In some circumstances, extraordinarily long instruments in excess of 10 to 14 inches may be opened and added to the long set-up for extremely obese patients. Placing the extra long instruments in the tray as a standard is not cost effective for the few times they will be used. In facilities where the extra long instruments are used frequently, it may be wise to establish a tray of extra long soft tissue instruments complete with its own count sheet for accountability.

Laparotomy Set

The laparotomy foundation set should be designed with the type of procedures performed at the facility in mind. The foundation set described here is intended to be a baseline for construction of a functional set that can be used for the majority of procedures performed within the open abdominal cavity. The design of this set should take into consideration that the weight of the wrapped set cannot exceed 17 pounds. If the set is more than 17 pounds wrapped weight it should be divided into two trays to prevent lifting strain on the scrub person and facilitate sterilization by steam under pressure.

Laparotomy Set – CLAMPS

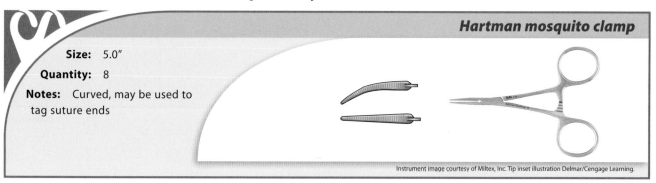

Hartman mosquito clamp

Size: 5.0"

Quantity: 8

Notes: Curved, may be used to tag suture ends

Instrument image courtesy of Miltex, Inc. Tip inset illustration Delmar/Cengage Learning.

FIGURE 5-65

Laparotomy Set – CLAMPS *continued*

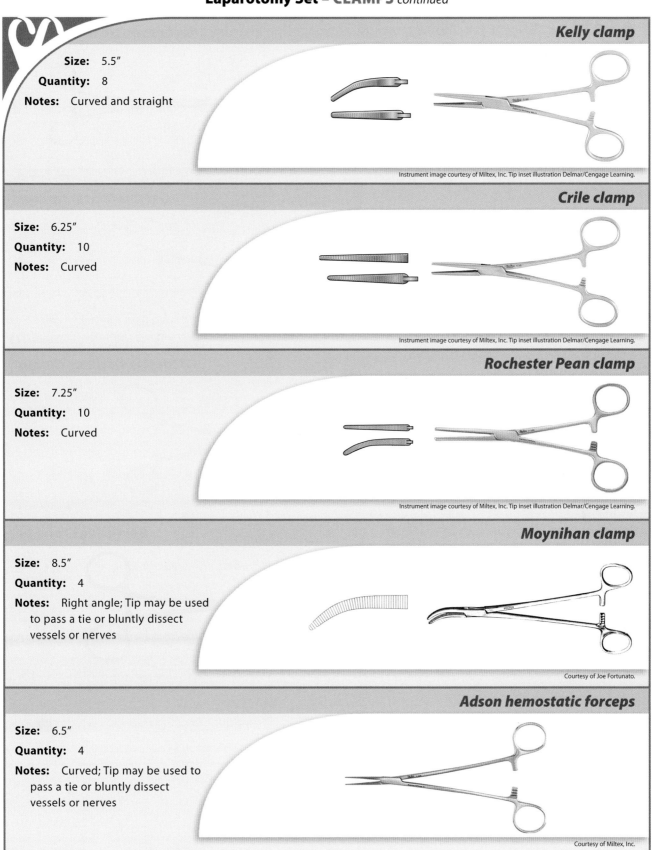

Kelly clamp

Size: 5.5″

Quantity: 8

Notes: Curved and straight

Instrument image courtesy of Miltex, Inc. Tip inset illustration Delmar/Cengage Learning.

FIGURE 5-66

Crile clamp

Size: 6.25″

Quantity: 10

Notes: Curved

Instrument image courtesy of Miltex, Inc. Tip inset illustration Delmar/Cengage Learning.

FIGURE 5-67

Rochester Pean clamp

Size: 7.25″

Quantity: 10

Notes: Curved

Instrument image courtesy of Miltex, Inc. Tip inset illustration Delmar/Cengage Learning.

FIGURE 5-68

Moynihan clamp

Size: 8.5″

Quantity: 4

Notes: Right angle; Tip may be used to pass a tie or bluntly dissect vessels or nerves

Courtesy of Joe Fortunato.

FIGURE 5-69

Adson hemostatic forceps

Size: 6.5″

Quantity: 4

Notes: Curved; Tip may be used to pass a tie or bluntly dissect vessels or nerves

Courtesy of Miltex, Inc.

FIGURE 5-70

continues

Laparotomy Set – CLAMPS *continued*

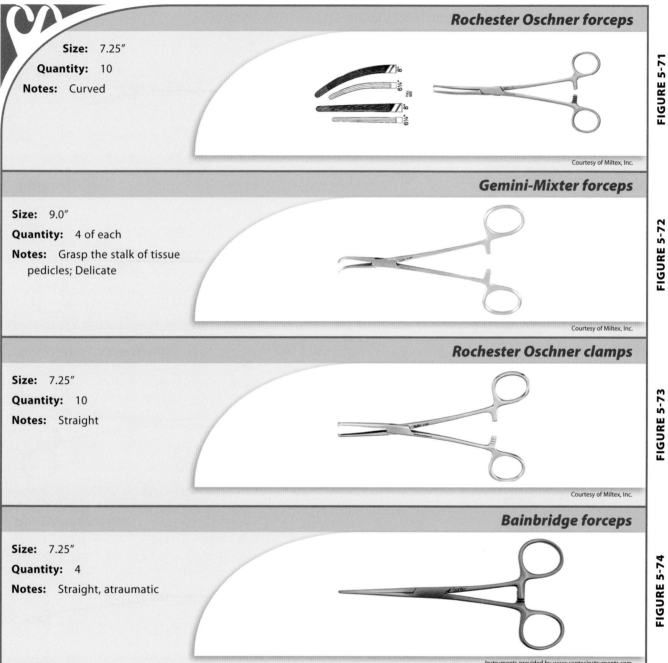

Rochester Oschner forceps

Size: 7.25"

Quantity: 10

Notes: Curved

Courtesy of Miltex, Inc.

FIGURE 5-71

Gemini-Mixter forceps

Size: 9.0"

Quantity: 4 of each

Notes: Grasp the stalk of tissue pedicles; Delicate

Courtesy of Miltex, Inc.

FIGURE 5-72

Rochester Oschner clamps

Size: 7.25"

Quantity: 10

Notes: Straight

Courtesy of Miltex, Inc.

FIGURE 5-73

Bainbridge forceps

Size: 7.25"

Quantity: 4

Notes: Straight, atraumatic

Instruments provided by www.sontecinstruments.com

FIGURE 5-74

Laparotomy Set – GRASPING FORCEPS

Allis tissue forceps

Size: 6.0"; 7.25"

Quantity: 10; 8

Notes: Straight, ring handle

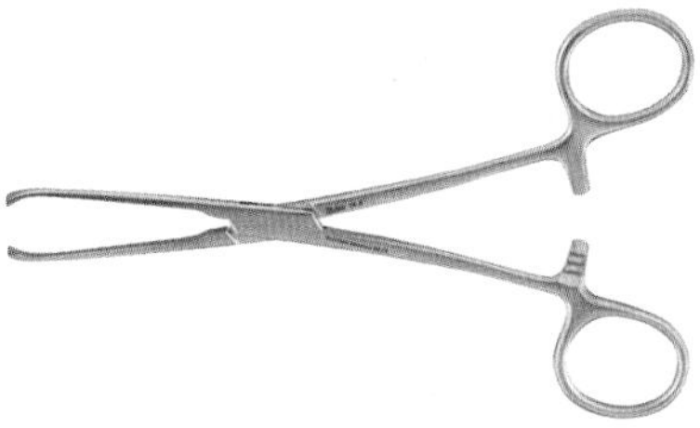

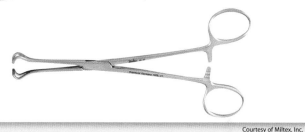

Courtesy of Miltex, Inc.

FIGURE 5-75

Babcock tissue forceps

Size: 8.25"

Quantity: 4

Notes: Use to grasp delicate tissues at the level of the peritoneum or bowel

Courtesy of Miltex, Inc.

FIGURE 5-76

Foerster sponge forceps

Size: 9.5"

Quantity: 4

Notes: Used to make sponge sticks for deep sponging for hemostasis and exposure; Can be used for blunt dissection

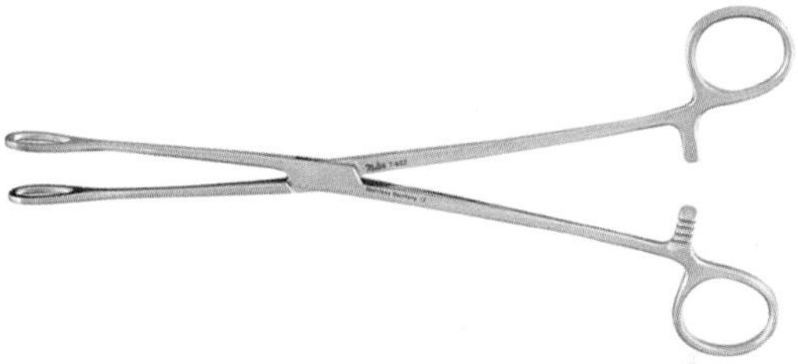

Courtesy of Miltex, Inc.

FIGURE 5-77

Adson tissue forceps

Size: 4.5"

Quantity: 2

Notes: Smooth, pick up; 1 × 2 teeth, pick up that will be used to approximate skin edges for closure with skin stapler

Courtesy of Miltex, Inc.

FIGURE 5-78

Gerald tissue forceps

Size: 7.0"

Quantity: 2

Notes: Fine straight tips with serrations for delicate tissue grasping

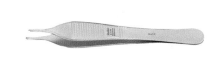
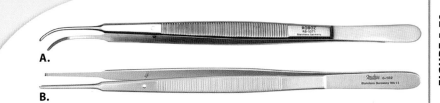

A.

B.

A. Copyright photo(s) courtesy of Roboz Surgical Instrument Co.
B. Courtesy of Miltex, Inc.

FIGURE 5-79

continues

Laparotomy Set – GRASPING FORCEPS *continued*

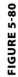

DeBakey tissue forceps

Size: 6.0″; 8.0″; 9.0″

Quantity: 2 of each

Notes: Fine teeth, pick up

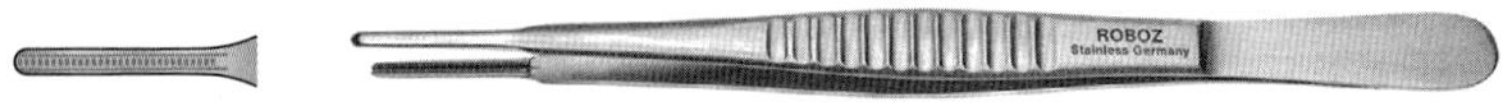

Copyright photo(s) courtesy of Roboz Surgical Instrument Co. Tip inset illustration Delmar/Cengage Learning.

FIGURE 5-80

Russian tissue forceps

Size: 9.0″

Quantity: 2

Notes: Circular serrated tips for handling intermediate to thick tissue layers or flaps; Atraumatic

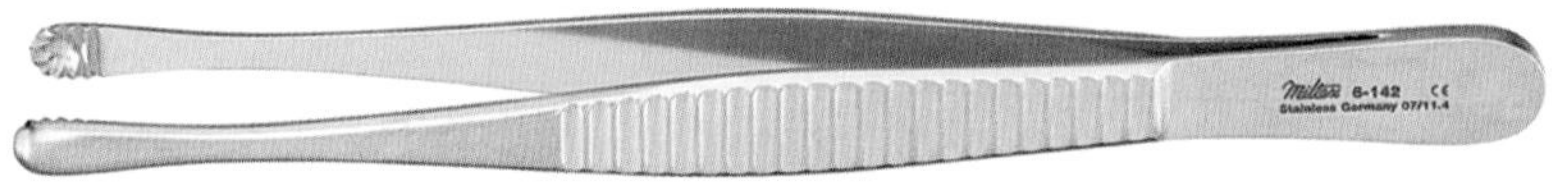

Courtesy of Miltex, Inc.

FIGURE 5-81

Dressing forceps

Size: 6.0″; 7.0″; 10.0″

Quantity: 2 of each

Notes: Fine serrations, pick up; Atraumatic; Can be used to place deep packing at the end of the case

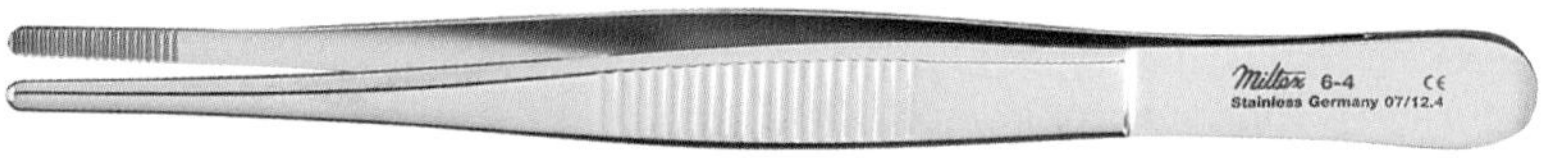

Courtesy of Miltex, Inc.

FIGURE 5-82

Tissue forceps

Size: 6.0″; 7.0″; 10.0″

Quantity: 2 of each

Notes: 1 × 2 teeth, pick up; Intermediate to heavy tissue handling

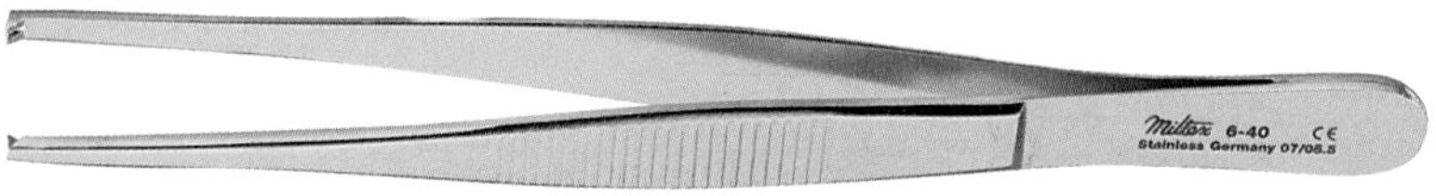

Courtesy of Miltex, Inc.

FIGURE 5-83

Laparotomy Set – DISSECTION INSTRUMENTS

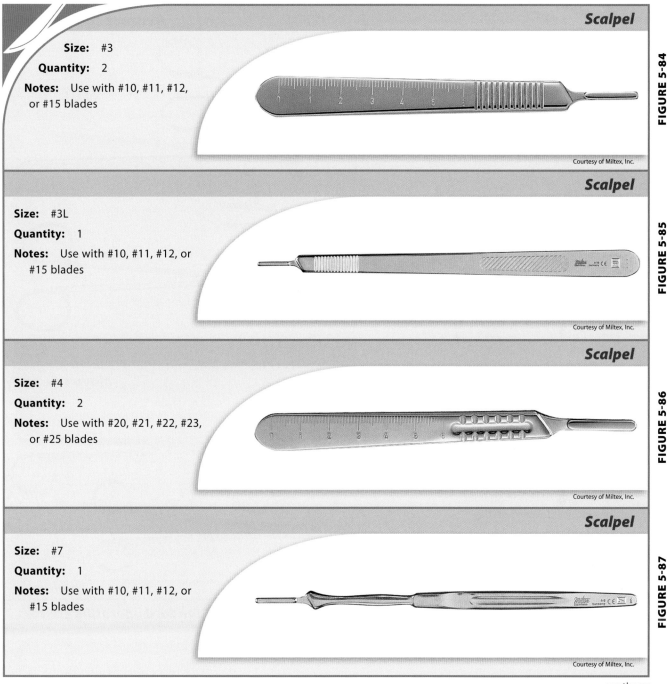

Scalpel

Size: #3
Quantity: 2
Notes: Use with #10, #11, #12, or #15 blades

Courtesy of Miltex, Inc.

FIGURE 5-84

Scalpel

Size: #3L
Quantity: 1
Notes: Use with #10, #11, #12, or #15 blades

Courtesy of Miltex, Inc.

FIGURE 5-85

Scalpel

Size: #4
Quantity: 2
Notes: Use with #20, #21, #22, #23, or #25 blades

Courtesy of Miltex, Inc.

FIGURE 5-86

Scalpel

Size: #7
Quantity: 1
Notes: Use with #10, #11, #12, or #15 blades

Courtesy of Miltex, Inc.

FIGURE 5-87

continues

Laparotomy Set – DISSECTION INSTRUMENTS *continued*

Metzenbaum scissors

Size: 7.0"; 9.0"; 11.0"

Quantity: 1 of each

Notes: Light to intermediate tissue dissection; Blunt-blunt tips

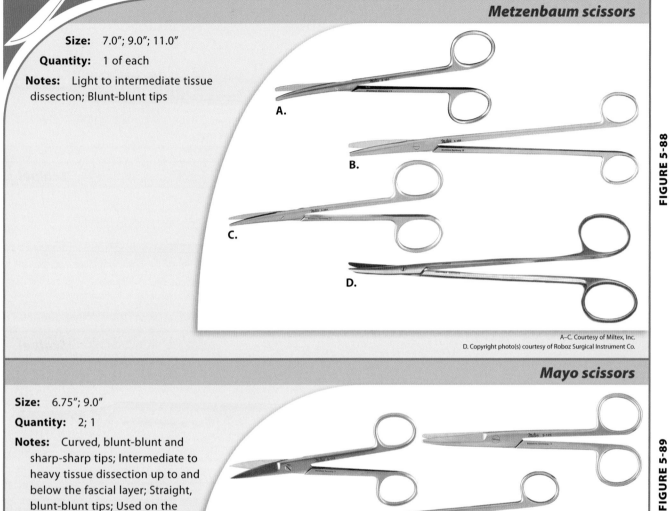

A.

B.

C.

D.

A–C. Courtesy of Miltex, Inc.
D. Copyright photo(s) courtesy of Roboz Surgical Instrument Co.

FIGURE 5-88

Mayo scissors

Size: 6.75"; 9.0"

Quantity: 2; 1

Notes: Curved, blunt-blunt and sharp-sharp tips; Intermediate to heavy tissue dissection up to and below the fascial layer; Straight, blunt-blunt tips; Used on the field to cut suture

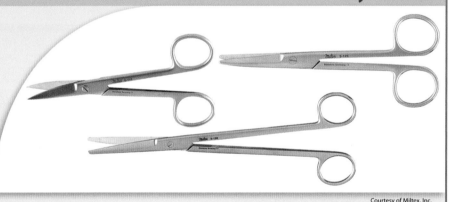

Courtesy of Miltex, Inc.

FIGURE 5-89

Standard operating scissors

Size: 5.0"

Quantity: 1

Notes: Straight, blunt-sharp tips; Used to trim suture ends

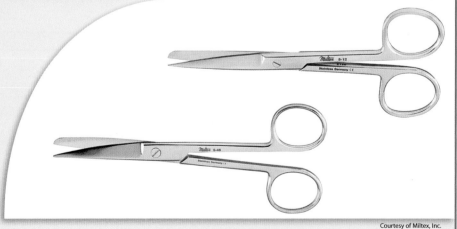

Courtesy of Miltex, Inc.

FIGURE 5-90

Laparotomy Set – DEBULKING INSTRUMENTS

None: Can be added if wound debridement is required

Laparotomy Set – PROBES AND DILATORS

None: Can be added if sinus tract or fistula is present

Laparotomy Set – EVACUATION AND INSTILLATION INSTRUMENTS

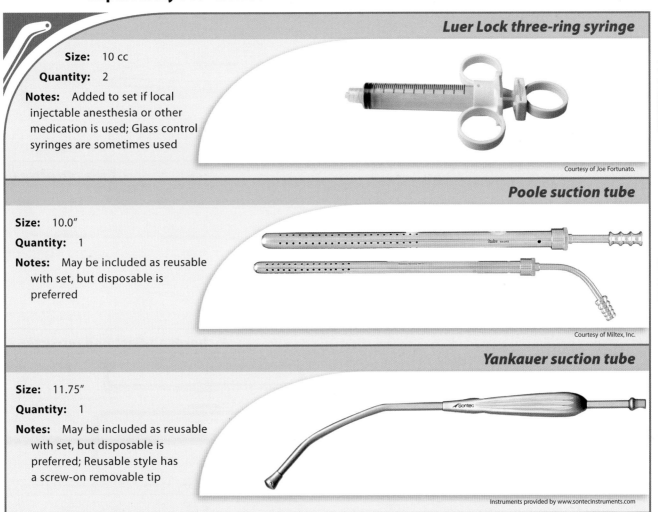

Luer Lock three-ring syringe

Size: 10 cc

Quantity: 2

Notes: Added to set if local injectable anesthesia or other medication is used; Glass control syringes are sometimes used

Courtesy of Joe Fortunato.

FIGURE 5-91

Poole suction tube

Size: 10.0"

Quantity: 1

Notes: May be included as reusable with set, but disposable is preferred

Courtesy of Miltex, Inc.

FIGURE 5-92

Yankauer suction tube

Size: 11.75"

Quantity: 1

Notes: May be included as reusable with set, but disposable is preferred; Reusable style has a screw-on removable tip

Instruments provided by www.sontecinstruments.com

FIGURE 5-93

Laparotomy Set – RETRACTION AND EXPOSURE INSTRUMENTS

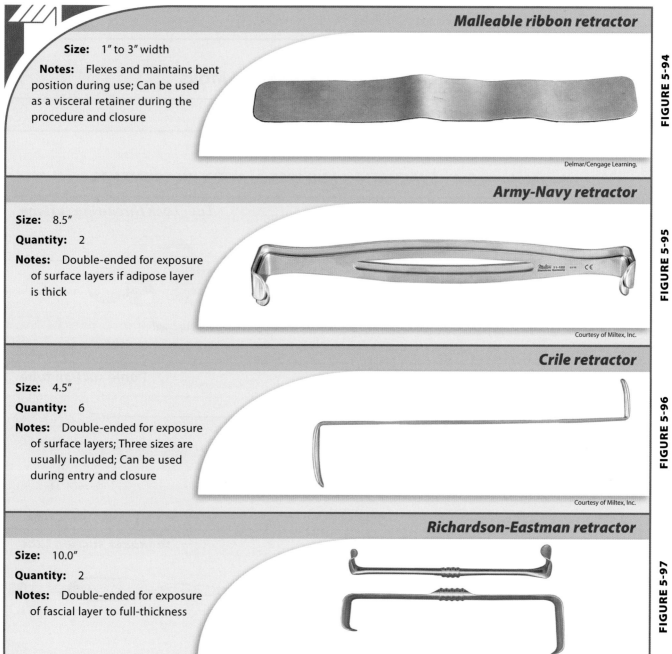

Malleable ribbon retractor

Size: 1" to 3" width

Notes: Flexes and maintains bent position during use; Can be used as a visceral retainer during the procedure and closure

Delmar/Cengage Learning.

FIGURE 5-94

Army-Navy retractor

Size: 8.5"

Quantity: 2

Notes: Double-ended for exposure of surface layers if adipose layer is thick

Courtesy of Miltex, Inc.

FIGURE 5-95

Crile retractor

Size: 4.5"

Quantity: 6

Notes: Double-ended for exposure of surface layers; Three sizes are usually included; Can be used during entry and closure

Courtesy of Miltex, Inc.

FIGURE 5-96

Richardson-Eastman retractor

Size: 10.0"

Quantity: 2

Notes: Double-ended for exposure of fascial layer to full-thickness

Courtesy of Jarit Surgical Instruments, a division of Integra LifeSciences Corporation.

FIGURE 5-97

Laparotomy Set – RETRACTION AND EXPOSURE INSTRUMENTS *continued*

Deaver retractor

Size: 12.0″

Quantity: 1

Notes: Width 1.0″

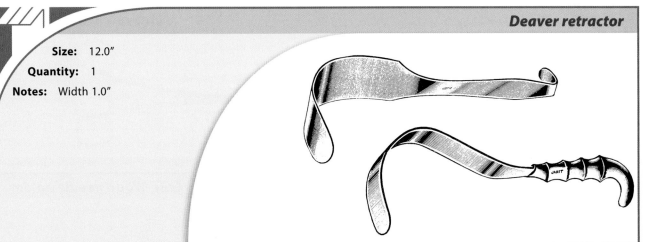

Courtesy of Jarit Surgical Instruments, a division of Integra LifeSciences Corporation.

FIGURE 5-98

Richardson retractor

Size: 9.5″

Quantity: In pairs; Usually 6

Notes: Usually there are three sets of graduated blade sizes; These are used in matched pairs for retraction in opposition of each other

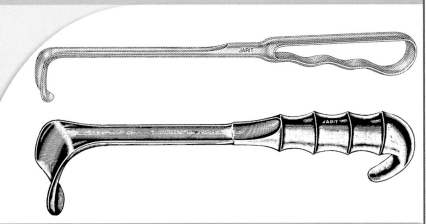

Courtesy of Jarit Surgical Instruments, a division of Integra LifeSciences Corporation.

FIGURE 5-99

Balfour self-retaining retractor

Size: 10.0″

Quantity: 1 set

Notes: Expandable arms with one bladder retraction blade; This retractor can be wrapped separately; Many other types of self-retaining retractors provide varying amounts of exposure and may be more advantageous to use; Some Balfour retractors have interchangeable side body wall blade assemblies

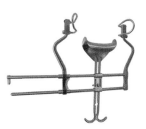

Instruments provided by www.sontecinstruments.com

FIGURE 5-100

Laparotomy Set – APPROXIMATION AND CLOSURE INSTRUMENTS

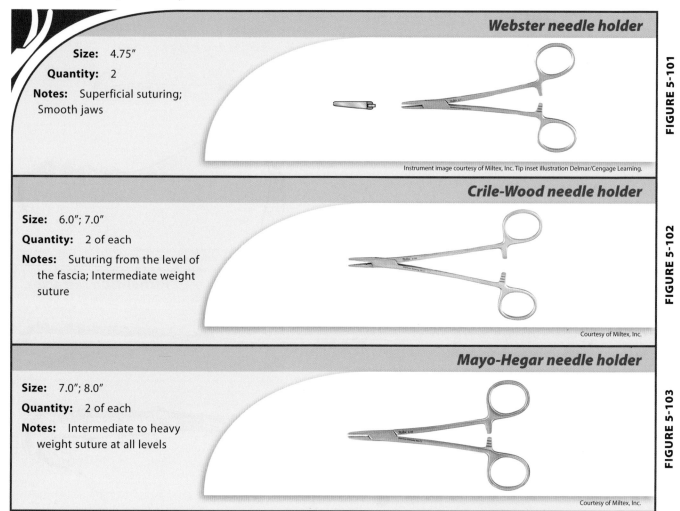

Webster needle holder

Size: 4.75″

Quantity: 2

Notes: Superficial suturing; Smooth jaws

Instrument image courtesy of Miltex, Inc. Tip inset illustration Delmar/Cengage Learning.

FIGURE 5-101

Crile-Wood needle holder

Size: 6.0″; 7.0″

Quantity: 2 of each

Notes: Suturing from the level of the fascia; Intermediate weight suture

Courtesy of Miltex, Inc.

FIGURE 5-102

Mayo-Hegar needle holder

Size: 7.0″; 8.0″

Quantity: 2 of each

Notes: Intermediate to heavy weight suture at all levels

Courtesy of Miltex, Inc.

FIGURE 5-103

Laparotomy Set – SPECIALTY SPECIFIC INSTRUMENTS

Note: Self-retaining retractor of surgeon's choice should be added if Balfour retractor does not provide the needed exposure.

Extra Long "Add-On" Set

Patients with deep adipose tissue pose a particularly complex problem. With the advent of bariatric procedures, more manufacturers are producing longer instrumentation for open surgery. When using a long foundation set for an open procedure on an obese patient, this grid may provide suggestions for the creation of an extra long add-on set.

Extra Long "Add-On" Set – CLAMPS

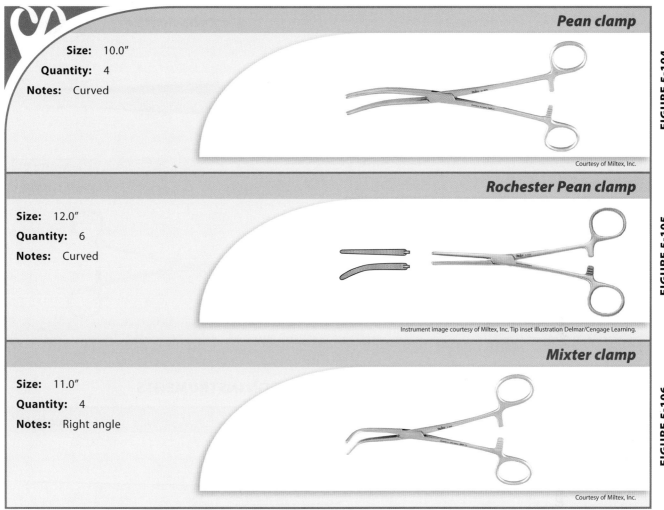

Pean clamp

Size: 10.0"
Quantity: 4
Notes: Curved

Courtesy of Miltex, Inc.

FIGURE 5-104

Rochester Pean clamp

Size: 12.0"
Quantity: 6
Notes: Curved

Instrument image courtesy of Miltex, Inc. Tip inset illustration Delmar/Cengage Learning.

FIGURE 5-105

Mixter clamp

Size: 11.0"
Quantity: 4
Notes: Right angle

Courtesy of Miltex, Inc.

FIGURE 5-106

Extra Long "Add-On" Set – GRASPING FORCEPS

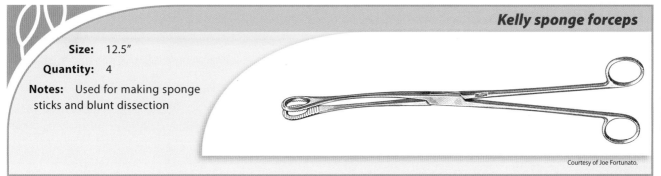

Kelly sponge forceps

Size: 12.5"
Quantity: 4
Notes: Used for making sponge sticks and blunt dissection

Courtesy of Joe Fortunato.

FIGURE 5-107

continues

Extra Long "Add-On" Set – GRASPING FORCEPS *continued*

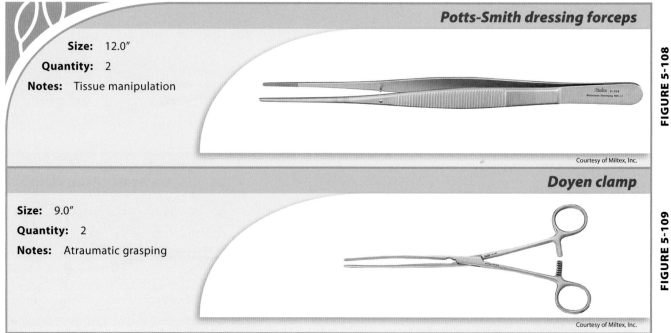

Potts-Smith dressing forceps

Size: 12.0"

Quantity: 2

Notes: Tissue manipulation

Courtesy of Miltex, Inc.

FIGURE 5-108

Doyen clamp

Size: 9.0"

Quantity: 2

Notes: Atraumatic grasping

Courtesy of Miltex, Inc.

FIGURE 5-109

Extra Long "Add-On" Set – DISSECTION INSTRUMENTS

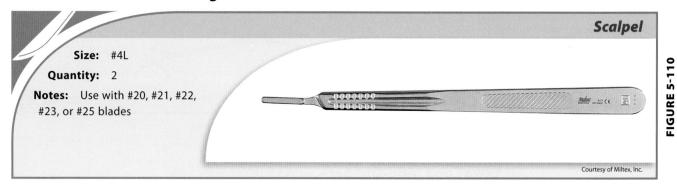

Scalpel

Size: #4L

Quantity: 2

Notes: Use with #20, #21, #22, #23, or #25 blades

Courtesy of Miltex, Inc.

FIGURE 5-110

Extra Long "Add-On" Set – DISSECTION INSTRUMENTS *continued*

Metzenbaum scissors

Size: 11.0"; 14.5"

Quantity: 2; 2

Notes: Curved and straight

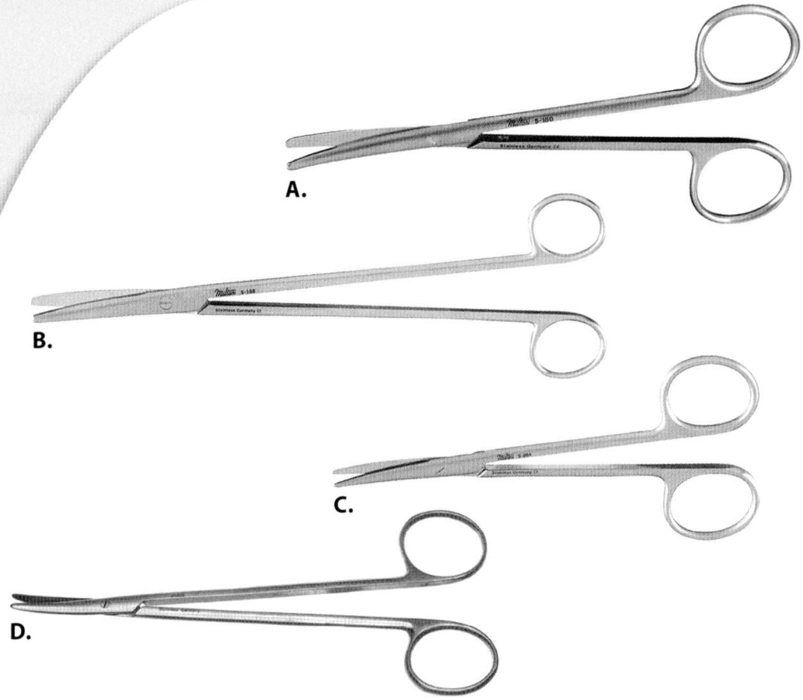

A.

B.

C.

D.

A-C. Courtesy of Miltex, Inc.
D. Copyright photo(s) courtesy of Roboz Surgical Instrument Co.

FIGURE 5-111

Harrington scissors

Size: 11.0"

Quantity: 1

Notes: Curved; Blunt-blunt tips

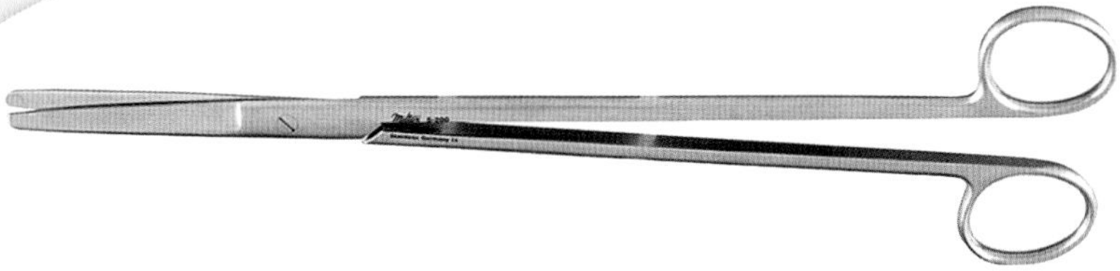

Courtesy of Miltex, Inc.

FIGURE 5-112

Extra Long "Add-On" Set – RETRACTION AND EXPOSURE INSTRUMENTS

Deaver retractor

Size: 12.0"

Quantity: 2

Notes: Extra wide blades 3.0" and 4.0"

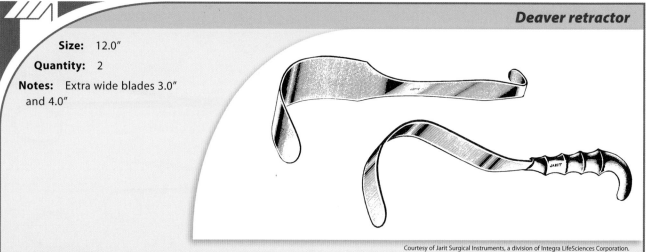

Courtesy of Jarit Surgical Instruments, a division of Integra LifeSciences Corporation.

FIGURE 5-113

Kelly retractor

Size: 10.0"

Quantity: 2

Notes: Long wide blades

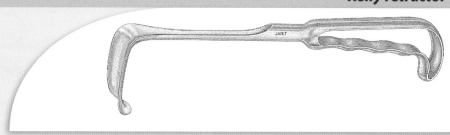

Courtesy of Jarit Surgical Instruments, a division of Integra LifeSciences Corporation.

FIGURE 5-114

Foss retractor

Size: 10.0"

Notes: Hollow grip handle with 1.75 inch blade; Used for large organ retraction

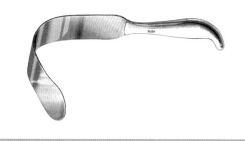

Courtesy of Joe Fortunato.

FIGURE 5-115

Extra Long "Add-On" Set – APPROXIMATION AND CLOSURE INSTRUMENTS

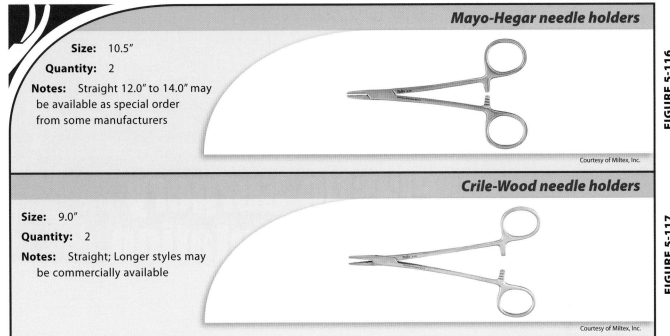

Mayo-Hegar needle holders

Size: 10.5"

Quantity: 2

Notes: Straight 12.0" to 14.0" may be available as special order from some manufacturers

Courtesy of Miltex, Inc.

FIGURE 5-116

Crile-Wood needle holders

Size: 9.0"

Quantity: 2

Notes: Straight; Longer styles may be commercially available

Courtesy of Miltex, Inc.

FIGURE 5-117

SUMMARY

Selection of the correct foundation set can be beneficial to the patient, surgeon, and team. The baseline instrumentation is determined by the depth of the target tissue and, in some circumstances, the depth of the patient's tissues. Constructing foundation sets with the appropriate quantities of instruments of varying types will differ between facilities and surgeon' s preferences. The foundation sets represented in this chapter are designed to be cost effective and manageable by the scrub person and are not intended to be the only groupings used by the surgical team. Each facility should have a committee of scrub personnel and circulating nurses to determine groupings that best represent the practices of the majority of surgeons and procedures. Establishing foundation sets can be useful for training new personnel and standardizing count sheets.

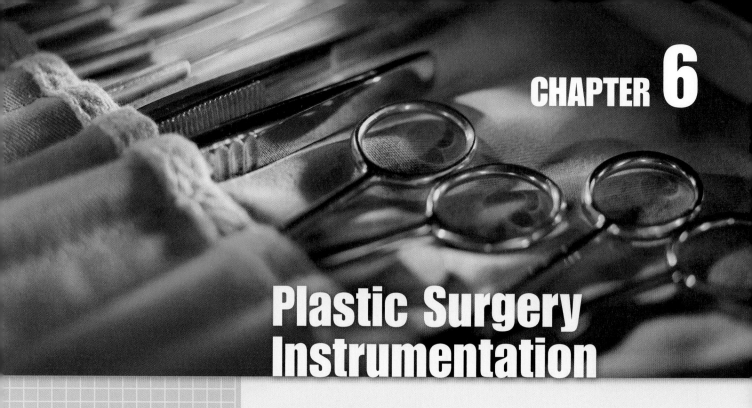

Plastic Surgery Instrumentation

INTRODUCTION

Plastic surgery requires predominantly delicate instrumentation that provides the surgeon the ability to work with fine tissues without causing damage at the cellular level. Meticulous handling of the tissues gives the patient the best chance for aesthetic healing. Patients who go to a plastic surgeon are seeking an improvement or restoration of form, function, or both. The main thing patients see at the end of the procedure is the closure and the overall external appearance. Although some plastic surgeons use microsurgery in their plastic surgical practices, microsurgery is covered in a separate chapter because it is shared with other specialties, such as neurosurgery and gynecology.

BASIC PLASTIC SURGERY INSTRUMENTATION

Basic plastic surgery sets have some of the common elements found in the soft tissue foundation sets. The soft tissue foundation sets have several instruments that are not commonly used in plastic surgery; therefore, it may be more functional to assemble a basic plastic surgery set that serves as the foundation for plastic surgical cases. Infrequently used instruments or highly specialized collections can be packaged together as procedure-specific add-on sets, such as for facelifts. The rationale for having add-on instrumentation is multi-fold:

1. Specialty instruments are very expensive. To package all of the instruments in one tray would require extensive duplication of instruments that are not commonly used for most cases.

2. Plastic surgery instruments are very delicate. The more they are processed and handled, the greater the risk to their tiny points and tips.

3. Steam sterilization causes sharp edges to dull. Repeated exposure to steam causes the metal instruments to soften over time. The blades will not hold a sharp edge. Dull scissors tear and rip tissue. This damages wound edges and causes irregular scars.

4. Unused instruments cause clutter on the field. The risk for retained foreign objects is increased when there are extraneous items within the sterile field.

5. The maintenance of the instrumentation is time consuming. Many instruments need tip protectors in place during sterilization. More instruments mean more tips. Extremely delicate instruments are sometimes wrapped individually within the assembled tray.

The predominant instrumentation for plastic surgery consists of gentle grasping, delicate dissection, and meticulous closure of soft tissue. Modification of bony tissue is discussed in a later chapter. Hemostasis is accomplished with fine-tipped clamps and needle-point cautery. Some surgeons believe that cautery leaves devitalized tissue in the wound that causes increased inflammation and potentiates infection. Surgeons who do not prefer cautery frequently use 2/0, 3/0, or 4/0 silk or absorbable synthetic ties for hemostasis.

Basic Plastic Surgery Instrumentation – CLAMPS

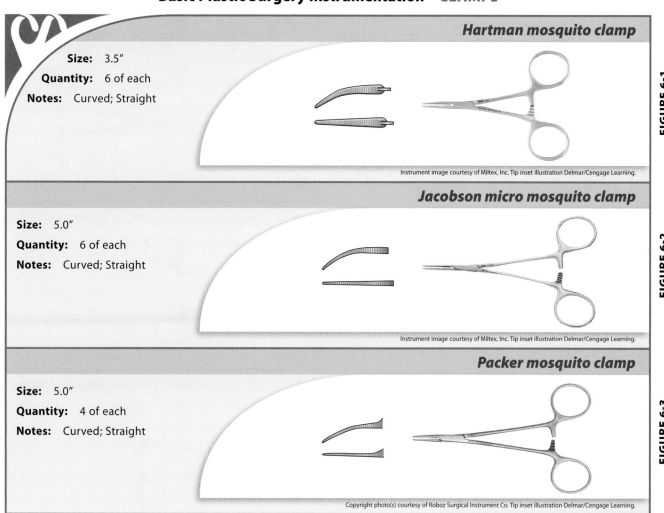

Hartman mosquito clamp

Size: 3.5″
Quantity: 6 of each
Notes: Curved; Straight

Instrument image courtesy of Miltex, Inc. Tip inset illustration Delmar/Cengage Learning.

FIGURE 6-1

Jacobson micro mosquito clamp

Size: 5.0″
Quantity: 6 of each
Notes: Curved; Straight

Instrument image courtesy of Miltex, Inc. Tip inset illustration Delmar/Cengage Learning.

FIGURE 6-2

Packer mosquito clamp

Size: 5.0″
Quantity: 4 of each
Notes: Curved; Straight

Copyright photo(s) courtesy of Roboz Surgical Instrument Co. Tip inset illustration Delmar/Cengage Learning.

FIGURE 6-3

continues

Basic Plastic Surgery Instrumentation – CLAMPS *continued*

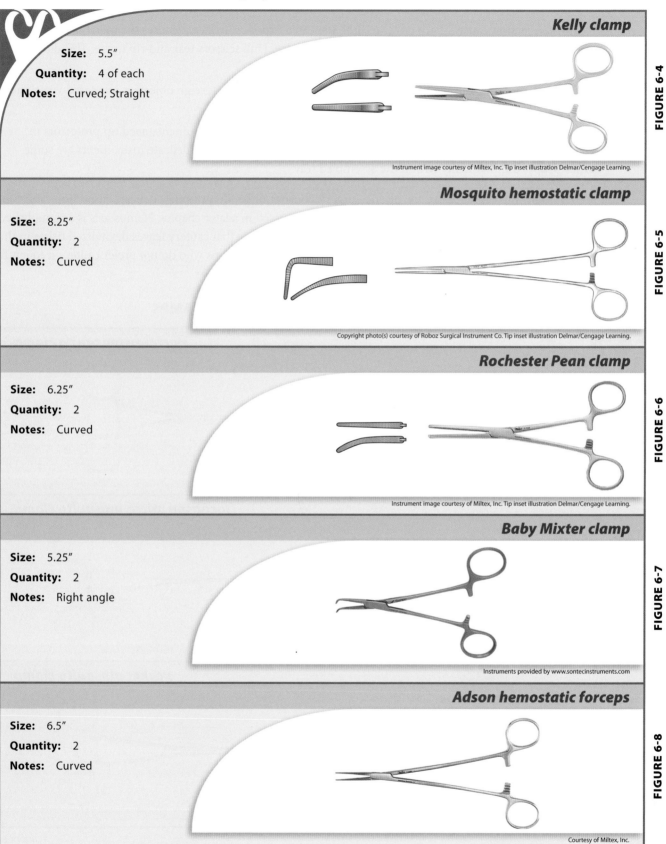

Kelly clamp

Size: 5.5"

Quantity: 4 of each

Notes: Curved; Straight

Instrument image courtesy of Miltex, Inc. Tip inset illustration Delmar/Cengage Learning.

FIGURE 6-4

Mosquito hemostatic clamp

Size: 8.25"

Quantity: 2

Notes: Curved

Copyright photo(s) courtesy of Roboz Surgical Instrument Co. Tip inset illustration Delmar/Cengage Learning.

FIGURE 6-5

Rochester Pean clamp

Size: 6.25"

Quantity: 2

Notes: Curved

Instrument image courtesy of Miltex, Inc. Tip inset illustration Delmar/Cengage Learning.

FIGURE 6-6

Baby Mixter clamp

Size: 5.25"

Quantity: 2

Notes: Right angle

Instruments provided by www.sontecinstruments.com

FIGURE 6-7

Adson hemostatic forceps

Size: 6.5"

Quantity: 2

Notes: Curved

Courtesy of Miltex, Inc.

FIGURE 6-8

Basic Plastic Surgery Instrumentation – CLAMPS *continued*

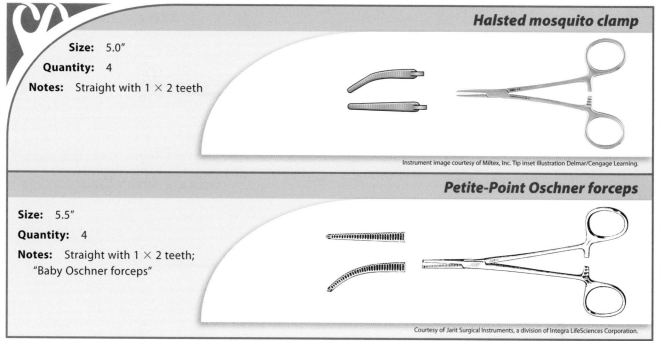

Halsted mosquito clamp

Size: 5.0"

Quantity: 4

Notes: Straight with 1 × 2 teeth

Instrument image courtesy of Miltex, Inc. Tip inset illustration Delmar/Cengage Learning.

FIGURE 6-9

Petite-Point Oschner forceps

Size: 5.5"

Quantity: 4

Notes: Straight with 1 × 2 teeth; "Baby Oschner forceps"

Courtesy of Jarit Surgical Instruments, a division of Integra LifeSciences Corporation.

FIGURE 6-10

Basic Plastic Surgery Instrumentation – GRASPING FORCEPS

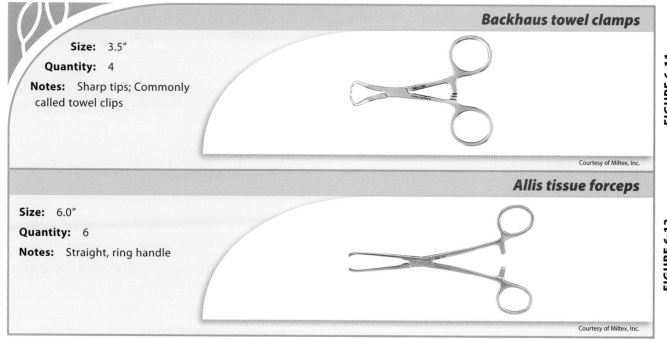

Backhaus towel clamps

Size: 3.5"

Quantity: 4

Notes: Sharp tips; Commonly called towel clips

Courtesy of Miltex, Inc.

FIGURE 6-11

Allis tissue forceps

Size: 6.0"

Quantity: 6

Notes: Straight, ring handle

Courtesy of Miltex, Inc.

FIGURE 6-12

continues

Basic Plastic Surgery Instrumentation – GRASPING FORCEPS *continued*

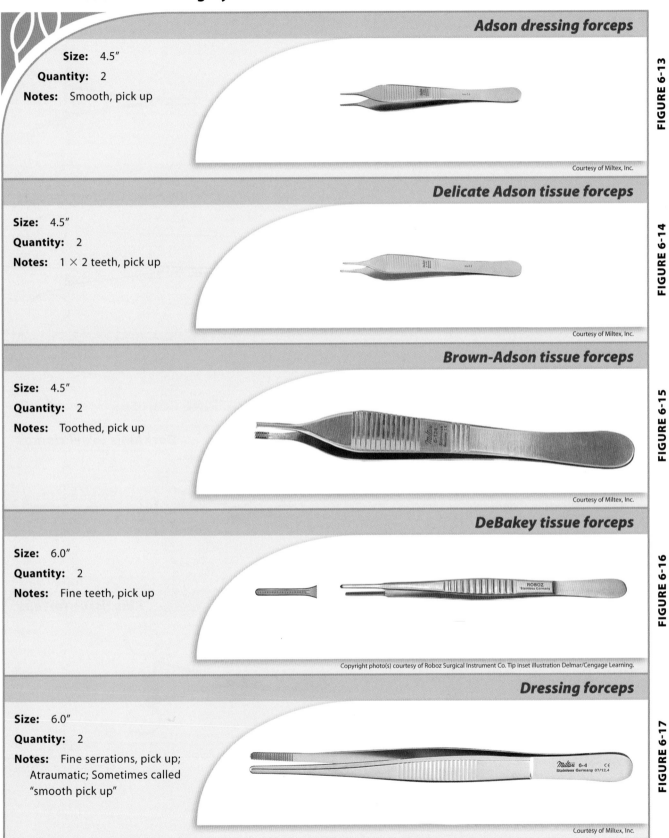

Adson dressing forceps

Size: 4.5"

Quantity: 2

Notes: Smooth, pick up

Courtesy of Miltex, Inc.

FIGURE 6-13

Delicate Adson tissue forceps

Size: 4.5"

Quantity: 2

Notes: 1 × 2 teeth, pick up

Courtesy of Miltex, Inc.

FIGURE 6-14

Brown-Adson tissue forceps

Size: 4.5"

Quantity: 2

Notes: Toothed, pick up

Courtesy of Miltex, Inc.

FIGURE 6-15

DeBakey tissue forceps

Size: 6.0"

Quantity: 2

Notes: Fine teeth, pick up

Copyright photo(s) courtesy of Roboz Surgical Instrument Co. Tip inset illustration Delmar/Cengage Learning.

FIGURE 6-16

Dressing forceps

Size: 6.0"

Quantity: 2

Notes: Fine serrations, pick up; Atraumatic; Sometimes called "smooth pick up"

Courtesy of Miltex, Inc.

FIGURE 6-17

Basic Plastic Surgery Instrumentation – GRASPING FORCEPS *continued*

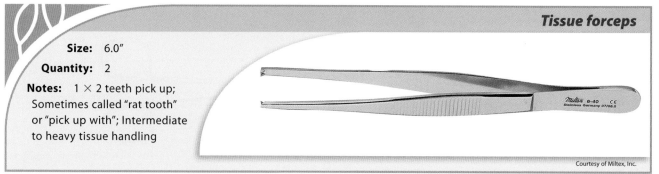

Tissue forceps

Size: 6.0"

Quantity: 2

Notes: 1 × 2 teeth pick up; Sometimes called "rat tooth" or "pick up with"; Intermediate to heavy tissue handling

Courtesy of Miltex, Inc.

FIGURE 6-18

Basic Plastic Surgery Instrumentation – DISSECTION INSTRUMENTS

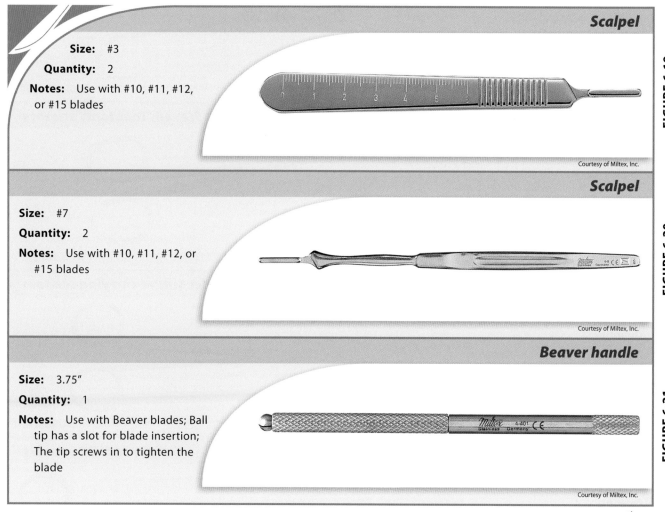

Scalpel

Size: #3

Quantity: 2

Notes: Use with #10, #11, #12, or #15 blades

Courtesy of Miltex, Inc.

FIGURE 6-19

Scalpel

Size: #7

Quantity: 2

Notes: Use with #10, #11, #12, or #15 blades

Courtesy of Miltex, Inc.

FIGURE 6-20

Beaver handle

Size: 3.75"

Quantity: 1

Notes: Use with Beaver blades; Ball tip has a slot for blade insertion; The tip screws in to tighten the blade

Courtesy of Miltex, Inc.

FIGURE 6-21

continues

Basic Plastic Surgery Instrumentation – DISSECTION INSTRUMENTS continued

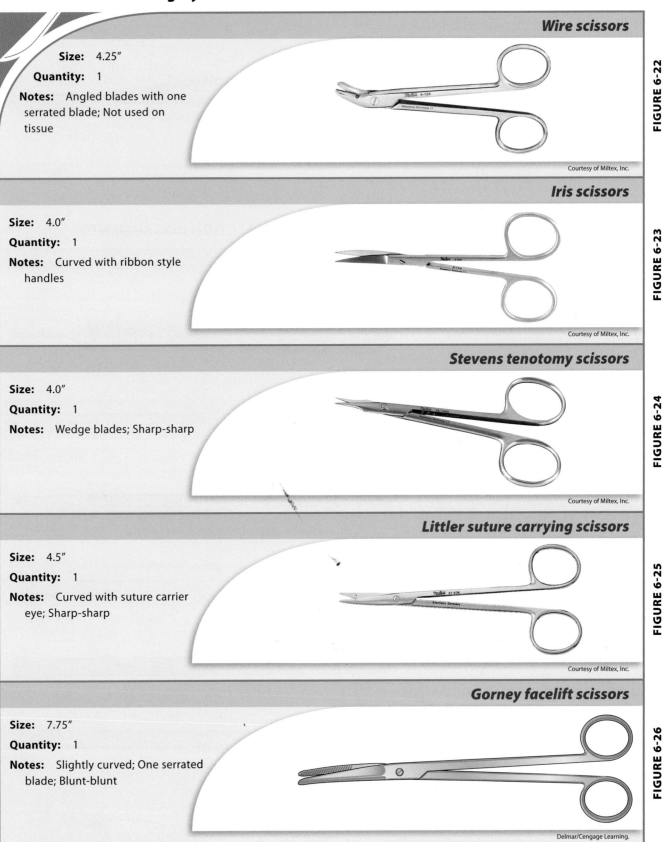

Wire scissors

Size: 4.25"

Quantity: 1

Notes: Angled blades with one serrated blade; Not used on tissue

Courtesy of Miltex, Inc.

FIGURE 6-22

Iris scissors

Size: 4.0"

Quantity: 1

Notes: Curved with ribbon style handles

Courtesy of Miltex, Inc.

FIGURE 6-23

Stevens tenotomy scissors

Size: 4.0"

Quantity: 1

Notes: Wedge blades; Sharp-sharp

Courtesy of Miltex, Inc.

FIGURE 6-24

Littler suture carrying scissors

Size: 4.5"

Quantity: 1

Notes: Curved with suture carrier eye; Sharp-sharp

Courtesy of Miltex, Inc.

FIGURE 6-25

Gorney facelift scissors

Size: 7.75"

Quantity: 1

Notes: Slightly curved; One serrated blade; Blunt-blunt

Delmar/Cengage Learning.

FIGURE 6-26

Basic Plastic Surgery Instrumentation – DISSECTION INSTRUMENTS continued

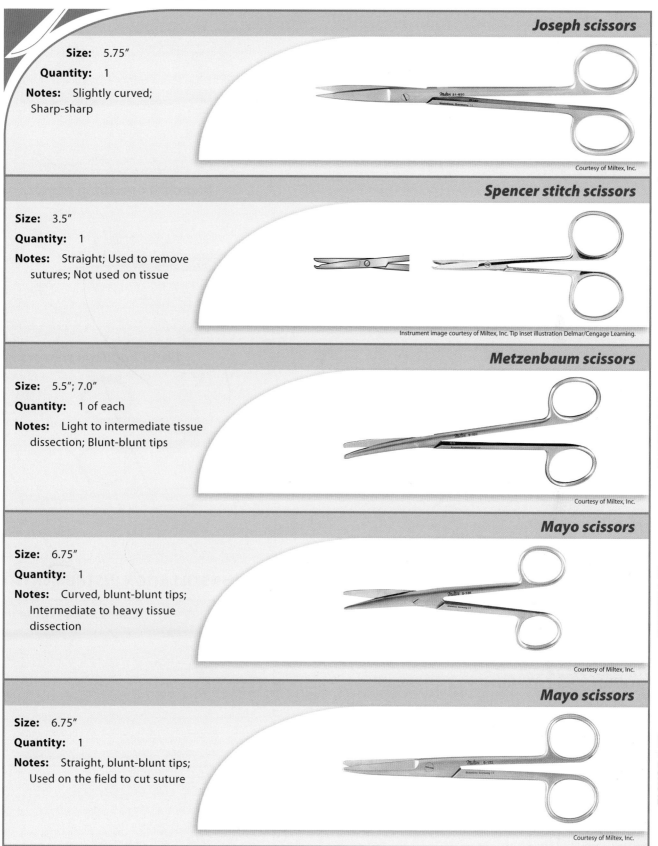

Joseph scissors

Size:	5.75″
Quantity:	1
Notes:	Slightly curved; Sharp-sharp

FIGURE 6-27

Courtesy of Miltex, Inc.

Spencer stitch scissors

Size: 3.5″

Quantity: 1

Notes: Straight; Used to remove sutures; Not used on tissue

FIGURE 6-28

Instrument image courtesy of Miltex, Inc. Tip inset illustration Delmar/Cengage Learning.

Metzenbaum scissors

Size: 5.5″; 7.0″

Quantity: 1 of each

Notes: Light to intermediate tissue dissection; Blunt-blunt tips

FIGURE 6-29

Courtesy of Miltex, Inc.

Mayo scissors

Size: 6.75″

Quantity: 1

Notes: Curved, blunt-blunt tips; Intermediate to heavy tissue dissection

FIGURE 6-30

Courtesy of Miltex, Inc.

Mayo scissors

Size: 6.75″

Quantity: 1

Notes: Straight, blunt-blunt tips; Used on the field to cut suture

FIGURE 6-31

Courtesy of Miltex, Inc.

continues

Basic Plastic Surgery Instrumentation – DISSECTION INSTRUMENTS *continued*

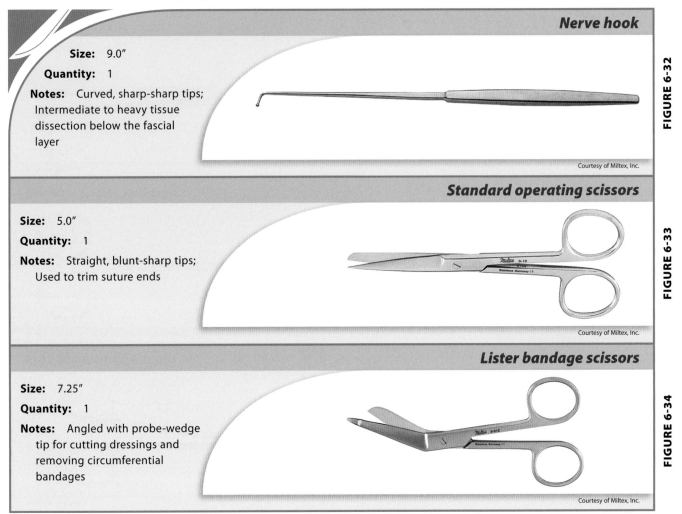

Nerve hook

Size: 9.0"

Quantity: 1

Notes: Curved, sharp-sharp tips; Intermediate to heavy tissue dissection below the fascial layer

Courtesy of Miltex, Inc.

FIGURE 6-32

Standard operating scissors

Size: 5.0"

Quantity: 1

Notes: Straight, blunt-sharp tips; Used to trim suture ends

Courtesy of Miltex, Inc.

FIGURE 6-33

Lister bandage scissors

Size: 7.25"

Quantity: 1

Notes: Angled with probe-wedge tip for cutting dressings and removing circumferential bandages

Courtesy of Miltex, Inc.

FIGURE 6-34

Basic Plastic Surgery Instrumentation – EVACUATION AND INSTILLATION INSTRUMENTS

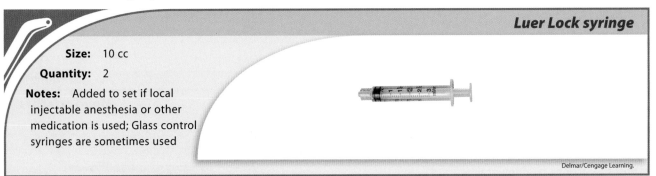

Luer Lock syringe

Size: 10 cc

Quantity: 2

Notes: Added to set if local injectable anesthesia or other medication is used; Glass control syringes are sometimes used

Delmar/Cengage Learning.

FIGURE 6-35

Basic Plastic Surgery Instrumentation – EVACUATION AND INSTILLATION INSTRUMENTS *continued*

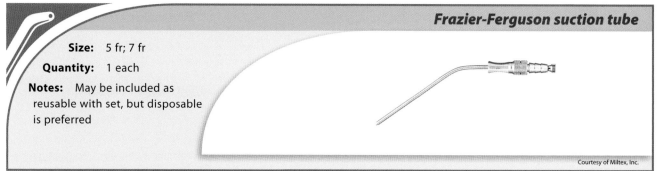

Frazier-Ferguson suction tube

Size: 5 fr; 7 fr

Quantity: 1 each

Notes: May be included as reusable with set, but disposable is preferred

Courtesy of Miltex, Inc.

FIGURE 6-36

Basic Plastic Surgery Instrumentation – RETRACTION AND EXPOSURE INSTRUMENTS

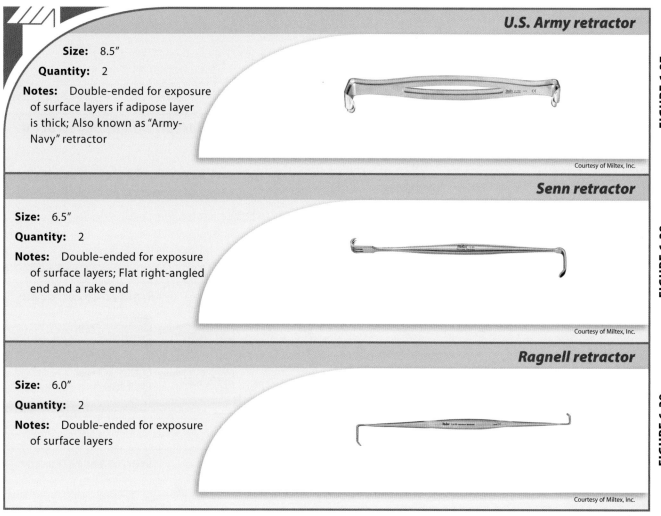

U.S. Army retractor

Size: 8.5″

Quantity: 2

Notes: Double-ended for exposure of surface layers if adipose layer is thick; Also known as "Army-Navy" retractor

Courtesy of Miltex, Inc.

FIGURE 6-37

Senn retractor

Size: 6.5″

Quantity: 2

Notes: Double-ended for exposure of surface layers; Flat right-angled end and a rake end

Courtesy of Miltex, Inc.

FIGURE 6-38

Ragnell retractor

Size: 6.0″

Quantity: 2

Notes: Double-ended for exposure of surface layers

Courtesy of Miltex, Inc.

FIGURE 6-39

continues

Basic Plastic Surgery Instrumentation – RETRACTION AND EXPOSURE INSTRUMENTS *continued*

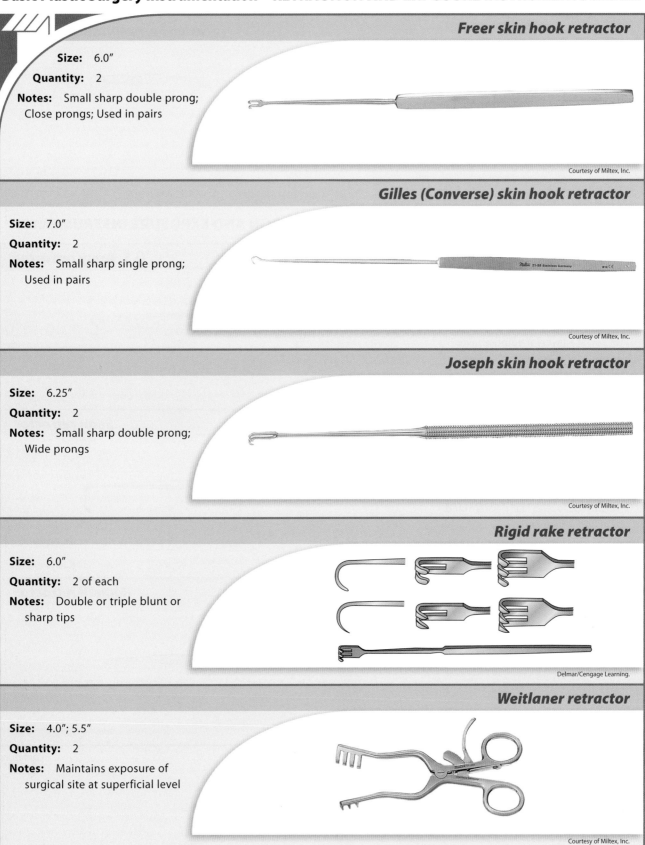

Freer skin hook retractor

Size: 6.0"

Quantity: 2

Notes: Small sharp double prong; Close prongs; Used in pairs

Courtesy of Miltex, Inc.

FIGURE 6-40

Gilles (Converse) skin hook retractor

Size: 7.0"

Quantity: 2

Notes: Small sharp single prong; Used in pairs

Courtesy of Miltex, Inc.

FIGURE 6-41

Joseph skin hook retractor

Size: 6.25"

Quantity: 2

Notes: Small sharp double prong; Wide prongs

Courtesy of Miltex, Inc.

FIGURE 6-42

Rigid rake retractor

Size: 6.0"

Quantity: 2 of each

Notes: Double or triple blunt or sharp tips

Delmar/Cengage Learning.

FIGURE 6-43

Weitlaner retractor

Size: 4.0"; 5.5"

Quantity: 2

Notes: Maintains exposure of surgical site at superficial level

Courtesy of Miltex, Inc.

FIGURE 6-44

Basic Plastic Surgery Instrumentation – APPROXIMATION AND CLOSURE INSTRUMENTS

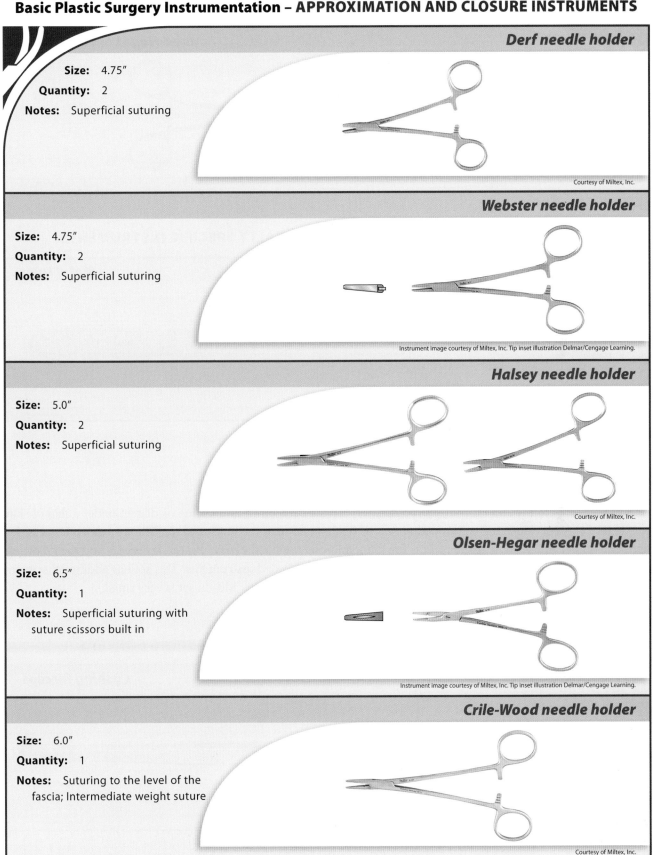

Derf needle holder

Size: 4.75″

Quantity: 2

Notes: Superficial suturing

Courtesy of Miltex, Inc.

FIGURE 6-45

Webster needle holder

Size: 4.75″

Quantity: 2

Notes: Superficial suturing

Instrument image courtesy of Miltex, Inc. Tip inset illustration Delmar/Cengage Learning.

FIGURE 6-46

Halsey needle holder

Size: 5.0″

Quantity: 2

Notes: Superficial suturing

Courtesy of Miltex, Inc.

FIGURE 6-47

Olsen-Hegar needle holder

Size: 6.5″

Quantity: 1

Notes: Superficial suturing with suture scissors built in

Instrument image courtesy of Miltex, Inc. Tip inset illustration Delmar/Cengage Learning.

FIGURE 6-48

Crile-Wood needle holder

Size: 6.0″

Quantity: 1

Notes: Suturing to the level of the fascia; Intermediate weight suture

Courtesy of Miltex, Inc.

FIGURE 6-49

continues

Basic Plastic Surgery Instrumentation – APPROXIMATION AND CLOSURE INSTRUMENTS continued

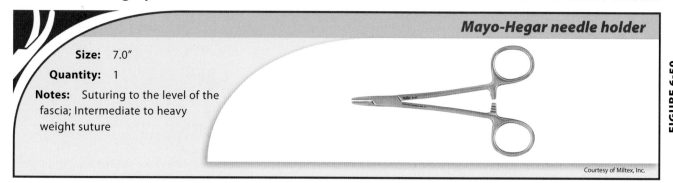

Mayo-Hegar needle holder

Size: 7.0"

Quantity: 1

Notes: Suturing to the level of the fascia; Intermediate to heavy weight suture

Courtesy of Miltex, Inc.

FIGURE 6-50

Basic Plastic Surgery Instrumentation – SPECIALTY SPECIFIC INSTRUMENTS

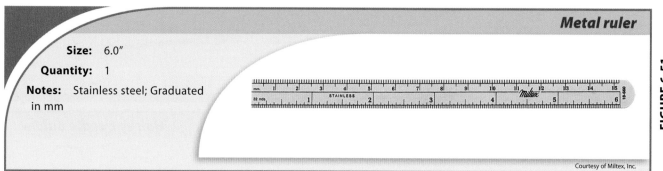

Metal ruler

Size: 6.0"

Quantity: 1

Notes: Stainless steel; Graduated in mm

Courtesy of Miltex, Inc.

FIGURE 6-51

Rhytidectomy-Browlift Add-On Instrumentation

Facelift, or *rhytidectomy* and browlift procedures, require the surgeon to undermine or dissect under a flap of skin on the face without damaging vessels and nerves to tighten and firm the outer surface. The instrumentation is designed to tunnel and separate tissue planes. The foundation set used is the basic plastic surgery set and the following instrumentation is opened to complete the complement of the needed instruments. This set has additional scissors and retractors that are useful for undermining and controlling a flap. This add-on set is very small.

Rhytidectomy-Browlift Add-On Instrumentation – GRASPING FORCEPS

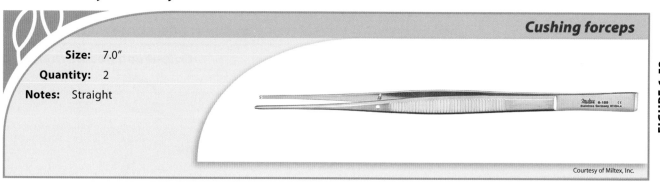

Cushing forceps

Size: 7.0"

Quantity: 2

Notes: Straight

Courtesy of Miltex, Inc.

FIGURE 6-52

Rhytidectomy-Browlift Add-On Instrumentation – DISSECTION INSTRUMENTS

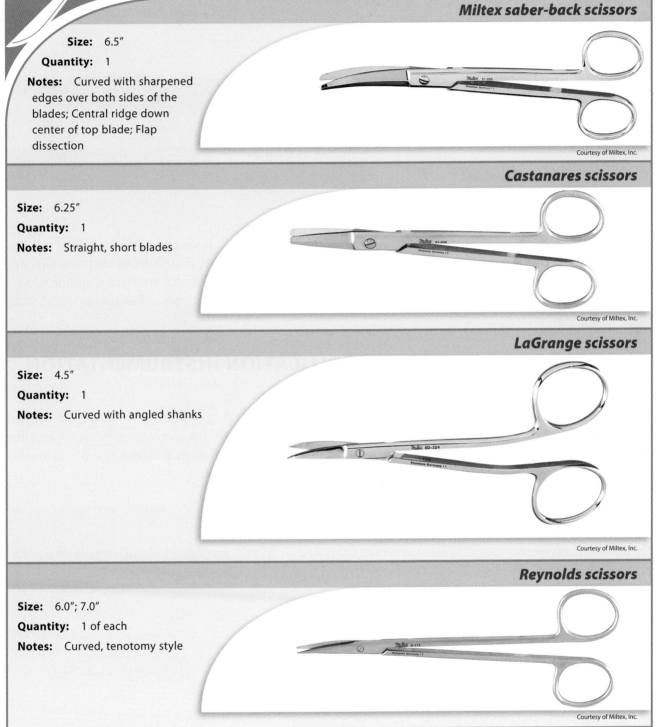

Miltex saber-back scissors

Size: 6.5"

Quantity: 1

Notes: Curved with sharpened edges over both sides of the blades; Central ridge down center of top blade; Flap dissection

Courtesy of Miltex, Inc.

FIGURE 6-53

Castanares scissors

Size: 6.25"

Quantity: 1

Notes: Straight, short blades

Courtesy of Miltex, Inc.

FIGURE 6-54

LaGrange scissors

Size: 4.5"

Quantity: 1

Notes: Curved with angled shanks

Courtesy of Miltex, Inc.

FIGURE 6-55

Reynolds scissors

Size: 6.0"; 7.0"

Quantity: 1 of each

Notes: Curved, tenotomy style

Courtesy of Miltex, Inc.

FIGURE 6-56

Rhytidectomy-Browlift Add-On Instrumentation – RETRACTION AND EXPOSURE INSTRUMENTS

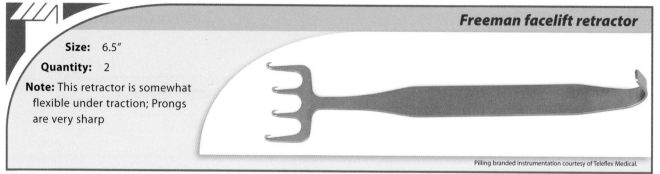

Freeman facelift retractor

Size: 6.5"

Quantity: 2

Note: This retractor is somewhat flexible under traction; Prongs are very sharp

Pilling branded instrumentation courtesy of Teleflex Medical.

FIGURE 6-57

Blepharoplasty Add-On Instrumentation

Blepharoplasty is a procedure that removes excess skin and subsurface fat pads from around the periorbital rim. The incisions are marked preoperatively and the tissue is excised by fine #15 scalpel blades during the procedure. The basic plastic set is sufficient for this procedure, although some surgeons have additional preferences for fine scissors or retractors. The use of plastic or metallic corneal shields is advised to prevent corneal abrasions during lid tissue dissection and excision.

SURFACE AND SUBSURFACE MODIFICATION INSTRUMENTATION

The outer and inner layers of skin are subject to modification during plastic surgery procedures. Some modifications are aesthetic and others are restorative. Loss of external body covering can be serious and requires prompt restoration to prevent permanent disfigurement or death. Excess subsurface tissue can cause external deformity and is commonly removed by debulking by liposuction.

Surface Modification Instruments for Skin Grafting

These instruments are used in combination with the basic plastic set. Most departments have each type of dermatome wrapped separately. It would not be cost effective to have all types of dermatomes in one set.

Surface Modification Instruments for Skin Grafting – DISSECTION INSTRUMENTS

Manual skin graft knives

Size: 12.0"

Quantity: 1

Notes: Several styles; Watson knife has a smooth surface; Blair-Brown knife has a smooth surface; Cobbett knife has a grooved surface; Silver's miniature knife is 3.5" with a double edge

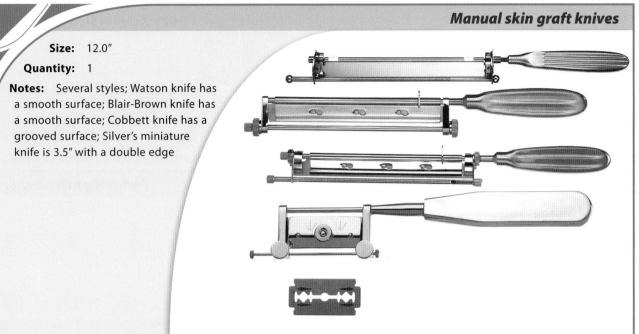

Courtesy of Integra LifeSciences Corporation.

FIGURE 6-58

Padgett air dermatome

Quantity: 1

Notes: Graft is cut 1 5/6th wide; Nitrogen power: Operates at 90 psi

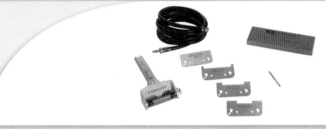

Courtesy of Padgett Surgical Instruments, a division of Integra LifeSciences Corporation.

FIGURE 6-59

Padgett electric dermatome

Quantity: 1

Notes: Uses electric power. Width of graft can be 2.0", 3.0", and 4.0"; Depth is adjustable to 1/1000 of an inch; Autoclavable with cord

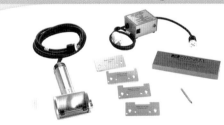

Courtesy of Padgett Surgical Instruments, a division of Integra LifeSciences Corporation.

FIGURE 6-60

continues

Surface Modification Instruments for Skin Grafting – DISSECTION INSTRUMENTS *continued*

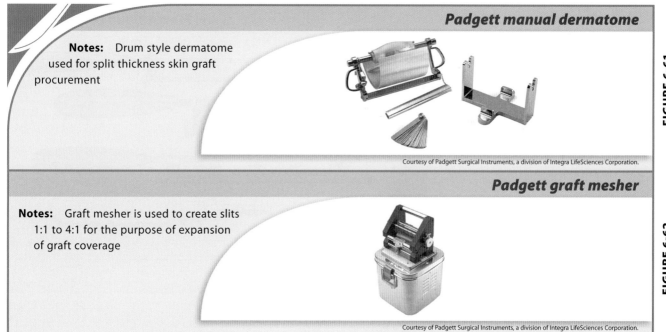

Padgett manual dermatome

Notes: Drum style dermatome used for split thickness skin graft procurement

Courtesy of Padgett Surgical Instruments, a division of Integra LifeSciences Corporation.

FIGURE 6-61

Padgett graft mesher

Notes: Graft mesher is used to create slits 1:1 to 4:1 for the purpose of expansion of graft coverage

Courtesy of Padgett Surgical Instruments, a division of Integra LifeSciences Corporation.

FIGURE 6-62

Debridement Instrumentation

Surface debridement involves trimming devitalized tissue with curettes or other sharp dissector. Special instruments are not commonly used for this procedure. The basic plastic set or the soft tissue foundation set can be used for smaller areas of debridement. If large amounts of surface and subsurface tissue will be removed by curettage it is advisable to have the dermatomes of the surgeon's choice and skin mesher available if an autograft may be necessary. Large volumes of tissue may require procurement of a full thickness flap to cover the defeat. This flap may require the use of a plastics and a short foundation set.

Liposuction

Subsurface adipose tissue can be removed with minimal surface tissue disruption. Preparation of adipose tissue for removal is performed by instilling 1 liter of sterile normal saline or Ringers lactate solution mixed with 30 to 50 ml 1% lidocaine and 1 to 2 ml epinephrine 1:1000 followed by modulated cannulated suction. The tumescent solution dosage will be dependent on the patient's physiology and surgeon's preference. The use of lidocaine minimizes postoperative pain and the epinephrine causes vasoconstriction to prevent excessive blood loss. Several liters can be mixed and used. Care is taken not to use more than 7 mg/kg of 1% lidocaine or 500 mg of 1% lidocaine, as that dose is considered potentially toxic.

The fluid can be injected manually or by an infusion pump machine. The instilled fluid creates tumescence (referred to as "wet technique") to fluff up the adipose for removal. The amount of adipose tissue mixed with tumescence removed will be double the amount of instilled fluid. Debulking the subsurface adipose tissue with sharpened cannulae causes the surface to have a more regular configuration. Adipose removal can be performed with vacuum suction alone or by ultrasonic-assisted technology. Results are dependent on the elasticity of the skin and its resiliency for remodeling.

Most of this instrumentation is disposable; however, many surgeons prefer to use reusable cannulas for the surgical procedure. Tiny 1-cm skin incisions are made with #11 or #15 blades using a #7 scalpel from the basic plastic set. Retractors and clamps are not used. Most areas of the body are subject to liposuction. The instrumentation ranges from heavy to delicate caliber suction tips. The tiny incisions are sutured using Webster needle holders and 3/0 or 4/0 nylon or other nonabsorbable sutures. The use of absorbable sutures is not advised because the wounds tend to seep fluid for several days, hastening the absorption or hydrolization of the suture. Tensile strength is then lost.

Subsurface Modification Instruments – DEBULKING INSTRUMENTS

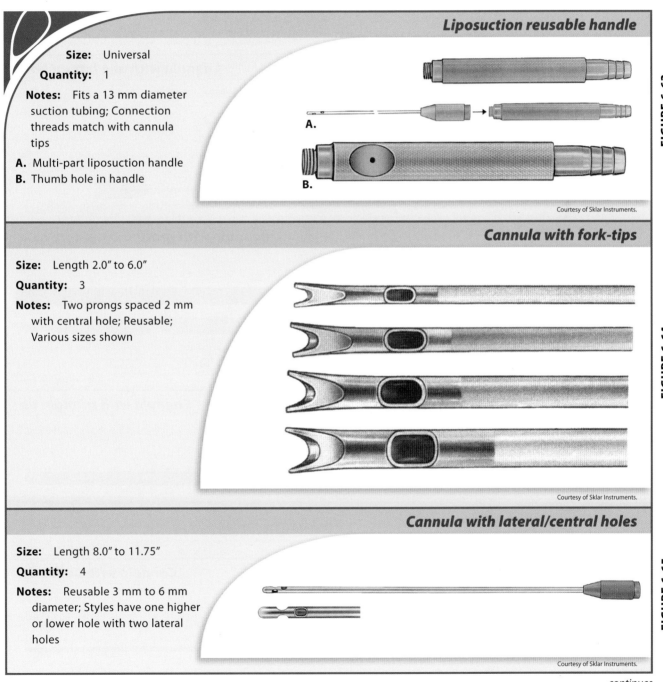

Liposuction reusable handle

Size: Universal

Quantity: 1

Notes: Fits a 13 mm diameter suction tubing; Connection threads match with cannula tips

A. Multi-part liposuction handle
B. Thumb hole in handle

A.

B.

Courtesy of Sklar Instruments.

FIGURE 6-63

Cannula with fork-tips

Size: Length 2.0″ to 6.0″

Quantity: 3

Notes: Two prongs spaced 2 mm with central hole; Reusable; Various sizes shown

Courtesy of Sklar Instruments.

FIGURE 6-64

Cannula with lateral/central holes

Size: Length 8.0″ to 11.75″

Quantity: 4

Notes: Reusable 3 mm to 6 mm diameter; Styles have one higher or lower hole with two lateral holes

Courtesy of Sklar Instruments.

FIGURE 6-65

continues

Subsurface Modification Instruments – DEBULKING INSTRUMENTS *continued*

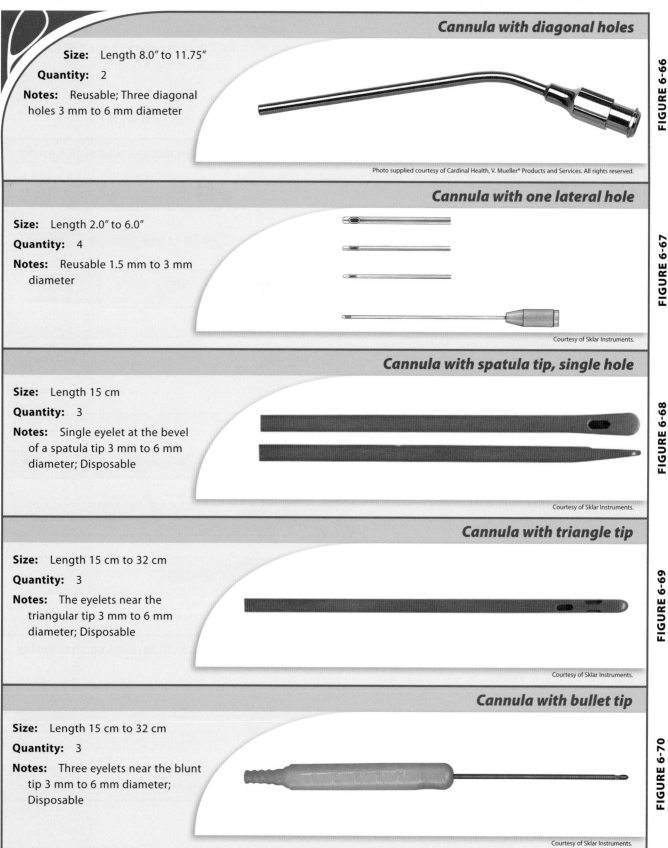

Cannula with diagonal holes

Size: Length 8.0" to 11.75"

Quantity: 2

Notes: Reusable; Three diagonal holes 3 mm to 6 mm diameter

FIGURE 6-66

Cannula with one lateral hole

Size: Length 2.0" to 6.0"

Quantity: 4

Notes: Reusable 1.5 mm to 3 mm diameter

FIGURE 6-67

Cannula with spatula tip, single hole

Size: Length 15 cm

Quantity: 3

Notes: Single eyelet at the bevel of a spatula tip 3 mm to 6 mm diameter; Disposable

FIGURE 6-68

Cannula with triangle tip

Size: Length 15 cm to 32 cm

Quantity: 3

Notes: The eyelets near the triangular tip 3 mm to 6 mm diameter; Disposable

FIGURE 6-69

Cannula with bullet tip

Size: Length 15 cm to 32 cm

Quantity: 3

Notes: Three eyelets near the blunt tip 3 mm to 6 mm diameter; Disposable

FIGURE 6-70

Subsurface Modification Instruments –
EVACUATION AND INSTILLATION INSTRUMENTS

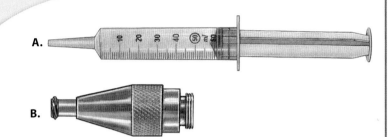

Plastic surgery slip-tip syringe instillation set

Size: 60 cc

Quantity: 2

Notes: For manual instillation of tumescence fluid; Aluminum stop prevents loss of pressure or vacuum in the syringe; Adaptor is available to fit other manufacturer's cannula; Disposable

A. Slip tip syringe
B. Luer lock adaptor

Courtesy of Sklar Instruments.

FIGURE 6-71

Suction tubing

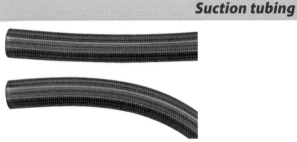

Size: 8 feet

Quantity: 1

Notes: Thick wall to prevent collapse of tubing during intense suctioning; Long enough to reach between the vacuum machine and the surface places of the patient; Disposable

Courtesy of Sklar Instruments.

FIGURE 6-72

Peristaltic pump infiltration tubing

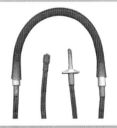

Size: 10 feet

Quantity: 1

Notes: Used to deliver large volumes of fluid under pressure to create tumescence; Disposable

Courtesy of Sklar Instruments.

FIGURE 6-73

Infiltration syringe

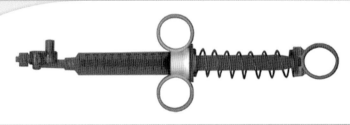

Size: 10 cc

Quantity: 2

Notes: Can deliver 10 cc of tumescence at one injection; Disposable

Courtesy of Sklar Instruments.

FIGURE 6-74

BREAST INSTRUMENTATION

Breast procedures are performed to restore, increase, or decrease the size of the breasts. Most of the procedure involves soft tissue incision and dissection. Plastic surgeons are concerned with the breast's form and external appearance so they utilize delicate tissue handling with fine instrumentation. Most surgeons will use the basic plastic set as the foundation for breast procedures. If a mastectomy is performed before reconstruction, additional soft tissue instrumentation with heavier hemostatic clamps will be needed.

Augmentation-Reduction Instrumentation

This instrumentation is an add-on to the basic plastic set. The contents of this set are used to dissect a tissue pocket for an implant or create a pattern for reconstruction after reduction mammoplasty.

Augmentation-Reduction Instrumentation – RETRACTION AND EXPOSURE INSTRUMENTS

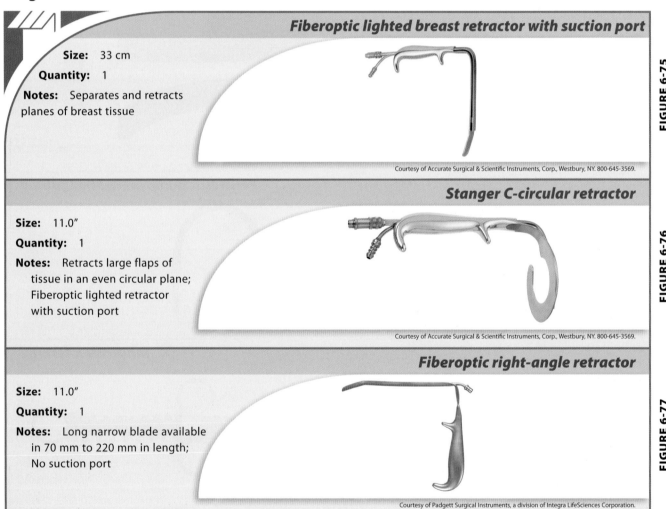

Fiberoptic lighted breast retractor with suction port

Size: 33 cm

Quantity: 1

Notes: Separates and retracts planes of breast tissue

Courtesy of Accurate Surgical & Scientific Instruments, Corp., Westbury, NY. 800-645-3569.

FIGURE 6-75

Stanger C-circular retractor

Size: 11.0″

Quantity: 1

Notes: Retracts large flaps of tissue in an even circular plane; Fiberoptic lighted retractor with suction port

Courtesy of Accurate Surgical & Scientific Instruments, Corp., Westbury, NY. 800-645-3569.

FIGURE 6-76

Fiberoptic right-angle retractor

Size: 11.0″

Quantity: 1

Notes: Long narrow blade available in 70 mm to 220 mm in length; No suction port

Courtesy of Padgett Surgical Instruments, a division of Integra LifeSciences Corporation.

FIGURE 6-77

Augmentation-Reduction Instrumentation – RETRACTION AND EXPOSURE INSTRUMENTS *continued*

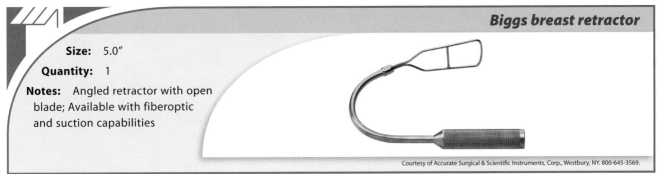

Biggs breast retractor

Size: 5.0"

Quantity: 1

Notes: Angled retractor with open blade; Available with fiberoptic and suction capabilities

Courtesy of Accurate Surgical & Scientific Instruments, Corp., Westbury, NY. 800-645-3569.

FIGURE 6-78

Augmentation-Reduction Instrumentation – SPECIALTY SPECIFIC INSTRUMENTS

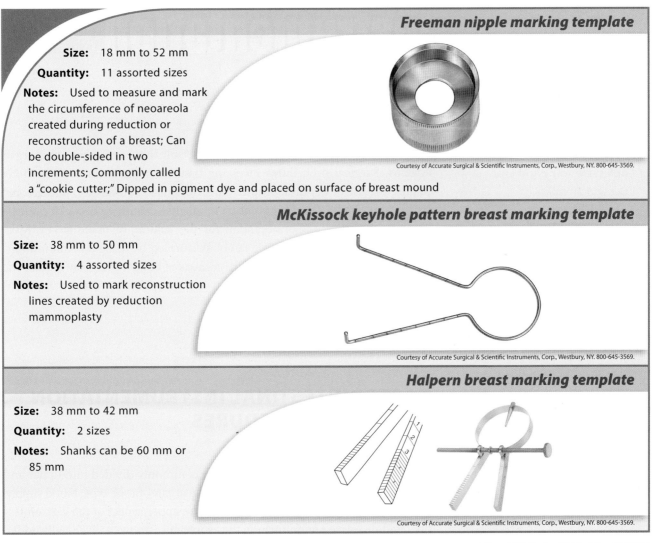

Freeman nipple marking template

Size: 18 mm to 52 mm

Quantity: 11 assorted sizes

Notes: Used to measure and mark the circumference of neoareola created during reduction or reconstruction of a breast; Can be double-sided in two increments; Commonly called a "cookie cutter;" Dipped in pigment dye and placed on surface of breast mound

Courtesy of Accurate Surgical & Scientific Instruments, Corp., Westbury, NY. 800-645-3569.

FIGURE 6-79

McKissock keyhole pattern breast marking template

Size: 38 mm to 50 mm

Quantity: 4 assorted sizes

Notes: Used to mark reconstruction lines created by reduction mammoplasty

Courtesy of Accurate Surgical & Scientific Instruments, Corp., Westbury, NY. 800-645-3569.

FIGURE 6-80

Halpern breast marking template

Size: 38 mm to 42 mm

Quantity: 2 sizes

Notes: Shanks can be 60 mm or 85 mm

Courtesy of Accurate Surgical & Scientific Instruments, Corp., Westbury, NY. 800-645-3569.

FIGURE 6-81

SUMMARY

Plastic surgery is essentially a process of soft tissue modification for the purpose of improving form and function. Compact tissue modification, not described here, can sometimes be part of a plastic surgery procedure and will be discussed in subsequent chapters.

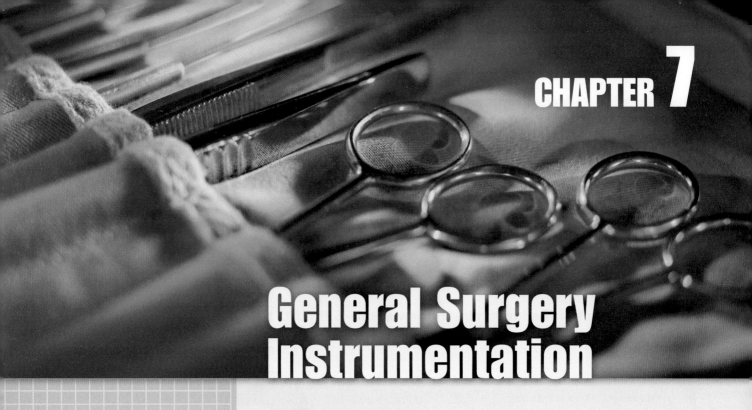

General Surgery Instrumentation

INTRODUCTION

General surgery involves procedures of the soft tissues of organs and organ systems. Surgical procedures involving tissues on the surface of the body require the use of depth-appropriate instruments. For example, mastectomy (removal of a breast and adjacent components) can differ between patients based on breast size. Consideration for the volume of tissue is key. Most surface, or external, procedures can be performed by using a medium foundation set. However, patients with large areas of bulky tissue may require the addition of individual long dissection and grasping instruments for areas such as the axilla.

GASTROINTESTINAL INSTRUMENTATION FOR OPEN PROCEDURES

Organs in the gastrointestinal system are commonly divided into upper and lower sections according to the depth of the organs, tissue type, blood supply, innervation, and disease state. Organs in the upper aspect of the gastrointestinal and digestive region include the esophagus, stomach, liver, gallbladder, pancreas, spleen, and inferior diaphragm. Preparation for procedures in the upper gastrointestinal compartment requires the use of the medium and long foundation sets described in Chapter 5. Superficial and preperitoneal procedures on an adult, such as herniorrhaphy, utilize the medium foundation set unless the patient is extremely obese.

Organs in the lower gastrointestinal region include the small bowel, large bowel, appendix, mesentery, omentum, rectum, and anus. Most of the lower gastrointestinal organ depth ranges from intraperitoneal to below the pelvic rim. Preparations for procedures in the lower gastrointestinal area require the use of medium, long, and possibly the extra long foundation sets described in Chapter 5.

Cholecystectomy Add-Ons

Cholecystectomy Add-Ons – CLAMPS

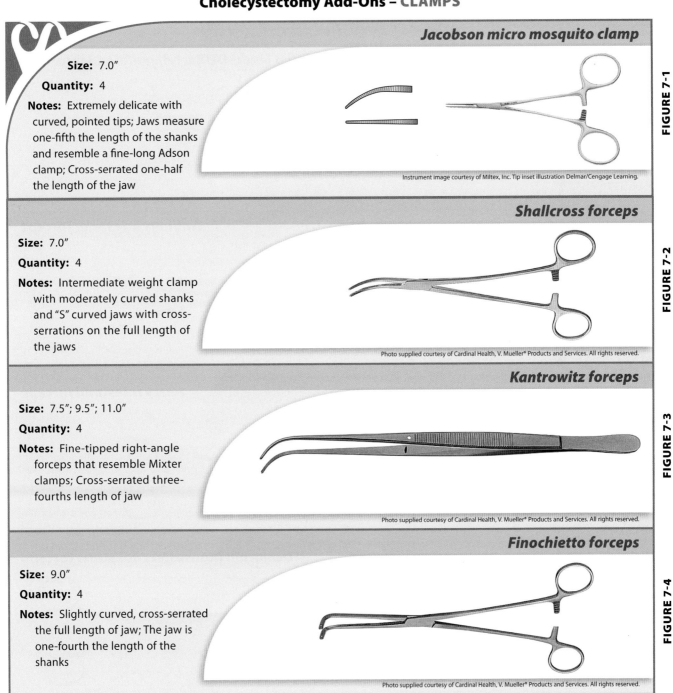

Jacobson micro mosquito clamp

Size: 7.0"

Quantity: 4

Notes: Extremely delicate with curved, pointed tips; Jaws measure one-fifth the length of the shanks and resemble a fine-long Adson clamp; Cross-serrated one-half the length of the jaw

FIGURE 7-1

Shallcross forceps

Size: 7.0"

Quantity: 4

Notes: Intermediate weight clamp with moderately curved shanks and "S" curved jaws with cross-serrations on the full length of the jaws

FIGURE 7-2

Kantrowitz forceps

Size: 7.5"; 9.5"; 11.0"

Quantity: 4

Notes: Fine-tipped right-angle forceps that resemble Mixter clamps; Cross-serrated three-fourths length of jaw

FIGURE 7-3

Finochietto forceps

Size: 9.0"

Quantity: 4

Notes: Slightly curved, cross-serrated the full length of jaw; The jaw is one-fourth the length of the shanks

FIGURE 7-4

Cholecystectomy Add-Ons – GRASPING FORCEPS

Lovelace gallbladder forceps

Size: 7.25"

Quantity: 1

Notes: Ring-handled forceps with angled shaft and open cross-serrated, 1.0" triangular tips; Locks with ratchets

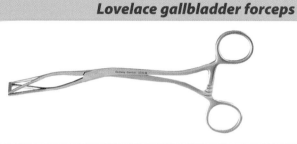

FIGURE 7-5

Collin (Judd-DeMartel) gallbladder forceps

Size: 6.0"

Quantity: 1

Notes: Straight; Ring-handled wide oval open-tipped forceps; Locks with ratchets

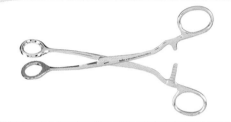

FIGURE 7-6

Williams intestinal forceps

Size: 6.5"

Quantity: 1

Notes: Straight, oval-tipped forceps with ratchets; Ring handles; Cross-serrated jaws

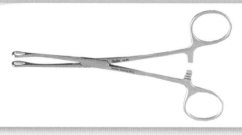

FIGURE 7-7

Percy intestinal forceps

Size: 6.0"

Quantity: 1

Notes: Straight, tiny open round tips with serrated jaws

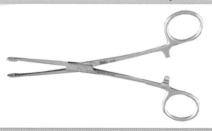

FIGURE 7-8

Desjardin (Rochester) gallstone forceps

Size: 9.0"

Quantity: 1

Notes: Long oval-tipped forceps; Ring handles; No ratchets; Slightly curved shanks

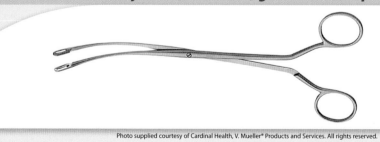

FIGURE 7-9

Cholecystectomy Add-Ons – GRASPING FORCEPS *continued*

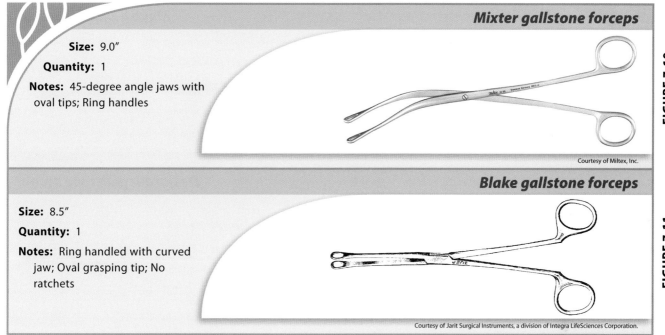

Mixter gallstone forceps

Size: 9.0"

Quantity: 1

Notes: 45-degree angle jaws with oval tips; Ring handles

Courtesy of Miltex, Inc.

FIGURE 7-10

Blake gallstone forceps

Size: 8.5"

Quantity: 1

Notes: Ring handled with curved jaw; Oval grasping tip; No ratchets

Courtesy of Jarit Surgical Instruments, a division of Integra LifeSciences Corporation.

FIGURE 7-11

Cholecystectomy Add-Ons – PROBES AND DILATORS

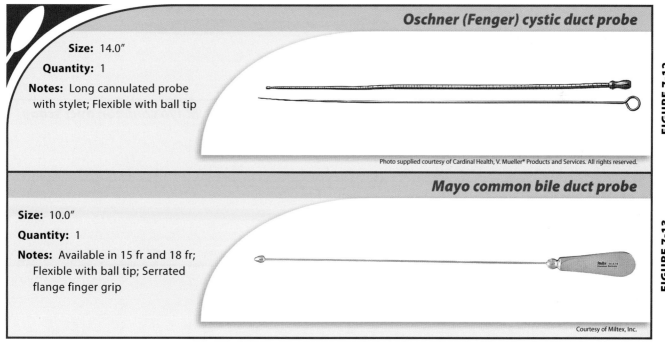

Oschner (Fenger) cystic duct probe

Size: 14.0"

Quantity: 1

Notes: Long cannulated probe with stylet; Flexible with ball tip

Photo supplied courtesy of Cardinal Health, V. Mueller® Products and Services. All rights reserved.

FIGURE 7-12

Mayo common bile duct probe

Size: 10.0"

Quantity: 1

Notes: Available in 15 fr and 18 fr; Flexible with ball tip; Serrated flange finger grip

Courtesy of Miltex, Inc.

FIGURE 7-13

continues

Cholecystectomy Add-Ons – PROBES AND DILATORS *continued*

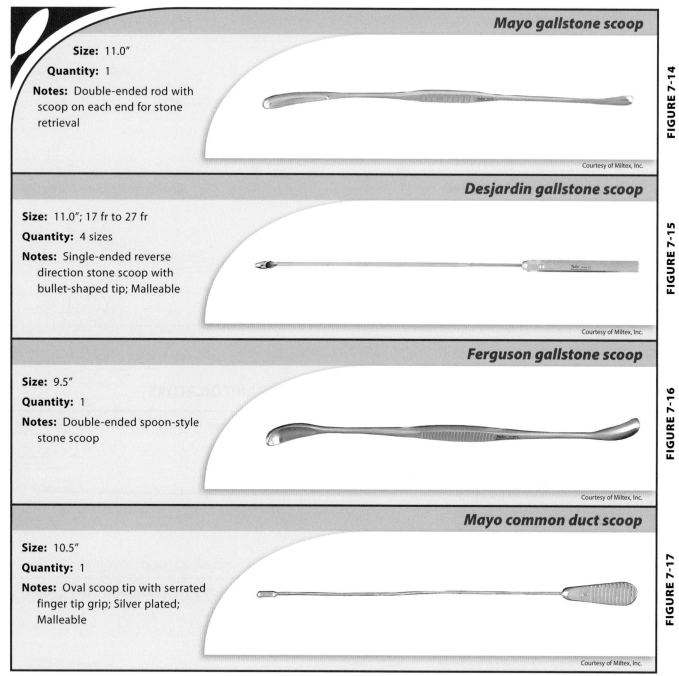

Mayo gallstone scoop

Size: 11.0"

Quantity: 1

Notes: Double-ended rod with scoop on each end for stone retrieval

Courtesy of Miltex, Inc.

FIGURE 7-14

Desjardin gallstone scoop

Size: 11.0"; 17 fr to 27 fr

Quantity: 4 sizes

Notes: Single-ended reverse direction stone scoop with bullet-shaped tip; Malleable

Courtesy of Miltex, Inc.

FIGURE 7-15

Ferguson gallstone scoop

Size: 9.5"

Quantity: 1

Notes: Double-ended spoon-style stone scoop

Courtesy of Miltex, Inc.

FIGURE 7-16

Mayo common duct scoop

Size: 10.5"

Quantity: 1

Notes: Oval scoop tip with serrated finger tip grip; Silver plated; Malleable

Courtesy of Miltex, Inc.

FIGURE 7-17

Cholecystectomy Add-Ons – EVACUATION AND INSTILLATION INSTRUMENTS

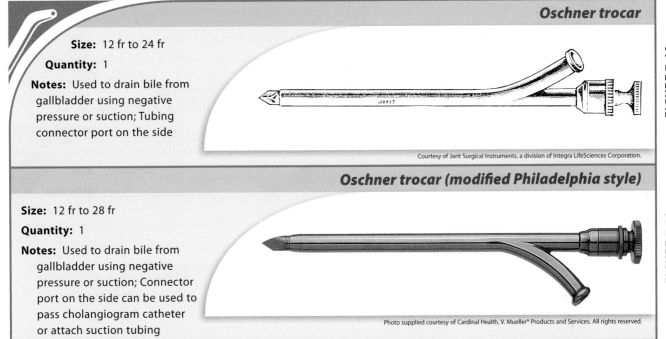

Oschner trocar

Size: 12 fr to 24 fr

Quantity: 1

Notes: Used to drain bile from gallbladder using negative pressure or suction; Tubing connector port on the side

Oschner trocar (modified Philadelphia style)

Size: 12 fr to 28 fr

Quantity: 1

Notes: Used to drain bile from gallbladder using negative pressure or suction; Connector port on the side can be used to pass cholangiogram catheter or attach suction tubing

FIGURE 7-18
FIGURE 7-19

Liver and Stomach Add-Ons

These instruments can be wrapped individually or collectively as preferential specialty sets. Each facility will have various procedures and procedural modifications that require the use of individual instruments. Pediatric facilities, for example, will use smaller or lighter versions of similar instruments. Patient individuality will indicate instrumentation based on body habitus, disease states, and anomalies. The following list is a collection of instrumentation primarily used in the adult population. Pediatric application will be designated as appropriate. Instrumentation in this list is not all-inclusive and can be modified as needed.

Right-angled clamps from the cholecystectomy may be added to this collection for controlled dissection of nerves and fine vessels. Splenectomy and pancreatic procedures use a combination of cholecystectomy and liver/stomach add-ons.

Liver and Stomach Add-Ons – CLAMPS

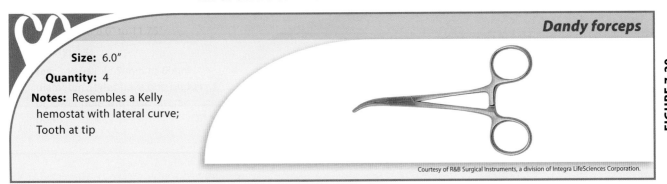

Dandy forceps

Size: 6.0″

Quantity: 4

Notes: Resembles a Kelly hemostat with lateral curve; Tooth at tip

FIGURE 7-20

continues

Liver and Stomach Add-Ons – CLAMPS *continued*

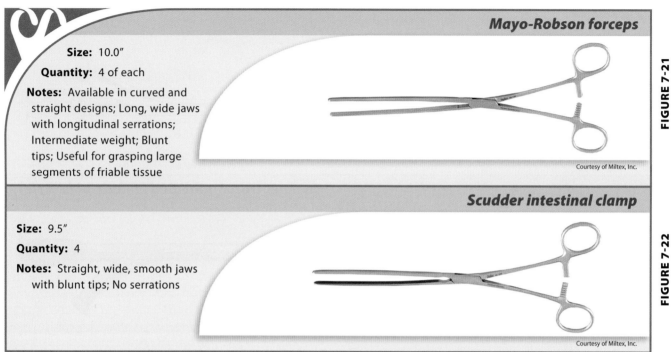

Mayo-Robson forceps

Size: 10.0"

Quantity: 4 of each

Notes: Available in curved and straight designs; Long, wide jaws with longitudinal serrations; Intermediate weight; Blunt tips; Useful for grasping large segments of friable tissue

Courtesy of Miltex, Inc.

FIGURE 7-21

Scudder intestinal clamp

Size: 9.5"

Quantity: 4

Notes: Straight, wide, smooth jaws with blunt tips; No serrations

Courtesy of Miltex, Inc.

FIGURE 7-22

Liver and Stomach Add-Ons – DISSECTION INSTRUMENTS

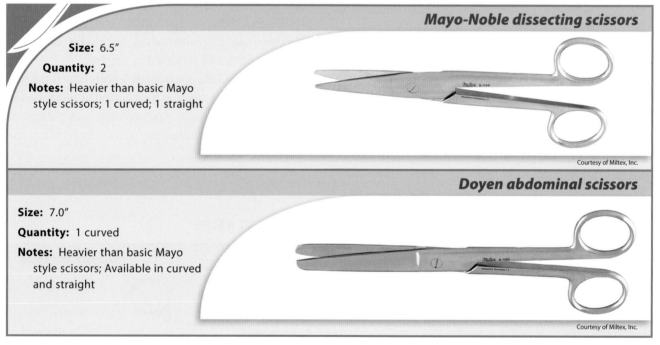

Mayo-Noble dissecting scissors

Size: 6.5"

Quantity: 2

Notes: Heavier than basic Mayo style scissors; 1 curved; 1 straight

Courtesy of Miltex, Inc.

FIGURE 7-23

Doyen abdominal scissors

Size: 7.0"

Quantity: 1 curved

Notes: Heavier than basic Mayo style scissors; Available in curved and straight

Courtesy of Miltex, Inc.

FIGURE 7-24

Liver and Stomach Add-Ons – PROBES AND DILATORS

Benson pylorus dilator

Size: 5.75"

Quantity: 1

Notes: Ring handle with right angle blunt tips; Separation of the ring handles spreads the tips

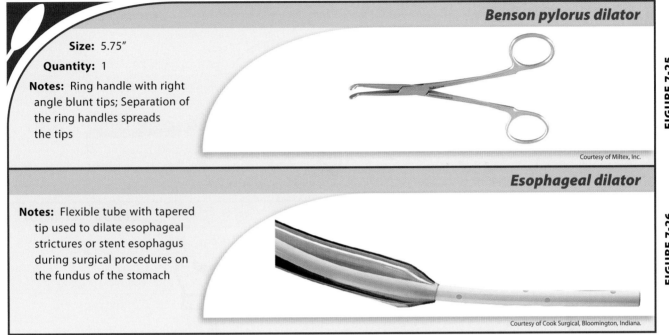

Courtesy of Miltex, Inc.

FIGURE 7-25

Esophageal dilator

Notes: Flexible tube with tapered tip used to dilate esophageal strictures or stent esophagus during surgical procedures on the fundus of the stomach

Courtesy of Cook Surgical, Bloomington, Indiana.

FIGURE 7-26

Liver and Stomach Add-Ons – RETRACTION AND EXPOSURE INSTRUMENTS

Murphy rake retractor

Size: 10.5"

Quantity: 2

Notes: Blunt, right angle, slightly malleable, 1.25" or 2.0" blade width; Solid handle

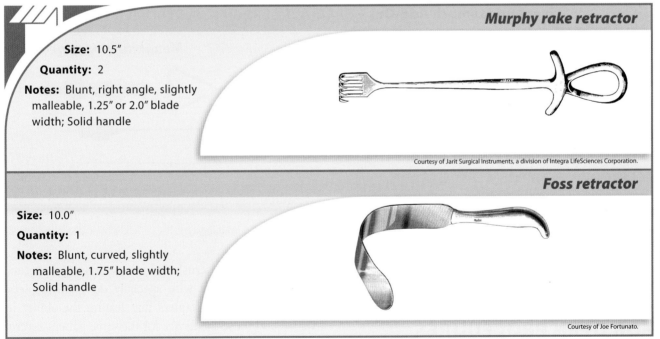

Courtesy of Jarit Surgical Instruments, a division of Integra LifeSciences Corporation.

FIGURE 7-27

Foss retractor

Size: 10.0"

Quantity: 1

Notes: Blunt, curved, slightly malleable, 1.75" blade width; Solid handle

Courtesy of Joe Fortunato.

FIGURE 7-28

continues

Liver and Stomach Add-Ons – RETRACTION AND EXPOSURE INSTRUMENTS *continued*

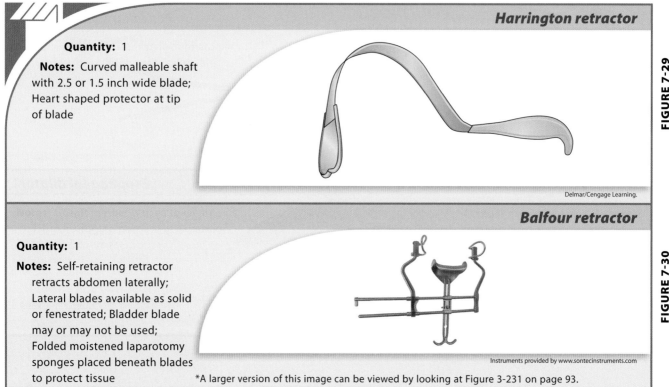

Harrington retractor

Quantity: 1

Notes: Curved malleable shaft with 2.5 or 1.5 inch wide blade; Heart shaped protector at tip of blade

Delmar/Cengage Learning.

FIGURE 7-29

Balfour retractor

Quantity: 1

Notes: Self-retaining retractor retracts abdomen laterally; Lateral blades available as solid or fenestrated; Bladder blade may or may not be used; Folded moistened laparotomy sponges placed beneath blades to protect tissue

Instruments provided by www.sontecinstruments.com

*A larger version of this image can be viewed by looking at Figure 3-231 on page 93.

FIGURE 7-30

Liver and Stomach Add-Ons – SPECIALTY SPECIFIC INSTRUMENTS

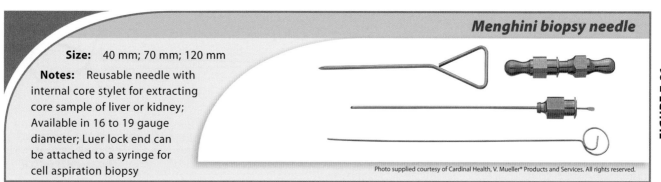

Menghini biopsy needle

Size: 40 mm; 70 mm; 120 mm

Notes: Reusable needle with internal core stylet for extracting core sample of liver or kidney; Available in 16 to 19 gauge diameter; Luer lock end can be attached to a syringe for cell aspiration biopsy

Photo supplied courtesy of Cardinal Health, V. Mueller® Products and Services. All rights reserved.

FIGURE 7-31

LOWER GASTROINTESTINAL INSTRUMENTATION FOR OPEN PROCEDURES

Bowel Resection Add-Ons

Lower bowel procedures involve traumatic or atraumatic occlusion of bowel segments. Selection of instruments includes consideration for adequate numbers of crushing and non-crushing clamps. Intestinal anastomosis is performed with specially designed staplers. Some facilities use staplers that feature the ability to reload and reuse the device for the same patient several times before disposal. Other facilities use a disposable instrument for each use. Regardless of which style of stapler is planned for use, the device is never opened and dispensed or flipped to the sterile field. The impact of hitting the metal table causes the staples to misalign and possibly can cause a misfire that would be harmful to the patient. The sterile package should be opened and its contents handed directly to the scrub person using sterile technique.

Instrumentation specific to bowel surgery can be added directly to the set-up with medium and long foundation sets. Some procedures will require a sec-ond sterile table when the approach requires entrance through the abdomen and perineum simultaneously. Contamination of the sterile abdominal table can occur when the same instruments are used for the rectal part of the procedure.

Bowel Resection Add-Ons – CLAMPS

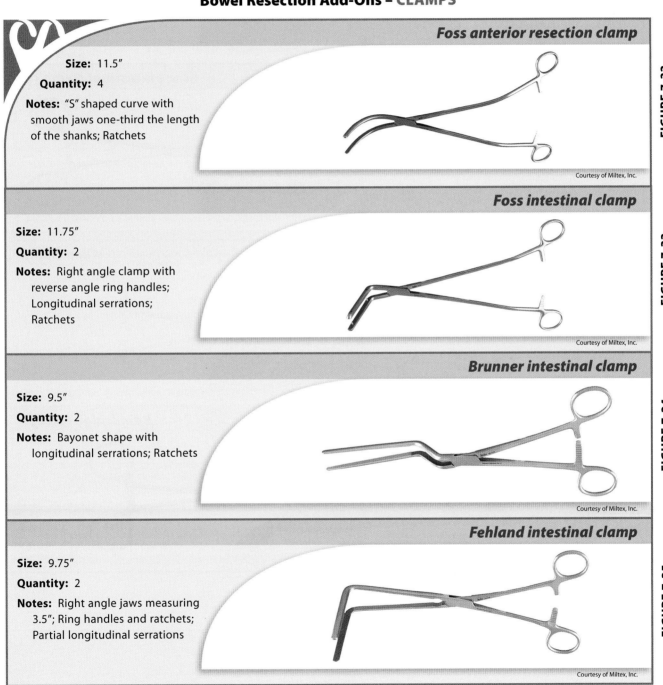

Foss anterior resection clamp

Size: 11.5″

Quantity: 4

Notes: "S" shaped curve with smooth jaws one-third the length of the shanks; Ratchets

Courtesy of Miltex, Inc.

FIGURE 7-32

Foss intestinal clamp

Size: 11.75″

Quantity: 2

Notes: Right angle clamp with reverse angle ring handles; Longitudinal serrations; Ratchets

Courtesy of Miltex, Inc.

FIGURE 7-33

Brunner intestinal clamp

Size: 9.5″

Quantity: 2

Notes: Bayonet shape with longitudinal serrations; Ratchets

Courtesy of Miltex, Inc.

FIGURE 7-34

Fehland intestinal clamp

Size: 9.75″

Quantity: 2

Notes: Right angle jaws measuring 3.5″; Ring handles and ratchets; Partial longitudinal serrations

Courtesy of Miltex, Inc.

FIGURE 7-35

continues

Bowel Resection Add-Ons – CLAMPS *continued*

Payr clamp

Size: 6.0"; 8.0"; 11.0"; 13.75"

Quantity: 1

Notes: Cushing bowel clamp used during resection; Long dolphin-shaped jaw with blunt tip; Locks by double action hinges

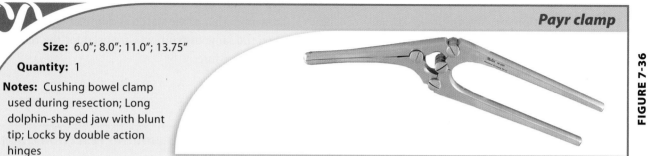

FIGURE 7-36

Stone intestinal clamp set

Size: 3.0"; 4.0"

Quantity: One of each size

Notes: Right angle "V"-shaped device that is closed over a segment of bowel for occlusion with a ring-handled forceps; Tip extends beyond edge of tissue and is secured with screw clamp locking device

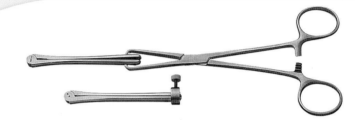

FIGURE 7-37

Allen clamp

Size: 8"

Quantity: 4

Notes: Longitudinal serrations with 1 × 2 teeth; Straight

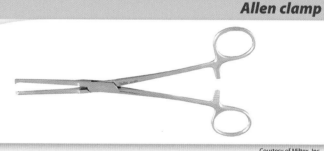

FIGURE 7-38

Bainbridge forceps

Size: 6.0"; 7.25"

Quantity: 2

Notes: Ring handle with ratchets; Longitudinal serrations with cross-serrations at the tip; Straight or curved

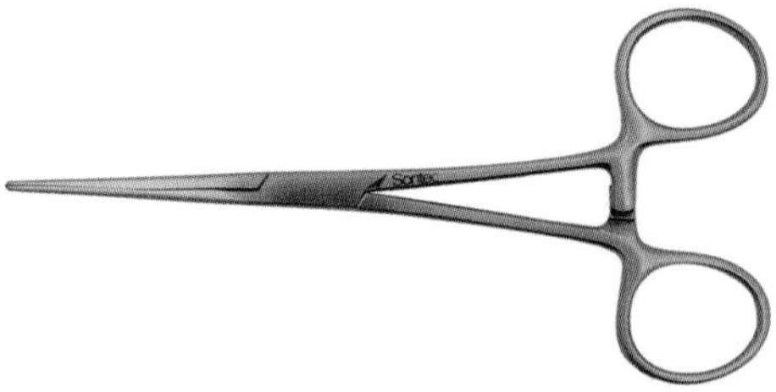

FIGURE 7-39

Bowel Resection Add-Ons – DISSECTION INSTRUMENTS

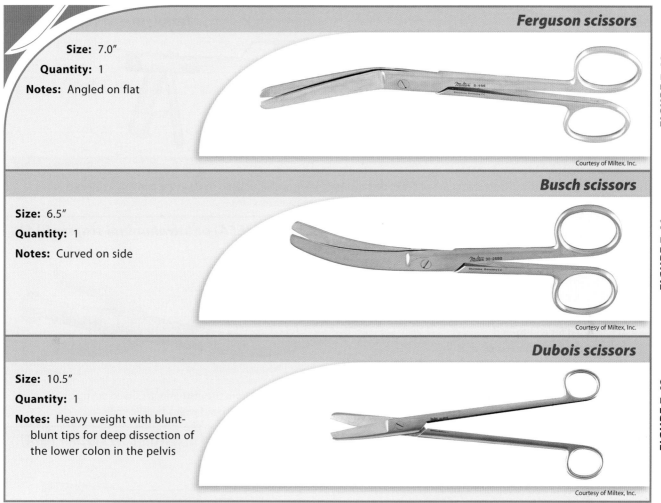

Ferguson scissors

Size: 7.0"

Quantity: 1

Notes: Angled on flat

Courtesy of Miltex, Inc.

FIGURE 7-40

Busch scissors

Size: 6.5"

Quantity: 1

Notes: Curved on side

Courtesy of Miltex, Inc.

FIGURE 7-41

Dubois scissors

Size: 10.5"

Quantity: 1

Notes: Heavy weight with blunt-blunt tips for deep dissection of the lower colon in the pelvis

Courtesy of Miltex, Inc.

FIGURE 7-42

Bowel Resection Add-Ons – RETRACTION AND EXPOSURE INSTRUMENTS

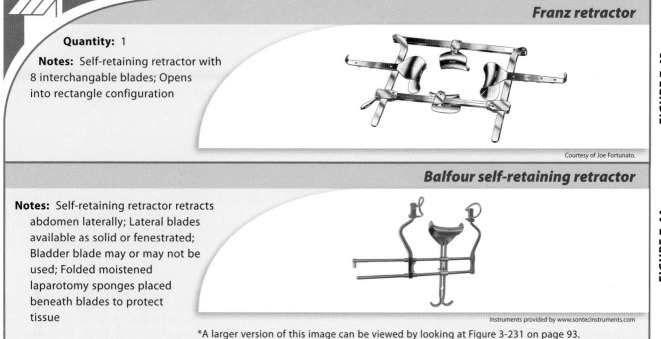

Franz retractor

Quantity: 1

Notes: Self-retaining retractor with 8 interchangable blades; Opens into rectangle configuration

Courtesy of Joe Fortunato.

FIGURE 7-43

Balfour self-retaining retractor

Notes: Self-retaining retractor retracts abdomen laterally; Lateral blades available as solid or fenestrated; Bladder blade may or may not be used; Folded moistened laparotomy sponges placed beneath blades to protect tissue

Instruments provided by www.sontecinstruments.com

FIGURE 7-44

*A larger version of this image can be viewed by looking at Figure 3-231 on page 93.

Bowel Resection Add-Ons – APPROXIMATION AND CLOSURE INSTRUMENTS

Terminal end stapler (TA)

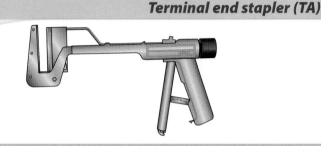

Size: 30 mm; 45 mm; 55 mm; 90 mm

Quantity: One of each available; Can be disposable with a rotating stapler head

Notes: Right angle stapler with pistol style hand grip; Cartridges with needed size of staples are opened and used with the reusable applicator; Three sizes; Disposable styles of preloaded applicators are available; Used to close the terminal angle of a tube with a linear double row of titanium staples; Also called terminal anastamosis (TA)

Delmar/Cengage Learning.

FIGURE 7-45

End-to-end anastomosis stapler (EEA) or Intraluminal stapler (ILS)

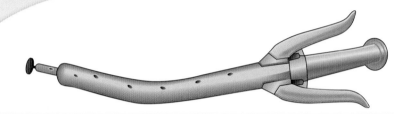

Size: 21 mm to 34 mm diameter

Quantity: One of each available; Can be disposable

Notes: Long cylindrical circular stapler used for end-to-end anastomosis of a tube; A circular knife trims the anastomotic rim when the wing-shaped hand grips are depressed; The excised tissue should be intact circles when removed from the instrument; Curved or straight; Multifire instrument can be loaded with 25 mm, 28 mm, or 31 mm circular stapling head with a built-in knife

Delmar/Cengage Learning.

FIGURE 7-46

Gastrointestinal anastomosis stapler (GIA)

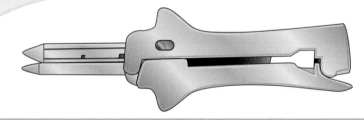

Size: 50 mm; 60 mm; 90 mm

Quantity: One of each available; Can be disposable with a rotating stapler

Notes: Two-piece linear stapler that is used to staple a transected tube in a side-to-side fashion; Reusable instrument can be reloaded with cartridges; Has a two-step function; GIA has a central knife that is used to open the tubes after stapling; SGIA staples a side-to-side anastomosis without a central knife

Delmar/Cengage Learning.

FIGURE 7-47

RECTAL-ANAL INSTRUMENTS

Hemorrhoidectomy and Rectal Excision

Procedures of the rectum and anus are commonly performed with the patient in the prone position and the patient's midsection elevated on a bolster or positioning device. Some rectal procedures on female patients are performed in the lithotomy position.

Hemorrhoidectomy and Rectal Excision – CLAMPS

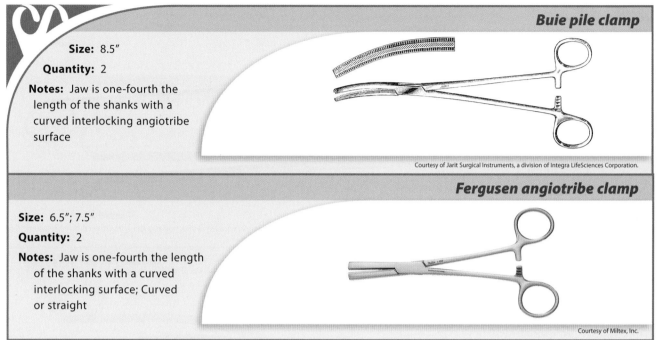

Buie pile clamp

Size: 8.5"

Quantity: 2

Notes: Jaw is one-fourth the length of the shanks with a curved interlocking angiotribe surface

Courtesy of Jarit Surgical Instruments, a division of Integra LifeSciences Corporation.

FIGURE 7-48

Fergusen angiotribe clamp

Size: 6.5"; 7.5"

Quantity: 2

Notes: Jaw is one-fourth the length of the shanks with a curved interlocking surface; Curved or straight

Courtesy of Miltex, Inc.

FIGURE 7-49

Hemorrhoidectomy and Rectal Excision – GRASPING FORCEPS

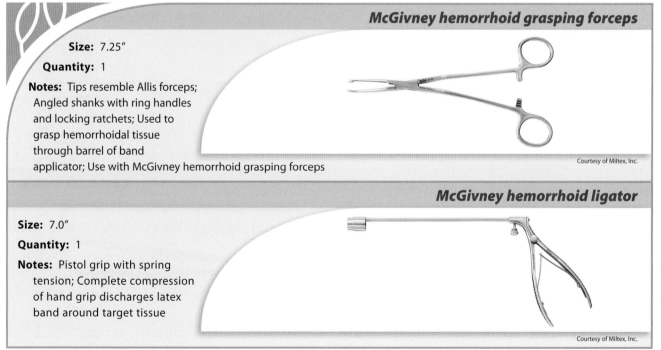

McGivney hemorrhoid grasping forceps

Size: 7.25"

Quantity: 1

Notes: Tips resemble Allis forceps; Angled shanks with ring handles and locking ratchets; Used to grasp hemorrhoidal tissue through barrel of band applicator; Use with McGivney hemorrhoid grasping forceps

Courtesy of Miltex, Inc.

FIGURE 7-50

McGivney hemorrhoid ligator

Size: 7.0"

Quantity: 1

Notes: Pistol grip with spring tension; Complete compression of hand grip discharges latex band around target tissue

Courtesy of Miltex, Inc.

FIGURE 7-51

Hemorrhoidectomy and Rectal Excision – DISSECTION INSTRUMENTS

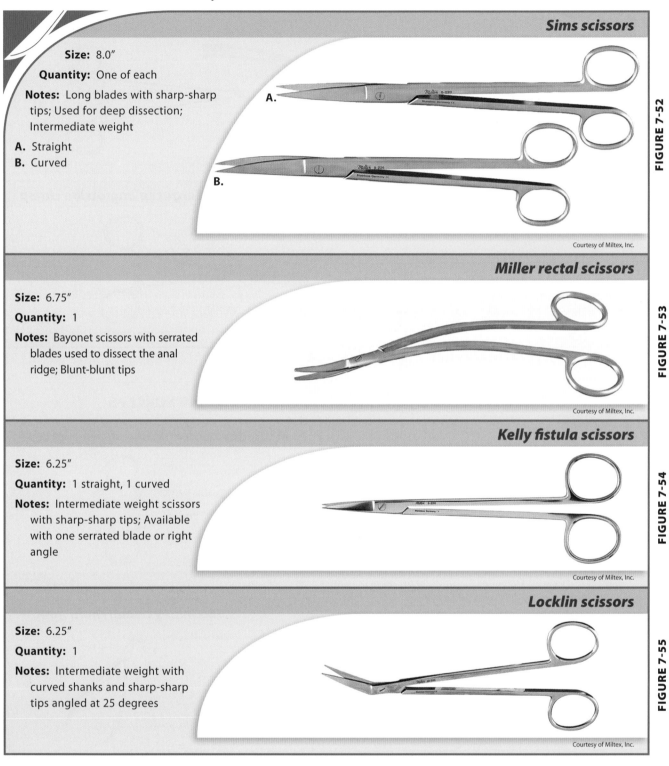

Sims scissors

Size: 8.0"

Quantity: One of each

Notes: Long blades with sharp-sharp tips; Used for deep dissection; Intermediate weight

A. Straight
B. Curved

A.

B.

Courtesy of Miltex, Inc.

FIGURE 7-52

Miller rectal scissors

Size: 6.75"

Quantity: 1

Notes: Bayonet scissors with serrated blades used to dissect the anal ridge; Blunt-blunt tips

Courtesy of Miltex, Inc.

FIGURE 7-53

Kelly fistula scissors

Size: 6.25"

Quantity: 1 straight, 1 curved

Notes: Intermediate weight scissors with sharp-sharp tips; Available with one serrated blade or right angle

Courtesy of Miltex, Inc.

FIGURE 7-54

Locklin scissors

Size: 6.25"

Quantity: 1

Notes: Intermediate weight with curved shanks and sharp-sharp tips angled at 25 degrees

Courtesy of Miltex, Inc.

FIGURE 7-55

Hemorrhoidectomy and Rectal Excision – DISSECTION INSTRUMENTS *continued*

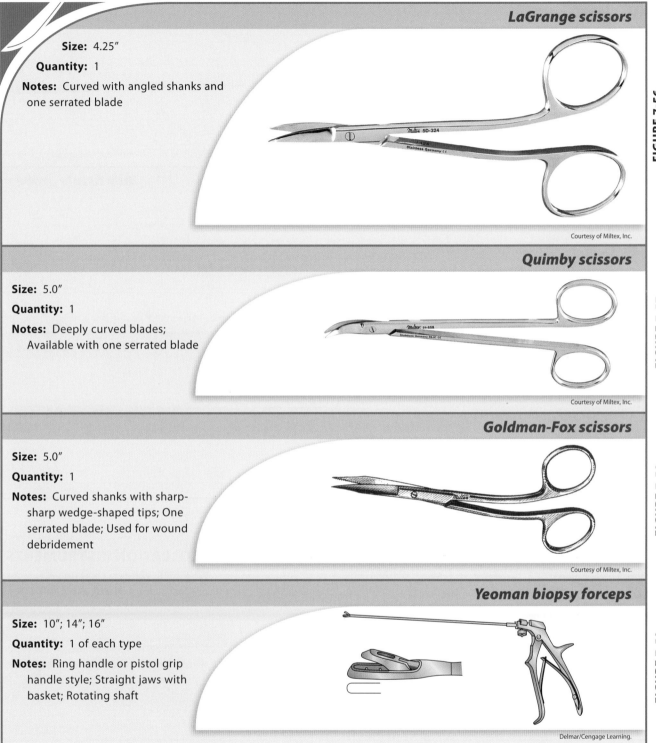

LaGrange scissors

Size: 4.25"

Quantity: 1

Notes: Curved with angled shanks and one serrated blade

Courtesy of Miltex, Inc.

FIGURE 7-56

Quimby scissors

Size: 5.0"

Quantity: 1

Notes: Deeply curved blades; Available with one serrated blade

Courtesy of Miltex, Inc.

FIGURE 7-57

Goldman-Fox scissors

Size: 5.0"

Quantity: 1

Notes: Curved shanks with sharp-sharp wedge-shaped tips; One serrated blade; Used for wound debridement

Courtesy of Miltex, Inc.

FIGURE 7-58

Yeoman biopsy forceps

Size: 10"; 14"; 16"

Quantity: 1 of each type

Notes: Ring handle or pistol grip handle style; Straight jaws with basket; Rotating shaft

Delmar/Cengage Learning.

FIGURE 7-59

Hemorrhoidectomy and Rectal Excision – PROBES AND DILATORS

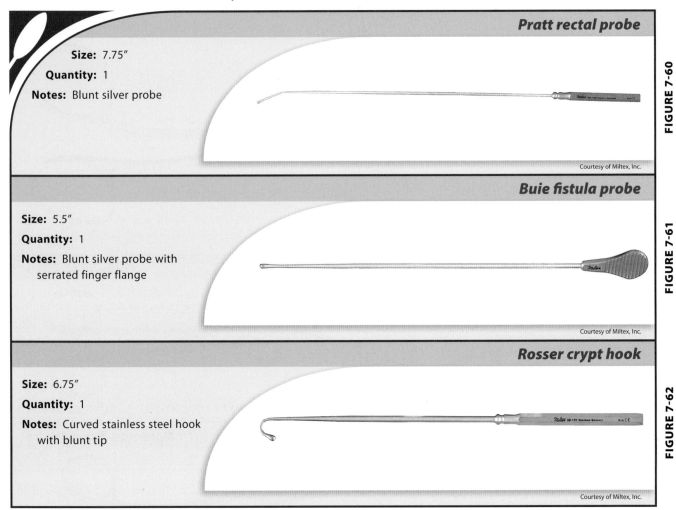

Pratt rectal probe

Size: 7.75"

Quantity: 1

Notes: Blunt silver probe

Courtesy of Miltex, Inc.

FIGURE 7-60

Buie fistula probe

Size: 5.5"

Quantity: 1

Notes: Blunt silver probe with serrated finger flange

Courtesy of Miltex, Inc.

FIGURE 7-61

Rosser crypt hook

Size: 6.75"

Quantity: 1

Notes: Curved stainless steel hook with blunt tip

Courtesy of Miltex, Inc.

FIGURE 7-62

Hemorrhoidectomy and Rectal Excision – EVACUATION AND INSTILLATION INSTRUMENTS

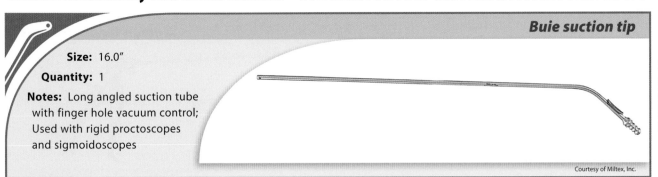

Buie suction tip

Size: 16.0"

Quantity: 1

Notes: Long angled suction tube with finger hole vacuum control; Used with rigid proctoscopes and sigmoidoscopes

Courtesy of Miltex, Inc.

FIGURE 7-63

Hemorrhoidectomy and Rectal Excision – RETRACTION AND EXPOSURE INSTRUMENTS

Hill-Ferguson manual retractor

Size: 8.5"

Quantity: 2

Notes: Scoop-shaped blade in right angle measuring 2.2 cm × 6.4 cm

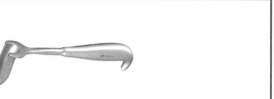

FIGURE 7-64

Sawyer retractor

Size: 11.0"

Quantity: 2

Notes Scoop-shaped blade measuring 7/8" × 2.5" in moderate right angle; Available in three size blades

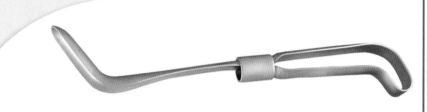

FIGURE 7-65

Fansler-Ives anoscope

Size: 3.25"

Quantity: 1

Notes: Circumferential speculum with central plastic obturator; 1.25" outer diameter

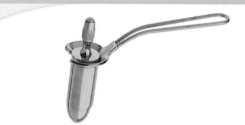

FIGURE 7-66

Hirschman anoscope

Size: 2.25"; 2.80"; 3.5"

Quantity: 1

Notes: Circumferential speculum with central metallic obturator; Available in three sizes

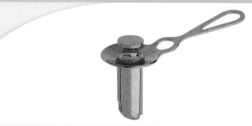

FIGURE 7-67

Hirschman proctoscope

Size: 5.5"

Quantity: 1

Notes Circumferential speculum with narrow 7/8" lumen for examination of the rectum; Metallic obturator

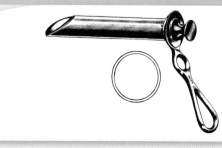

FIGURE 7-68

continues

Hemorrhoidectomy and Rectal Excision – RETRACTION AND EXPOSURE INSTRUMENTS *continued*

Rigid sigmoidoscope

Size: 25 cm

Quantity: 1

Notes: Circumferential speculum with 15 mm lumen; Used for examination to the level of the sigmoid colon; Metallic obturator

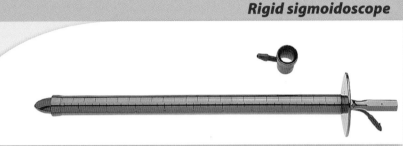

FIGURE 7-69

Chelsea-Eaton anal speculum

Size: 2.75″

Quantity: 1

Notes: Single blade retractor with solid metallic obturator

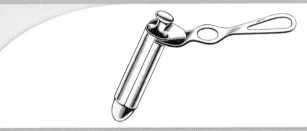

FIGURE 7-70

Barr anal self-retaining retractor

Size: 8.0″; Opens to 2.75″ × 7/8″

Quantity: 1

Notes: Ring handled with bilateral scooped blades that retract with locking ratchets

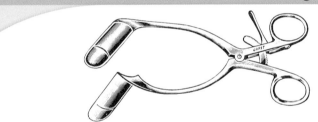

FIGURE 7-71

Gosset self-retaining retractor

Size: Opens to 3.5″; 4.0″; 5.0″

Quantity: 1

Notes: Available in three sizes; Smallest is used in pediatrics; Two open side blades that extend laterally for exposure

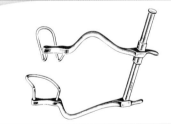

FIGURE 7-72

Pratt rectal speculum

Size: 8.0″

Quantity: 1

Notes: Blades measure 3.5″ × 1.0″; Locks open with a set screw

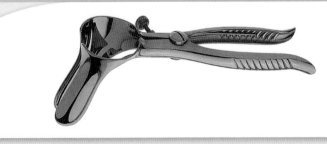

FIGURE 7-73

Hemorrhoidectomy and Rectal Excision – RETRACTION AND EXPOSURE INSTRUMENTS *continued*

Sims rectal speculum

Size: 6.0″

Quantity: 1

Notes: Fenestrated blades measure 3.5″ × 5/8″; Locks open with a set screw; Long narrow

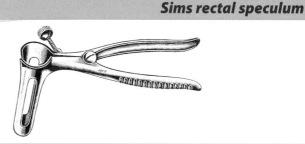

Courtesy of Jarit Surgical Instruments, a division of Integra LifeSciences Corporation.

FIGURE 7-74

Bodenhammer rectal speculum

Size: 6.0″

Quantity: 1

Notes: Solid blades measure 3.5″ × 0.75″; Useful for small or stenosed orifices

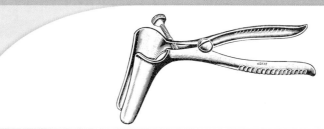

Courtesy of Jarit Surgical Instruments, a division of Integra LifeSciences Corporation.

FIGURE 7-75

Mayo-Adams self-retaining retractor

Size: Opens to 6.75″

Quantity: 1

Notes: Lateral open blades with posterior distracting blade held by a wing nut; Ring handles with locking ratchets

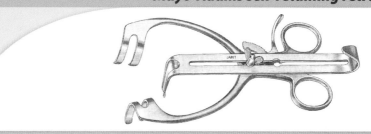

Courtesy of Jarit Surgical Instruments, a division of Integra LifeSciences Corporation.

FIGURE 7-76

Smith (Buie) anal retractor

Size: Opens to 4.0″

Quantity: 1

Notes: In two sizes: 2.5″ or 4.0″ blades; Opens on sliding bar without ratchets; Blades swivel to permit displacement of securing slide bar

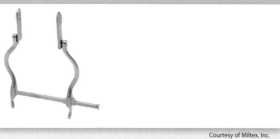

Courtesy of Miltex, Inc.

FIGURE 7-77

SUMMARY

Procedures on the gastrointestinal system will commonly require the use of both medium and long foundation sets in addition to specialty instrumentation. Most of the clamps and graspers are common to many services, but they are the most important instruments associated with general surgery.

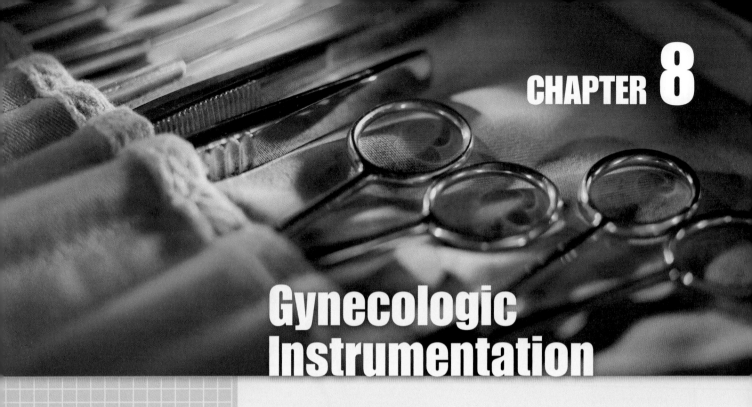

CHAPTER **8**

Gynecologic Instrumentation

INTRODUCTION

Gynecologic procedures can be performed by an abdominal incision, vaginal incision, laparoscopic procedure, or other endoscopic method through the cervix. This chapter will explore instrumentation for abdominal and vaginal procedures. Laparoscopic instrumentation will be discussed in Chapter 15.

OPEN ABDOMINAL GYNECOLOGIC INSTRUMENTATION

Open abdominal instrumentations for gynecologic surgery are used to perform procedures on the female reproductive system through an abdominal incision.

Abdominal Hysterectomy Instrumentation

The abdominal hysterectomy instrumentations is based on the long and medium foundation sets from Chapter 5 with the addition of the following add-on instruments. Abdominal hysterectomy is performed to remove the uterus and sometimes the ovaries and fallopian tubes.

Abdominal Hysterectomy Instrumentation – CLAMPS

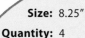

Heaney hysterectomy forceps

Size: 8.25"

Quantity: 4

Notes: Curved with cross-serrations; One grasping tooth is located 1.5 cm from tip

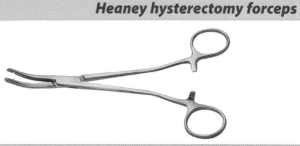

FIGURE 8-1

Heaney-Ballentine clamp

Size: 8.50"

Quantity: 4 of each

Notes: Curved or straight with short jaw and longitudinal serrations

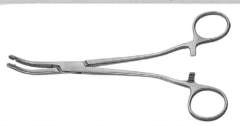

FIGURE 8-2

Long hysterectomy clamp

Size: 7.25"

Quantity: 6

Notes: Slightly curved clamp with longitudinal serrations; 1 × 2 teeth at the tip for secure grasp; Commonly used to grasp the uterine cervix

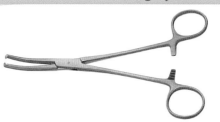

FIGURE 8-3

Phaneuf uterine artery clamp

Size: 8.0"

Quantity: 4 straight and 4 curved

Notes: Straight (shown) or angled clamp with 1 × 2 teeth at tip; Horizontal serrations

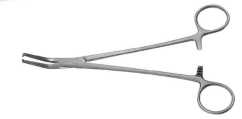

FIGURE 8-4

Wertheim pedicle clamp

Size: 9.75"

Quantity: 4

Notes: Curved short jaw with horizontal serrations

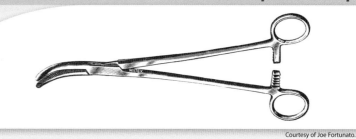

FIGURE 8-5

continues

Abdominal Hysterectomy Istrumentation – CLAMPS *continued*

Wertheim-Cullen pedicle clamp

Size: 8.5″

Quantity: 2

Notes: Sharply angled 2.0″ jaw with longitudinal serrations; Used to hold wide ligaments and vascular tissue during removal of the uterus

Photo supplied courtesy of Cardinal Health, V. Mueller® Products and Services. All rights reserved.

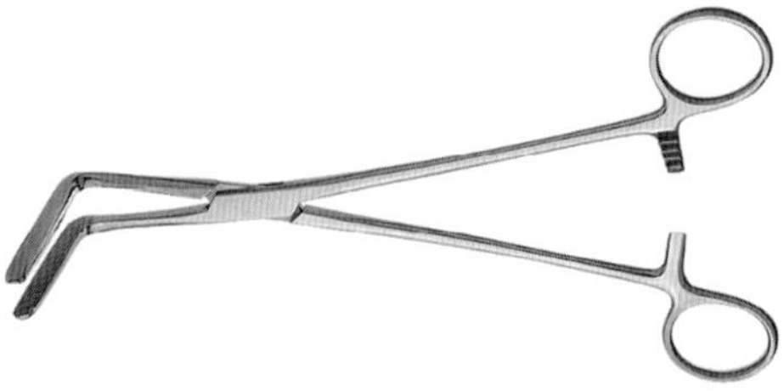

FIGURE 8-6

Pean hysterectomy forceps

Size: 9″; 10.25″

Quantity: 4

Notes: Curved with longitudinal serrations; Sometimes referred to as long Kellys

Courtesy of Miltex, Inc.

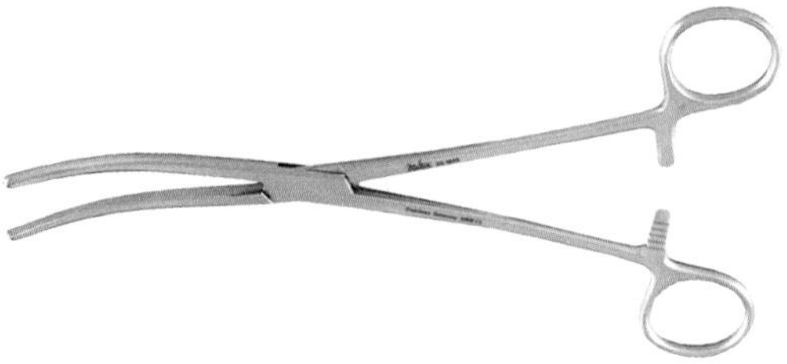

FIGURE 8-7

Abdominal Hysterectomy Instrumentation – GRASPING FORCEPS

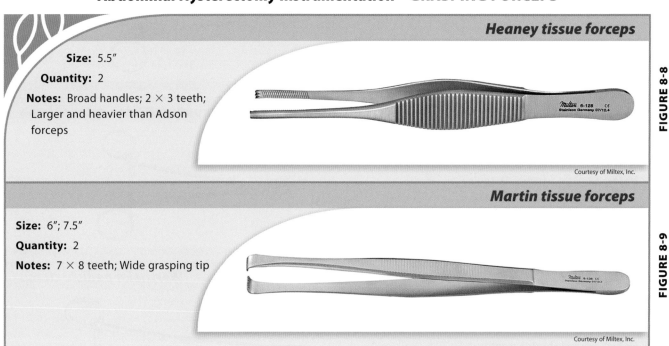

Heaney tissue forceps

Size: 5.5″

Quantity: 2

Notes: Broad handles; 2 × 3 teeth; Larger and heavier than Adson forceps

Courtesy of Miltex, Inc.

FIGURE 8-8

Martin tissue forceps

Size: 6″; 7.5″

Quantity: 2

Notes: 7 × 8 teeth; Wide grasping tip

Courtesy of Miltex, Inc.

FIGURE 8-9

Abdominal Hysterectomy Instrumentation – GRASPING FORCEPS *continued*

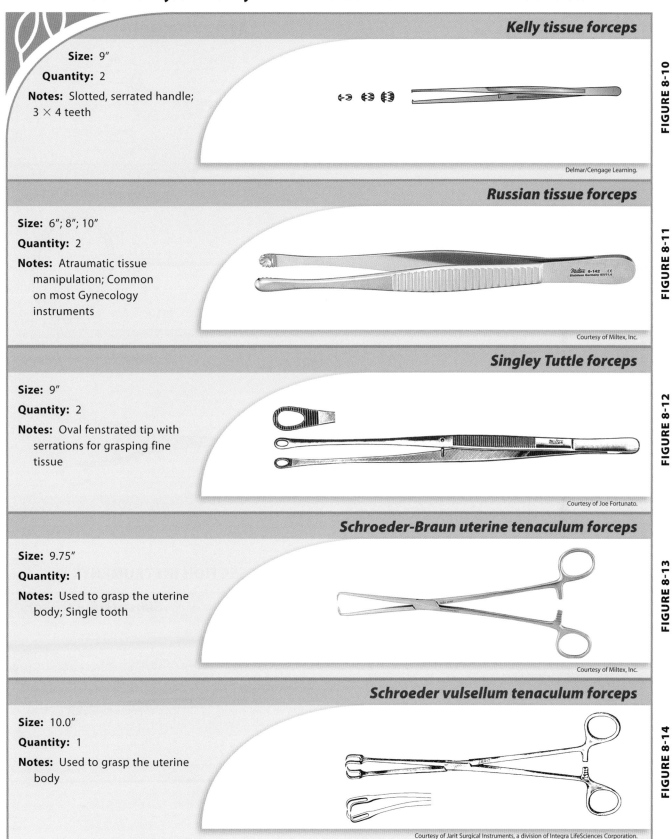

Kelly tissue forceps

Size: 9″

Quantity: 2

Notes: Slotted, serrated handle; 3 × 4 teeth

Delmar/Cengage Learning.

FIGURE 8-10

Russian tissue forceps

Size: 6″; 8″; 10″

Quantity: 2

Notes: Atraumatic tissue manipulation; Common on most Gynecology instruments

Courtesy of Miltex, Inc.

FIGURE 8-11

Singley Tuttle forceps

Size: 9″

Quantity: 2

Notes: Oval fenstrated tip with serrations for grasping fine tissue

Courtesy of Joe Fortunato.

FIGURE 8-12

Schroeder-Braun uterine tenaculum forceps

Size: 9.75″

Quantity: 1

Notes: Used to grasp the uterine body; Single tooth

Courtesy of Miltex, Inc.

FIGURE 8-13

Schroeder vulsellum tenaculum forceps

Size: 10.0″

Quantity: 1

Notes: Used to grasp the uterine body

Courtesy of Jarit Surgical Instruments, a division of Integra LifeSciences Corporation.

FIGURE 8-14

continues

Abdominal Hysterectomy Instrumentation – GRASPING FORCEPS *continued*

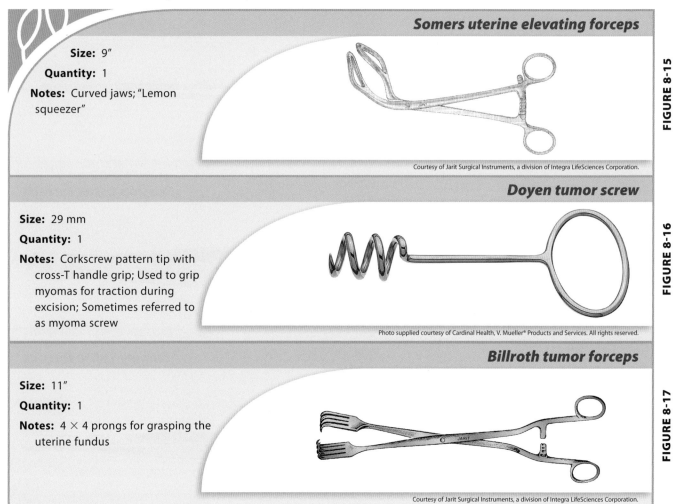

Somers uterine elevating forceps

Size: 9″

Quantity: 1

Notes: Curved jaws; "Lemon squeezer"

FIGURE 8-15

Doyen tumor screw

Size: 29 mm

Quantity: 1

Notes: Corkscrew pattern tip with cross-T handle grip; Used to grip myomas for traction during excision; Sometimes referred to as myoma screw

FIGURE 8-16

Billroth tumor forceps

Size: 11″

Quantity: 1

Notes: 4 × 4 prongs for grasping the uterine fundus

FIGURE 8-17

Abdominal Hysterectomy Instrumentation – DISSECTION INSTRUMENTS

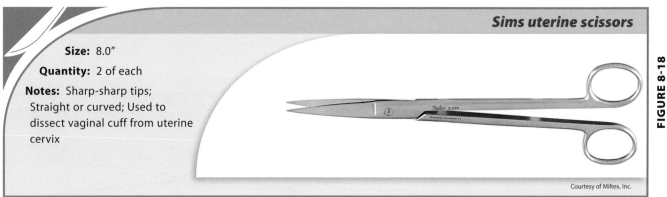

Sims uterine scissors

Size: 8.0″

Quantity: 2 of each

Notes: Sharp-sharp tips; Straight or curved; Used to dissect vaginal cuff from uterine cervix

FIGURE 8-18

Abdominal Hysterectomy Instrumentation – DISSECTION INSTRUMENTS *continued*

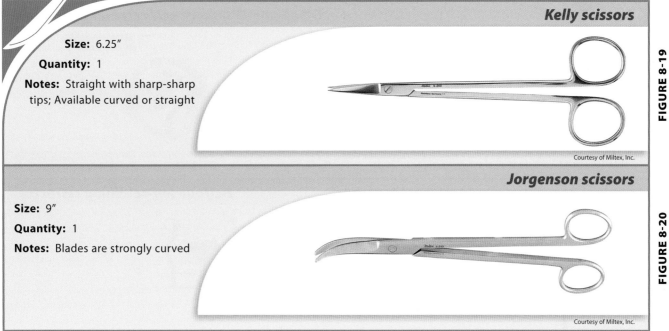

Kelly scissors

FIGURE 8-19

Size: 6.25"

Quantity: 1

Notes: Straight with sharp-sharp tips; Available curved or straight

Courtesy of Miltex, Inc.

Jorgenson scissors

FIGURE 8-20

Size: 9"

Quantity: 1

Notes: Blades are strongly curved

Courtesy of Miltex, Inc.

Abdominal Hysterectomy Instrumentation – EVACUATION AND INSTILLATION INSTRUMENTS

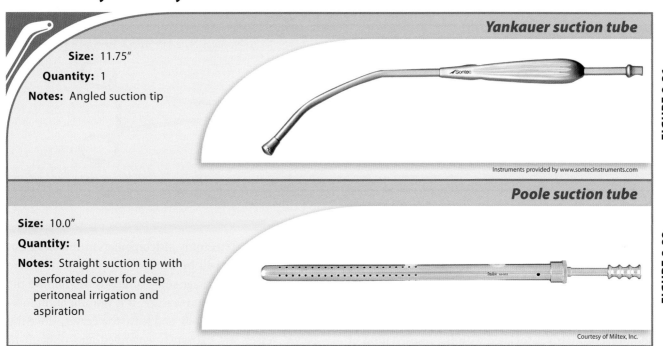

Yankauer suction tube

FIGURE 8-21

Size: 11.75"

Quantity: 1

Notes: Angled suction tip

Instruments provided by www.sontecinstruments.com

Poole suction tube

FIGURE 8-22

Size: 10.0"

Quantity: 1

Notes: Straight suction tip with perforated cover for deep peritoneal irrigation and aspiration

Courtesy of Miltex, Inc.

Abdominal Hysterectomy Instrumentation – RETRACTION AND EXPOSURE INSTRUMENTS

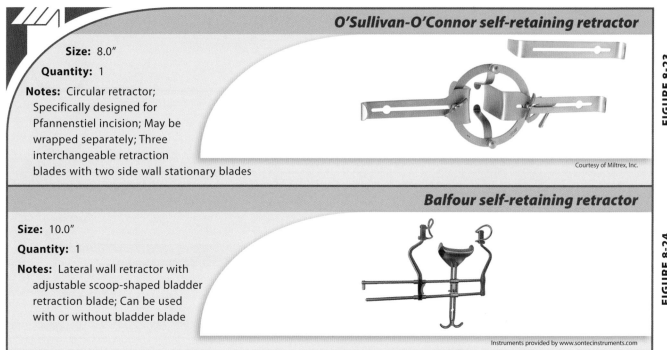

O'Sullivan-O'Connor self-retaining retractor

Size: 8.0″

Quantity: 1

Notes: Circular retractor; Specifically designed for Pfannenstiel incision; May be wrapped separately; Three interchangeable retraction blades with two side wall stationary blades

Courtesy of Miltrex, Inc.

FIGURE 8-23

Balfour self-retaining retractor

Size: 10.0″

Quantity: 1

Notes: Lateral wall retractor with adjustable scoop-shaped bladder retraction blade; Can be used with or without bladder blade

Instruments provided by www.sontecinstruments.com

FIGURE 8-24

Abdominal Hysterectomy Instrumentation – APPROXIMATION AND CLOSURE INSTRUMENTS

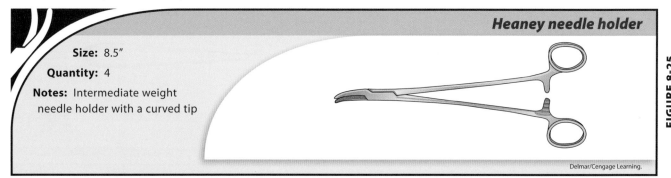

Heaney needle holder

Size: 8.5″

Quantity: 4

Notes: Intermediate weight needle holder with a curved tip

Delmar/Cengage Learning.

FIGURE 8-25

Cesarean Section Instrumentation

Cesarean section is the procedure performed for the surgical delivery of a baby through an abdominal incision. The primary instruments used are the medium and long foundation instruments with a few specialty additions primarily associated with the resuscitation of the baby after removal from the mother's uterus.

In the rare event that the uterus must be removed during the cesarean birth the full medium set, long set, abdominal hysterectomy instrumentation, and cesarean instrumentation will be needed. In the case of severe infection or hemorrhage some surgeons will remove the uterus as a life-saving measure. It is not uncommon to remove the uterine body and leave the cervix, since the pelvic vessels are extremely engorged and difficult to manage in the deeper aspects below the pelvic rim. This is referred to as a supracervical cesarean hysterectomy. The woman is rendered sterile by this procedure.

Cesarean Section Instrumentation – CLAMPS

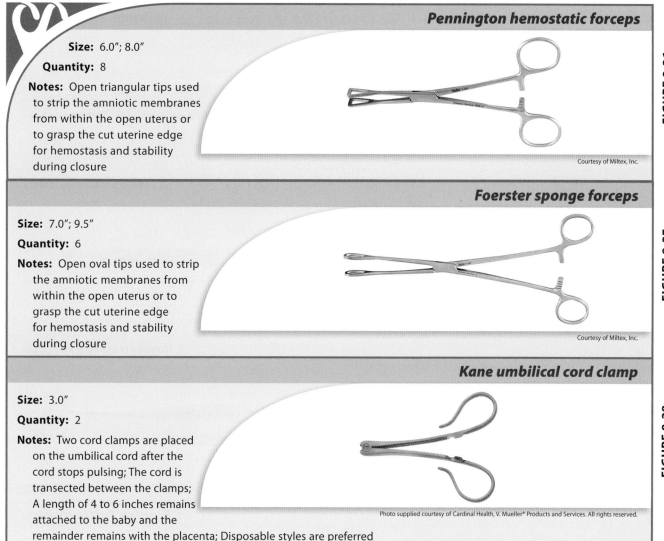

Pennington hemostatic forceps

Size: 6.0"; 8.0"

Quantity: 8

Notes: Open triangular tips used to strip the amniotic membranes from within the open uterus or to grasp the cut uterine edge for hemostasis and stability during closure

Courtesy of Miltex, Inc.

FIGURE 8-26

Foerster sponge forceps

Size: 7.0"; 9.5"

Quantity: 6

Notes: Open oval tips used to strip the amniotic membranes from within the open uterus or to grasp the cut uterine edge for hemostasis and stability during closure

Courtesy of Miltex, Inc.

FIGURE 8-27

Kane umbilical cord clamp

Size: 3.0"

Quantity: 2

Notes: Two cord clamps are placed on the umbilical cord after the cord stops pulsing; The cord is transected between the clamps; A length of 4 to 6 inches remains attached to the baby and the remainder remains with the placenta; Disposable styles are preferred

Photo supplied courtesy of Cardinal Health, V. Mueller® Products and Services. All rights reserved.

FIGURE 8-28

Cesarean Section Instrumentation – GRASPING FORCEPS

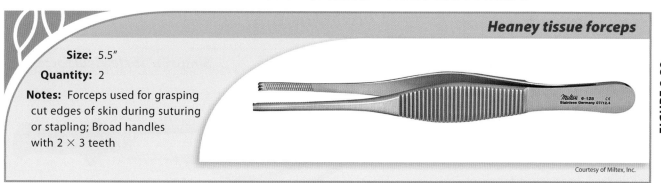

Heaney tissue forceps

Size: 5.5"

Quantity: 2

Notes: Forceps used for grasping cut edges of skin during suturing or stapling; Broad handles with 2 × 3 teeth

Courtesy of Miltex, Inc.

FIGURE 8-29

continues

Cesarean Section Insrumentation – GRASPING FORCEPS *continued*

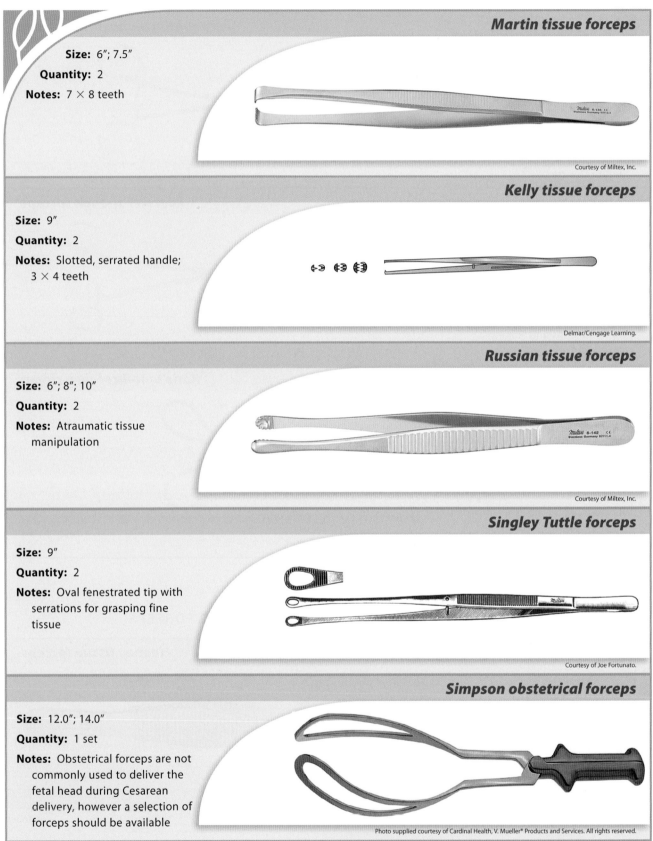

Martin tissue forceps

Size: 6"; 7.5"

Quantity: 2

Notes: 7 × 8 teeth

FIGURE 8-30

Kelly tissue forceps

Size: 9"

Quantity: 2

Notes: Slotted, serrated handle; 3 × 4 teeth

FIGURE 8-31

Russian tissue forceps

Size: 6"; 8"; 10"

Quantity: 2

Notes: Atraumatic tissue manipulation

FIGURE 8-32

Singley Tuttle forceps

Size: 9"

Quantity: 2

Notes: Oval fenestrated tip with serrations for grasping fine tissue

FIGURE 8-33

Simpson obstetrical forceps

Size: 12.0"; 14.0"

Quantity: 1 set

Notes: Obstetrical forceps are not commonly used to deliver the fetal head during Cesarean delivery, however a selection of forceps should be available

FIGURE 8-34

Cesarean Section Instrumentation– GRASPING FORCEPS *continued*

Elliott obstetrical forceps

Size: 12.5″

Quantity: 1

Notes: Used to grasp the fetal head for delivery; Open blades

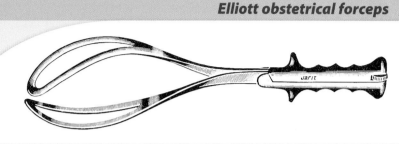

Courtesy of Jarit Surgical Instruments, a division of Integra LifeSciences Corporation.

FIGURE 8-35

Piper obstetrical forceps

Size: 17.5″

Quantity: 1

Notes: Used to grasp the fetal head for delivery; Reverse angle forceps; Open blades

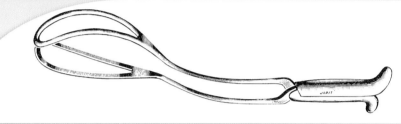

Courtesy of Jarit Surgical Instruments, a division of Integra LifeSciences Corporation.

FIGURE 8-36

Kielland obstetrical forceps

Size: 15.5″

Quantity: 1

Notes: Used to grasp the fetal head for delivery; Straight angle forceps; Handle is narrow and smooth; Open blades

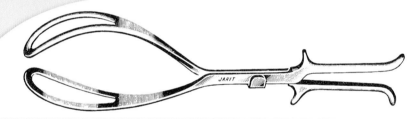

Courtesy of Jarit Surgical Instruments, a division of Integra LifeSciences Corporation.

FIGURE 8-37

Luikart obstetrical forceps

Size: 15.5″

Quantity: 1

Notes: Used to grasp the fetal head for delivery; Closed blades

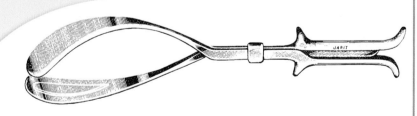

Courtesy of Jarit Surgical Instruments, a division of Integra LifeSciences Corporation.

FIGURE 8-38

Simpson–Luikart obstetrical forceps

Size: 14.0″

Quantity: 1

Notes: Used to grasp the fetal head for delivery; Closed blades

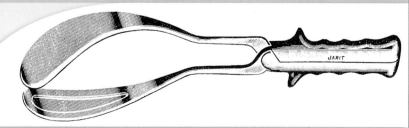

Courtesy of Jarit Surgical Instruments, a division of Integra LifeSciences Corporation.

FIGURE 8-39

continues

Cesarean Section Instrumentation – GRASPING FORCEPS *continued*

McLean-Luikart obstetrical forceps

Size: 15.25"

Quantity: 1

Notes: Used to grasp the fetal head for delivery; Closed blades

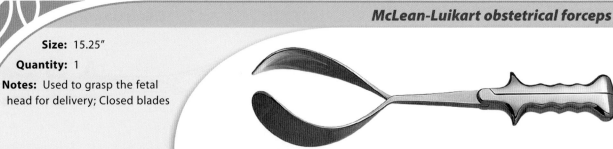

FIGURE 8-40

McLean-Tucker-Luikart Tucker obstetrical forceps

Size: 15.75"

Quantity: 1

Notes: Used to grasp the fetal head for delivery; Closed blades

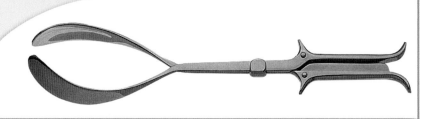

FIGURE 8-41

Bill traction handle

Quantity: 1 handle

Notes: Used to securely hold obstetrical forceps with a non-slip grip

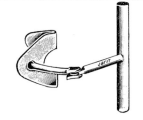

FIGURE 8-42

Iowa membrane puncturing forceps

Size: 10.25"

Quantity: 1

Notes: Used to rupture the amniotic sac; Double curved 6 × 6 teeth

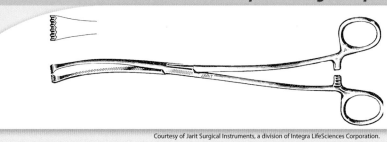

FIGURE 8-43

Cesarean Section Instrumentation – EVACUATION AND INSTILLATION INSTRUMENTS

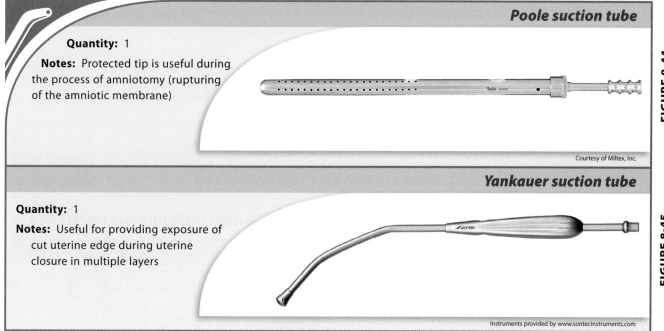

Poole suction tube

Quantity: 1

Notes: Protected tip is useful during the process of amniotomy (rupturing of the amniotic membrane)

Courtesy of Miltex, Inc.

FIGURE 8-44

Yankauer suction tube

Quantity: 1

Notes: Useful for providing exposure of cut uterine edge during uterine closure in multiple layers

Instruments provided by www.sontecinstruments.com

FIGURE 8-45

Cesarean Section Instrumentation – RETRACTION AND EXPOSURE INSTRUMENTS

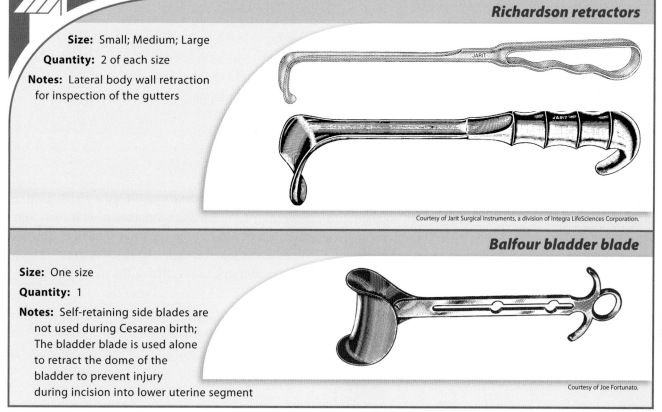

Richardson retractors

Size: Small; Medium; Large

Quantity: 2 of each size

Notes: Lateral body wall retraction for inspection of the gutters

Courtesy of Jarit Surgical Instruments, a division of Integra LifeSciences Corporation.

FIGURE 8-46

Balfour bladder blade

Size: One size

Quantity: 1

Notes: Self-retaining side blades are not used during Cesarean birth; The bladder blade is used alone to retract the dome of the bladder to prevent injury during incision into lower uterine segment

Courtesy of Joe Fortunato.

FIGURE 8-47

continues

Cesarean Section Instrumentation – RETRACTION AND EXPOSURE INSTRUMENTS *continued*

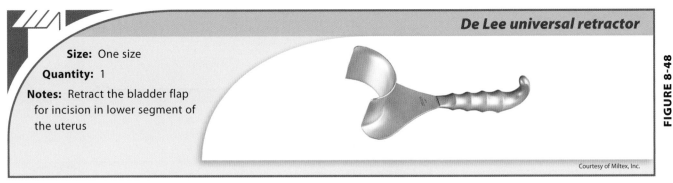

De Lee universal retractor

Size: One size

Quantity: 1

Notes: Retract the bladder flap for incision in lower segment of the uterus

Courtesy of Miltex, Inc.

FIGURE 8-48

Cesarean Section Instrumentation – APPROXIMATION AND CLOSURE INSTRUMENTS

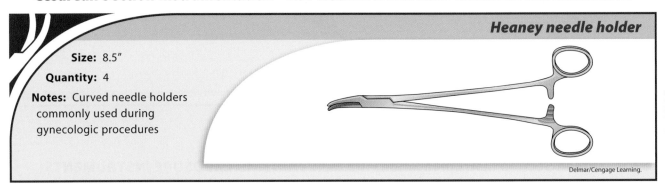

Heaney needle holder

Size: 8.5″

Quantity: 4

Notes: Curved needle holders commonly used during gynecologic procedures

Delmar/Cengage Learning.

FIGURE 8-49

VAGINAL INSTRUMENTATION

Vaginal sets commonly use long curved instruments because the vaginal outlet obscures the observation of the instrument tip.

Vaginal-Perineal Instrumentation

Vaginoplastic procedures involve working with the vaginal mucosa. A medium foundation set is used with the addition of the instruments in the following group for vaginal-perineal procedures. The medium foundation set is used alone for incision and drainage of infected Skene's or Bartholin glands. Colporrhaphy of the vagina is sometimes referred to as anterior or posterior repair for correction of herniation of the bladder into the vagina (cystocele), urethral laxity (urethrocele), rectal herniation into the vagina (rectocele), or a combination relaxed vaginal outlet (enterocele).

Vaginal-Perineal Instrumentation – GRASPING FORCEPS

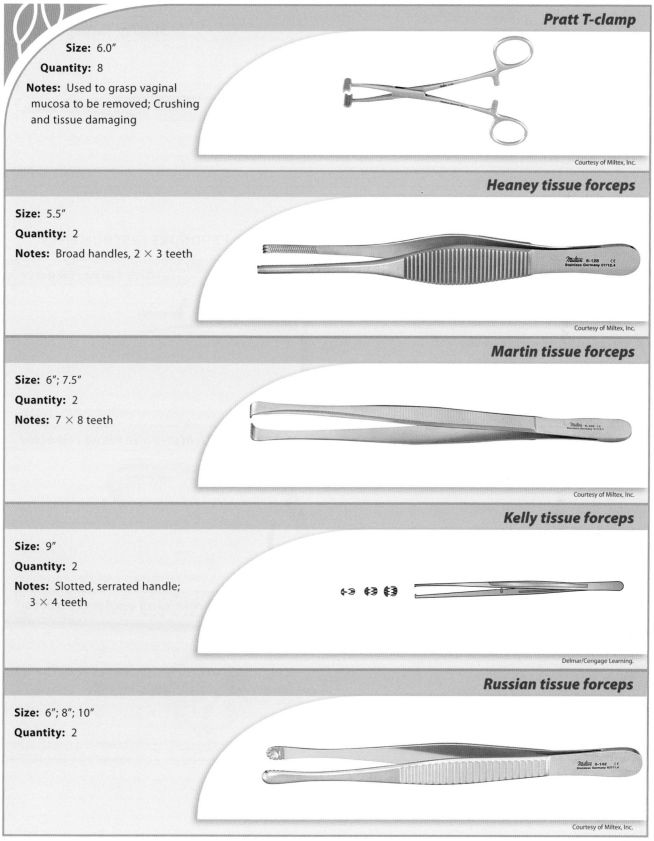

Pratt T-clamp

Size: 6.0"

Quantity: 8

Notes: Used to grasp vaginal mucosa to be removed; Crushing and tissue damaging

Courtesy of Miltex, Inc.

FIGURE 8-50

Heaney tissue forceps

Size: 5.5"

Quantity: 2

Notes: Broad handles, 2 × 3 teeth

Courtesy of Miltex, Inc.

FIGURE 8-51

Martin tissue forceps

Size: 6"; 7.5"

Quantity: 2

Notes: 7 × 8 teeth

Courtesy of Miltex, Inc.

FIGURE 8-52

Kelly tissue forceps

Size: 9"

Quantity: 2

Notes: Slotted, serrated handle; 3 × 4 teeth

Delmar/Cengage Learning.

FIGURE 8-53

Russian tissue forceps

Size: 6"; 8"; 10"

Quantity: 2

Courtesy of Miltex, Inc.

FIGURE 8-54

continues

Vaginal-Perineal Instrumentation – GRASPING FORCEPS *continued*

Singley Tuttle forceps

Size: 9"

Quantity: 2

Notes: Fenestrated jaws; Slotted grooved handles

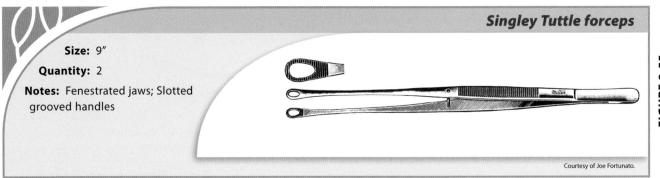

Courtesy of Joe Fortunato.

FIGURE 8-55

Vaginal-Perineal Instrumentation – RETRACTION AND EXPOSURE INSTRUMENTS

Richter vulva retractor

Size: 18 cm

Quantity: 1

Notes: Fenestrated self-retaining retractor used to separate the labia for perineal procedures; Ring handles with locking ratchets; Single tooth

Courtesy of Joe Fortunato.

FIGURE 8-56

Richter-Stille vulva retractor

Size: 18 cm

Quantity: 1

Notes: Fenestrated self-retaining retractor used to separate the labia for perineal procedures; Ring handles with locking ratchets; Allis serrations on tips

Courtesy of Surgical Tools, Inc.

FIGURE 8-57

O'Sullivan-O'Connor self-retaining vaginal retractor

Size: 3.5" depth

Quantity: 1

Notes: Four blades; Exposure is anterior-posterior and both side walls

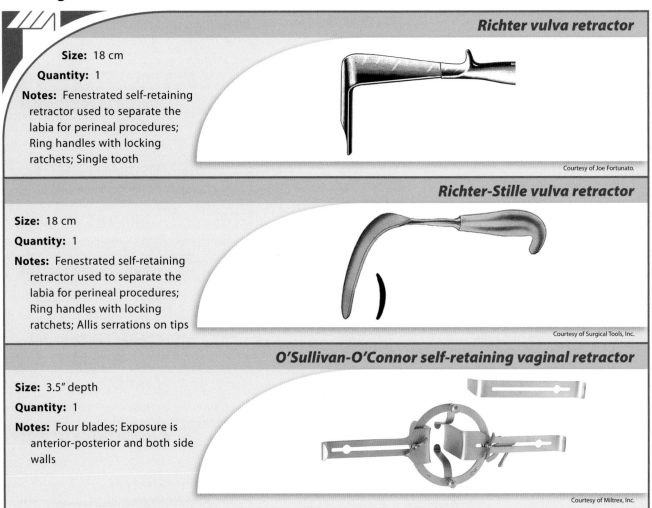

Courtesy of Miltrex, Inc.

FIGURE 8-58

Vaginal-Perineal Instrumentation – RETRACTION AND EXPOSURE INSTRUMENTS *continued*

Lateral self-retaining vaginal retractor

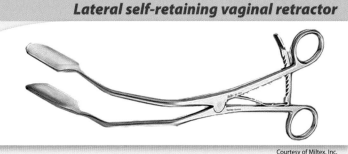

Size: 8.25″

Quantity: 1

Notes: Side wall retractor with ring handles and locking ratchets

FIGURE 8-59

Graves vaginal speculum

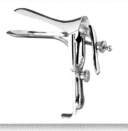

Size: Small; Medium; Large

Quantity: 1

Notes: Speculum opens anterior-posterior with thumb lever and thumb screw; Available in right angle or 45-degree angle with side opening; Standard model is stainless steel; Ebonized is available for laser applications

FIGURE 8-60

Pederson vaginal speculum

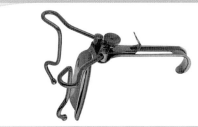

Size: Small; Medium; Large

Quantity: 1

Notes: Narrow blades for anterior-posterior exposure; Similar to Graves speculum

FIGURE 8-61

Gutmann vaginal speculum

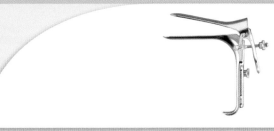

Size: 4.0″

Quantity: 1

Notes: Anterior-posterior retraction in three planes; Self-retaining with a thumb screw

FIGURE 8-62

Sims vaginal retractor

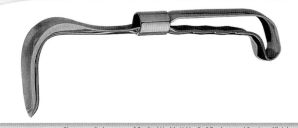

Size: Small; Medium; Large

Quantity: 1

Notes: Single-ended retractor with scoop-blunt edge

FIGURE 8-63

continues

Vaginal-Perineal Instrumentation – RETRACTION AND EXPOSURE INSTRUMENTS *continued*

Sims vaginal retractor double end

Size: Small; Medium; Large

Quantity: 1

Notes: Scoop-blunt edge; Both blades face same direction

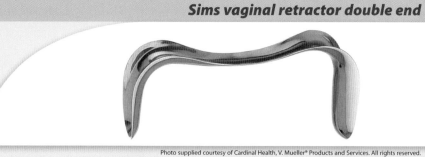

FIGURE 8-64

Auvard weighted vaginal speculum

Size: 2 lbs; 2.5 lbs; 3.0 lbs

Quantity: 1

Notes: Single-end vaginal retractor with weight on dependent edge; Blade is available as straight, angled, and extra long; Sterile glove can be applied over weight to collect blood and drainage

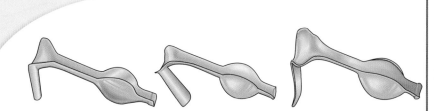

Delmar/Cengage Learning.

FIGURE 8-65

Weissbarth vaginal speculum

Size: 21 cm

Quantity: 1

Notes: Right angle weighted speculum with removable collection chamber

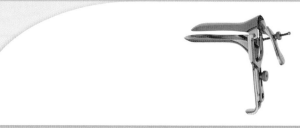

FIGURE 8-66

Jackson vaginal retractor

Size: 7.0"

Quantity: 1

Notes: Single end with straight edge

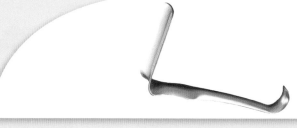

Courtesy of Miltex, Inc.

FIGURE 8-67

Eastman vaginal retractor

Size: 7.0"

Quantity: 1

Notes: Single end with angled edge

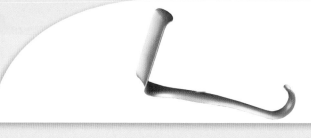

Courtesy of Miltex, Inc.

FIGURE 8-68

Vaginal-Perineal Instrumentation – RETRACTION AND EXPOSURE INSTRUMENTS *continued*

Heaney retractor

Size: 10.5"

Quantity: 2

Notes: Single end with straight edge; Serrated finger grip

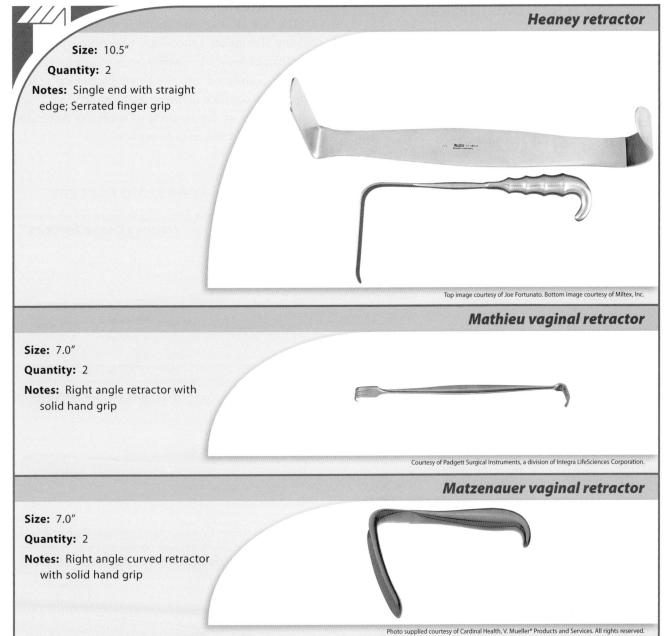

FIGURE 8-69

Mathieu vaginal retractor

Size: 7.0"

Quantity: 2

Notes: Right angle retractor with solid hand grip

FIGURE 8-70

Matzenauer vaginal retractor

Size: 7.0"

Quantity: 2

Notes: Right angle curved retractor with solid hand grip

FIGURE 8-71

Breisky vaginal retractor

Size: 70 mm

Quantity: 2

Notes: Bayonet side wall retractor; Sometimes referred to as "shovels"

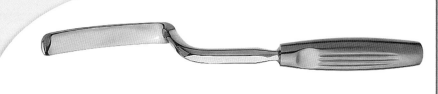

FIGURE 8-72

Dilation and Curettage-Cervix Procedural Instrumentation

Debulking the uterine cavity is performed by scraping the endometrial walls with sharp or blunt curettes. The endometrium is peeled away and sent to pathology for analysis.

Removing lesions from the uterine cervix by electrosurgery is done with instrumentation prefaced with LEEP (Loop Electrical Excisional Procedure) or LLETZ (Large Loop Excision of the Transformational Zone).

The use of vaginal-uterine instrumentation can facilitate abdominal gynecologic procedures by allowing pelvic exposure by uterine manipulation. The instrument is inserted into the cervix by vaginal access. Cannulae in place for uterine manipulation can be used for instillation of dye or contrast media to determine tubal patency during fertility studies.

Dilation and Curettage-Cervix Procedural Instrumentation – GRASPING FORCEPS

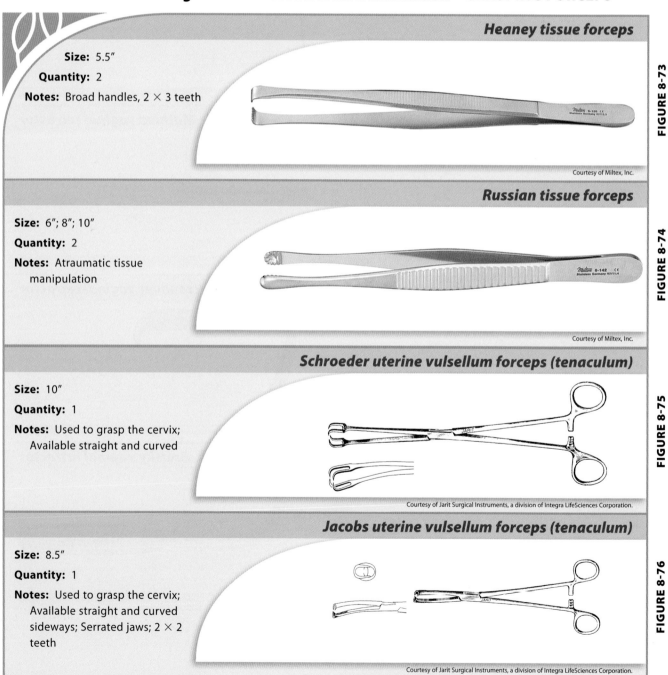

Heaney tissue forceps

Size: 5.5"

Quantity: 2

Notes: Broad handles, 2 × 3 teeth

Courtesy of Miltex, Inc.

FIGURE 8-73

Russian tissue forceps

Size: 6"; 8"; 10"

Quantity: 2

Notes: Atraumatic tissue manipulation

Courtesy of Miltex, Inc.

FIGURE 8-74

Schroeder uterine vulsellum forceps (tenaculum)

Size: 10"

Quantity: 1

Notes: Used to grasp the cervix; Available straight and curved

Courtesy of Jarit Surgical Instruments, a division of Integra LifeSciences Corporation.

FIGURE 8-75

Jacobs uterine vulsellum forceps (tenaculum)

Size: 8.5"

Quantity: 1

Notes: Used to grasp the cervix; Available straight and curved sideways; Serrated jaws; 2 × 2 teeth

Courtesy of Jarit Surgical Instruments, a division of Integra LifeSciences Corporation.

FIGURE 8-76

Dilation and Curettage-Cervix Procedural Instrumentation – GRASPING FORCEPS *continued*

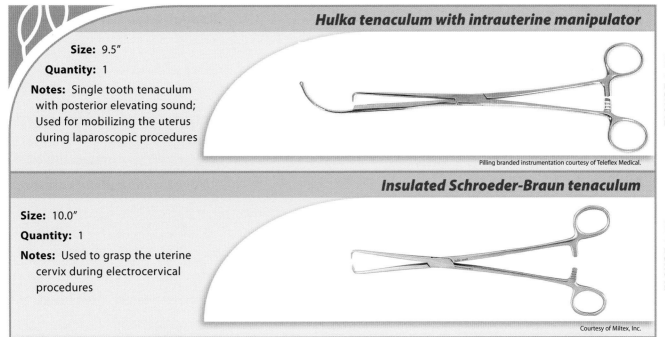

Hulka tenaculum with intrauterine manipulator

Size: 9.5"

Quantity: 1

Notes: Single tooth tenaculum with posterior elevating sound; Used for mobilizing the uterus during laparoscopic procedures

Pilling branded instrumentation courtesy of Teleflex Medical.

FIGURE 8-77

Insulated Schroeder-Braun tenaculum

Size: 10.0"

Quantity: 1

Notes: Used to grasp the uterine cervix during electrocervical procedures

Courtesy of Miltex, Inc.

FIGURE 8-78

Dilation and Curettage-Cervix Procedural Instrumentation – DEBULKING INSTRUMENTS

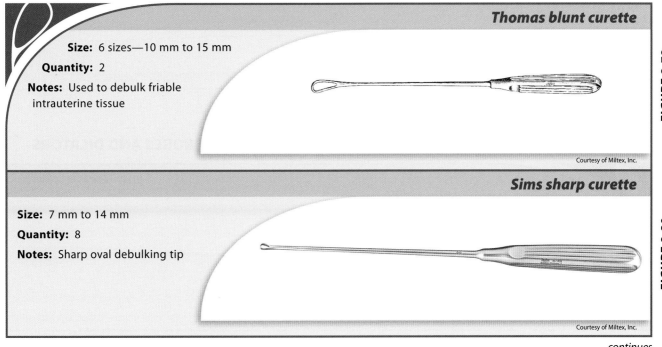

Thomas blunt curette

Size: 6 sizes—10 mm to 15 mm

Quantity: 2

Notes: Used to debulk friable intrauterine tissue

Courtesy of Miltex, Inc.

FIGURE 8-79

Sims sharp curette

Size: 7 mm to 14 mm

Quantity: 8

Notes: Sharp oval debulking tip

Courtesy of Miltex, Inc.

FIGURE 8-80

continues

Dilation and Curettage-Cervix Procedural Instrumentation – DEBULKING INSTRUMENTS *continued*

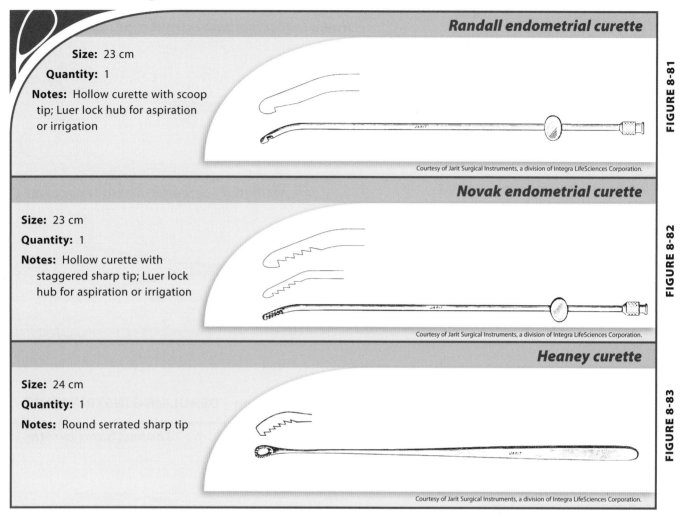

Randall endometrial curette

Size: 23 cm

Quantity: 1

Notes: Hollow curette with scoop tip; Luer lock hub for aspiration or irrigation

Courtesy of Jarit Surgical Instruments, a division of Integra LifeSciences Corporation.

FIGURE 8-81

Novak endometrial curette

Size: 23 cm

Quantity: 1

Notes: Hollow curette with staggered sharp tip; Luer lock hub for aspiration or irrigation

Courtesy of Jarit Surgical Instruments, a division of Integra LifeSciences Corporation.

FIGURE 8-82

Heaney curette

Size: 24 cm

Quantity: 1

Notes: Round serrated sharp tip

Courtesy of Jarit Surgical Instruments, a division of Integra LifeSciences Corporation.

FIGURE 8-83

Dilation and Curettage-Cervix Procedural Instrumentation – PROBES AND DILATORS

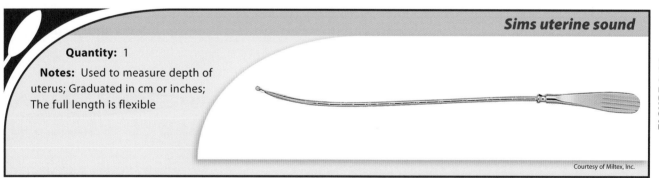

Sims uterine sound

Quantity: 1

Notes: Used to measure depth of uterus; Graduated in cm or inches; The full length is flexible

Courtesy of Miltex, Inc.

FIGURE 8-84

Dilation and Curettage-Cervix Procedural Instrumentation – PROBES AND DILATORS *continued*

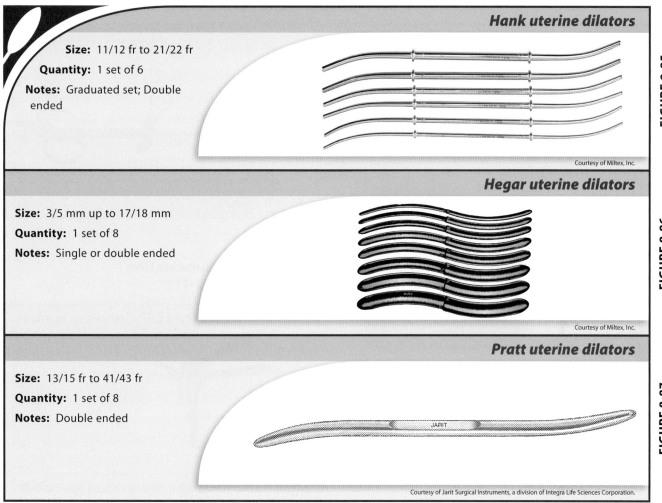

Hank uterine dilators

Size: 11/12 fr to 21/22 fr

Quantity: 1 set of 6

Notes: Graduated set; Double ended

Courtesy of Miltex, Inc.

FIGURE 8-85

Hegar uterine dilators

Size: 3/5 mm up to 17/18 mm

Quantity: 1 set of 8

Notes: Single or double ended

Courtesy of Miltex, Inc.

FIGURE 8-86

Pratt uterine dilators

Size: 13/15 fr to 41/43 fr

Quantity: 1 set of 8

Notes: Double ended

JARIT

Courtesy of Jarit Surgical Instruments, a division of Integra Life Sciences Corporation.

FIGURE 8-87

Dilation and Curettage-Cervix Procedural Instrumentation – EVACUATION AND INSTILLATION INSTRUMENTS

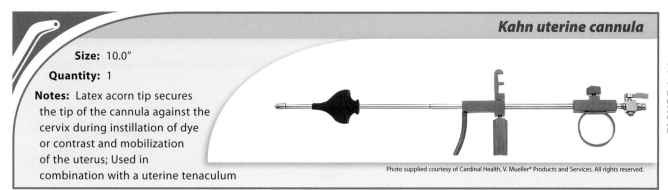

Kahn uterine cannula

Size: 10.0"

Quantity: 1

Notes: Latex acorn tip secures the tip of the cannula against the cervix during instillation of dye or contrast and mobilization of the uterus; Used in combination with a uterine tenaculum

Photo supplied courtesy of Cardinal Health, V. Mueller® Products and Services. All rights reserved.

FIGURE 8-88

continues

Dilation and Curettage-Cervix Procedural Instrumentation –
EVACUATION AND INSTILLATION INSTRUMENTS *continued*

Jarco uterine cannula

Size: 10.0"

Quantity: 1

Notes: Latex acorn tip secures the tip of the cannula against the cervix during instillation of dye or contrast and mobilization of the uterus; Used in combination with a uterine tenaculum; Has a self-retaining support that attaches to the ring handles of the uterine tenaculum

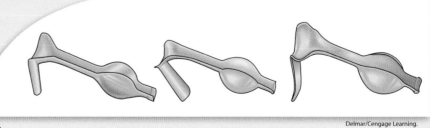

FIGURE 8-89

Dilation and Curettage-Cervix Procedural Instrumentation –
RETRACTION AND EXPOSURE INSTRUMENTS

Insulated LEEP Graves speculum

Size: Small; Medium; Large

Quantity: 1

Notes: Used with electrosurgical procedures of the vagina and cervix; Smoke evacuation port

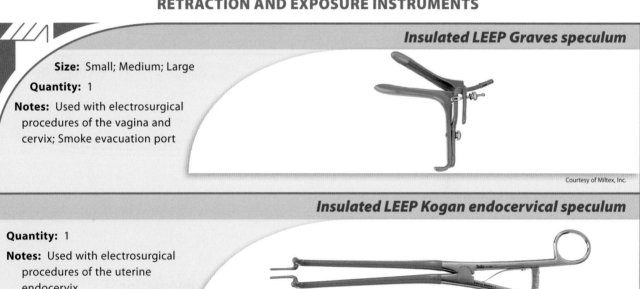

FIGURE 8-90

Insulated LEEP Kogan endocervical speculum

Quantity: 1

Notes: Used with electrosurgical procedures of the uterine endocervix

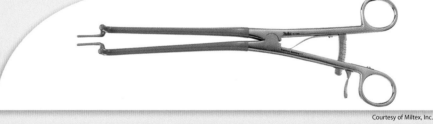

FIGURE 8-91

Auvard weighted vaginal speculum

Size: 2 lbs; 2.5 lbs; 3.0 lbs

Quantity: 1

Notes: Single-end vaginal retractor with weight on dependent edge; Blade is available straight, angled, and extra long; Sterile glove can be applied over weight to collect blood and drainage

FIGURE 8-92

Dilation and Curettage-Cervix Procedural Instrumentation –
RETRACTION AND EXPOSURE INSTRUMENTS *continued*

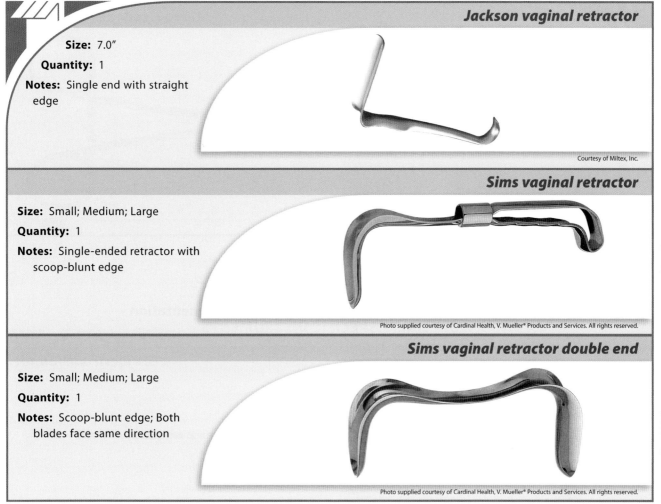

Jackson vaginal retractor

Size: 7.0″

Quantity: 1

Notes: Single end with straight edge

FIGURE 8-93

Sims vaginal retractor

Size: Small; Medium; Large

Quantity: 1

Notes: Single-ended retractor with scoop-blunt edge

FIGURE 8-94

Sims vaginal retractor double end

Size: Small; Medium; Large

Quantity: 1

Notes: Scoop-blunt edge; Both blades face same direction

FIGURE 8-95

Dilation and Curettage-Cervix Procedural Instrumentation –
APPROXIMATION AND CLOSURE INSTRUMENTS

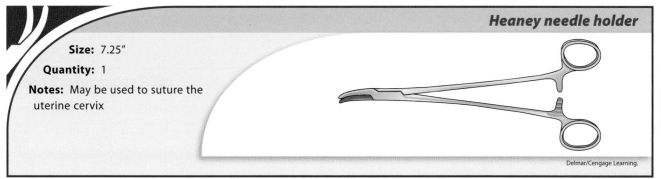

Heaney needle holder

Size: 7.25″

Quantity: 1

Notes: May be used to suture the uterine cervix

FIGURE 8-96

continues

Dilation and Curettage-Cervix Procedural Instrumentation – **APPROXIMATION AND CLOSURE INSTRUMENTS** *continued*

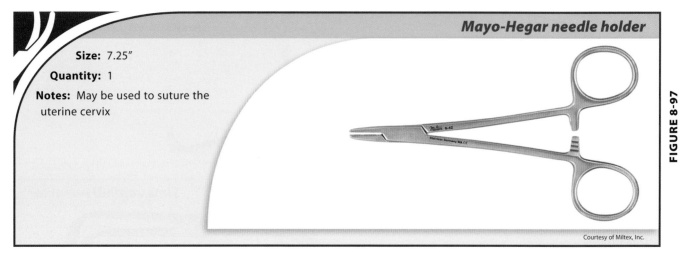

Mayo-Hegar needle holder

Size: 7.25″

Quantity: 1

Notes: May be used to suture the uterine cervix

Courtesy of Miltex, Inc.

FIGURE 8-97

Dilation and Curettage-Cervix Procedural Instrumentation – **SPECIALTY SPECIFIC INSTRUMENTS**

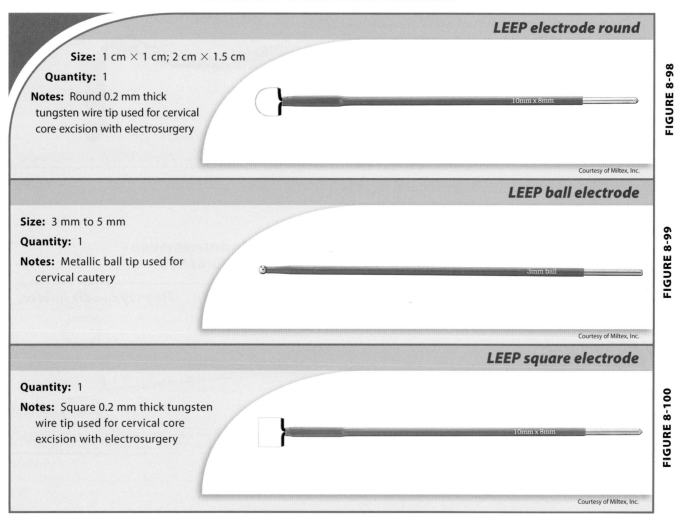

LEEP electrode round

Size: 1 cm × 1 cm; 2 cm × 1.5 cm

Quantity: 1

Notes: Round 0.2 mm thick tungsten wire tip used for cervical core excision with electrosurgery

10mm x 8mm

Courtesy of Miltex, Inc.

FIGURE 8-98

LEEP ball electrode

Size: 3 mm to 5 mm

Quantity: 1

Notes: Metallic ball tip used for cervical cautery

3mm ball

Courtesy of Miltex, Inc.

FIGURE 8-99

LEEP square electrode

Quantity: 1

Notes: Square 0.2 mm thick tungsten wire tip used for cervical core excision with electrosurgery

10mm x 8mm

Courtesy of Miltex, Inc.

FIGURE 8-100

Vaginal Hysterectomy Instrumentation

Vaginal hysterectomy instruments are usually long and curved. The long fundamental set with added vaginal retractors provides the exposure and manipulation needed to remove the uterus and ovaries as appropriate.

Vaginal Hysterectomy Instrumentation – CLAMPS

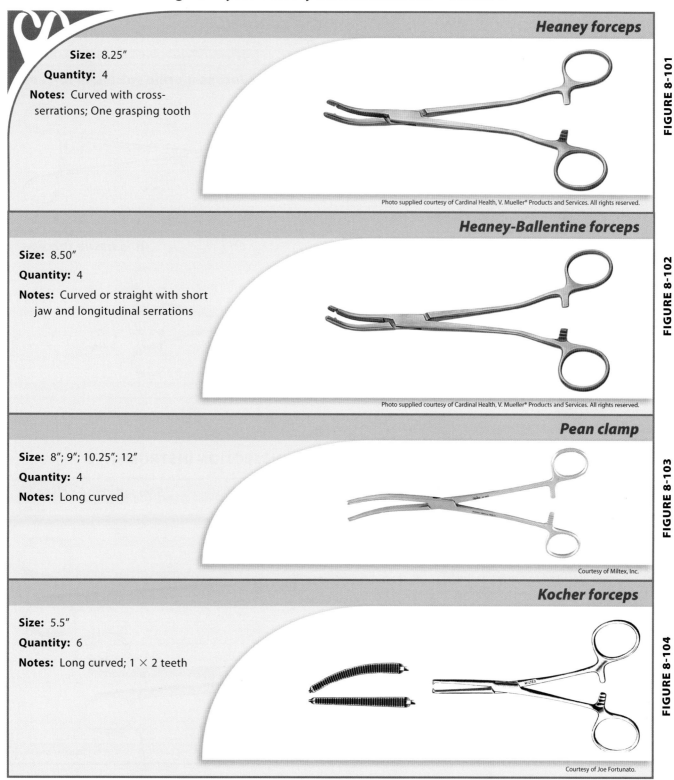

Heaney forceps

Size: 8.25″

Quantity: 4

Notes: Curved with cross-serrations; One grasping tooth

Photo supplied courtesy of Cardinal Health, V. Mueller® Products and Services. All rights reserved.

FIGURE 8-101

Heaney-Ballentine forceps

Size: 8.50″

Quantity: 4

Notes: Curved or straight with short jaw and longitudinal serrations

Photo supplied courtesy of Cardinal Health, V. Mueller® Products and Services. All rights reserved.

FIGURE 8-102

Pean clamp

Size: 8″; 9″; 10.25″; 12″

Quantity: 4

Notes: Long curved

Courtesy of Miltex, Inc.

FIGURE 8-103

Kocher forceps

Size: 5.5″

Quantity: 6

Notes: Long curved; 1 × 2 teeth

Courtesy of Joe Fortunato.

FIGURE 8-104

Vaginal Hysterectomy Instrumentation – GRASPING FORCEPS

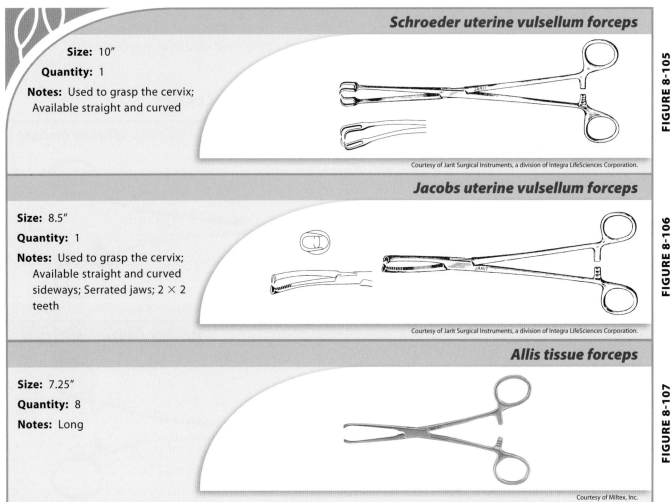

Schroeder uterine vulsellum forceps

Size: 10"

Quantity: 1

Notes: Used to grasp the cervix; Available straight and curved

Courtesy of Jarit Surgical Instruments, a division of Integra LifeSciences Corporation.

FIGURE 8-105

Jacobs uterine vulsellum forceps

Size: 8.5"

Quantity: 1

Notes: Used to grasp the cervix; Available straight and curved sideways; Serrated jaws; 2 × 2 teeth

Courtesy of Jarit Surgical Instruments, a division of Integra LifeSciences Corporation.

FIGURE 8-106

Allis tissue forceps

Size: 7.25"

Quantity: 8

Notes: Long

Courtesy of Miltex, Inc.

FIGURE 8-107

Vaginal Hysterectomy Instrumentation – DISSECTION INSTRUMENTS

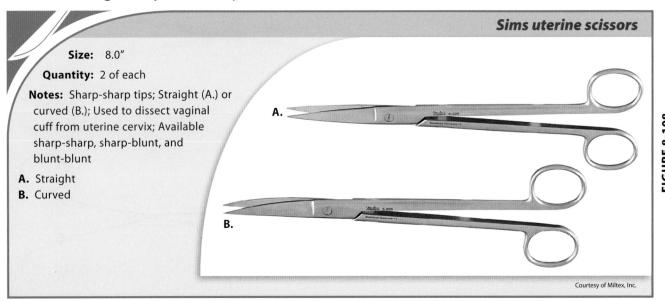

Sims uterine scissors

Size: 8.0"

Quantity: 2 of each

Notes: Sharp-sharp tips; Straight (A.) or curved (B.); Used to dissect vaginal cuff from uterine cervix; Available sharp-sharp, sharp-blunt, and blunt-blunt

A. Straight
B. Curved

Courtesy of Miltex, Inc.

FIGURE 8-108

Vaginal Hysterectomy Instrumentation – DISSECTION INSTRUMENTS *continued*

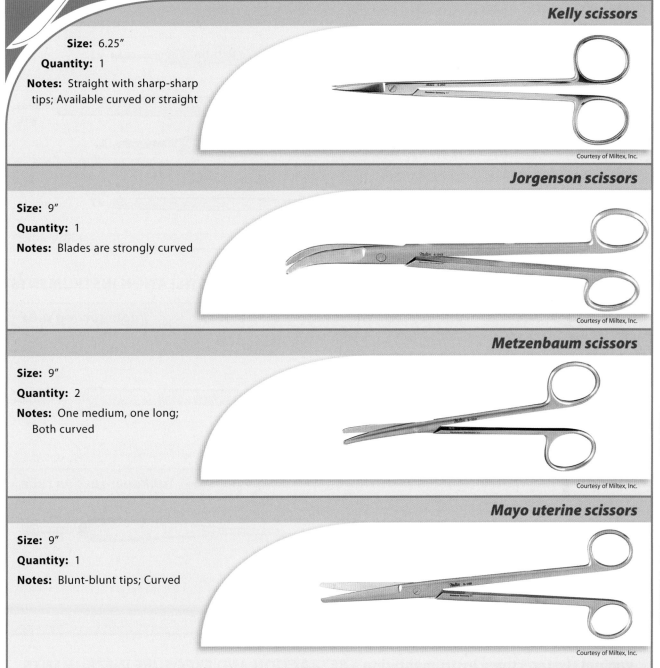

Kelly scissors

Size: 6.25″

Quantity: 1

Notes: Straight with sharp-sharp tips; Available curved or straight

Courtesy of Miltex, Inc.

FIGURE 8-109

Jorgenson scissors

Size: 9″

Quantity: 1

Notes: Blades are strongly curved

Courtesy of Miltex, Inc.

FIGURE 8-110

Metzenbaum scissors

Size: 9″

Quantity: 2

Notes: One medium, one long; Both curved

Courtesy of Miltex, Inc.

FIGURE 8-111

Mayo uterine scissors

Size: 9″

Quantity: 1

Notes: Blunt-blunt tips; Curved

Courtesy of Miltex, Inc.

FIGURE 8-112

continues

Vaginal Hysterectomy Instrumentation – DISSECTION INSTRUMENTS *continued*

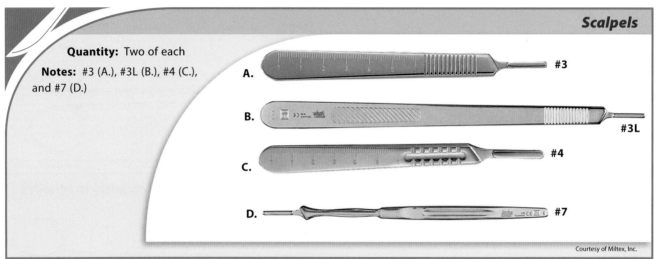

Scalpels

Quantity: Two of each

Notes: #3 (A.), #3L (B.), #4 (C.), and #7 (D.)

A. #3

B. #3L

C. #4

D. #7

Courtesy of Miltex, Inc.

FIGURE 8-113

Vaginal Hysterectomy Instrumentation – EVACUATION AND INSTILLATION INSTRUMENTS

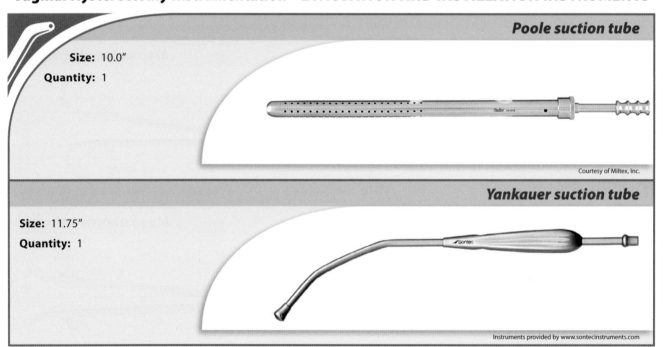

Poole suction tube

Size: 10.0"

Quantity: 1

Courtesy of Miltex, Inc.

FIGURE 8-114

Yankauer suction tube

Size: 11.75"

Quantity: 1

Instruments provided by www.sontecinstruments.com

FIGURE 8-115

Vaginal Hysterectomy Instrumentation – RETRACTION AND EXPOSURE INSTRUMENTS

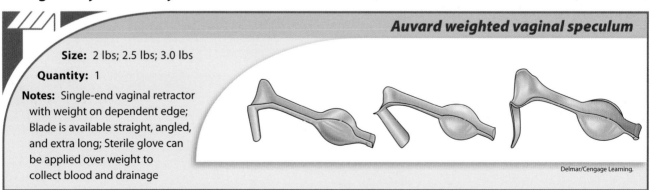

Auvard weighted vaginal speculum

Size: 2 lbs; 2.5 lbs; 3.0 lbs

Quantity: 1

Notes: Single-end vaginal retractor with weight on dependent edge; Blade is available straight, angled, and extra long; Sterile glove can be applied over weight to collect blood and drainage

Delmar/Cengage Learning.

FIGURE 8-116

Vaginal Hysterectomy Instrumentation – RETRACTION AND EXPOSURE INSTRUMENTS *continued*

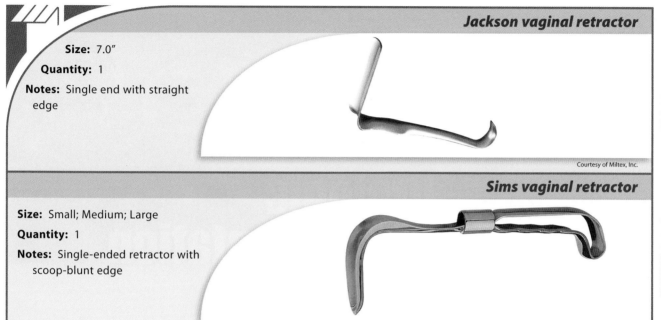

Jackson vaginal retractor

Size: 7.0"

Quantity: 1

Notes: Single end with straight edge

Courtesy of Miltex, Inc.

FIGURE 8-117

Sims vaginal retractor

Size: Small; Medium; Large

Quantity: 1

Notes: Single-ended retractor with scoop-blunt edge

Photo supplied courtesy of Cardinal Health, V. Mueller® Products and Services. All rights reserved.

FIGURE 8-118

Vaginal Hysterectomy Instrumentation – APPROXIMATION AND CLOSURE INSTRUMENTS

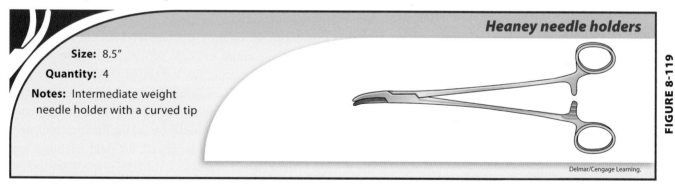

Heaney needle holders

Size: 8.5"

Quantity: 4

Notes: Intermediate weight needle holder with a curved tip

Delmar/Cengage Learning.

FIGURE 8-119

SUMMARY

Gynecologic procedures require many of the same instruments as are commonly used in other intra-abdominal surgical procedures—such as general surgery—with the exception of heavy hemostatic clamps and graspers. The surgical approach can involve open and endoscopic methods that complement each other and can be used in combination to remove, repair, or remodel the female reproductive system. Keep in mind that the surgeon may need to perform an intravaginal procedure as part of an abdominal open or endoscopic surgery. Preparation of dilation and curettage (D&C) instrumentation may be necessary. In select surgeries it may be advisable to have a D&C set available on the case cart just in case.

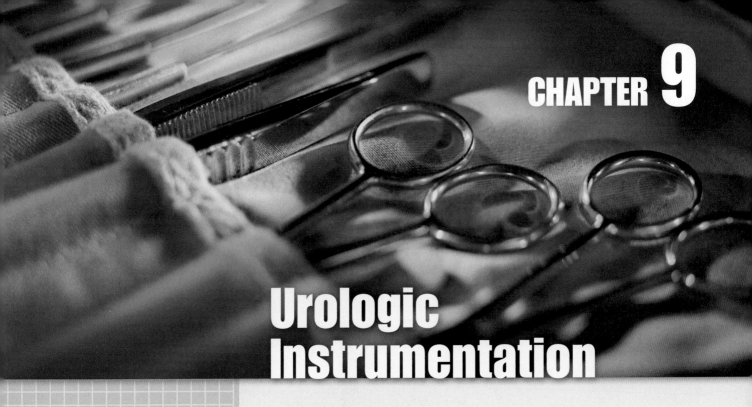

CHAPTER **9**

Urologic Instrumentation

INTRODUCTION

Urologic surgical procedures commonly use multiple modalities. Soft tissue surgery associated with urology will require the use of medium and long foundation sets with the addition of dilation and probing instruments if the tubular anatomic components, such as the ureters or urethra, are entered.

An endoscopic cystoscopy set up on a separate table should be prepared and maintained throughout the entire urologic procedure because periodic examination of the continuity and integrity of the urinary system will be performed. The table should be pushed to the side when not in use and left intact until the case is completed. The circulating nurse will keep an accurate record of the fluid expansion medium (commonly sterile water) instilled and returned. This is important because the patient may be at risk for fluid retention and overload if the urinary system has an occult leak into the preperitoneum, intraperitoneal cavity, or retroperitoneum. The peritoneal membrane can absorb and diffuse electrolytes, causing an imbalance in the patient. Severe imbalances can cause the susceptible patient to develop congestive heart failure.

OPEN UROLOGY INSTRUMENTATION

Open surgical procedures performed on the urinary system require the use of clamps and graspers that are angled or curved to accommodate the position and shape of the target organs. Male genitourinary procedures are commonly included in the urologic specialty service. In addition, most female reproductive organ procedures are included in the gynecologic specialty service described in Chapter 8. Endoscopic instrumentation for the genitourinary systems of both sexes is described in Chapter 15.

Nephrectomy, Cystectomy, and Prostatectomy Instrumentation

Surgical procedures involving the kidneys, bladder, and prostate are performed using the medium and long foundation sets from Chapter 5 with the inclusion of the following add-on set. Patients with a large body habitus may require the use of the optional extra long add-on set.

Nephrectomy, Cystectomy, and Prostatectomy Instrumentation – CLAMPS

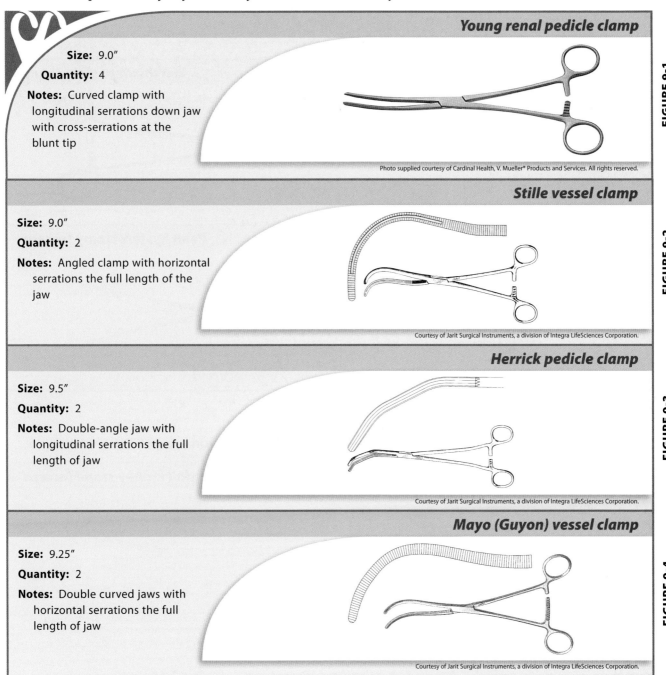

Young renal pedicle clamp

Size: 9.0″

Quantity: 4

Notes: Curved clamp with longitudinal serrations down jaw with cross-serrations at the blunt tip

FIGURE 9-1

Stille vessel clamp

Size: 9.0″

Quantity: 2

Notes: Angled clamp with horizontal serrations the full length of the jaw

FIGURE 9-2

Herrick pedicle clamp

Size: 9.5″

Quantity: 2

Notes: Double-angle jaw with longitudinal serrations the full length of jaw

FIGURE 9-3

Mayo (Guyon) vessel clamp

Size: 9.25″

Quantity: 2

Notes: Double curved jaws with horizontal serrations the full length of jaw

FIGURE 9-4

continues

Nephrectomy, Cystectomy, and Prostatectomy Instrumentation – CLAMPS *continued*

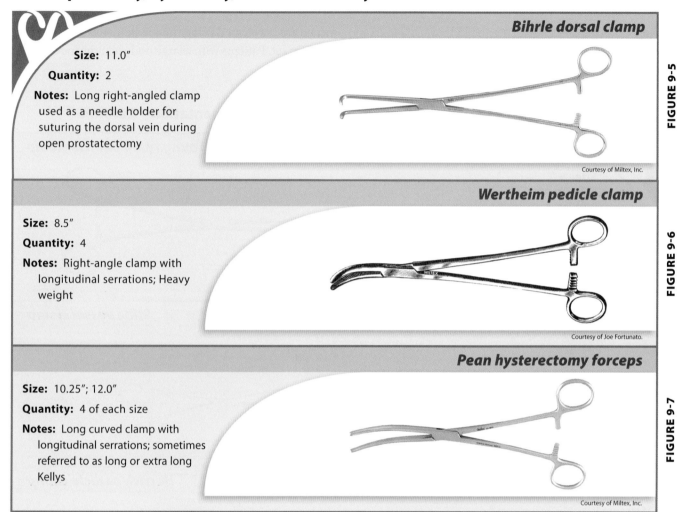

Bihrle dorsal clamp

Size: 11.0″

Quantity: 2

Notes: Long right-angled clamp used as a needle holder for suturing the dorsal vein during open prostatectomy

Courtesy of Miltex, Inc.

FIGURE 9-5

Wertheim pedicle clamp

Size: 8.5″

Quantity: 4

Notes: Right-angle clamp with longitudinal serrations; Heavy weight

Courtesy of Joe Fortunato.

FIGURE 9-6

Pean hysterectomy forceps

Size: 10.25″; 12.0″

Quantity: 4 of each size

Notes: Long curved clamp with longitudinal serrations; sometimes referred to as long or extra long Kellys

Courtesy of Miltex, Inc.

FIGURE 9-7

Nephrectomy, Cystectomy, and Prostatectomy Instrumentation – GRASPING FORCEPS

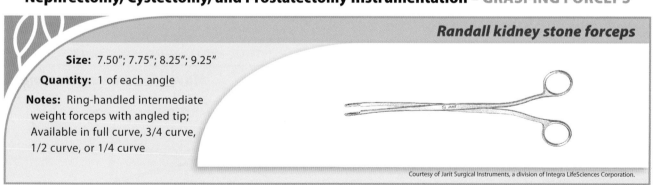

Randall kidney stone forceps

Size: 7.50″; 7.75″; 8.25″; 9.25″

Quantity: 1 of each angle

Notes: Ring-handled intermediate weight forceps with angled tip; Available in full curve, 3/4 curve, 1/2 curve, or 1/4 curve

Courtesy of Jarit Surgical Instruments, a division of Integra LifeSciences Corporation.

FIGURE 9-8

Nephrectomy, Cystectomy, and Prostatectomy Instrumentation – GRASPING FORCEPS *continued*

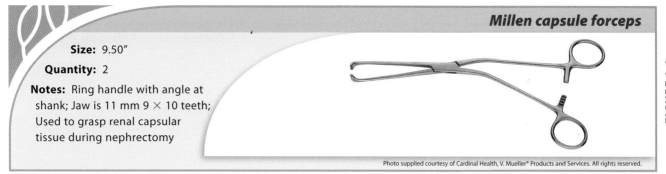

Millen capsule forceps

Size: 9.50″

Quantity: 2

Notes: Ring handle with angle at shank; Jaw is 11 mm 9 × 10 teeth; Used to grasp renal capsular tissue during nephrectomy

FIGURE 9-9

Nephrectomy, Cystectomy, and Prostatectomy Instrumentation – DISSECTION INSTRUMENTS

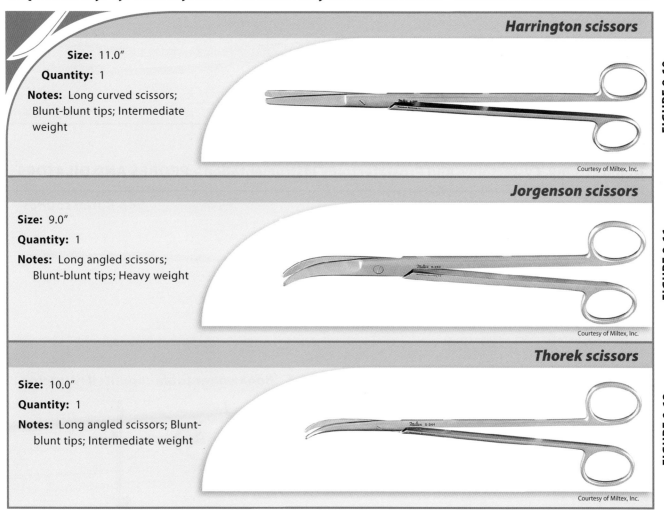

Harrington scissors

Size: 11.0″

Quantity: 1

Notes: Long curved scissors; Blunt-blunt tips; Intermediate weight

FIGURE 9-10

Jorgenson scissors

Size: 9.0″

Quantity: 1

Notes: Long angled scissors; Blunt-blunt tips; Heavy weight

FIGURE 9-11

Thorek scissors

Size: 10.0″

Quantity: 1

Notes: Long angled scissors; Blunt-blunt tips; Intermediate weight

FIGURE 9-12

continues

Nephrectomy, Cystectomy, and Prostatectomy Instrumentation –
DISSECTION INSTRUMENTS *continued*

Metzenbaum-Nelson scissors

Size: 11.0"; 14.0"

Quantity: 1 of each size

Notes: Long curved scissors; Blunt-blunt tips; Light weight

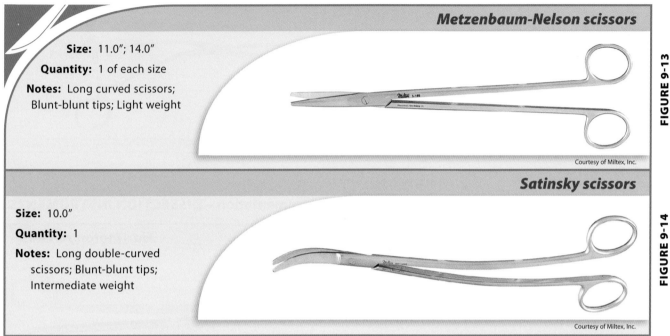

Courtesy of Miltex, Inc.

FIGURE 9-13

Satinsky scissors

Size: 10.0"

Quantity: 1

Notes: Long double-curved scissors; Blunt-blunt tips; Intermediate weight

Courtesy of Miltex, Inc.

FIGURE 9-14

Nephrectomy, Cystectomy, and Prostatectomy Instrumentation – PROBES AND DILATORS

Van Buren sounds

Size: 11.0"; Set of 12 Sized 8 fr to 30 fr

Quantity: 1 set

Notes: Used in male patients; Can be used to probe the prostatic urethra from the inferior or superior angle during open prostatectomy; Curved, single-ended

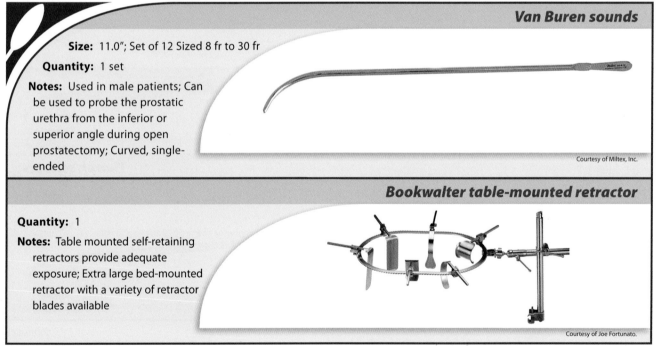

Courtesy of Miltex, Inc.

FIGURE 9-15

Bookwalter table-mounted retractor

Quantity: 1

Notes: Table mounted self-retaining retractors provide adequate exposure; Extra large bed-mounted retractor with a variety of retractor blades available

Courtesy of Joe Fortunato.

FIGURE 9-16

Nephrectomy, Cystectomy, and Prostatectomy Instrumentation –
RETRACTION AND EXPOSURE INSTRUMENTS

Masson-Judd bladder retractor

Quantity: 1

Notes: Self-retaining bladder retractor with two 1" swivel blades 1" center blade available

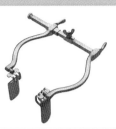

FIGURE 9-17

Table-mounted retractor ring with blades

Notes: Any large table-mounted retractor with a variety of blades such as Kelly, Harrington, Deaver, and malleable

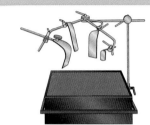

Delmar/Cengage Learning.

FIGURE 9-18

Kelly retractor

Size: 10.0"

Quantity: 2

Notes: Wide right-angle manual body wall retractor; Finger ridge handle; Heavy weight; Resembles a Richardson retractor

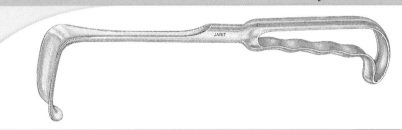

FIGURE 9-19

Foss retractor

Size: 10.0"

Quantity: 1

Notes: Wide curved manual body wall retractor; Malleable 1.75" wide blade

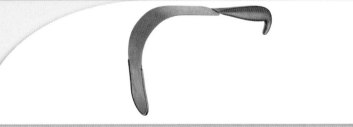

FIGURE 9-20

Harrington retractor

Size: 12.0"

Quantity: 2

Notes: Wide curved manual body wall retractor; Malleable 2.5" wide blade with blunted heart-shaped tip

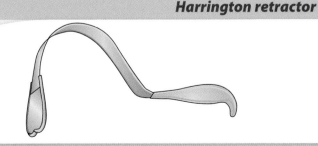

Delmar/Cengage Learning.

FIGURE 9-21

continues

Nephrectomy, Cystectomy, and Prostatectomy Instrumentation – RETRACTION AND EXPOSURE INSTRUMENTS *continued*

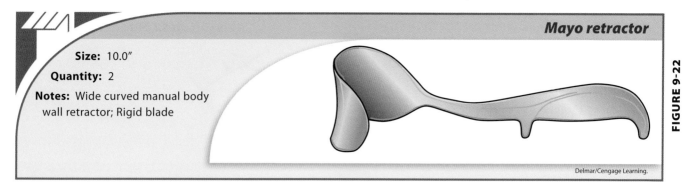

Mayo retractor

Size: 10.0"

Quantity: 2

Notes: Wide curved manual body wall retractor; Rigid blade

Delmar/Cengage Learning.

FIGURE 9-22

Nephrectomy, Cystectomy, and Prostatectomy Instrumentation – APPROXIMATION AND CLOSURE INSTRUMENTS

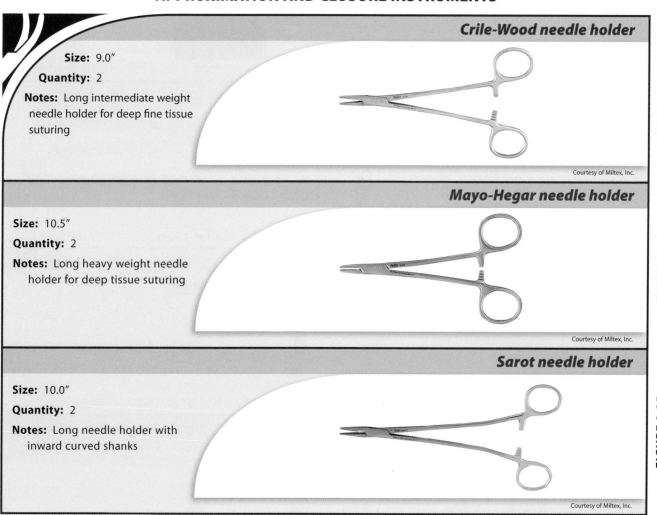

Crile-Wood needle holder

Size: 9.0"

Quantity: 2

Notes: Long intermediate weight needle holder for deep fine tissue suturing

Courtesy of Miltex, Inc.

FIGURE 9-23

Mayo-Hegar needle holder

Size: 10.5"

Quantity: 2

Notes: Long heavy weight needle holder for deep tissue suturing

Courtesy of Miltex, Inc.

FIGURE 9-24

Sarot needle holder

Size: 10.0"

Quantity: 2

Notes: Long needle holder with inward curved shanks

Courtesy of Miltex, Inc.

FIGURE 9-25

Nephrectomy, Cystectomy, and Prostatectomy Instrumentation –
APPROXIMATION AND CLOSURE INSTRUMENTS *continued*

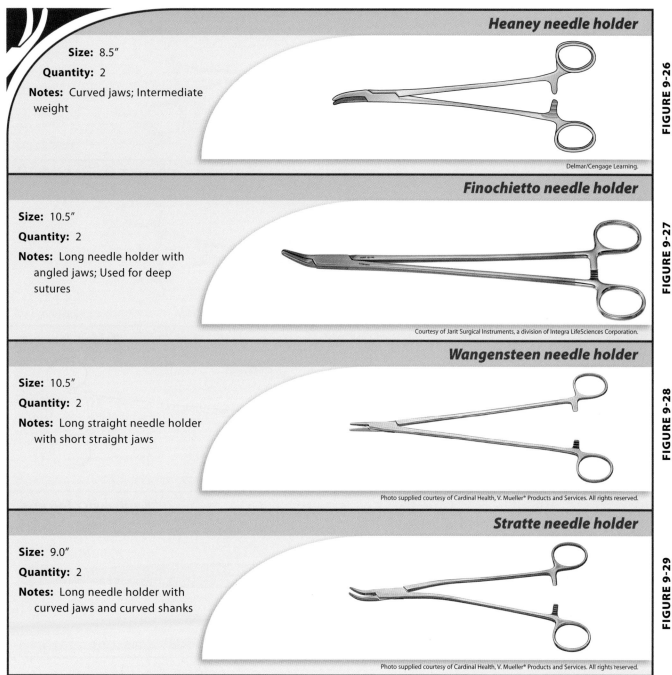

Heaney needle holder

Size: 8.5″

Quantity: 2

Notes: Curved jaws; Intermediate weight

Delmar/Cengage Learning.

FIGURE 9-26

Finochietto needle holder

Size: 10.5″

Quantity: 2

Notes: Long needle holder with angled jaws; Used for deep sutures

Courtesy of Jarit Surgical Instruments, a division of Integra LifeSciences Corporation.

FIGURE 9-27

Wangensteen needle holder

Size: 10.5″

Quantity: 2

Notes: Long straight needle holder with short straight jaws

Photo supplied courtesy of Cardinal Health, V. Mueller® Products and Services. All rights reserved.

FIGURE 9-28

Stratte needle holder

Size: 9.0″

Quantity: 2

Notes: Long needle holder with curved jaws and curved shanks

Photo supplied courtesy of Cardinal Health, V. Mueller® Products and Services. All rights reserved.

FIGURE 9-29

Testicular Instrumentation

Testicular procedures do not require long instrumentation unless there is crypt orchidism or neoplasm involving the deep inguinal lymph nodes. Short and medium foundation sets have adequate instrumentation for most testicular procedures. This particularly includes orchiectomy and vasectomy, which are commonly performed in most ORs. Dissection may require the addition of the following instrumentation.

Testicular Instrumentation – CLAMPS

Hartman Lee mosquito clamp

Size: 3.5"

Quantity: 4

Notes: Mosquito style clamp with angled shanks used for tagging suture at the level of the tunica

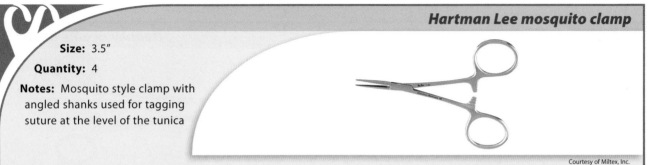

Courtesy of Miltex, Inc.

FIGURE 9-30

Pratt T-shape forceps

Size: 6.0"

Quantity: 6

Notes: Ring-handled clamp with multi-toothed tip used for holding tissue edges

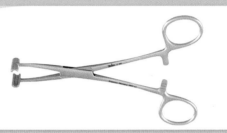

Courtesy of Miltex, Inc.

FIGURE 9-31

Bridge forceps

Size: 11.0"

Quantity: 2

Notes: Long curved clamp; Intermediate weight; Short serrated jaw; Used for deeper grasping

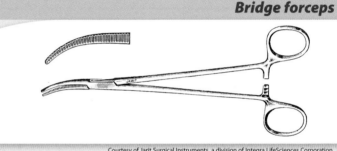

Courtesy of Jarit Surgical Instruments, a division of Integra LifeSciences Corporation.

FIGURE 9-32

Kantrowitz forceps

Size: 11.0"

Quantity: 2

Notes: Long right angle clamp; Intermediate weight; Short serrated jaw; Used for deeper grasping or passing ties

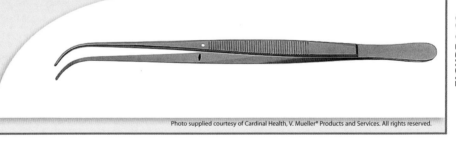

Photo supplied courtesy of Cardinal Health, V. Mueller® Products and Services. All rights reserved.

FIGURE 9-33

Testicular Instrumentation – SPECIALTY SPECIFIC INSTRUMENTS

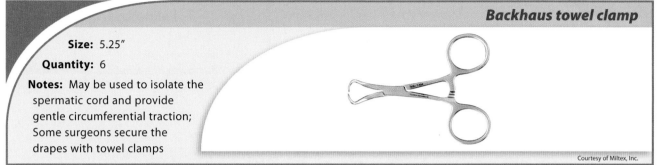

Backhaus towel clamp

Size: 5.25″

Quantity: 6

Notes: May be used to isolate the spermatic cord and provide gentle circumferential traction; Some surgeons secure the drapes with towel clamps

Courtesy of Miltex, Inc.

FIGURE 9-34

Uroplasty Instrumentation

Uroplasty involves repair or reconstruction of the meatus and/or the full length of the urethra. The extent of the procedure and the body size of the patient will determine the type of instrumentation necessary for the procedure. The short foundation set is usually all that is needed for meatal procedures. However, if the full urethra is involved, such as in hypospadius, then the surgeon may need elements of the medium or long foundation sets. The following instruments are useful additions for open urethroplasty. The surgeon may want an assortment of Robinson and Foley catheters on the sterile field. Endoscopic instrumentation for cystoscopy is described in Chapter 15.

Uroplasty Instrumentation – PROBES AND DILATORS

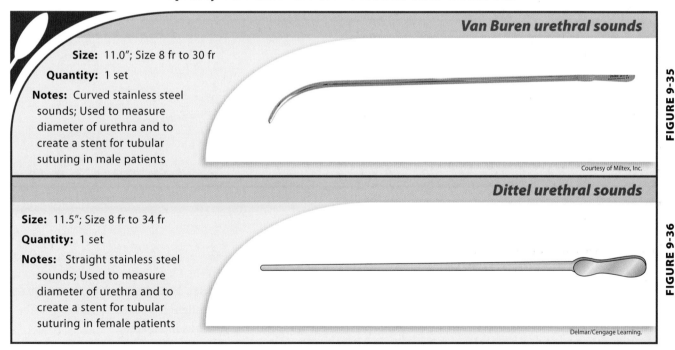

Van Buren urethral sounds

Size: 11.0″; Size 8 fr to 30 fr

Quantity: 1 set

Notes: Curved stainless steel sounds; Used to measure diameter of urethra and to create a stent for tubular suturing in male patients

Courtesy of Miltex, Inc.

FIGURE 9-35

Dittel urethral sounds

Size: 11.5″; Size 8 fr to 34 fr

Quantity: 1 set

Notes: Straight stainless steel sounds; Used to measure diameter of urethra and to create a stent for tubular suturing in female patients

Delmar/Cengage Learning.

FIGURE 9-36

continues

Uroplasty Instrumentation – PROBES AND DILATORS *continued*

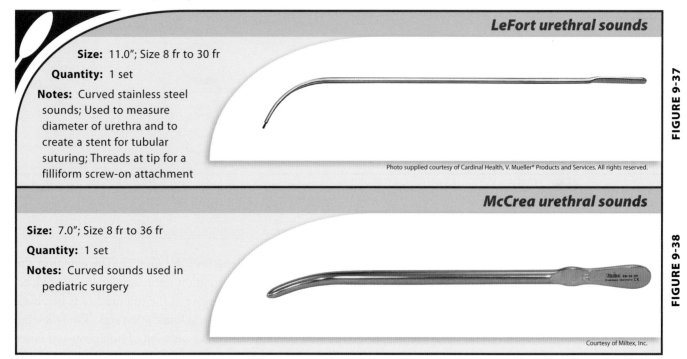

LeFort urethral sounds

Size: 11.0"; Size 8 fr to 30 fr

Quantity: 1 set

Notes: Curved stainless steel sounds; Used to measure diameter of urethra and to create a stent for tubular suturing; Threads at tip for a filliform screw-on attachment

Photo supplied courtesy of Cardinal Health, V. Mueller® Products and Services. All rights reserved.

FIGURE 9-37

McCrea urethral sounds

Size: 7.0"; Size 8 fr to 36 fr

Quantity: 1 set

Notes: Curved sounds used in pediatric surgery

Courtesy of Miltex, Inc.

FIGURE 9-38

Uroplasty Instrumentation – APPROXIMATION AND CLOSURE INSTRUMENTS

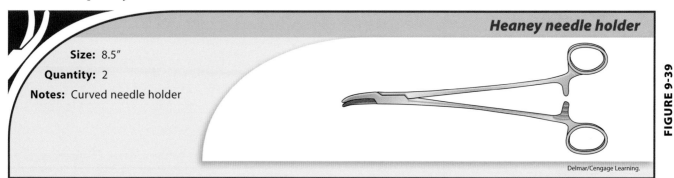

Heaney needle holder

Size: 8.5"

Quantity: 2

Notes: Curved needle holder

Delmar/Cengage Learning.

FIGURE 9-39

Circumcision

Adult circumcision of the male foreskin requires the use of a short foundation set. Pediatric circumcision utilizes minimal instrumentation with the exception of a glans cover, a hemostat or two, straight iris scissors, and a #7 scalpel with a #15 blade. Circumcision in older children is performed in a similar manner as in an adult.

Circumcision – PROBES AND DILATORS

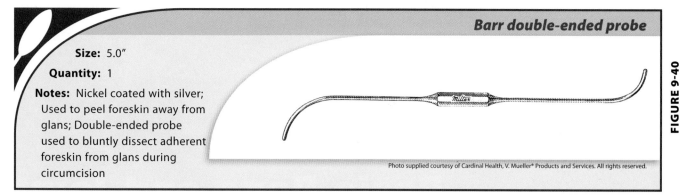

Barr double-ended probe

Size: 5.0″

Quantity: 1

Notes: Nickel coated with silver; Used to peel foreskin away from glans; Double-ended probe used to bluntly dissect adherent foreskin from glans during circumcision

FIGURE 9-40

Circumcision – SPECIALTY SPECIFIC INSTRUMENTS

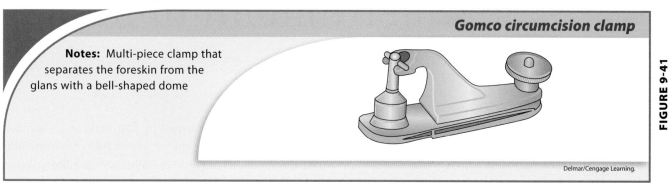

Gomco circumcision clamp

Notes: Multi-piece clamp that separates the foreskin from the glans with a bell-shaped dome

FIGURE 9-41

SUMMARY

Urologic surgery can combine open and endoscopic approaches during the same procedure. The importance of accuracy in procedural scheduling by the surgeon facilitates adequate preparation by the surgical team. When an open urologic procedure is scheduled without listing the need for a cystoscopy set-up, it is advisable to check with the surgeon before the case is started in order to prepare one. If checking with the surgeon in advance is not possible, a cystoscopy set with the necessary illumination source and expansion medium can be placed on the case cart as "have available" items and not opened unless actually needed. This saves valuable time if the set is suddenly needed by preventing the gathering of last minute supplies by the circulating nurse.

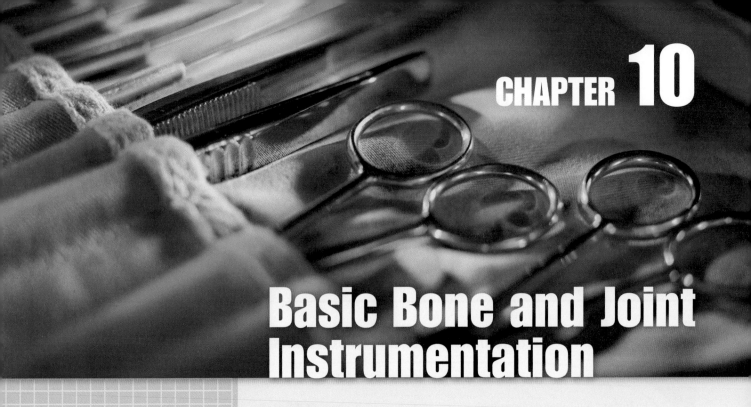

CHAPTER **10**

Basic Bone and Joint Instrumentation

INTRODUCTION

Basic bone and joint procedures are performed by first making an incision into the overlying soft tissues. This requires the use of soft tissue instrumentation that is appropriate for the depth of tissue to be incised and the position and type of the target bony or compact tissue. Endoscopic instrumentation is not included in this chapter.

Compact bone is also referred to as cortical bone by many manufacturers. This type of bone is very solid and hard. In contrast, cancellous bone is softer and requires the use of specific instruments. Bone fragments are not permitted to remain in the surgical site at closure because they can become a barrier to wound healing. Irrigation is supplied during drilling to maintain clear vision and cooling of the bone. Casting materials are commonly used as rigid support of bone postoperatively.

PLASTER INSTRUMENTATION

Plaster and fiberglass casting material is commonly used for rigid stabilization of bone. Large or small quantities of this material require instrumentation with the ability to shape, restore, or remove the hard casing from the surgical site. Standard instrumentation is not adequate for the task. The following chart depicts the most common cast instrumentation that is not used for patient tissues. These items may be present or added to any compact or cancellous bone set.

Plaster Instrumentation – SPECIALTY SPECIFIC INSTRUMENTS

Lister bandage scissors

Size: 5.5"; 7.5"

Quantity: 1 of each

Notes: For cutting plaster or fabric; Protective tip

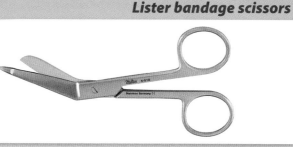

Courtesy of Miltex, Inc.

FIGURE 10-1

Utility scissors

Size: 7.5"

Quantity: 1

Notes: For cutting heavy non-metallic materials; Protective tip and larger thumb handle

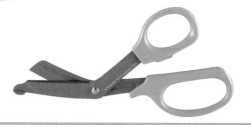

Courtesy of Miltex, Inc.

FIGURE 10-2

Hercules scissors

Size: 7.5"

Quantity: 1

Notes: Heavy scissors with serrations for cutting aluminum and plaster cast

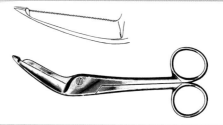

K-Medic branded instrumentation courtesy of Teleflex Medical, Inc.

FIGURE 10-3

Bruns shears

Size: 9.25"

Quantity: 1

Notes: Heavy shears with larger thumb handle and serrated lower blade

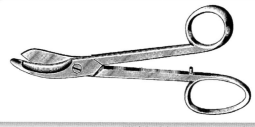

K-Medic branded instrumentation courtesy of Teleflex Medical, Inc.

FIGURE 10-4

Engel plaster saw

Size: 6.0"

Quantity: 1

Notes: Loop handle manual saw for cutting dried plaster cast; Stainless steel blade with chrome-plated handle

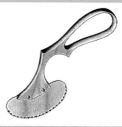

K-Medic branded instrumentation courtesy of Teleflex Medical, Inc.

FIGURE 10-5

continues

Plaster Instrumentation – SPECIALTY SPECIFIC INSTRUMENTS *continued*

Reiner plaster knife

Size: 7.0"

Quantity: 1

Notes: Angled knife used to slice section of dried plaster cast

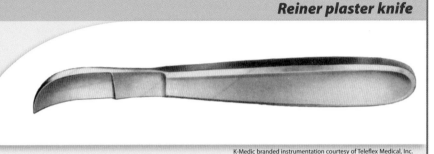

K-Medic branded instrumentation courtesy of Teleflex Medical, Inc.

FIGURE 10-6

Pediatric cast breaker

Size: 7.0"

Quantity: 1

Notes: Serrated duckbill tips on a spring handle used to trim cast edges

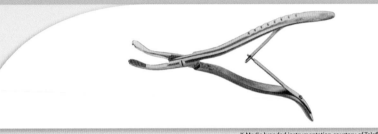

K-Medic branded instrumentation courtesy of Teleflex Medical, Inc.

FIGURE 10-7

Wolff-Boehler plaster breaker

Size: 7.0"; 9.0"

Quantity: 1

Notes: Heavier serrated tips on spring handle used to trim and break away cast edges

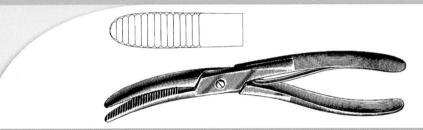

K-Medic branded instrumentation courtesy of Teleflex Medical, Inc.

FIGURE 10-8

Walton cast spreader

Size: 9.0"

Quantity: 1

Notes: Three-pronged opposition tips used with one hand to spread and remove cast; Serrated tips for traction on surface

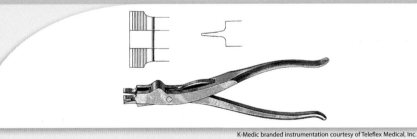

K-Medic branded instrumentation courtesy of Teleflex Medical, Inc.

FIGURE 10-9

Hennig plaster spreader

Size: 11.0"

Quantity: 1

Notes: Manual cast spreader used with one hand in opposition to opening in cast; Large casts

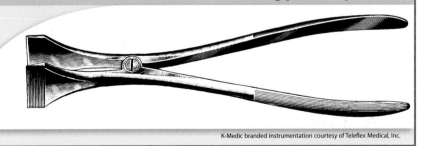

K-Medic branded instrumentation courtesy of Teleflex Medical, Inc.

FIGURE 10-10

Plaster Instrumentation – SPECIALTY SPECIFIC INSTRUMENTS *continued*

Stille plaster shears

Size: 15.0"

Quantity: 1

Notes: Two-hand operation; Cuts large casts with scissors-like action with one serrated and one sharp blade; Good for body casts

Courtesy of Jarit Surgical Instruments, a division of Integra LifeSciences Corporation.

FIGURE 10-11

PLATES AND SCREWS

Generic plates and screws are described here only for style. Each manufacturer has specific attributes and materials suitable for patient bone fixation, such as stainless steel or titanium. Most facilities and surgeons refer to these collective materials as "hardware." Keep in mind that the use of plates and screws requires instrumentation for measuring, positioning, tapping, drilling, inserting, countersinking, and affixing the implanted device regardless of site. The number and configuration of threads on the screws will vary according to type and size.

Removal of the implanted hardware will in turn require the use of specific screwdrivers or removal instrumentation appropriate for the type of implant in place. Use of the wrong removal tools can result in broken or stuck screws. The retained hardware can act as a mechanical barrier to surgical site healing.

Plates and screws are treated as implants because they are retained for a prolonged period of time within the patient's body. Biological monitoring is essential for in-house assembled sets of plates and screws. Infection around an implanted site can lead to osteomyelitis and failure to heal. Prepackaged screws and plates that have been sterilized by the manufacturer are preferred. The following chart lists commonly used styles of implants and their associated instrumentation without preference for one brand over the other.

Pins and Wires – SPECIALTY SPECIFIC INSTRUMENTS

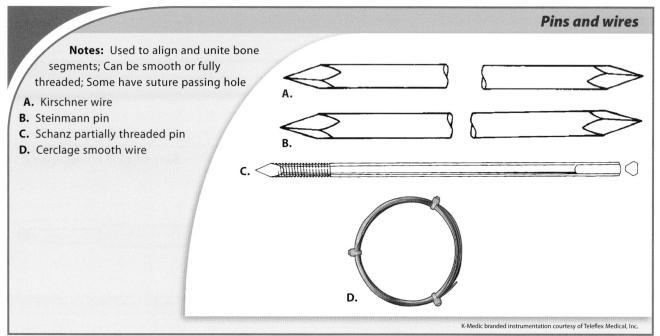

Pins and wires

Notes: Used to align and unite bone segments; Can be smooth or fully threaded; Some have suture passing hole

A. Kirschner wire
B. Steinmann pin
C. Schanz partially threaded pin
D. Cerclage smooth wire

A.

B.

C.

D.

K-Medic branded instrumentation courtesy of Teleflex Medical, Inc.

FIGURE 10-12

Other Devices – SPECIALTY SPECIFIC INSTRUMENTS

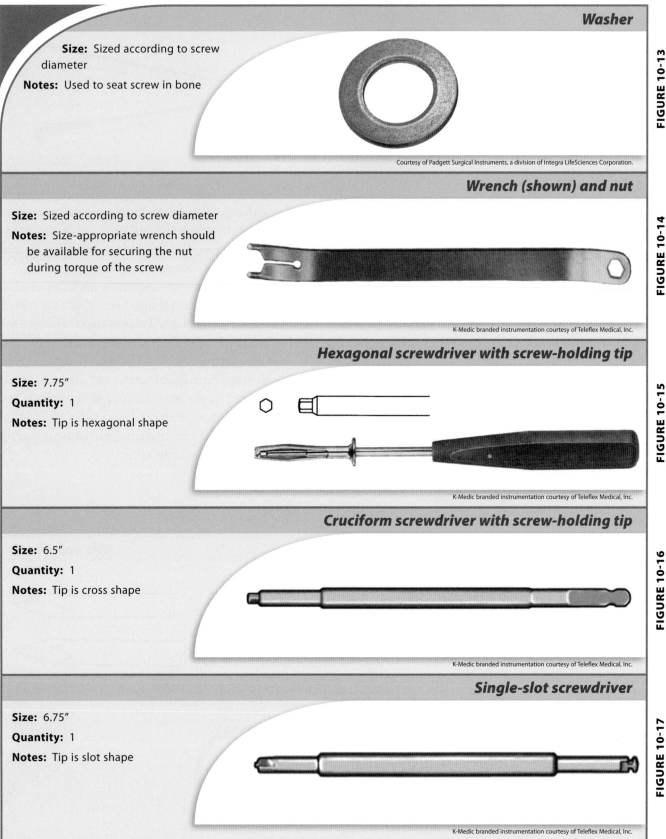

Washer

Size: Sized according to screw diameter

Notes: Used to seat screw in bone

Courtesy of Padgett Surgical Instruments, a division of Integra LifeSciences Corporation.

FIGURE 10-13

Wrench (shown) and nut

Size: Sized according to screw diameter

Notes: Size-appropriate wrench should be available for securing the nut during torque of the screw

K-Medic branded instrumentation courtesy of Teleflex Medical, Inc.

FIGURE 10-14

Hexagonal screwdriver with screw-holding tip

Size: 7.75"

Quantity: 1

Notes: Tip is hexagonal shape

K-Medic branded instrumentation courtesy of Teleflex Medical, Inc.

FIGURE 10-15

Cruciform screwdriver with screw-holding tip

Size: 6.5"

Quantity: 1

Notes: Tip is cross shape

K-Medic branded instrumentation courtesy of Teleflex Medical, Inc.

FIGURE 10-16

Single-slot screwdriver

Size: 6.75"

Quantity: 1

Notes: Tip is slot shape

K-Medic branded instrumentation courtesy of Teleflex Medical, Inc.

FIGURE 10-17

Other Devices – SPECIALTY SPECIFIC INSTRUMENTS *continued*

Plate-bending iron

Size: 5.0"; 5.5"; 9.5"

Quantity: 2 of each size

Notes: Used for custom bending of implantable plate on the sterile field

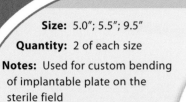
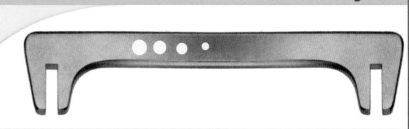

K-Medic branded instrumentation courtesy of Teleflex Medical, Inc.

FIGURE 10-18

Plate-bending pliers

Size: 5.0"

Quantity: 2

Notes: Pliers with flat tip for bending plates

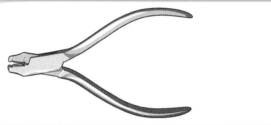

K-Medic branded instrumentation courtesy of Teleflex Medical, Inc.

FIGURE 10-19

Large plate-bending pliers

Size: 10.0"

Quantity: 2

Notes: Manual plate bending

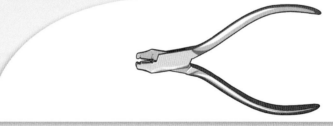

K-Medic branded instrumentation courtesy of Teleflex Medical, Inc.

FIGURE 10-20

Plate-bending pliers with interchangeable anvils

Size: 10.0"

Quantity: 2

Notes: Locking plate-bending pliers with interchangeable tips for wide or narrow plates

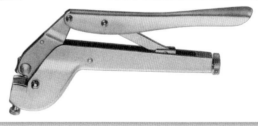

K-Medic branded instrumentation courtesy of Teleflex Medical, Inc.

FIGURE 10-21

French rod shaper

Size: 11.5"

Quantity: 2

Notes: Used to bend rods on the sterile field

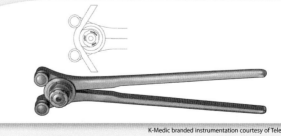

K-Medic branded instrumentation courtesy of Teleflex Medical, Inc.

FIGURE 10-22

continues

Other Devices – SPECIALTY SPECIFIC INSTRUMENTS *continued*

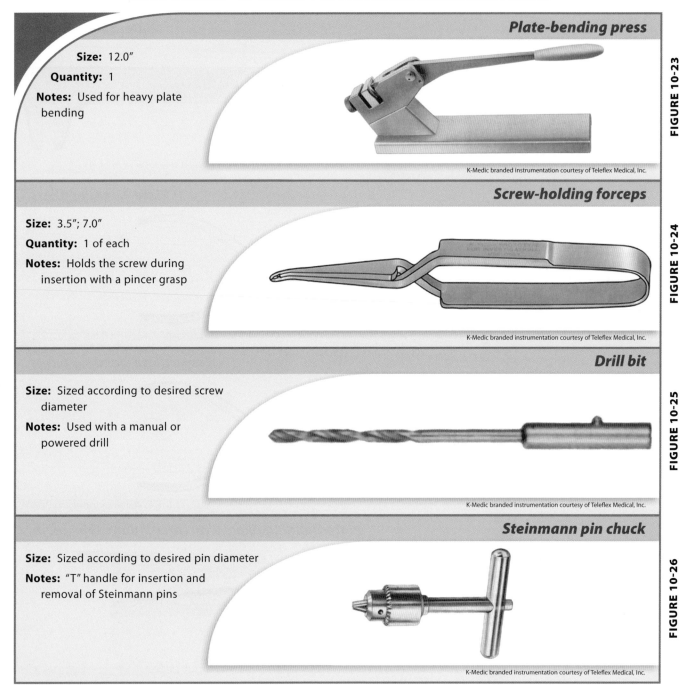

Plate-bending press

Size: 12.0″

Quantity: 1

Notes: Used for heavy plate bending

K-Medic branded instrumentation courtesy of Teleflex Medical, Inc.

FIGURE 10-23

Screw-holding forceps

Size: 3.5″; 7.0″

Quantity: 1 of each

Notes: Holds the screw during insertion with a pincer grasp

K-Medic branded instrumentation courtesy of Teleflex Medical, Inc.

FIGURE 10-24

Drill bit

Size: Sized according to desired screw diameter

Notes: Used with a manual or powered drill

K-Medic branded instrumentation courtesy of Teleflex Medical, Inc.

FIGURE 10-25

Steinmann pin chuck

Size: Sized according to desired pin diameter

Notes: "T" handle for insertion and removal of Steinmann pins

K-Medic branded instrumentation courtesy of Teleflex Medical, Inc.

FIGURE 10-26

MANUAL DRILLS AND DEVICES

Some surgeons prefer to use manual drills to create holes for pins, wire, and screws. Cleaning, sterilization, and lubrication of these complex devices is performed according to manufacturer's recommendations.

Manual Drills and Devices – SPECIALTY SPECIFIC INSTRUMENTS

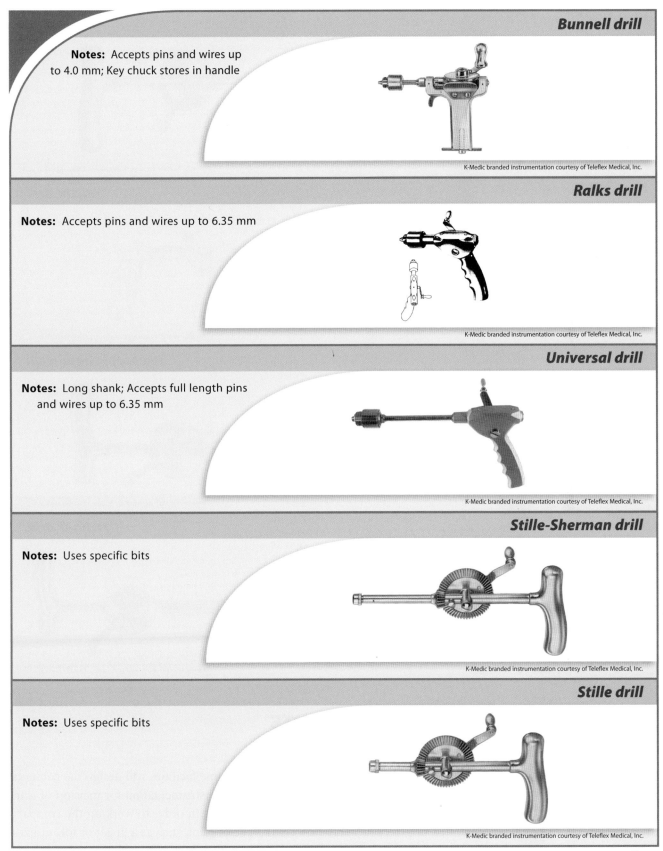

Bunnell drill

Notes: Accepts pins and wires up to 4.0 mm; Key chuck stores in handle

K-Medic branded instrumentation courtesy of Teleflex Medical, Inc.

FIGURE 10-27

Ralks drill

Notes: Accepts pins and wires up to 6.35 mm

K-Medic branded instrumentation courtesy of Teleflex Medical, Inc.

FIGURE 10-28

Universal drill

Notes: Long shank; Accepts full length pins and wires up to 6.35 mm

K-Medic branded instrumentation courtesy of Teleflex Medical, Inc.

FIGURE 10-29

Stille-Sherman drill

Notes: Uses specific bits

K-Medic branded instrumentation courtesy of Teleflex Medical, Inc.

FIGURE 10-30

Stille drill

Notes: Uses specific bits

K-Medic branded instrumentation courtesy of Teleflex Medical, Inc.

FIGURE 10-31

continues

Manual Drills and Devices – SPECIALTY SPECIFIC INSTRUMENTS *continued*

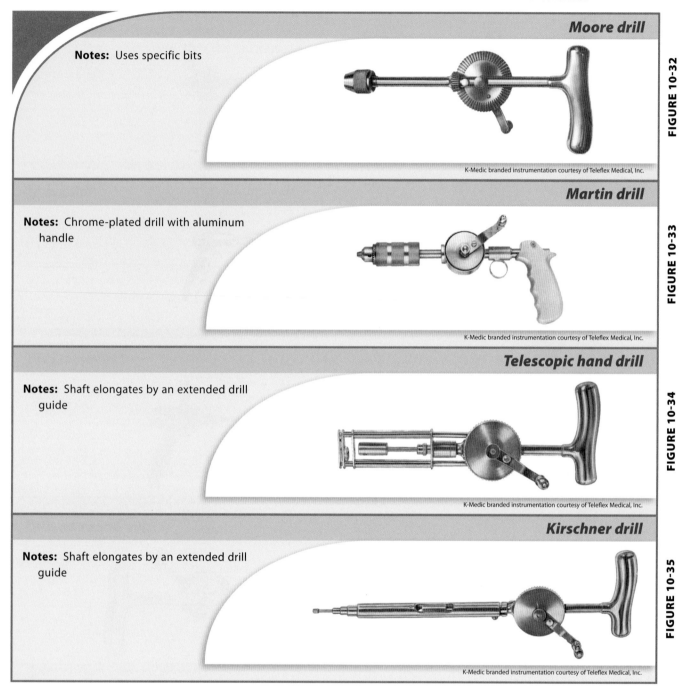

Moore drill

Notes: Uses specific bits

K-Medic branded instrumentation courtesy of Teleflex Medical, Inc.

FIGURE 10-32

Martin drill

Notes: Chrome-plated drill with aluminum handle

K-Medic branded instrumentation courtesy of Teleflex Medical, Inc.

FIGURE 10-33

Telescopic hand drill

Notes: Shaft elongates by an extended drill guide

K-Medic branded instrumentation courtesy of Teleflex Medical, Inc.

FIGURE 10-34

Kirschner drill

Notes: Shaft elongates by an extended drill guide

K-Medic branded instrumentation courtesy of Teleflex Medical, Inc.

FIGURE 10-35

SMALL BONE AND JOINT INSTRUMENTS

Small bones and joints can be accessed by the use of a short foundation set. Some facilities will design the contents of the small bone and joint sets to include the necessary soft tissue dissection instrumentation for incision of skin to periosteum. All soft tissue is incised to the level of the deepest periosteal layer in order to work on the compact and cancellous bony tissue. The intended surgical procedure on a small bone or joint, such as a finger or toe, utilizes instrumentation specialized for holding and grasping, debulking, cutting, probing, retracting, distracting, and approximating. The following chart lists a set designed for use as a basic small hand and foot bone and joint set. This collection can be used with an additional tray of soft tissue instruments.

Small Bone and Joint Instruments – CLAMPS

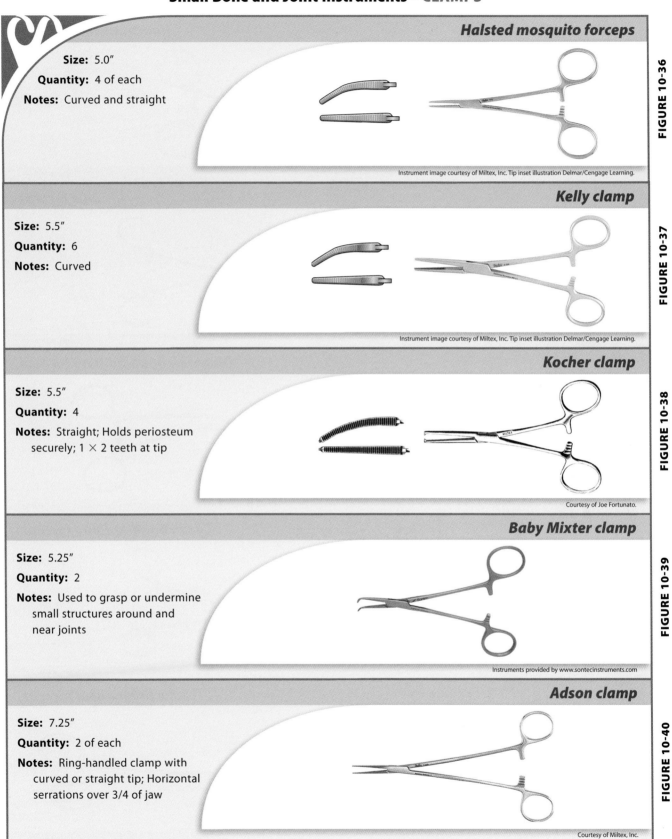

Halsted mosquito forceps

Size: 5.0"

Quantity: 4 of each

Notes: Curved and straight

Instrument image courtesy of Miltex, Inc. Tip inset illustration Delmar/Cengage Learning.

FIGURE 10-36

Kelly clamp

Size: 5.5"

Quantity: 6

Notes: Curved

Instrument image courtesy of Miltex, Inc. Tip inset illustration Delmar/Cengage Learning.

FIGURE 10-37

Kocher clamp

Size: 5.5"

Quantity: 4

Notes: Straight; Holds periosteum securely; 1 × 2 teeth at tip

Courtesy of Joe Fortunato.

FIGURE 10-38

Baby Mixter clamp

Size: 5.25"

Quantity: 2

Notes: Used to grasp or undermine small structures around and near joints

Instruments provided by www.sontecinstruments.com

FIGURE 10-39

Adson clamp

Size: 7.25"

Quantity: 2 of each

Notes: Ring-handled clamp with curved or straight tip; Horizontal serrations over 3/4 of jaw

Courtesy of Miltex, Inc.

FIGURE 10-40

Small Bone and Joint Instruments – GRASPING FORCEPS

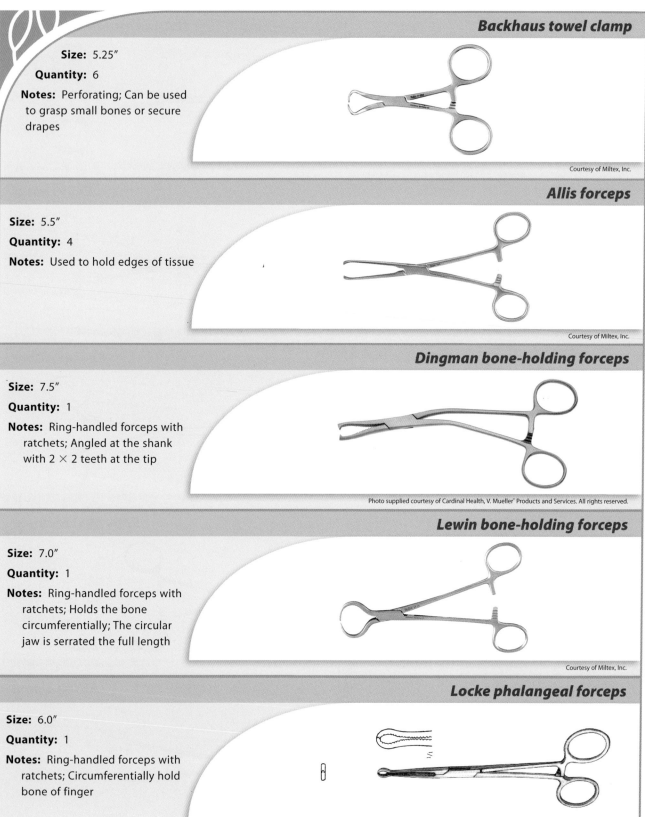

Backhaus towel clamp

Size: 5.25"

Quantity: 6

Notes: Perforating; Can be used to grasp small bones or secure drapes

Courtesy of Miltex, Inc.

FIGURE 10-41

Allis forceps

Size: 5.5"

Quantity: 4

Notes: Used to hold edges of tissue

Courtesy of Miltex, Inc.

FIGURE 10-42

Dingman bone-holding forceps

Size: 7.5"

Quantity: 1

Notes: Ring-handled forceps with ratchets; Angled at the shank with 2 × 2 teeth at the tip

Photo supplied courtesy of Cardinal Health, V. Mueller® Products and Services. All rights reserved.

FIGURE 10-43

Lewin bone-holding forceps

Size: 7.0"

Quantity: 1

Notes: Ring-handled forceps with ratchets; Holds the bone circumferentially; The circular jaw is serrated the full length

Courtesy of Miltex, Inc.

FIGURE 10-44

Locke phalangeal forceps

Size: 6.0"

Quantity: 1

Notes: Ring-handled forceps with ratchets; Circumferentially hold bone of finger

K-Medic branded instrumentation courtesy of Teleflex Medical, Inc.

FIGURE 10-45

Small Bone and Joint Instruments – GRASPING FORCEPS *continued*

Sesamoidectomy clamp

Size: 6.5"

Quantity: 1

Notes: Ring-handled clamp used to grasp small bony segments in small joints

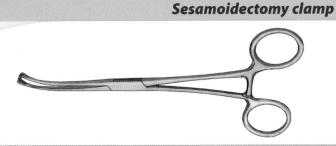

K-Medic branded instrumentation courtesy of Teleflex Medical, Inc.

FIGURE 10-46

Vogen sesamoid clamp

Size: 4.0"

Quantity: 1

Notes: Pistol grip with finger rings; Opposition pin and prong tip is used to secure sesamoid bones for removal

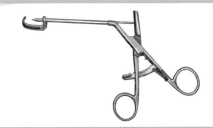

K-Medic branded instrumentation courtesy of Teleflex Medical, Inc.

FIGURE 10-47

Plate forceps

Size: 4.75"

Quantity: 1

Notes: Ring-handled forceps with prong and plate configuration at tip for holding mini plates

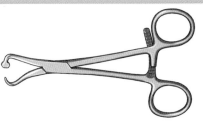

K-Medic branded instrumentation courtesy of Teleflex Medical, Inc.

FIGURE 10-48

Verbrugge bone-holding forceps

Size: 6.75"

Quantity: 1

Notes: Ring-handled forceps with locking ratchet; Lateral angle with curved serrated jaws

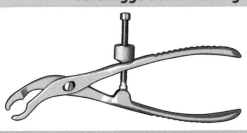

K-Medic branded instrumentation courtesy of Teleflex Medical, Inc.

FIGURE 10-49

Kern bone-holding forceps

Size: 6.0"

Quantity: 1

Notes: Serrated grasping jaws; Available with a ratchet

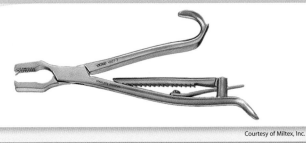

Courtesy of Miltex, Inc.

FIGURE 10-50

continues

Small Bone and Joint Instruments – GRASPING FORCEPS *continued*

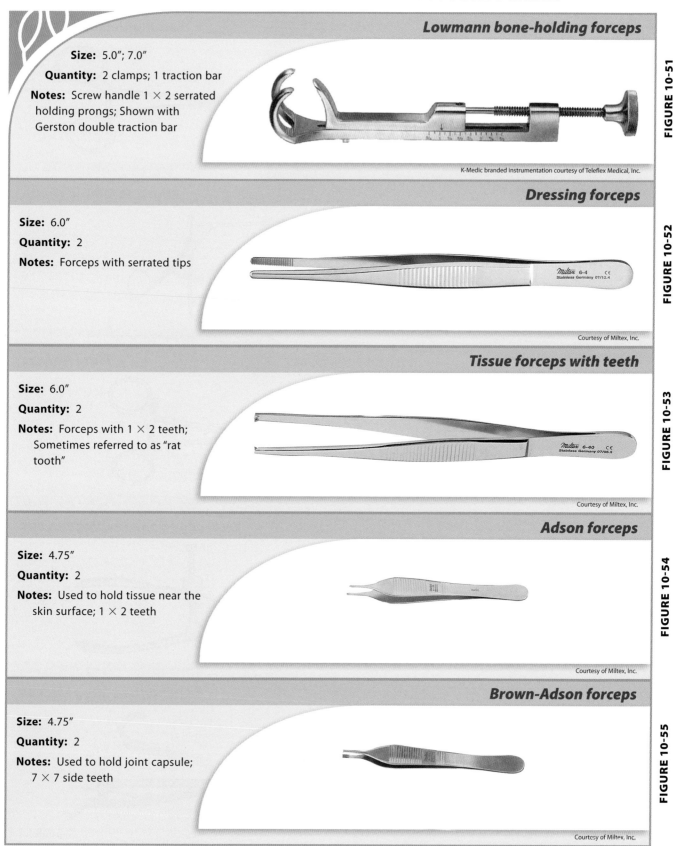

Lowmann bone-holding forceps

Size: 5.0"; 7.0"

Quantity: 2 clamps; 1 traction bar

Notes: Screw handle 1 × 2 serrated holding prongs; Shown with Gerston double traction bar

K-Medic branded instrumentation courtesy of Teleflex Medical, Inc.

FIGURE 10-51

Dressing forceps

Size: 6.0"

Quantity: 2

Notes: Forceps with serrated tips

Courtesy of Miltex, Inc.

FIGURE 10-52

Tissue forceps with teeth

Size: 6.0"

Quantity: 2

Notes: Forceps with 1 × 2 teeth; Sometimes referred to as "rat tooth"

Courtesy of Miltex, Inc.

FIGURE 10-53

Adson forceps

Size: 4.75"

Quantity: 2

Notes: Used to hold tissue near the skin surface; 1 × 2 teeth

Courtesy of Miltex, Inc.

FIGURE 10-54

Brown-Adson forceps

Size: 4.75"

Quantity: 2

Notes: Used to hold joint capsule; 7 × 7 side teeth

Courtesy of Miltex, Inc.

FIGURE 10-55

Small Bone and Joint Instruments – GRASPING FORCEPS *continued*

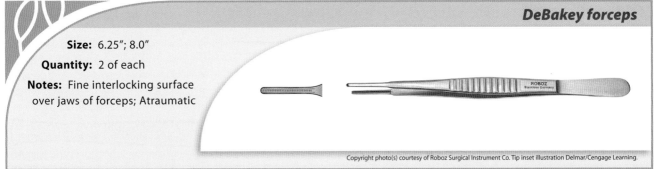

DeBakey forceps

Size: 6.25"; 8.0"

Quantity: 2 of each

Notes: Fine interlocking surface over jaws of forceps; Atraumatic

Copyright photo(s) courtesy of Roboz Surgical Instrument Co. Tip inset illustration Delmar/Cengage Learning.

FIGURE 10-56

Small Bone and Joint Instruments – DISSECTION INSTRUMENTS

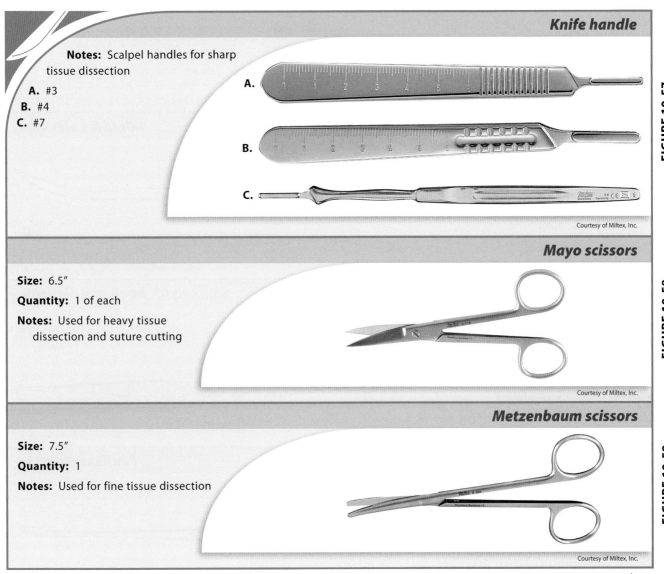

Knife handle

Notes: Scalpel handles for sharp tissue dissection

A. #3
B. #4
C. #7

Courtesy of Miltex, Inc.

FIGURE 10-57

Mayo scissors

Size: 6.5"

Quantity: 1 of each

Notes: Used for heavy tissue dissection and suture cutting

Courtesy of Miltex, Inc.

FIGURE 10-58

Metzenbaum scissors

Size: 7.5"

Quantity: 1

Notes: Used for fine tissue dissection

Courtesy of Miltex, Inc.

FIGURE 10-59

continues

Small Bone and Joint Instruments – DISSECTION INSTRUMENTS *continued*

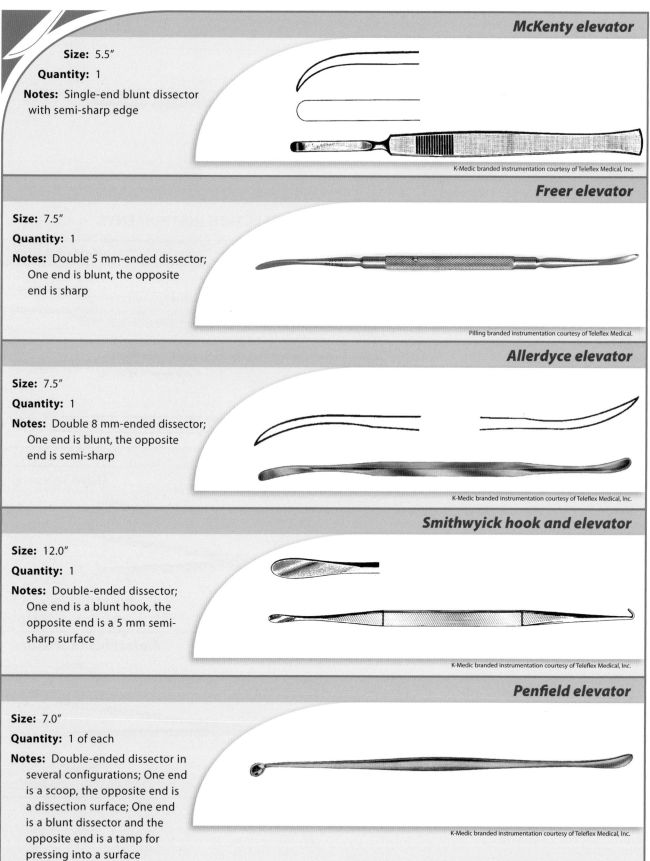

McKenty elevator

Size: 5.5"

Quantity: 1

Notes: Single-end blunt dissector with semi-sharp edge

K-Medic branded instrumentation courtesy of Teleflex Medical, Inc.

FIGURE 10-60

Freer elevator

Size: 7.5"

Quantity: 1

Notes: Double 5 mm-ended dissector; One end is blunt, the opposite end is sharp

Pilling branded instrumentation courtesy of Teleflex Medical.

FIGURE 10-61

Allerdyce elevator

Size: 7.5"

Quantity: 1

Notes: Double 8 mm-ended dissector; One end is blunt, the opposite end is semi-sharp

K-Medic branded instrumentation courtesy of Teleflex Medical, Inc.

FIGURE 10-62

Smithwyick hook and elevator

Size: 12.0"

Quantity: 1

Notes: Double-ended dissector; One end is a blunt hook, the opposite end is a 5 mm semi-sharp surface

K-Medic branded instrumentation courtesy of Teleflex Medical, Inc.

FIGURE 10-63

Penfield elevator

Size: 7.0"

Quantity: 1 of each

Notes: Double-ended dissector in several configurations; One end is a scoop, the opposite end is a dissection surface; One end is a blunt dissector and the opposite end is a tamp for pressing into a surface

K-Medic branded instrumentation courtesy of Teleflex Medical, Inc.

FIGURE 10-64

Small Bone and Joint Instruments – DISSECTION INSTRUMENTS *continued*

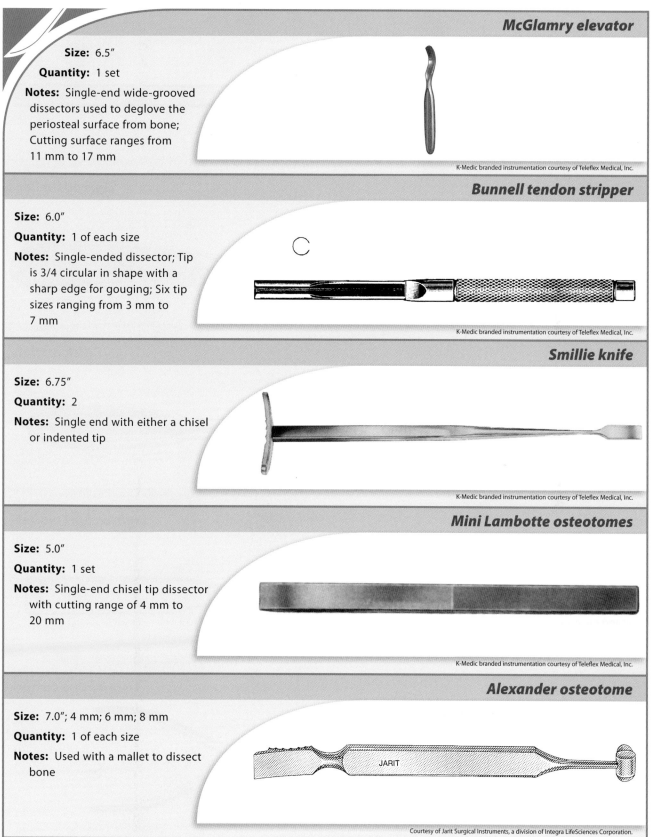

McGlamry elevator

Size: 6.5"

Quantity: 1 set

Notes: Single-end wide-grooved dissectors used to deglove the periosteal surface from bone; Cutting surface ranges from 11 mm to 17 mm

K-Medic branded instrumentation courtesy of Teleflex Medical, Inc.

FIGURE 10-65

Bunnell tendon stripper

Size: 6.0"

Quantity: 1 of each size

Notes: Single-ended dissector; Tip is 3/4 circular in shape with a sharp edge for gouging; Six tip sizes ranging from 3 mm to 7 mm

K-Medic branded instrumentation courtesy of Teleflex Medical, Inc.

FIGURE 10-66

Smillie knife

Size: 6.75"

Quantity: 2

Notes: Single end with either a chisel or indented tip

K-Medic branded instrumentation courtesy of Teleflex Medical, Inc.

FIGURE 10-67

Mini Lambotte osteotomes

Size: 5.0"

Quantity: 1 set

Notes: Single-end chisel tip dissector with cutting range of 4 mm to 20 mm

K-Medic branded instrumentation courtesy of Teleflex Medical, Inc.

FIGURE 10-68

Alexander osteotome

Size: 7.0"; 4 mm; 6 mm; 8 mm

Quantity: 1 of each size

Notes: Used with a mallet to dissect bone

Courtesy of Jarit Surgical Instruments, a division of Integra LifeSciences Corporation.

FIGURE 10-69

continues

Small Bone and Joint Instruments – DISSECTION INSTRUMENTS *continued*

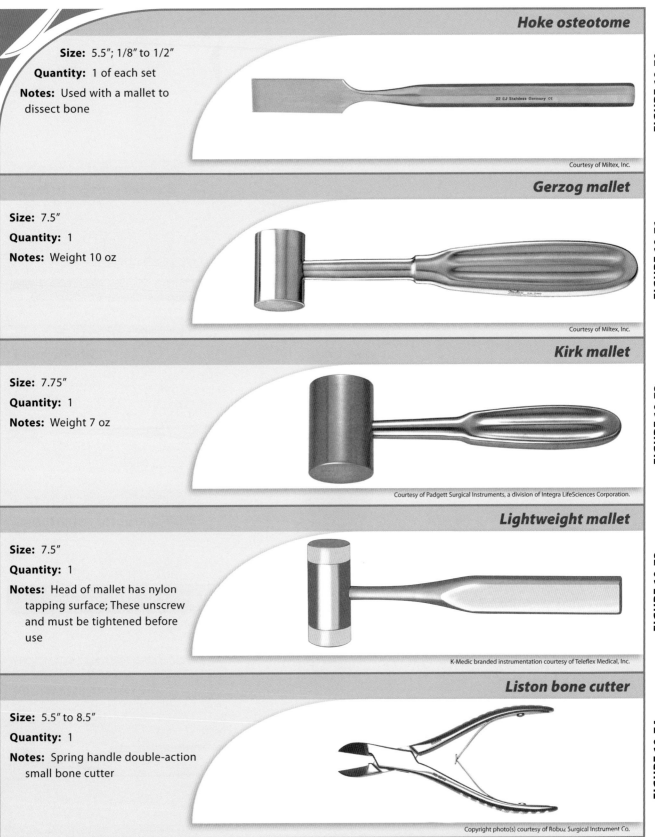

Hoke osteotome

Size: 5.5"; 1/8" to 1/2"

Quantity: 1 of each set

Notes: Used with a mallet to dissect bone

Courtesy of Miltex, Inc.

FIGURE 10-70

Gerzog mallet

Size: 7.5"

Quantity: 1

Notes: Weight 10 oz

Courtesy of Miltex, Inc.

FIGURE 10-71

Kirk mallet

Size: 7.75"

Quantity: 1

Notes: Weight 7 oz

Courtesy of Padgett Surgical Instruments, a division of Integra LifeSciences Corporation.

FIGURE 10-72

Lightweight mallet

Size: 7.5"

Quantity: 1

Notes: Head of mallet has nylon tapping surface; These unscrew and must be tightened before use

K-Medic branded instrumentation courtesy of Teleflex Medical, Inc.

FIGURE 10-73

Liston bone cutter

Size: 5.5" to 8.5"

Quantity: 1

Notes: Spring handle double-action small bone cutter

Copyright photo(s) courtesy of Robuz Surgical Instrument Co.

FIGURE 10-74

Small Bone and Joint Instruments – DISSECTION INSTRUMENTS *continued*

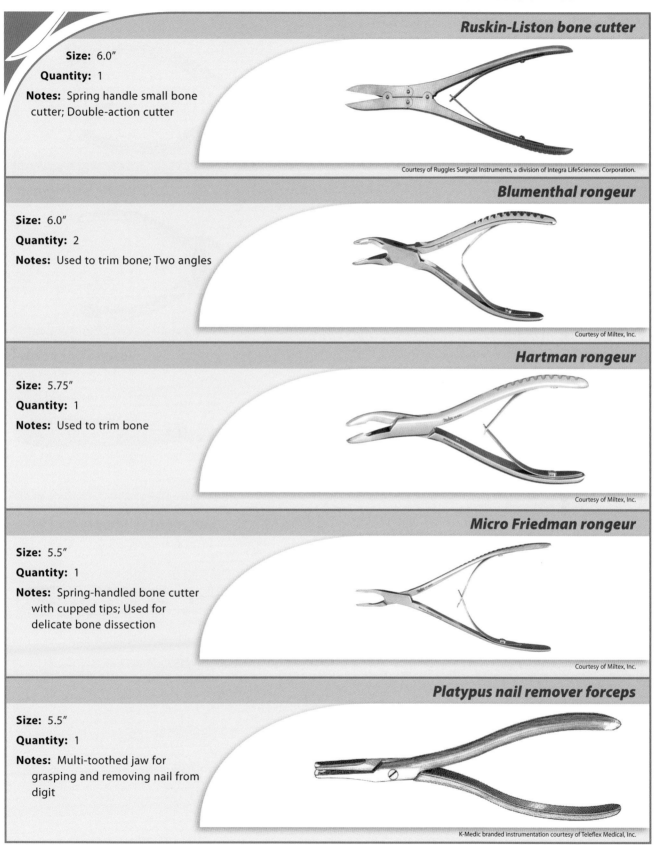

Ruskin-Liston bone cutter

Size: 6.0"

Quantity: 1

Notes: Spring handle small bone cutter; Double-action cutter

Courtesy of Ruggles Surgical Instruments, a division of Integra LifeSciences Corporation.

FIGURE 10-75

Blumenthal rongeur

Size: 6.0"

Quantity: 2

Notes: Used to trim bone; Two angles

Courtesy of Miltex, Inc.

FIGURE 10-76

Hartman rongeur

Size: 5.75"

Quantity: 1

Notes: Used to trim bone

Courtesy of Miltex, Inc.

FIGURE 10-77

Micro Friedman rongeur

Size: 5.5"

Quantity: 1

Notes: Spring-handled bone cutter with cupped tips; Used for delicate bone dissection

Courtesy of Miltex, Inc.

FIGURE 10-78

Platypus nail remover forceps

Size: 5.5"

Quantity: 1

Notes: Multi-toothed jaw for grasping and removing nail from digit

K-Medic branded instrumentation courtesy of Teleflex Medical, Inc.

FIGURE 10-79

continues

Small Bone and Joint Instruments – DISSECTION INSTRUMENTS *continued*

Nail nipper

Size: 5.5″

Quantity: 1

Notes: Spring-handled nippers with angled cutting surface; Locking handle to keep blades closed when not in use

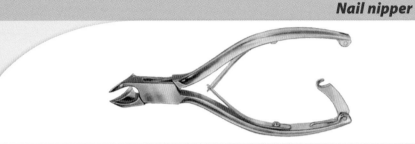

K-Medic branded instrumentation courtesy of Teleflex Medical, Inc.

FIGURE 10-80

Mycotic nail nipper

Size: 6.0″

Quantity: 1

Notes: Spring-handled nippers with heavy angled cutting surface for coarse and overgrown fungal nails; Locking handle to keep blades closed when not in use

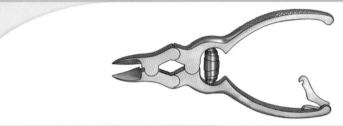

K-Medic branded instrumentation courtesy of Teleflex Medical, Inc.

FIGURE 10-81

Joseph bone saw

Size: 7.5″

Quantity: 1

Notes: Manual saw with straight or bayonet edge

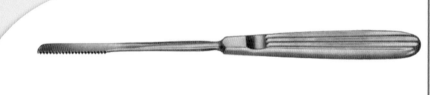

K-Medic branded instrumentation courtesy of Teleflex Medical, Inc.

FIGURE 10-82

Langenbeck metacarpal saw

Size: 9.0″

Quantity: 1

Notes: Straight small bone saw

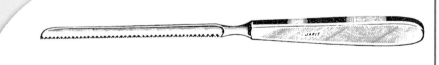

Courtesy of Jarit Surgical Instruments, a division of Integra LifeSciences Corporation.

FIGURE 10-83

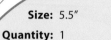

Small Bone and Joint Instruments – DEBULKING INSTRUMENTS

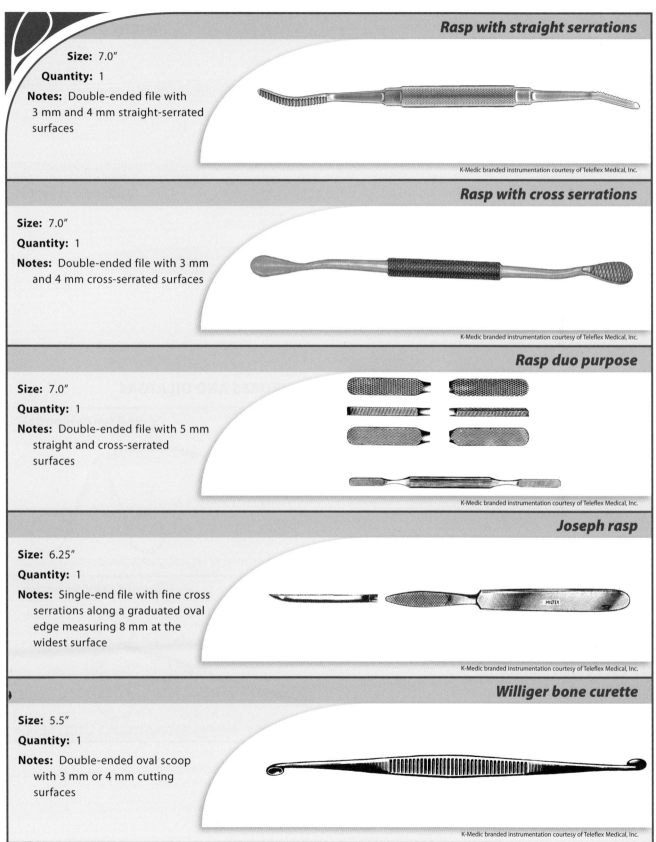

Rasp with straight serrations

Size: 7.0"

Quantity: 1

Notes: Double-ended file with 3 mm and 4 mm straight-serrated surfaces

K-Medic branded instrumentation courtesy of Teleflex Medical, Inc.

FIGURE 10-84

Rasp with cross serrations

Size: 7.0"

Quantity: 1

Notes: Double-ended file with 3 mm and 4 mm cross-serrated surfaces

K-Medic branded instrumentation courtesy of Teleflex Medical, Inc.

FIGURE 10-85

Rasp duo purpose

Size: 7.0"

Quantity: 1

Notes: Double-ended file with 5 mm straight and cross-serrated surfaces

K-Medic branded instrumentation courtesy of Teleflex Medical, Inc.

FIGURE 10-86

Joseph rasp

Size: 6.25"

Quantity: 1

Notes: Single-end file with fine cross serrations along a graduated oval edge measuring 8 mm at the widest surface

K-Medic branded instrumentation courtesy of Teleflex Medical, Inc.

FIGURE 10-87

Williger bone curette

Size: 5.5"

Quantity: 1

Notes: Double-ended oval scoop with 3 mm or 4 mm cutting surfaces

K-Medic branded instrumentation courtesy of Teleflex Medical, Inc.

FIGURE 10-88

continues

Small Bone and Joint Instruments – DEBULKING INSTRUMENTS *continued*

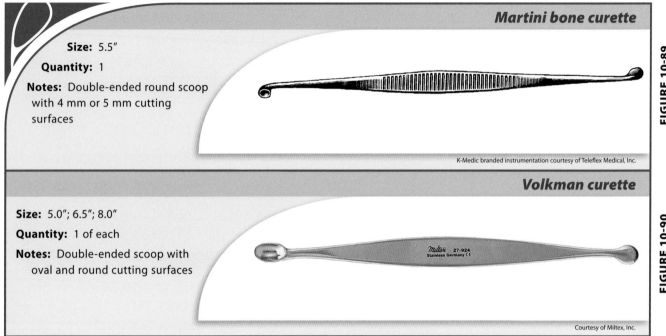

Martini bone curette

FIGURE 10-89

Size: 5.5″

Quantity: 1

Notes: Double-ended round scoop with 4 mm or 5 mm cutting surfaces

K-Medic branded instrumentation courtesy of Teleflex Medical, Inc.

Volkman curette

FIGURE 10-90

Size: 5.0″; 6.5″; 8.0″

Quantity: 1 of each

Notes: Double-ended scoop with oval and round cutting surfaces

Courtesy of Miltex, Inc.

Small Bone and Joint Instruments – PROBES AND DILATORS

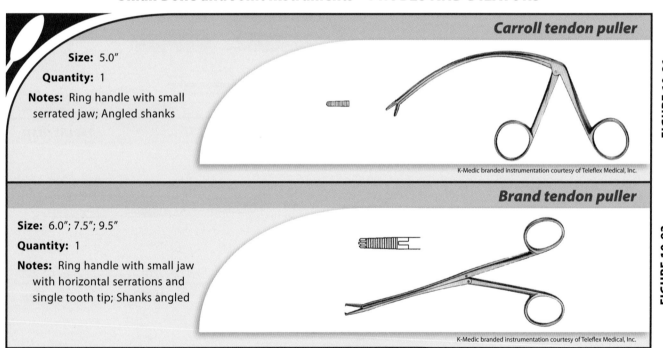

Carroll tendon puller

FIGURE 10-91

Size: 5.0″

Quantity: 1

Notes: Ring handle with small serrated jaw; Angled shanks

K-Medic branded instrumentation courtesy of Teleflex Medical, Inc.

Brand tendon puller

FIGURE 10-92

Size: 6.0″; 7.5″; 9.5″

Quantity: 1

Notes: Ring handle with small jaw with horizontal serrations and single tooth tip; Shanks angled

K-Medic branded instrumentation courtesy of Teleflex Medical, Inc.

Small Bone and Joint Instruments – PROBES AND DILATORS *continued*

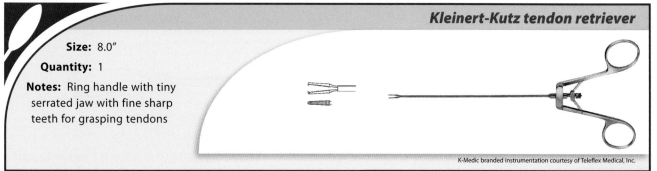

Kleinert-Kutz tendon retriever

Size: 8.0″

Quantity: 1

Notes: Ring handle with tiny serrated jaw with fine sharp teeth for grasping tendons

K-Medic branded instrumentation courtesy of Teleflex Medical, Inc.

FIGURE 10-93

Small Bone and Joint Instruments – EVACUATION AND INSTILLATION INSTRUMENTS

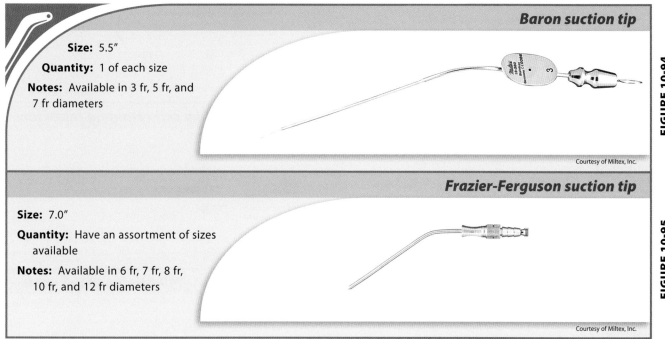

Baron suction tip

Size: 5.5″

Quantity: 1 of each size

Notes: Available in 3 fr, 5 fr, and 7 fr diameters

Courtesy of Miltex, Inc.

FIGURE 10-94

Frazier-Ferguson suction tip

Size: 7.0″

Quantity: Have an assortment of sizes available

Notes: Available in 6 fr, 7 fr, 8 fr, 10 fr, and 12 fr diameters

Courtesy of Miltex, Inc.

FIGURE 10-95

Small Bone and Joint Instruments – RETRACTION AND EXPOSURE INSTRUMENTS

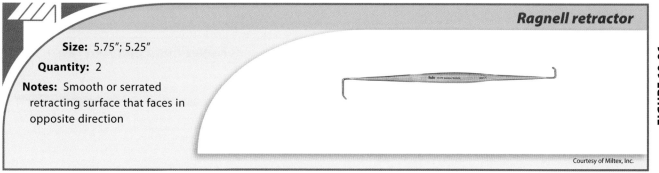

Ragnell retractor

Size: 5.75″; 5.25″

Quantity: 2

Notes: Smooth or serrated retracting surface that faces in opposite direction

Courtesy of Miltex, Inc.

FIGURE 10-96

continues

Small Bone and Joint Instruments – RETRACTION AND EXPOSURE INSTRUMENTS *continued*

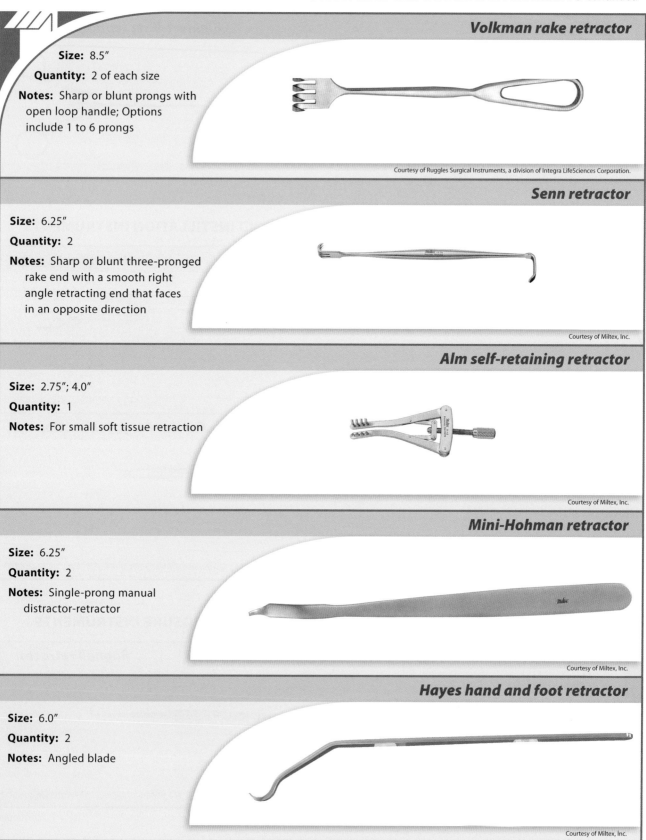

Volkman rake retractor

Size: 8.5″

Quantity: 2 of each size

Notes: Sharp or blunt prongs with open loop handle; Options include 1 to 6 prongs

Courtesy of Ruggles Surgical Instruments, a division of Integra LifeSciences Corporation.

FIGURE 10-97

Senn retractor

Size: 6.25″

Quantity: 2

Notes: Sharp or blunt three-pronged rake end with a smooth right angle retracting end that faces in an opposite direction

Courtesy of Miltex, Inc.

FIGURE 10-98

Alm self-retaining retractor

Size: 2.75″; 4.0″

Quantity: 1

Notes: For small soft tissue retraction

Courtesy of Miltex, Inc.

FIGURE 10-99

Mini-Hohman retractor

Size: 6.25″

Quantity: 2

Notes: Single-prong manual distractor-retractor

Courtesy of Miltex, Inc.

FIGURE 10-100

Hayes hand and foot retractor

Size: 6.0″

Quantity: 2

Notes: Angled blade

Courtesy of Miltex, Inc.

FIGURE 10-101

Small Bone and Joint Instruments – RETRACTION AND EXPOSURE INSTRUMENTS *continued*

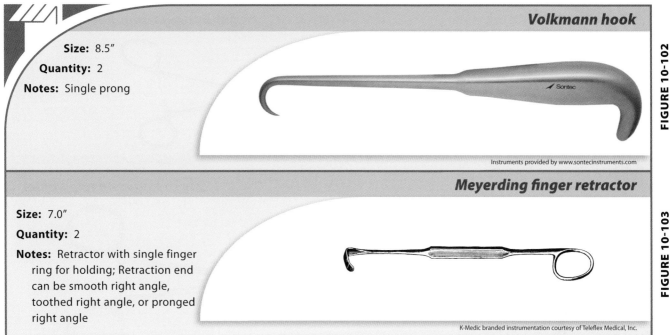

Volkmann hook

Size: 8.5″

Quantity: 2

Notes: Single prong

Instruments provided by www.sontecinstruments.com

FIGURE 10-102

Meyerding finger retractor

Size: 7.0″

Quantity: 2

Notes: Retractor with single finger ring for holding; Retraction end can be smooth right angle, toothed right angle, or pronged right angle

K-Medic branded instrumentation courtesy of Teleflex Medical, Inc.

FIGURE 10-103

Small Bone and Joint Instruments – APPROXIMATION AND CLOSURE INSTRUMENTS

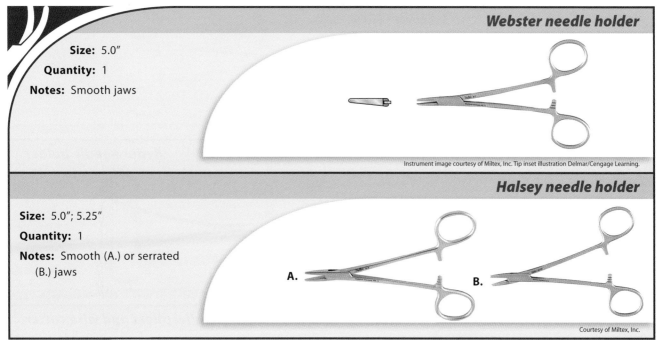

Webster needle holder

Size: 5.0″

Quantity: 1

Notes: Smooth jaws

Instrument image courtesy of Miltex, Inc. Tip inset illustration Delmar/Cengage Learning.

FIGURE 10-104

Halsey needle holder

Size: 5.0″; 5.25″

Quantity: 1

Notes: Smooth (A.) or serrated (B.) jaws

A. B.

Courtesy of Miltex, Inc.

FIGURE 10-105

continues

Small Bone and Joint Instruments – APPROXIMATION AND CLOSURE INSTRUMENTS *continued*

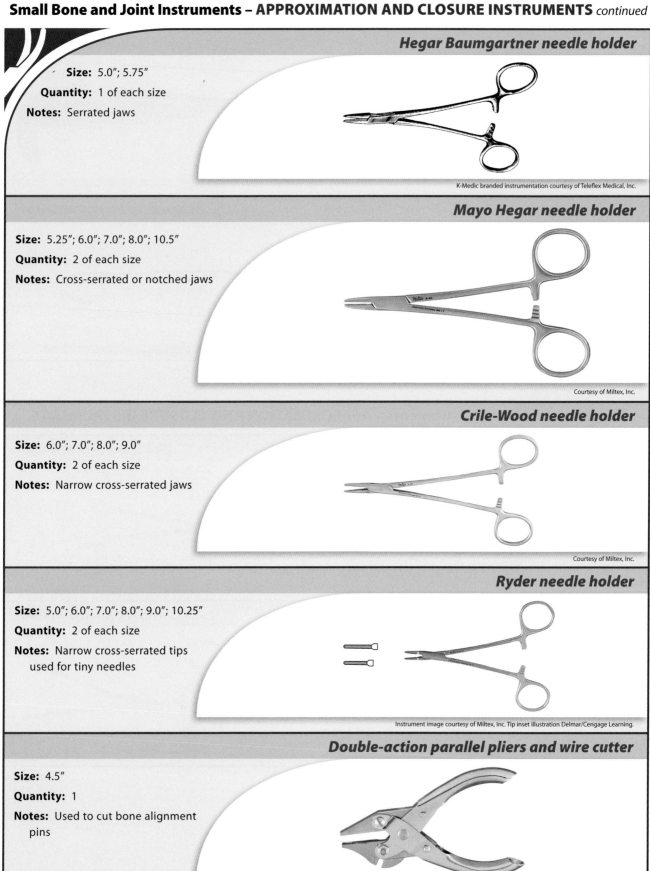

Hegar Baumgartner needle holder

Size: 5.0"; 5.75"

Quantity: 1 of each size

Notes: Serrated jaws

K-Medic branded instrumentation courtesy of Teleflex Medical, Inc.

FIGURE 10-106

Mayo Hegar needle holder

Size: 5.25"; 6.0"; 7.0"; 8.0"; 10.5"

Quantity: 2 of each size

Notes: Cross-serrated or notched jaws

Courtesy of Miltex, Inc.

FIGURE 10-107

Crile-Wood needle holder

Size: 6.0"; 7.0"; 8.0"; 9.0"

Quantity: 2 of each size

Notes: Narrow cross-serrated jaws

Courtesy of Miltex, Inc.

FIGURE 10-108

Ryder needle holder

Size: 5.0"; 6.0"; 7.0"; 8.0"; 9.0"; 10.25"

Quantity: 2 of each size

Notes: Narrow cross-serrated tips used for tiny needles

Instrument image courtesy of Miltex, Inc. Tip inset illustration Delmar/Cengage Learning.

FIGURE 10-109

Double-action parallel pliers and wire cutter

Size: 4.5"

Quantity: 1

Notes: Used to cut bone alignment pins

Courtesy of Miltex, Inc.

FIGURE 10-110

Small Bone and Joint Instruments – APPROXIMATION AND CLOSURE INSTRUMENTS *continued*

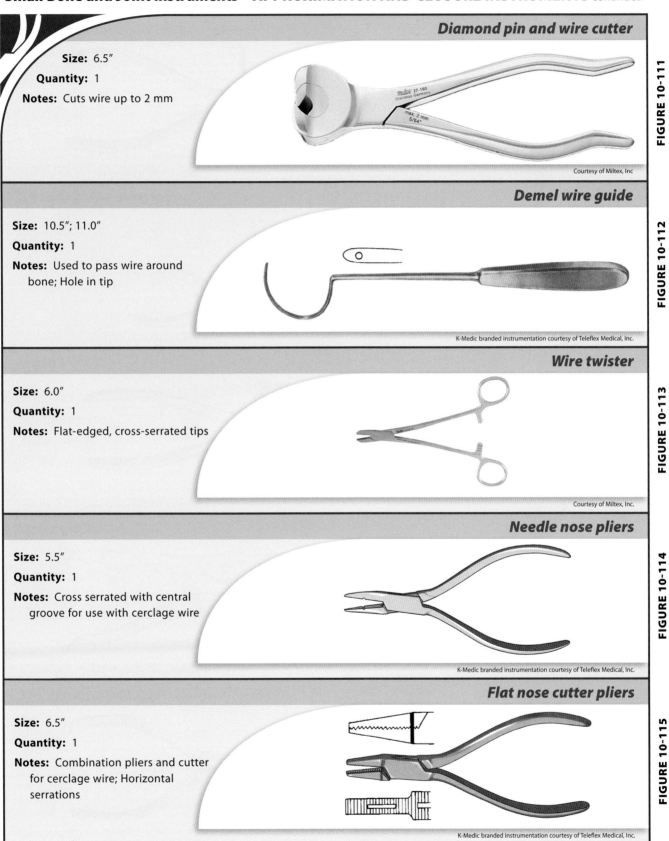

Diamond pin and wire cutter

Size: 6.5″

Quantity: 1

Notes: Cuts wire up to 2 mm

Courtesy of Miltex, Inc

FIGURE 10-111

Demel wire guide

Size: 10.5″; 11.0″

Quantity: 1

Notes: Used to pass wire around bone; Hole in tip

K-Medic branded instrumentation courtesy of Teleflex Medical, Inc.

FIGURE 10-112

Wire twister

Size: 6.0″

Quantity: 1

Notes: Flat-edged, cross-serrated tips

Courtesy of Miltex, Inc.

FIGURE 10-113

Needle nose pliers

Size: 5.5″

Quantity: 1

Notes: Cross serrated with central groove for use with cerclage wire

K-Medic branded instrumentation courtesy of Teleflex Medical, Inc.

FIGURE 10-114

Flat nose cutter pliers

Size: 6.5″

Quantity: 1

Notes: Combination pliers and cutter for cerclage wire; Horizontal serrations

K-Medic branded instrumentation courtesy of Teleflex Medical, Inc.

FIGURE 10-115

continues

Small Bone and Joint Instruments – APPROXIMATION AND CLOSURE INSTRUMENTS *continued*

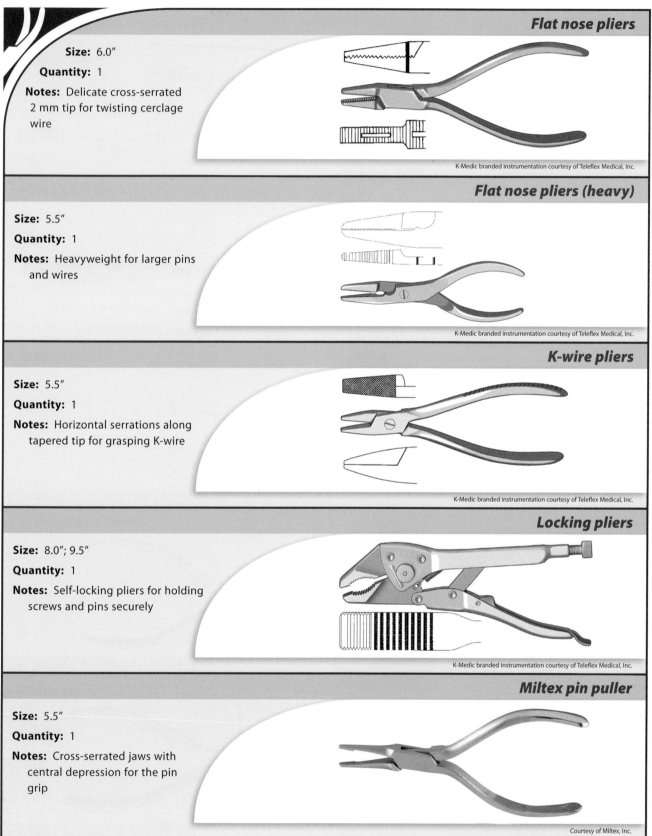

Flat nose pliers

Size: 6.0″

Quantity: 1

Notes: Delicate cross-serrated 2 mm tip for twisting cerclage wire

K-Medic branded instrumentation courtesy of Teleflex Medical, Inc.

FIGURE 10-116

Flat nose pliers (heavy)

Size: 5.5″

Quantity: 1

Notes: Heavyweight for larger pins and wires

K-Medic branded instrumentation courtesy of Teleflex Medical, Inc.

FIGURE 10-117

K-wire pliers

Size: 5.5″

Quantity: 1

Notes: Horizontal serrations along tapered tip for grasping K-wire

K-Medic branded instrumentation courtesy of Teleflex Medical, Inc.

FIGURE 10-118

Locking pliers

Size: 8.0″; 9.5″

Quantity: 1

Notes: Self-locking pliers for holding screws and pins securely

K-Medic branded instrumentation courtesy of Teleflex Medical, Inc.

FIGURE 10-119

Miltex pin puller

Size: 5.5″

Quantity: 1

Notes: Cross-serrated jaws with central depression for the pin grip

Courtesy of Miltex, Inc.

FIGURE 10-120

Small Bone and Joint Instruments – APPROXIMATION AND CLOSURE INSTRUMENTS *continued*

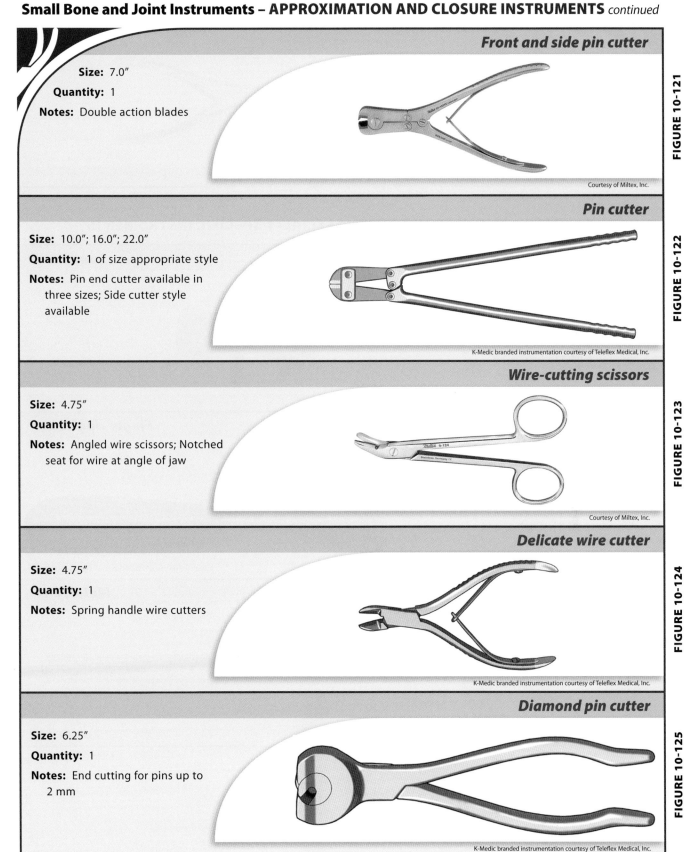

Front and side pin cutter

Size: 7.0″

Quantity: 1

Notes: Double action blades

Courtesy of Miltex, Inc.

FIGURE 10-121

Pin cutter

Size: 10.0″; 16.0″; 22.0″

Quantity: 1 of size appropriate style

Notes: Pin end cutter available in three sizes; Side cutter style available

K-Medic branded instrumentation courtesy of Teleflex Medical, Inc.

FIGURE 10-122

Wire-cutting scissors

Size: 4.75″

Quantity: 1

Notes: Angled wire scissors; Notched seat for wire at angle of jaw

Courtesy of Miltex, Inc.

FIGURE 10-123

Delicate wire cutter

Size: 4.75″

Quantity: 1

Notes: Spring handle wire cutters

K-Medic branded instrumentation courtesy of Teleflex Medical, Inc.

FIGURE 10-124

Diamond pin cutter

Size: 6.25″

Quantity: 1

Notes: End cutting for pins up to 2 mm

K-Medic branded instrumentation courtesy of Teleflex Medical, Inc.

FIGURE 10-125

continues

Small Bone and Joint Instruments – APPROXIMATION AND CLOSURE INSTRUMENTS *continued*

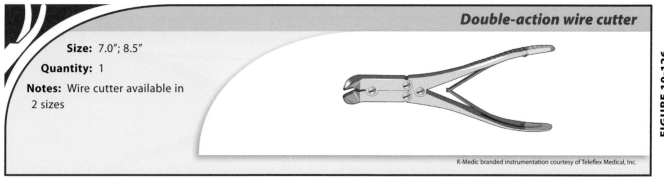

Double-action wire cutter

Size: 7.0″; 8.5″

Quantity: 1

Notes: Wire cutter available in 2 sizes

K-Medic branded instrumentation courtesy of Teleflex Medical, Inc.

FIGURE 10-126

Small Bone and Joint Instruments – SPECIALTY SPECIFIC INSTRUMENTS

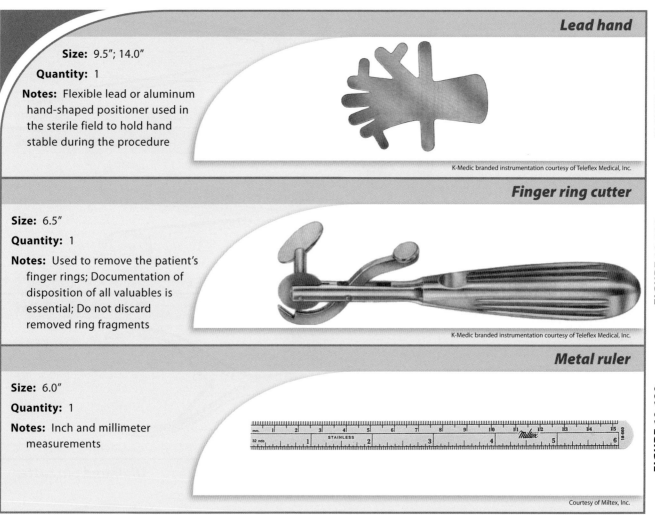

Lead hand

Size: 9.5″; 14.0″

Quantity: 1

Notes: Flexible lead or aluminum hand-shaped positioner used in the sterile field to hold hand stable during the procedure

K-Medic branded instrumentation courtesy of Teleflex Medical, Inc.

FIGURE 10-127

Finger ring cutter

Size: 6.5″

Quantity: 1

Notes: Used to remove the patient's finger rings; Documentation of disposition of all valuables is essential; Do not discard removed ring fragments

K-Medic branded instrumentation courtesy of Teleflex Medical, Inc.

FIGURE 10-128

Metal ruler

Size: 6.0″

Quantity: 1

Notes: Inch and millimeter measurements

Courtesy of Miltex, Inc.

FIGURE 10-129

Small Bone and Joint Instruments – SPECIALTY SPECIFIC INSTRUMENTS *continued*

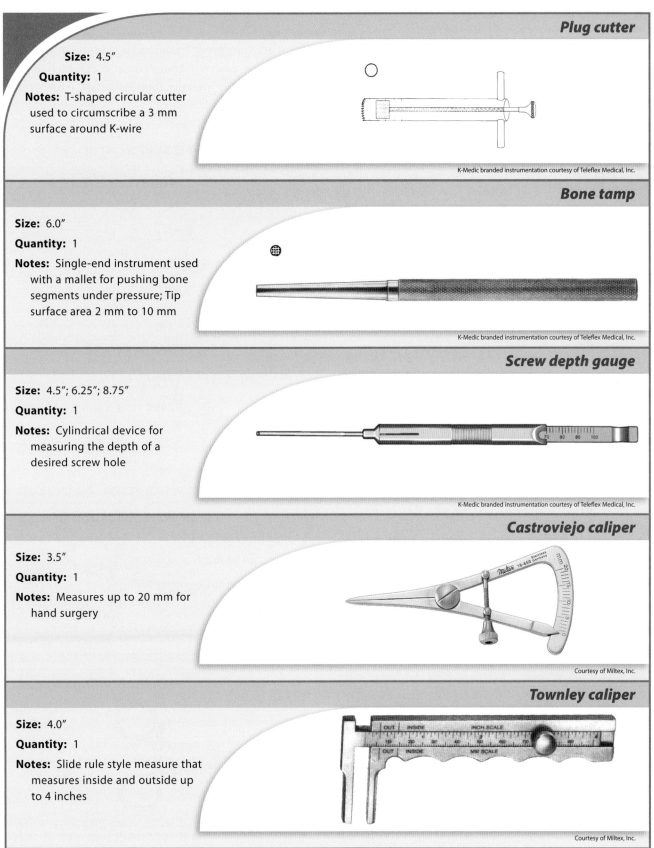

Plug cutter

Size: 4.5″

Quantity: 1

Notes: T-shaped circular cutter used to circumscribe a 3 mm surface around K-wire

K-Medic branded instrumentation courtesy of Teleflex Medical, Inc.

FIGURE 10-130

Bone tamp

Size: 6.0″

Quantity: 1

Notes: Single-end instrument used with a mallet for pushing bone segments under pressure; Tip surface area 2 mm to 10 mm

K-Medic branded instrumentation courtesy of Teleflex Medical, Inc.

FIGURE 10-131

Screw depth gauge

Size: 4.5″; 6.25″; 8.75″

Quantity: 1

Notes: Cylindrical device for measuring the depth of a desired screw hole

K-Medic branded instrumentation courtesy of Teleflex Medical, Inc.

FIGURE 10-132

Castroviejo caliper

Size: 3.5″

Quantity: 1

Notes: Measures up to 20 mm for hand surgery

Courtesy of Miltex, Inc.

FIGURE 10-133

Townley caliper

Size: 4.0″

Quantity: 1

Notes: Slide rule style measure that measures inside and outside up to 4 inches

Courtesy of Miltex, Inc.

FIGURE 10-134

LARGE BONE AND JOINT INSTRUMENTS

Instruments similar to those found in small bone instrumentation are commonly found in large bone sets in larger sizes. Before performing a procedure on larger bones and joints, it is necessary to transect soft tissue such as skin, muscle, fascia, and periosteum. Deeper tissues will require the initial use of a medium foundation set. Patients with a large body habitus will require the use of longer instrumentation.

Large Bone and Joint Instruments – GRASPING FORCEPS

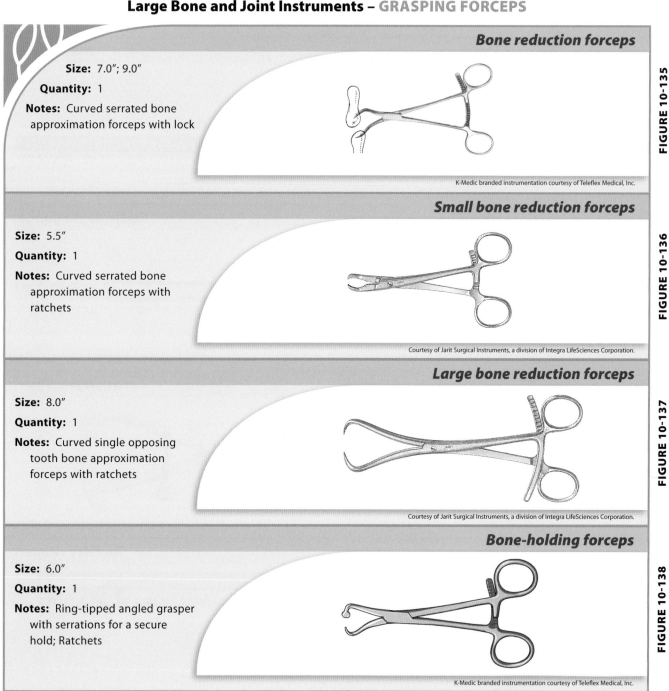

Bone reduction forceps

Size: 7.0"; 9.0"

Quantity: 1

Notes: Curved serrated bone approximation forceps with lock

K-Medic branded instrumentation courtesy of Teleflex Medical, Inc.

FIGURE 10-135

Small bone reduction forceps

Size: 5.5"

Quantity: 1

Notes: Curved serrated bone approximation forceps with ratchets

Courtesy of Jarit Surgical Instruments, a division of Integra LifeSciences Corporation.

FIGURE 10-136

Large bone reduction forceps

Size: 8.0"

Quantity: 1

Notes: Curved single opposing tooth bone approximation forceps with ratchets

Courtesy of Jarit Surgical Instruments, a division of Integra LifeSciences Corporation.

FIGURE 10-137

Bone-holding forceps

Size: 6.0"

Quantity: 1

Notes: Ring-tipped angled grasper with serrations for a secure hold; Ratchets

K-Medic branded instrumentation courtesy of Teleflex Medical, Inc.

FIGURE 10-138

Large Bone and Joint Instruments – GRASPING FORCEPS *continued*

Fergusson bone-holding forceps

Size: 8.25"

Quantity: 1

Notes: Quadruple toothed grasping surface; Pressure grip handle with no lock

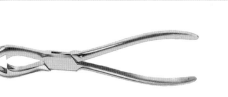

K-Medic branded instrumentation courtesy of Teleflex Medical, Inc.

FIGURE 10-139

Langenbeck bone-holding forceps

Size: 8.25"

Quantity: 1

Notes: Double-toothed grasping surface; Pressure grip handle with no lock

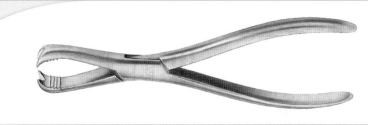

K-Medic branded instrumentation courtesy of Teleflex Medical, Inc.

FIGURE 10-140

Pelvic reduction forceps

Size: 7.25"; 9.5"; 10"

Quantity: 1 of each size

Notes: Double opposing sharp prong tips with ball stops in varied angles; Ring handle grip with screw lock

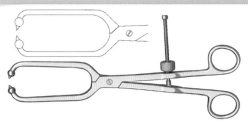

K-Medic branded instrumentation courtesy of Teleflex Medical, Inc.

FIGURE 10-141

Kern bone-holding forceps

Size: 8.5"

Quantity: 1

Notes: Toothed and serrated tips

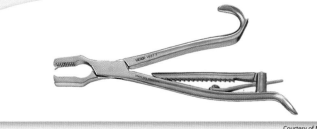

Courtesy of Miltex, Inc.

FIGURE 10-142

Lane bone-holding forceps

Size: 13.0"

Quantity: 1

Notes: Toothed and serrated tips; Non-locking and locking handles

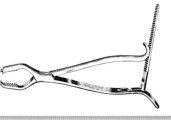

Courtesy of Jarit Surgical Instruments, a division of Integra LifeSciences Corporation.

FIGURE 10-143

continues

Large Bone and Joint Instruments – GRASPING FORCEPS *continued*

Parham-Martin bone-holding forceps

Size: 8.5"

Quantity: 1

Notes: Spring-loaded bone holder that uses disposable bands to hold bone fractures in alignment

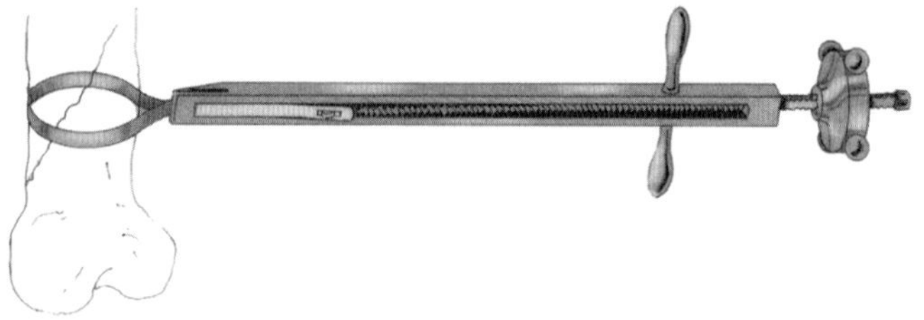

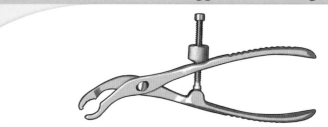

K-Medic branded instrumentation courtesy of Teleflex Medical, Inc.

FIGURE 10-144

Verbrugge bone-holding forceps

Size: 6.0"; 7.25"; 9.5"; 10.25"; 11.0"

Quantity: 1 of each size

Notes: Angled bone grasper with a prong on one jaw and serrations on the opposing jaw; Locks with a screw or ratchets

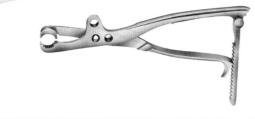

K-Medic branded instrumentation courtesy of Teleflex Medical, Inc.

FIGURE 10-145

Lambotte bone-holding forceps

Size: 8.0"; 10.5"; 11.5"

Quantity: 1

Notes: Circumferential serrated jaws that hold secure with ratchets; One swivel jaw

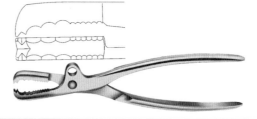

K-Medic branded instrumentation courtesy of Teleflex Medical, Inc.

FIGURE 10-146

Farabeuf bone-holding forceps

Size: 7.25"; 9.0"; 10.0"; 10.5"

Quantity: 1 of each size

Notes: Adjustable toothed jaw for larger bones; Non-locking, large locking, medium locking

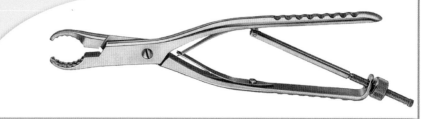

K-Medic branded instrumentation courtesy of Teleflex Medical, Inc.

FIGURE 10-147

Ulrich bone-holding forceps

Size: 11.0"

Quantity: 1

Notes: Speed lock with screw; One swivel serrated jaw

K-Medic branded instrumentation courtesy of Teleflex Medical, Inc.

FIGURE 10-148

Large Bone and Joint Instruments – DISSECTION INSTRUMENTS

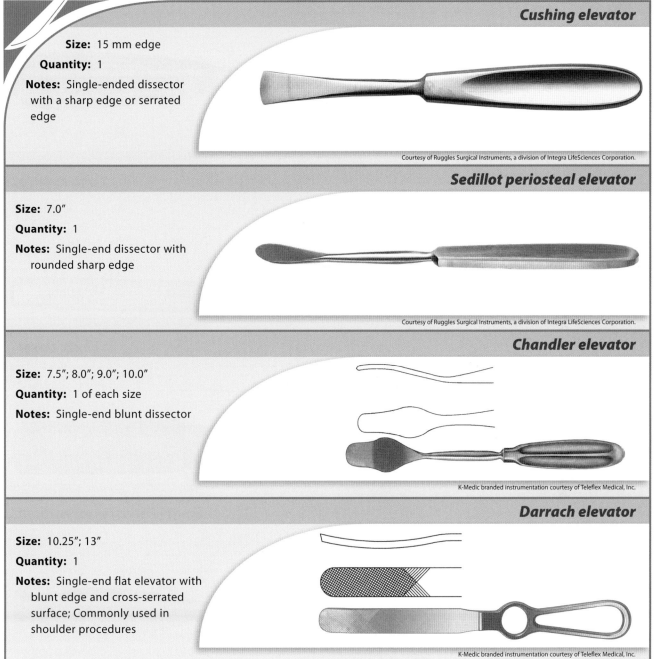

Cushing elevator

Size: 15 mm edge

Quantity: 1

Notes: Single-ended dissector with a sharp edge or serrated edge

Courtesy of Ruggles Surgical Instruments, a division of Integra LifeSciences Corporation.

FIGURE 10-149

Sedillot periosteal elevator

Size: 7.0″

Quantity: 1

Notes: Single-end dissector with rounded sharp edge

Courtesy of Ruggles Surgical Instruments, a division of Integra LifeSciences Corporation.

FIGURE 10-150

Chandler elevator

Size: 7.5″; 8.0″; 9.0″; 10.0″

Quantity: 1 of each size

Notes: Single-end blunt dissector

K-Medic branded instrumentation courtesy of Teleflex Medical, Inc.

FIGURE 10-151

Darrach elevator

Size: 10.25″; 13″

Quantity: 1

Notes: Single-end flat elevator with blunt edge and cross-serrated surface; Commonly used in shoulder procedures

K-Medic branded instrumentation courtesy of Teleflex Medical, Inc.

FIGURE 10-152

Large Bone and Joint Instruments – DEBULKING INSTRUMENTS

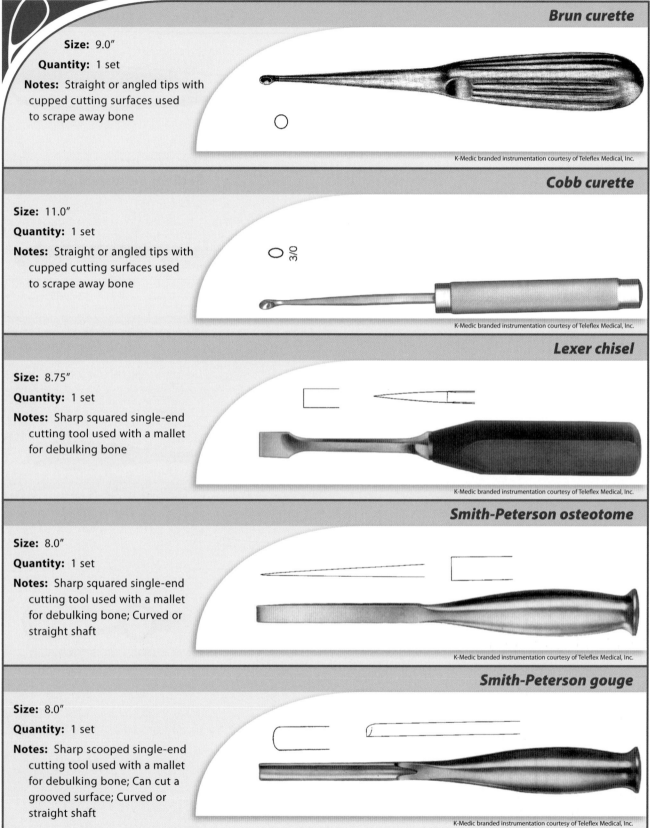

Brun curette

Size: 9.0″

Quantity: 1 set

Notes: Straight or angled tips with cupped cutting surfaces used to scrape away bone

FIGURE 10-153

K-Medic branded instrumentation courtesy of Teleflex Medical, Inc.

Cobb curette

Size: 11.0″

Quantity: 1 set

Notes: Straight or angled tips with cupped cutting surfaces used to scrape away bone

FIGURE 10-154

K-Medic branded instrumentation courtesy of Teleflex Medical, Inc.

Lexer chisel

Size: 8.75″

Quantity: 1 set

Notes: Sharp squared single-end cutting tool used with a mallet for debulking bone

FIGURE 10-155

K-Medic branded instrumentation courtesy of Teleflex Medical, Inc.

Smith-Peterson osteotome

Size: 8.0″

Quantity: 1 set

Notes: Sharp squared single-end cutting tool used with a mallet for debulking bone; Curved or straight shaft

FIGURE 10-156

K-Medic branded instrumentation courtesy of Teleflex Medical, Inc.

Smith-Peterson gouge

Size: 8.0″

Quantity: 1 set

Notes: Sharp scooped single-end cutting tool used with a mallet for debulking bone; Can cut a grooved surface; Curved or straight shaft

FIGURE 10-157

K-Medic branded instrumentation courtesy of Teleflex Medical, Inc.

Large Bone and Joint Instruments – DEBULKING INSTRUMENTS *continued*

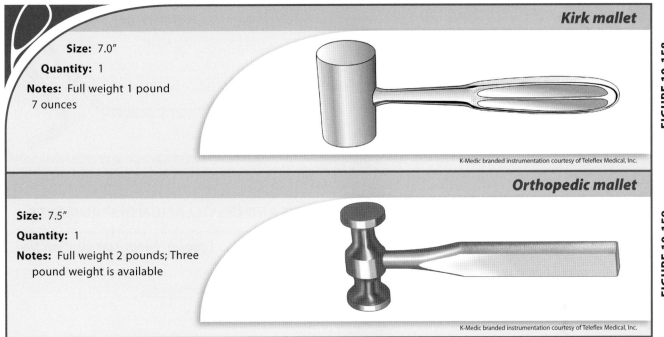

Kirk mallet

Size: 7.0″

Quantity: 1

Notes: Full weight 1 pound 7 ounces

FIGURE 10-158

K-Medic branded instrumentation courtesy of Teleflex Medical, Inc.

Orthopedic mallet

Size: 7.5″

Quantity: 1

Notes: Full weight 2 pounds; Three pound weight is available

FIGURE 10-159

K-Medic branded instrumentation courtesy of Teleflex Medical, Inc.

Large Bone and Joint Instruments – PROBES AND DILATORS

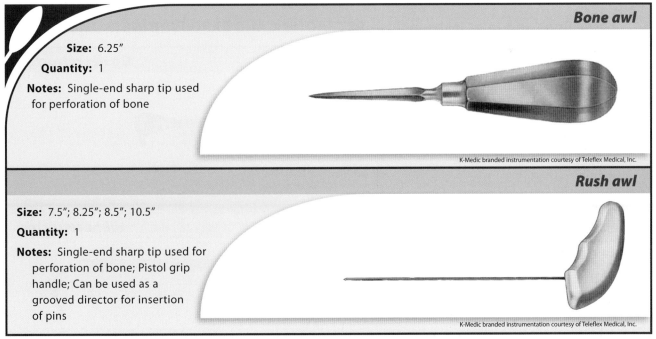

Bone awl

Size: 6.25″

Quantity: 1

Notes: Single-end sharp tip used for perforation of bone

FIGURE 10-160

K-Medic branded instrumentation courtesy of Teleflex Medical, Inc.

Rush awl

Size: 7.5″; 8.25″; 8.5″; 10.5″

Quantity: 1

Notes: Single-end sharp tip used for perforation of bone; Pistol grip handle; Can be used as a grooved director for insertion of pins

FIGURE 10-161

K-Medic branded instrumentation courtesy of Teleflex Medical, Inc.

continues

Large Bone and Joint Instruments – PROBES AND DILATORS *continued*

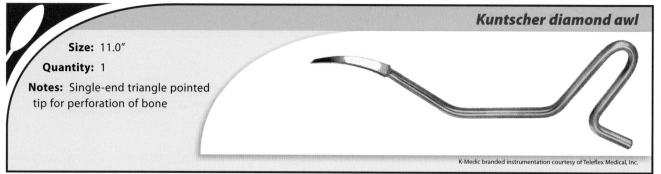

Kuntscher diamond awl

Size: 11.0"

Quantity: 1

Notes: Single-end triangle pointed tip for perforation of bone

K-Medic branded instrumentation courtesy of Teleflex Medical, Inc.

FIGURE 10-162

Large Bone and Joint Instruments – EVACUATION AND INSTILLATION INSTRUMENTS

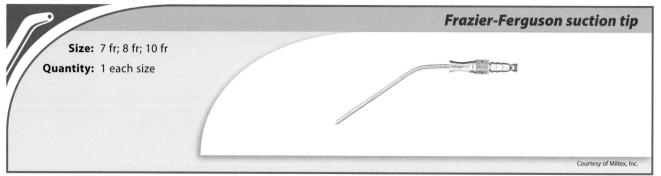

Frazier-Ferguson suction tip

Size: 7 fr; 8 fr; 10 fr

Quantity: 1 each size

Courtesy of Miltex, Inc.

FIGURE 10-163

Large Bone and Joint Instruments – RETRACTION AND EXPOSURE INSTRUMENTS

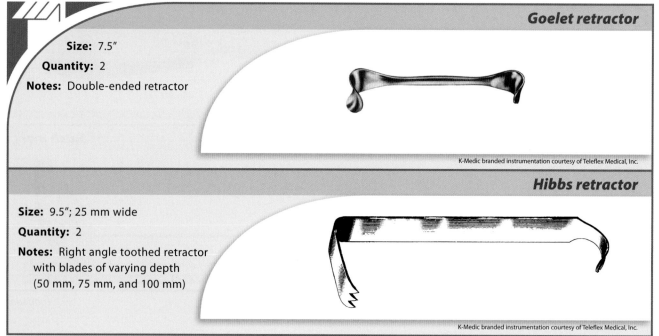

Goelet retractor

Size: 7.5"

Quantity: 2

Notes: Double-ended retractor

K-Medic branded instrumentation courtesy of Teleflex Medical, Inc.

FIGURE 10-164

Hibbs retractor

Size: 9.5"; 25 mm wide

Quantity: 2

Notes: Right angle toothed retractor with blades of varying depth (50 mm, 75 mm, and 100 mm)

K-Medic branded instrumentation courtesy of Teleflex Medical, Inc.

FIGURE 10-165

Large Bone and Joint Instruments – RETRACTION AND EXPOSURE INSTRUMENTS *continued*

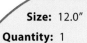

Murphy bone skid

Size: 12.0″

Quantity: 1

Notes: Scoop end retractor-distractor

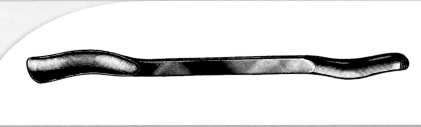

K-Medic branded instrumentation courtesy of Teleflex Medical, Inc.

FIGURE 10-166

Aufranc cobra retractor

Size: 10.5″

Quantity: 2

Notes: Serrated tip retractor-distractor with cobra-shaped end

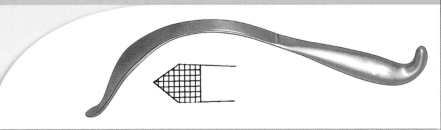

K-Medic branded instrumentation courtesy of Teleflex Medical, Inc.

FIGURE 10-167

Bennett bone elevator-retractor

Size: 10.0″

Quantity: 2

Notes: Wide end retractor with curved lip

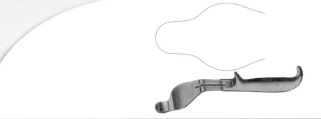

K-Medic branded instrumentation courtesy of Teleflex Medical, Inc.

FIGURE 10-168

Ollier rake retractor

Size: 9.0″

Quantity: 2

Notes: Four blunt prongs for retraction of heavy tissue; Similar to Israel rake

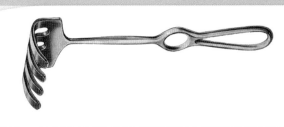

K-Medic branded instrumentation courtesy of Teleflex Medical, Inc.

FIGURE 10-169

Bristow Bankhart humeral retractor

Size: 102 mm deep

Quantity: 1

Notes: Double blunt prong for retractor and distraction of the shoulder joint

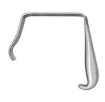

K-Medic branded instrumentation courtesy of Teleflex Medical, Inc.

FIGURE 10-170

continues

Large Bone and Joint Instruments – RETRACTION AND EXPOSURE INSTRUMENTS *continued*

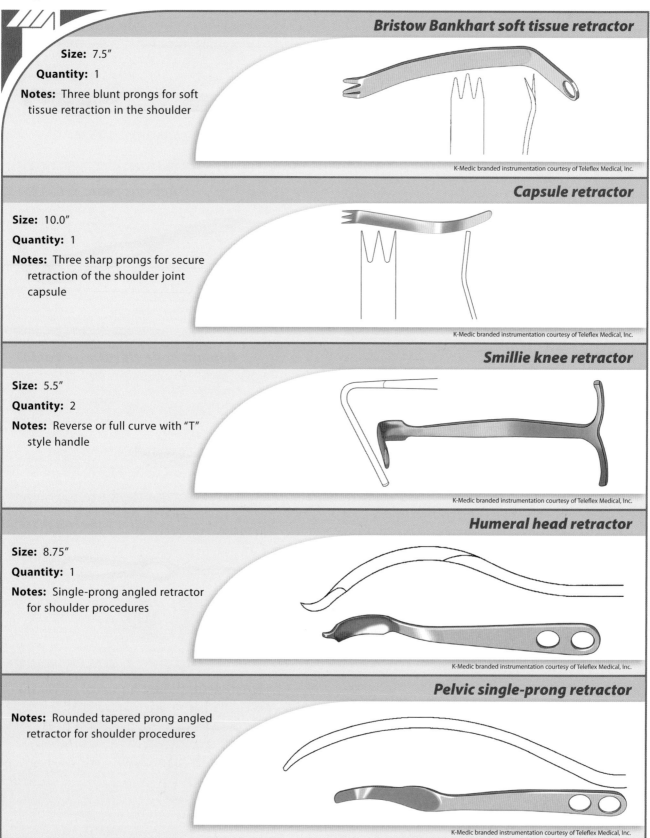

Bristow Bankhart soft tissue retractor

Size: 7.5"

Quantity: 1

Notes: Three blunt prongs for soft tissue retraction in the shoulder

K-Medic branded instrumentation courtesy of Teleflex Medical, Inc.

FIGURE 10-171

Capsule retractor

Size: 10.0"

Quantity: 1

Notes: Three sharp prongs for secure retraction of the shoulder joint capsule

K-Medic branded instrumentation courtesy of Teleflex Medical, Inc.

FIGURE 10-172

Smillie knee retractor

Size: 5.5"

Quantity: 2

Notes: Reverse or full curve with "T" style handle

K-Medic branded instrumentation courtesy of Teleflex Medical, Inc.

FIGURE 10-173

Humeral head retractor

Size: 8.75"

Quantity: 1

Notes: Single-prong angled retractor for shoulder procedures

K-Medic branded instrumentation courtesy of Teleflex Medical, Inc.

FIGURE 10-174

Pelvic single-prong retractor

Notes: Rounded tapered prong angled retractor for shoulder procedures

K-Medic branded instrumentation courtesy of Teleflex Medical, Inc.

FIGURE 10-175

Large Bone and Joint Instruments – RETRACTION AND EXPOSURE INSTRUMENTS *continued*

Blount retractor

Size: 10.5"; 7.0"

Quantity: 2

Notes: Pronged right angle retractors characterized by variance in style; Double-prong, single-prong, and knee-tapered single prong

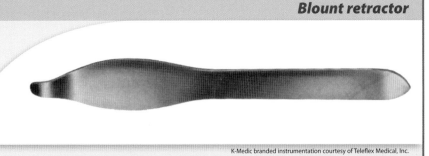

K-Medic branded instrumentation courtesy of Teleflex Medical, Inc.

FIGURE 10-176

Fukuda shoulder retractor

Size: 81 mm

Quantity: 1

Notes: "T" handle leverage retractor for shoulder procedures

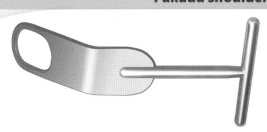

K-Medic branded instrumentation courtesy of Teleflex Medical, Inc.

FIGURE 10-177

Gelpi self-retaining retractor

Size: 7.5"

Quantity: 2

Notes: Sharp prongs hold tissue apart; Some styles have ball stops near the tip to prevent retractor from creating a button hole through the skin; Ring handles and ratchets

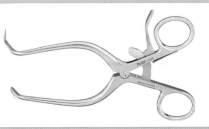

Courtesy of Miltex, Inc.

FIGURE 10-178

Weitlaner self-retaining retractor

Size: 6.5"

Quantity: 2

Notes: Ring handles and ratchets; Prongs can be sharp or blunt

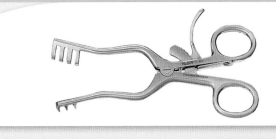

Courtesy of Miltex, Inc.

FIGURE 10-179

Bone hook

Size: 9.0"

Quantity: 2

Notes: Sharp hook to hold bone

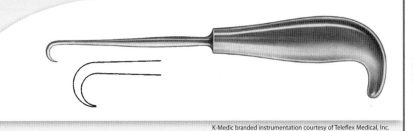

K-Medic branded instrumentation courtesy of Teleflex Medical, Inc.

FIGURE 10-180

continues

Large Bone and Joint Instruments – RETRACTION AND EXPOSURE INSTRUMENTS *continued*

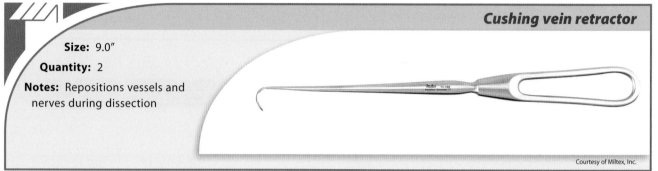

Cushing vein retractor

Size: 9.0″

Quantity: 2

Notes: Repositions vessels and nerves during dissection

Courtesy of Miltex, Inc.

FIGURE 10-181

Large Bone and Joint Instruments – APPROXIMATION AND CLOSURE INSTRUMENTS

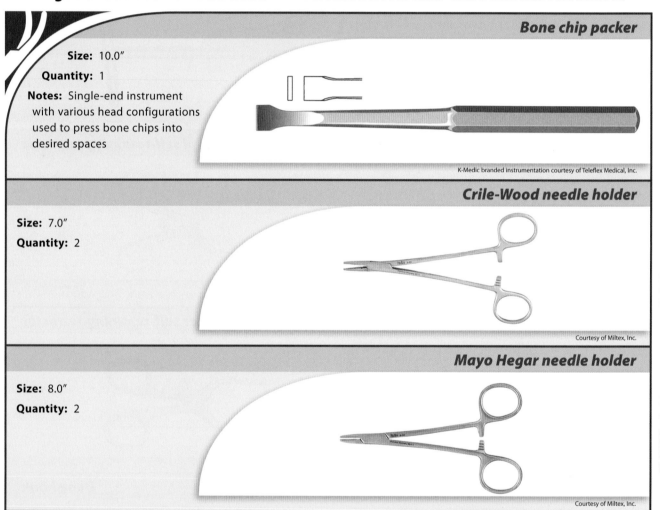

Bone chip packer

Size: 10.0″

Quantity: 1

Notes: Single-end instrument with various head configurations used to press bone chips into desired spaces

K-Medic branded instrumentation courtesy of Teleflex Medical, Inc.

FIGURE 10-182

Crile-Wood needle holder

Size: 7.0″

Quantity: 2

Courtesy of Miltex, Inc.

FIGURE 10-183

Mayo Hegar needle holder

Size: 8.0″

Quantity: 2

Courtesy of Miltex, Inc.

FIGURE 10-184

SUMMARY

Surgical services that perform procedures involving manipulation of bone that are not for specific orthopaedic purposes will utilize many of the instruments found in this chapter. Additional specialties, such as plastics or neurology that alter or manipulate bony tissue are described in other chapters.

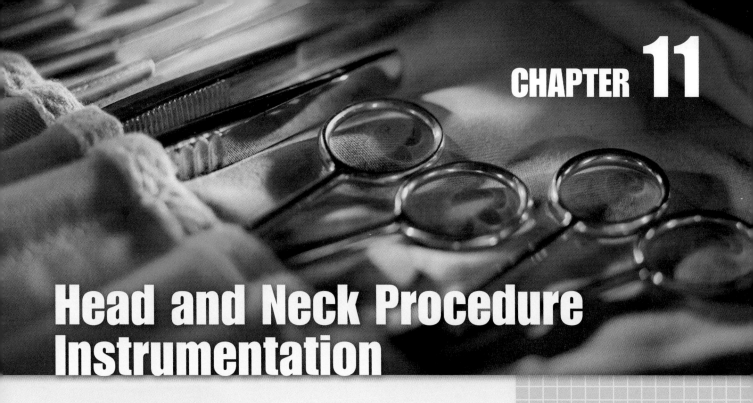

CHAPTER 11

Head and Neck Procedure Instrumentation

INTRODUCTION

Head and neck procedures involving soft tissues of the face, neck, and low anterior throat commonly require the use of soft tissue sets appropriate in length for the surgical site. Short and medium foundation sets easily offer the correct exposure and hemostasis for these procedures with the addition of a few specialty dissectors, graspers, or debulking instruments.

Specialty procedures such as ear, dental, and intraoral sites employ the use of instrumentation that performs like their larger counterparts, but have smaller than usual tips or jaws and have specially designed shanks and jaws. The reason for this is because the access point is smaller and less amenable to additional exposure by retraction when the operator's hand is in the field of vision.

EAR AND MASTOID INSTRUMENTATION

Ear instruments are highly specialized with smaller, shorter jaws and box lock angles. The handles are frequently offset so the user's hands and fingers do not obscure the target tissue. Instruments used in the intra-aural canal are described here. Microscopic instruments are listed in Chapter 14.

Ear Instrumentation

Ear Instrumentation – GRASPING FORCEPS

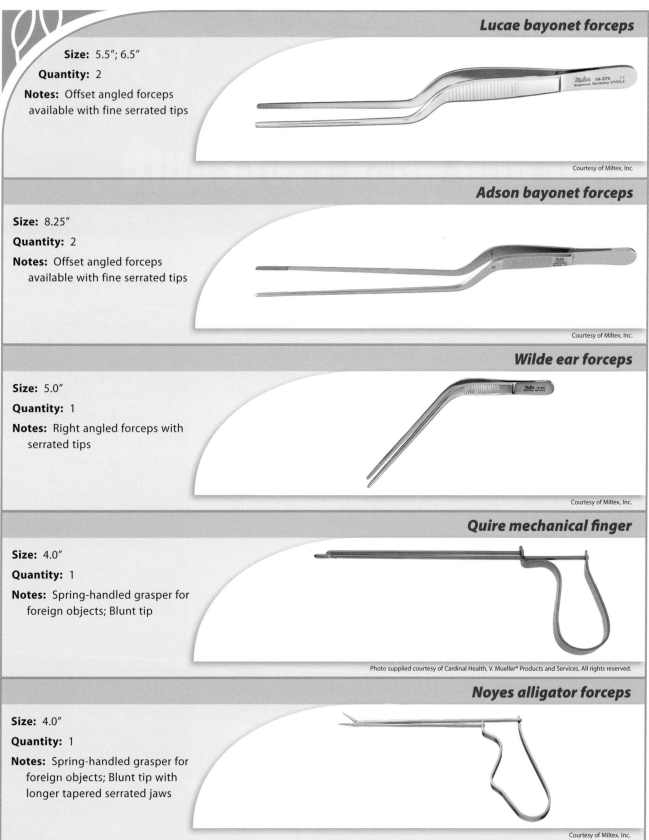

Lucae bayonet forceps

Size: 5.5″; 6.5″

Quantity: 2

Notes: Offset angled forceps available with fine serrated tips

Courtesy of Miltex, Inc.

FIGURE 11-1

Adson bayonet forceps

Size: 8.25″

Quantity: 2

Notes: Offset angled forceps available with fine serrated tips

Courtesy of Miltex, Inc.

FIGURE 11-2

Wilde ear forceps

Size: 5.0″

Quantity: 1

Notes: Right angled forceps with serrated tips

Courtesy of Miltex, Inc.

FIGURE 11-3

Quire mechanical finger

Size: 4.0″

Quantity: 1

Notes: Spring-handled grasper for foreign objects; Blunt tip

Photo supplied courtesy of Cardinal Health, V. Mueller® Products and Services. All rights reserved.

FIGURE 11-4

Noyes alligator forceps

Size: 4.0″

Quantity: 1

Notes: Spring-handled grasper for foreign objects; Blunt tip with longer tapered serrated jaws

Courtesy of Miltex, Inc.

FIGURE 11-5

Ear Instrumentation – GRASPING FORCEPS *continued*

Hartman-Herzfeld cup forceps

Size: 3.0"; 2 mm cup; 3 mm cup

Quantity: 1

Notes: Ring-handled right angled grasper; No ratchets; Small jaw

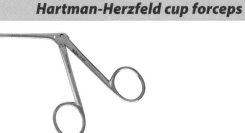

FIGURE 11-6

Weingartner ear forceps

Size: 3.0"

Quantity: 1

Notes: Ring-handled right angled grasper with concave serrated jaws

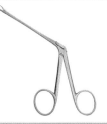

FIGURE 11-7

Struempel ear forceps

Size: 3.0"

Quantity: 1

Notes: Ring-handled right angled grasper with open oval spoon jaws with serrated edges

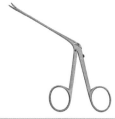

FIGURE 11-8

Hoffman ear forceps

Size: 3.0"

Quantity: 1

Notes: Ring-handled right angled grasper with open rounded cutting edged jaws

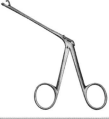

FIGURE 11-9

Wullenstein ear forceps

Size: 3.0"

Quantity: 1

Notes: Ring-handled angled forceps; Oval or round style cup jaws; 1 mm in diameter

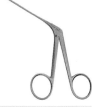

FIGURE 11-10

continues

Ear Instrumentation – GRASPING FORCEPS *continued*

Micro alligator ear forceps

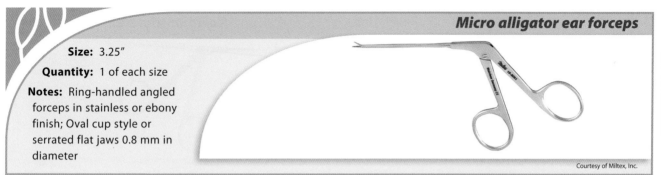

Size: 3.25"

Quantity: 1 of each size

Notes: Ring-handled angled forceps in stainless or ebony finish; Oval cup style or serrated flat jaws 0.8 mm in diameter

Courtesy of Miltex, Inc.

FIGURE 11-11

Ear Instrumentation – DISSECTION INSTRUMENTS

Myringotomy knife

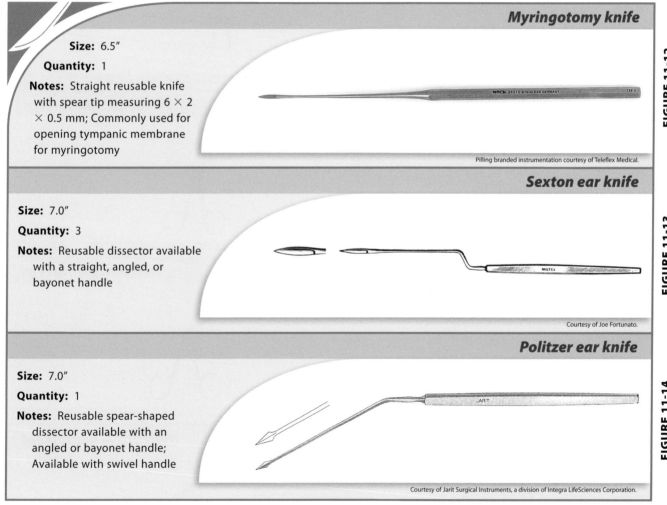

Size: 6.5"

Quantity: 1

Notes: Straight reusable knife with spear tip measuring 6 × 2 × 0.5 mm; Commonly used for opening tympanic membrane for myringotomy

Pilling branded instrumentation courtesy of Teleflex Medical.

FIGURE 11-12

Sexton ear knife

Size: 7.0"

Quantity: 3

Notes: Reusable dissector available with a straight, angled, or bayonet handle

Courtesy of Joe Fortunato.

FIGURE 11-13

Politzer ear knife

Size: 7.0"

Quantity: 1

Notes: Reusable spear-shaped dissector available with an angled or bayonet handle; Available with swivel handle

Courtesy of Jarit Surgical Instruments, a division of Integra LifeSciences Corporation.

FIGURE 11-14

Ear Instrumentation – DISSECTION INSTRUMENTS *continued*

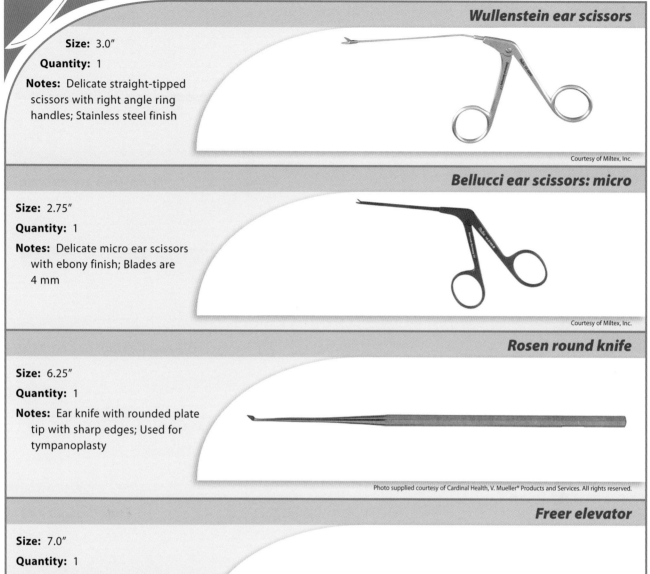

Wullenstein ear scissors

Size: 3.0″

Quantity: 1

Notes: Delicate straight-tipped scissors with right angle ring handles; Stainless steel finish

Courtesy of Miltex, Inc.

Bellucci ear scissors: micro

Size: 2.75″

Quantity: 1

Notes: Delicate micro ear scissors with ebony finish; Blades are 4 mm

Courtesy of Miltex, Inc.

Rosen round knife

Size: 6.25″

Quantity: 1

Notes: Ear knife with rounded plate tip with sharp edges; Used for tympanoplasty

Photo supplied courtesy of Cardinal Health, V. Mueller® Products and Services. All rights reserved.

Freer elevator

Size: 7.0″

Quantity: 1

Notes: Double-ended dissector; One end is sharp and the other end is blunt; Can have bright or satin finish; Cross-serrated hand-grip

Courtesy of Miltex, Inc.

Ear Instrumentation – DEBULKING INSTRUMENTS

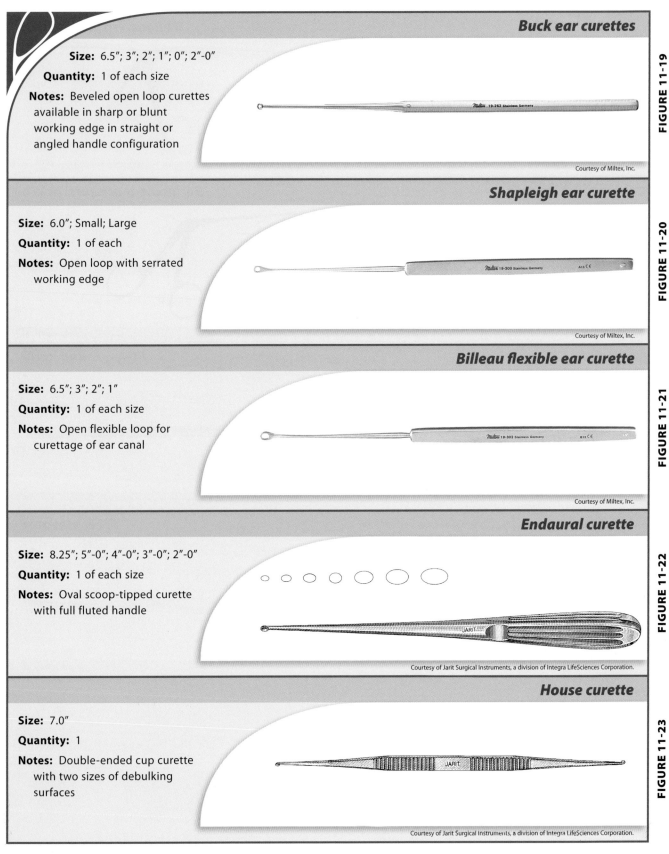

Buck ear curettes

Size: 6.5"; 3"; 2"; 1"; 0"; 2"-0"

Quantity: 1 of each size

Notes: Beveled open loop curettes available in sharp or blunt working edge in straight or angled handle configuration

Courtesy of Miltex, Inc.

FIGURE 11-19

Shapleigh ear curette

Size: 6.0"; Small; Large

Quantity: 1 of each

Notes: Open loop with serrated working edge

Courtesy of Miltex, Inc.

FIGURE 11-20

Billeau flexible ear curette

Size: 6.5"; 3"; 2"; 1"

Quantity: 1 of each size

Notes: Open flexible loop for curettage of ear canal

Courtesy of Miltex, Inc.

FIGURE 11-21

Endaural curette

Size: 8.25"; 5"-0"; 4"-0"; 3"-0"; 2"-0"

Quantity: 1 of each size

Notes: Oval scoop-tipped curette with full fluted handle

Courtesy of Jarit Surgical Instruments, a division of Integra LifeSciences Corporation.

FIGURE 11-22

House curette

Size: 7.0"

Quantity: 1

Notes: Double-ended cup curette with two sizes of debulking surfaces

Courtesy of Jarit Surgical Instruments, a division of Integra LifeSciences Corporation.

FIGURE 11-23

Ear Instrumentation – DEBULKING INSTRUMENTS *continued*

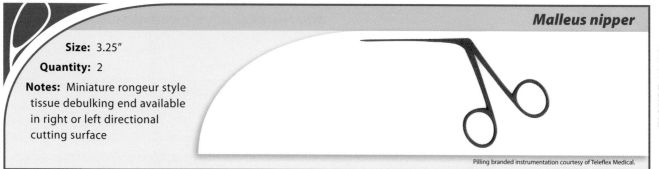

Malleus nipper

Size: 3.25"

Quantity: 2

Notes: Miniature rongeur style tissue debulking end available in right or left directional cutting surface

Pilling branded instrumentation courtesy of Teleflex Medical.

FIGURE 11-24

Ear Instrumentation – PROBES AND DILATORS

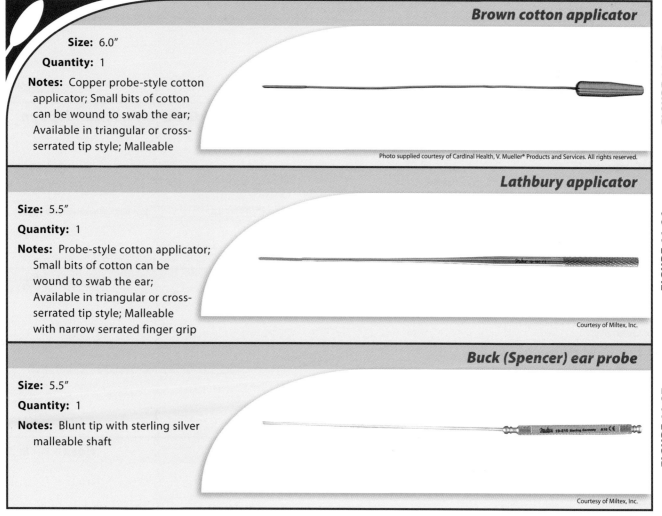

Brown cotton applicator

Size: 6.0"

Quantity: 1

Notes: Copper probe-style cotton applicator; Small bits of cotton can be wound to swab the ear; Available in triangular or cross-serrated tip style; Malleable

Photo supplied courtesy of Cardinal Health, V. Mueller® Products and Services. All rights reserved.

FIGURE 11-25

Lathbury applicator

Size: 5.5"

Quantity: 1

Notes: Probe-style cotton applicator; Small bits of cotton can be wound to swab the ear; Available in triangular or cross-serrated tip style; Malleable with narrow serrated finger grip

Courtesy of Miltex, Inc.

FIGURE 11-26

Buck (Spencer) ear probe

Size: 5.5"

Quantity: 1

Notes: Blunt tip with sterling silver malleable shaft

Courtesy of Miltex, Inc.

FIGURE 11-27

continues

Ear Instrumentation – PROBES AND DILATORS *continued*

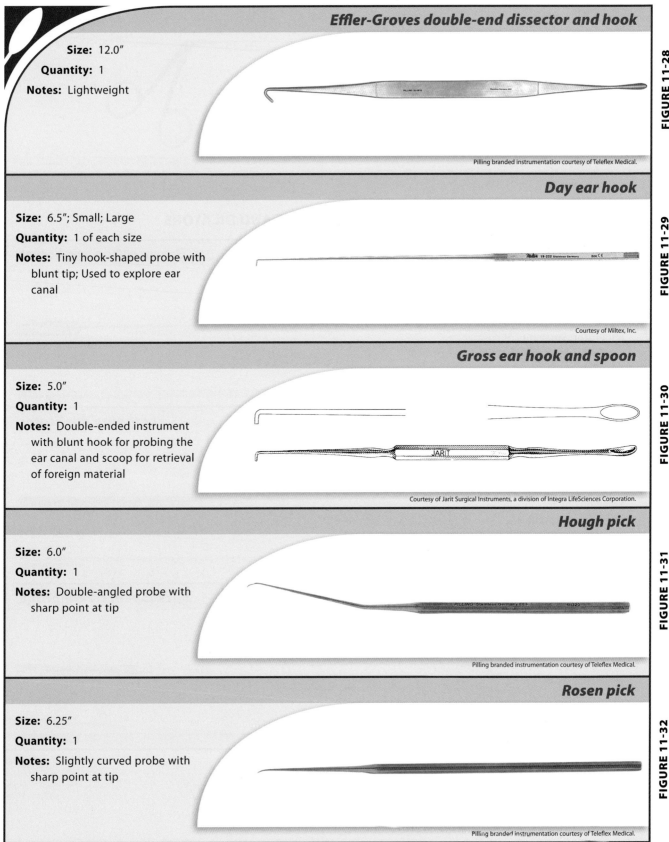

Effler-Groves double-end dissector and hook

Size: 12.0"

Quantity: 1

Notes: Lightweight

Pilling branded instrumentation courtesy of Teleflex Medical.

FIGURE 11-28

Day ear hook

Size: 6.5"; Small; Large

Quantity: 1 of each size

Notes: Tiny hook-shaped probe with blunt tip; Used to explore ear canal

Courtesy of Miltex, Inc.

FIGURE 11-29

Gross ear hook and spoon

Size: 5.0"

Quantity: 1

Notes: Double-ended instrument with blunt hook for probing the ear canal and scoop for retrieval of foreign material

Courtesy of Jarit Surgical Instruments, a division of Integra LifeSciences Corporation.

FIGURE 11-30

Hough pick

Size: 6.0"

Quantity: 1

Notes: Double-angled probe with sharp point at tip

Pilling branded instrumentation courtesy of Teleflex Medical.

FIGURE 11-31

Rosen pick

Size: 6.25"

Quantity: 1

Notes: Slightly curved probe with sharp point at tip

Pilling branded instrumentation courtesy of Teleflex Medical.

FIGURE 11-32

Ear Instrumentation – PROBES AND DILATORS *continued*

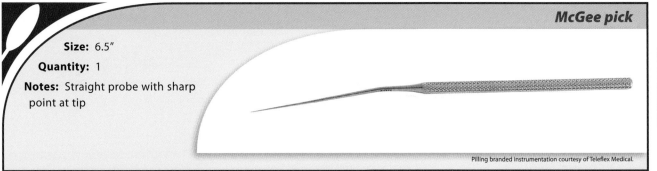

McGee pick

Size: 6.5″

Quantity: 1

Notes: Straight probe with sharp point at tip

Pilling branded instrumentation courtesy of Teleflex Medical.

FIGURE 11-33

Ear Instrumentation – EVACUATION AND INSTILLATION INSTRUMENTS

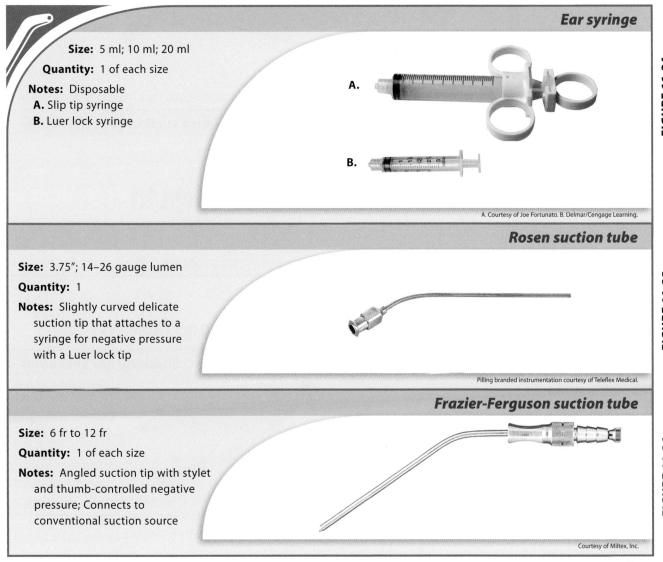

Ear syringe

Size: 5 ml; 10 ml; 20 ml

Quantity: 1 of each size

Notes: Disposable
A. Slip tip syringe
B. Luer lock syringe

A.

B.

A. Courtesy of Joe Fortunato. B. Delmar/Cengage Learning.

FIGURE 11-34

Rosen suction tube

Size: 3.75″; 14–26 gauge lumen

Quantity: 1

Notes: Slightly curved delicate suction tip that attaches to a syringe for negative pressure with a Luer lock tip

Pilling branded instrumentation courtesy of Teleflex Medical.

FIGURE 11-35

Frazier-Ferguson suction tube

Size: 6 fr to 12 fr

Quantity: 1 of each size

Notes: Angled suction tip with stylet and thumb-controlled negative pressure; Connects to conventional suction source

Courtesy of Miltex, Inc.

FIGURE 11-36

continues

Ear Instrumentation – EVACUATION AND INSTILLATION INSTRUMENTS *continued*

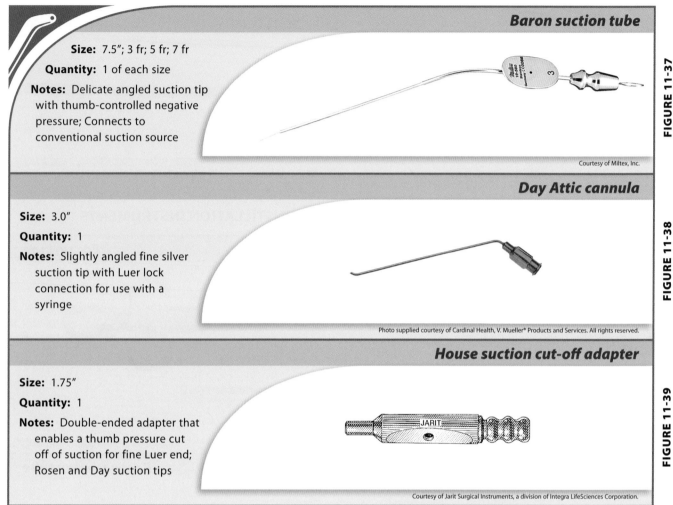

Baron suction tube

Size: 7.5"; 3 fr; 5 fr; 7 fr

Quantity: 1 of each size

Notes: Delicate angled suction tip with thumb-controlled negative pressure; Connects to conventional suction source

Courtesy of Miltex, Inc.

FIGURE 11-37

Day Attic cannula

Size: 3.0"

Quantity: 1

Notes: Slightly angled fine silver suction tip with Luer lock connection for use with a syringe

Photo supplied courtesy of Cardinal Health, V. Mueller® Products and Services. All rights reserved.

FIGURE 11-38

House suction cut-off adapter

Size: 1.75"

Quantity: 1

Notes: Double-ended adapter that enables a thumb pressure cut off of suction for fine Luer end; Rosen and Day suction tips

Courtesy of Jarit Surgical Instruments, a division of Integra LifeSciences Corporation.

FIGURE 11-39

Ear Instrumentation – RETRACTION AND EXPOSURE INSTRUMENTS

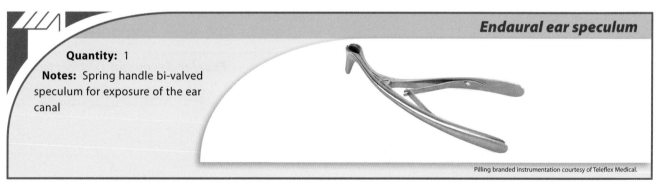

Endaural ear speculum

Quantity: 1

Notes: Spring handle bi-valved speculum for exposure of the ear canal

Pilling branded instrumentation courtesy of Teleflex Medical.

FIGURE 11-40

Ear Instrumentation – RETRACTION AND EXPOSURE INSTRUMENTS *continued*

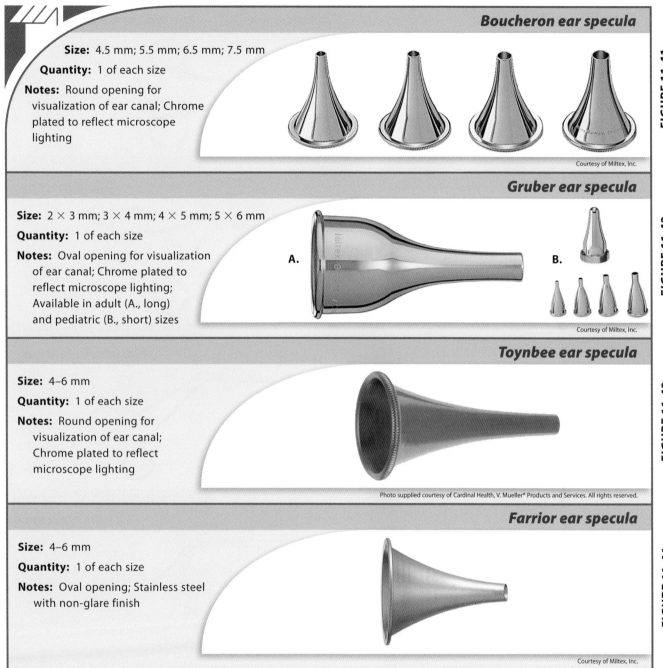

Boucheron ear specula

Size: 4.5 mm; 5.5 mm; 6.5 mm; 7.5 mm

Quantity: 1 of each size

Notes: Round opening for visualization of ear canal; Chrome plated to reflect microscope lighting

Courtesy of Miltex, Inc.

FIGURE 11-41

Gruber ear specula

Size: 2 × 3 mm; 3 × 4 mm; 4 × 5 mm; 5 × 6 mm

Quantity: 1 of each size

Notes: Oval opening for visualization of ear canal; Chrome plated to reflect microscope lighting; Available in adult (A., long) and pediatric (B., short) sizes

A.   B.

Courtesy of Miltex, Inc.

FIGURE 11-42

Toynbee ear specula

Size: 4–6 mm

Quantity: 1 of each size

Notes: Round opening for visualization of ear canal; Chrome plated to reflect microscope lighting

Photo supplied courtesy of Cardinal Health, V. Mueller® Products and Services. All rights reserved.

FIGURE 11-43

Farrior ear specula

Size: 4–6 mm

Quantity: 1 of each size

Notes: Oval opening; Stainless steel with non-glare finish

Courtesy of Miltex, Inc.

FIGURE 11-44

Mastoid Instrumentation

Mastoid procedures are a combination of compact and soft tissue surgery. The procedure involves incising epidermis and dermis with a short foundation set, cutting through bony areas, and debulking bony mastoid air cells. The following table lists several types of instruments that are commonly used during a mastoidectomy. These few instruments are added to the previously listed ear procedure instruments for a full complement of external and internal ear procedural needs.

Mastoid Instrumentation – GRASPING FORCEPS

House Gelfoam press

Size: 5.0"

Quantity: 1

Notes: Ring handle forceps with ratchets that use a snub-flat jaw for crushing Gelfoam pieces for expression of air and/or fluid

Pilling branded instrumentation courtesy of Teleflex Medical.

FIGURE 11-45

Tobey forceps

Size: 5.0"

Quantity: 1

Notes: Ring handle forceps with shanks in down angle to maintain visual perspective; No ratchet; Serrated narrow jaws

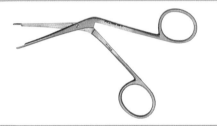

Pilling branded instrumentation courtesy of Teleflex Medical.

FIGURE 11-46

Hartmann forceps

Size: 5.0"

Quantity: 1

Notes: Ring handle forceps with shanks in down angle to maintain visual perspective; No ratchet; Serrated wider jaws

Courtesy of Ruggles Surgical Instruments, a division of Integra LifeSciences Corporation.

FIGURE 11-47

Littauer forceps

Size: 4.75"

Quantity: 1

Notes: Ring handle forceps with shanks in down angle to maintain visual perspective; No ratchet; Serrated delicate jaws

Pilling branded instrumentation courtesy of Teleflex Medical.

FIGURE 11-48

Noyes ear forceps

Size: 3.5"

Quantity: 1

Notes: Ring handle forceps with shanks in down angle to maintain visual perspective; No ratchet; Serrated up biting jaws

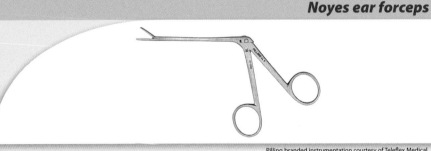

Pilling branded instrumentation courtesy of Teleflex Medical.

FIGURE 11-49

Mastoid Instrumentation – DISSECTION INSTRUMENTS

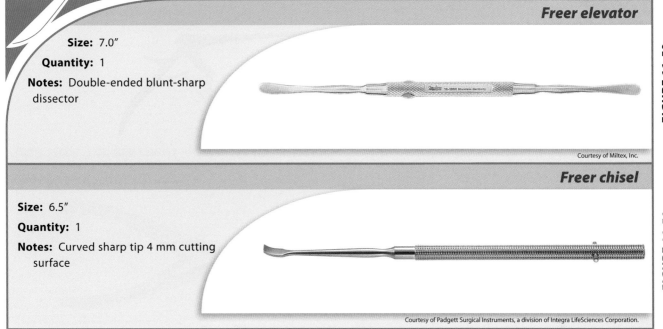

Freer elevator

Size: 7.0″

Quantity: 1

Notes: Double-ended blunt-sharp dissector

Courtesy of Miltex, Inc.

FIGURE 11-50

Freer chisel

Size: 6.5″

Quantity: 1

Notes: Curved sharp tip 4 mm cutting surface

Courtesy of Padgett Surgical Instruments, a division of Integra LifeSciences Corporation.

FIGURE 11-51

Mastoid Instrumentation – DEBULKING INSTRUMENTS

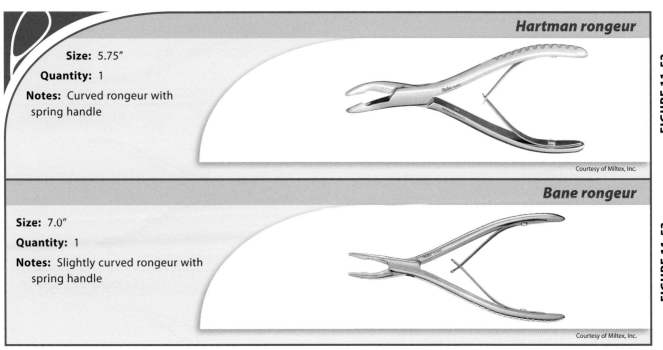

Hartman rongeur

Size: 5.75″

Quantity: 1

Notes: Curved rongeur with spring handle

Courtesy of Miltex, Inc.

FIGURE 11-52

Bane rongeur

Size: 7.0″

Quantity: 1

Notes: Slightly curved rongeur with spring handle

Courtesy of Miltex, Inc.

FIGURE 11-53

continues

Small Bone and Joint Instruments – DEBULKING INSTRUMENTS *continued*

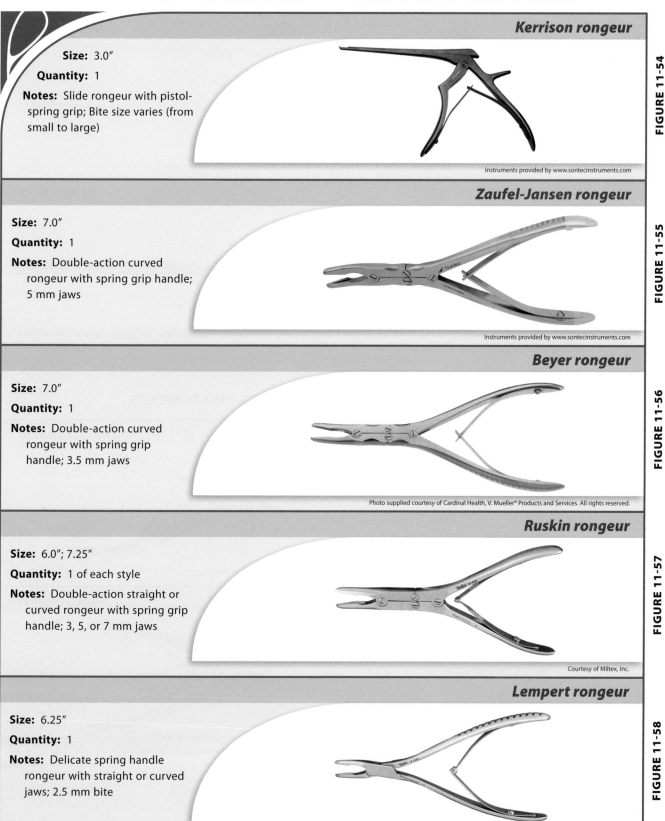

Kerrison rongeur

Size: 3.0"

Quantity: 1

Notes: Slide rongeur with pistol-spring grip; Bite size varies (from small to large)

Instruments provided by www.sontecinstruments.com

FIGURE 11-54

Zaufel-Jansen rongeur

Size: 7.0"

Quantity: 1

Notes: Double-action curved rongeur with spring grip handle; 5 mm jaws

Instruments provided by www.sontecinstruments.com

FIGURE 11-55

Beyer rongeur

Size: 7.0"

Quantity: 1

Notes: Double-action curved rongeur with spring grip handle; 3.5 mm jaws

Photo supplied courtesy of Cardinal Health, V. Mueller® Products and Services. All rights reserved.

FIGURE 11-56

Ruskin rongeur

Size: 6.0"; 7.25"

Quantity: 1 of each style

Notes: Double-action straight or curved rongeur with spring grip handle; 3, 5, or 7 mm jaws

Courtesy of Miltex, Inc.

FIGURE 11-57

Lempert rongeur

Size: 6.25"

Quantity: 1

Notes: Delicate spring handle rongeur with straight or curved jaws; 2.5 mm bite

Courtesy of Miltex, Inc.

FIGURE 11-58

Small Bone and Joint Instruments – DEBULKING INSTRUMENTS *continued*

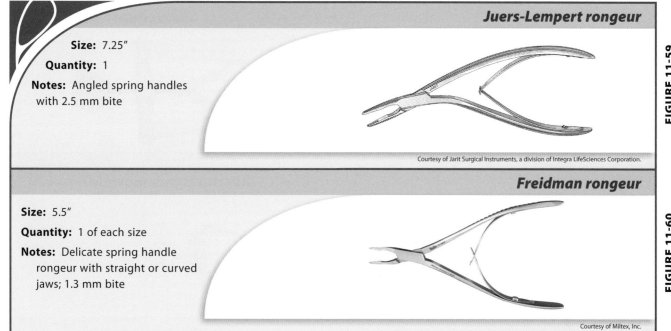

Juers-Lempert rongeur

Size: 7.25"

Quantity: 1

Notes: Angled spring handles with 2.5 mm bite

Courtesy of Jarit Surgical Instruments, a division of Integra LifeSciences Corporation.

FIGURE 11-59

Freidman rongeur

Size: 5.5"

Quantity: 1 of each size

Notes: Delicate spring handle rongeur with straight or curved jaws; 1.3 mm bite

Courtesy of Miltex, Inc.

FIGURE 11-60

Mastoid Instrumentation – RETRACTION AND EXPOSURE INSTRUMENTS

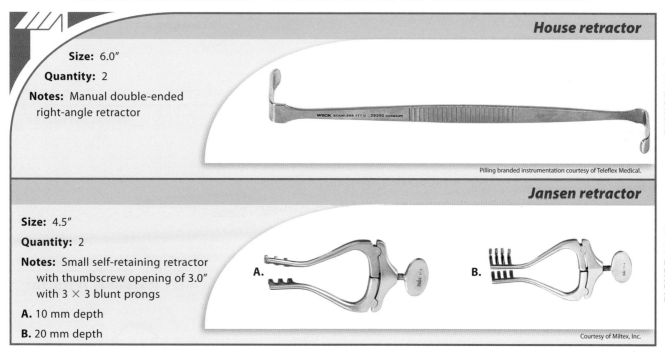

House retractor

Size: 6.0"

Quantity: 2

Notes: Manual double-ended right-angle retractor

Pilling branded instrumentation courtesy of Teleflex Medical.

FIGURE 11-61

Jansen retractor

Size: 4.5"

Quantity: 2

Notes: Small self-retaining retractor with thumbscrew opening of 3.0" with 3 × 3 blunt prongs

A. 10 mm depth

B. 20 mm depth

Courtesy of Miltex, Inc.

FIGURE 11-62

continues

Mastoid Instrumentation – RETRACTION AND EXPOSURE INSTRUMENTS *continued*

Allport mastoid retractor

Size: 4.0"

Quantity: 2

Notes: Self-retaining retractor with thumbscrew spread of 2.5"; Sharp 4 × 4 prongs

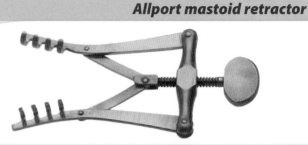

FIGURE 11-63

Jansen-Wagner mastoid retractor

Size: 5.0"

Quantity: 2

Notes: Self-retaining retractor with thumbscrew; Sharp prongs 5 × 5 on pivots for self-adjusting positioning

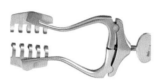

FIGURE 11-64

Alm retractor

Size: 2.75"; 3.75"

Quantity: 1

Notes: Small self-retaining retractor with thumbscrew and short 4 × 4 prongs

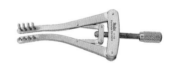

FIGURE 11-65

Heiss retractor

Size: 4.0"

Quantity: 2

Notes: Cross-action retractor with 4 × 4 prongs available in sharp or blunt styles

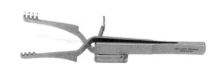

FIGURE 11-66

Weitlaner retractor

Size: 4.0"; 5.5"; 6.5"

Quantity: 2

Notes: Self-retaining retractor that locks with ratchets; Ring handles; Sharp or blunt prongs

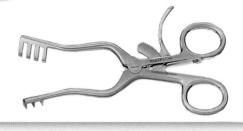

FIGURE 11-67

Mastoid Instrumentation – RETRACTION AND EXPOSURE INSTRUMENTS *continued*

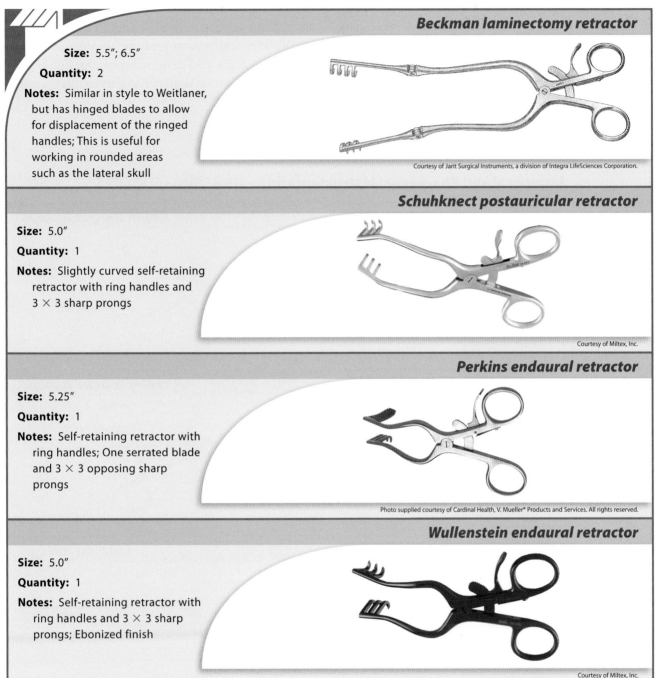

Beckman laminectomy retractor

FIGURE 11-68

Size: 5.5"; 6.5"

Quantity: 2

Notes: Similar in style to Weitlaner, but has hinged blades to allow for displacement of the ringed handles; This is useful for working in rounded areas such as the lateral skull

Courtesy of Jarit Surgical Instruments, a division of Integra LifeSciences Corporation.

Schuhknect postauricular retractor

FIGURE 11-69

Size: 5.0"

Quantity: 1

Notes: Slightly curved self-retaining retractor with ring handles and 3 × 3 sharp prongs

Courtesy of Miltex, Inc.

Perkins endaural retractor

FIGURE 11-70

Size: 5.25"

Quantity: 1

Notes: Self-retaining retractor with ring handles; One serrated blade and 3 × 3 opposing sharp prongs

Photo supplied courtesy of Cardinal Health, V. Mueller® Products and Services. All rights reserved.

Wullenstein endaural retractor

FIGURE 11-71

Size: 5.0"

Quantity: 1

Notes: Self-retaining retractor with ring handles and 3 × 3 sharp prongs; Ebonized finish

Courtesy of Miltex, Inc.

NOSE AND THROAT INSTRUMENTATION

Nasal procedures include internal and external components of soft and compact tissue modification. External tissue modification requires the use of a short foundation set. When external nasal procedures are combined with internal procedures the following instrumentation should be added to complete the set-up.

Internal nasal instruments commonly have ring handles, spring handles, or pistol-style grips. The working space limits the area available for instrument jaw mobility; therefore, the shanks will be narrow and the jaws and tips will be shorter. Some debulking instruments will have double-action hinges to minimize visual obstruction during tissue removal. Many of the instruments will be angled to prevent the user's hands from blocking the view of the surgical field. Scrub personnel should keep the suction immediately available to the site because of the vascular nature of nasal tissue and the anatomic structures. The nasopharynx is a direct path to the airway and could collect clots and tissue around the balloon of the endotracheal tube. If the sinuses are entered, the aspirated material could be purulent and heavily laden with microorganisms. The instrumentation in this section are used in the nasopharynx. The exterior neck instrumentation is described later in this chapter.

Intranasal and Pharyngeal Instrumentation

Intranasal and Pharyngeal Instrumentation – GRASPING FORCEPS

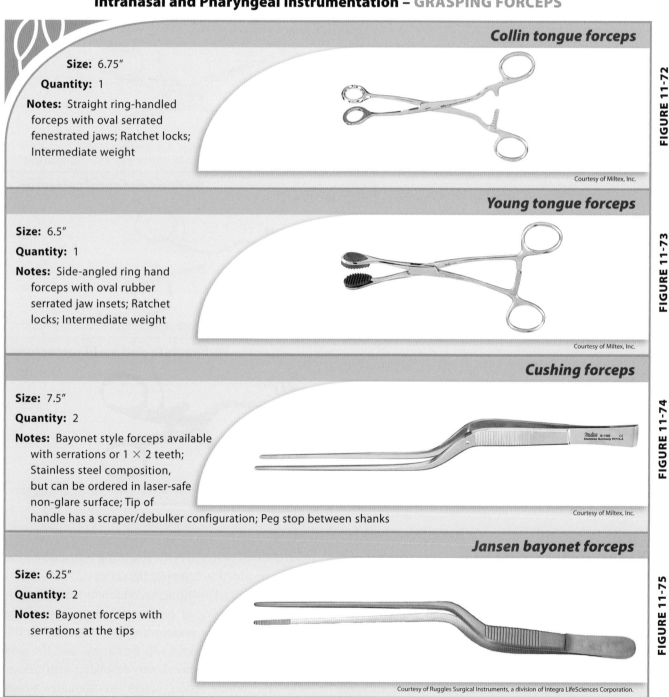

Collin tongue forceps

Size: 6.75"

Quantity: 1

Notes: Straight ring-handled forceps with oval serrated fenestrated jaws; Ratchet locks; Intermediate weight

Courtesy of Miltex, Inc.

FIGURE 11-72

Young tongue forceps

Size: 6.5"

Quantity: 1

Notes: Side-angled ring hand forceps with oval rubber serrated jaw insets; Ratchet locks; Intermediate weight

Courtesy of Miltex, Inc.

FIGURE 11-73

Cushing forceps

Size: 7.5"

Quantity: 2

Notes: Bayonet style forceps available with serrations or 1 × 2 teeth; Stainless steel composition, but can be ordered in laser-safe non-glare surface; Tip of handle has a scraper/debulker configuration; Peg stop between shanks

Courtesy of Miltex, Inc.

FIGURE 11-74

Jansen bayonet forceps

Size: 6.25"

Quantity: 2

Notes: Bayonet forceps with serrations at the tips

Courtesy of Ruggles Surgical Instruments, a division of Integra LifeSciences Corporation.

FIGURE 11-75

Intranasal and Pharyngeal Instrumentation – GRASPING FORCEPS *continued*

Adson bayonet forceps

Size: 8.25″

Quantity: 1

Notes: Longer bayonet forceps with serrations at the tip; Peg stop between shanks

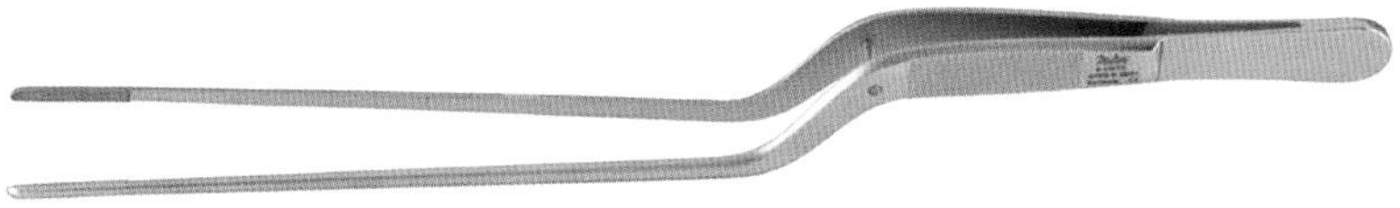

Courtesy of Miltex, Inc.

FIGURE 11-76

Hartman nasal forceps

Size: 7.0″; 7.25″

Quantity: 1

Notes: Ring handle angled grasper with long shanks, oval tips, and serrated jaws; Delicate weight available; No ratchets

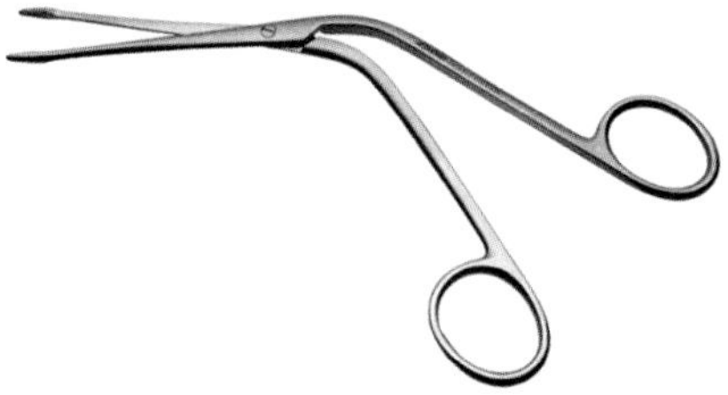

Instruments provided by www.sontecinstruments.com

FIGURE 11-77

Noyes alligator forceps

Size: 5.50″; 6.50″

Quantity: 1 of each size

Notes: Short serrated oval jaws with angled ring handles; 1 × 2 teeth available; No ratchets

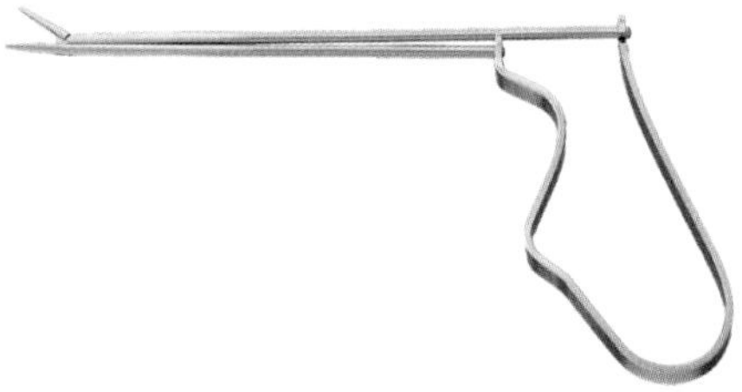

Courtesy of Miltex, Inc.

FIGURE 11-78

Knight nasal forceps

Size: 6.75″

Quantity: 1

Notes: Medium length serrated oval or cupped jaws with angled ring handles; No ratchets

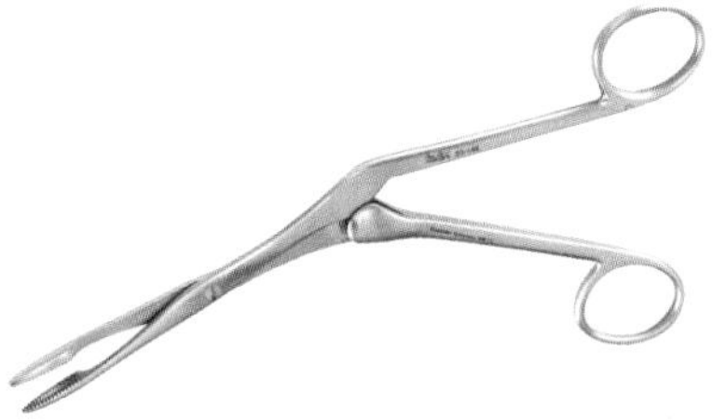

Courtesy of Miltex, Inc.

FIGURE 11-79

Museholdt nasal forceps

Size: 7.0″

Quantity: 1

Notes: Long narrow serrated jaws with angled ring handles; Hinge situated along shanks to minimize space needed for opening; No ratchets

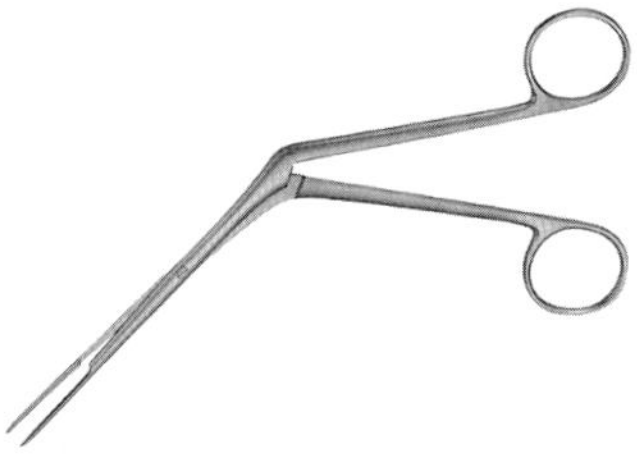

Photo supplied courtesy of Cardinal Health, V. Mueller® Products and Services. All rights reserved.

FIGURE 11-80

continues

Intranasal and Pharyngeal Instrumentation – GRASPING FORCEPS *continued*

Killian septum forceps

Size: 6.75"

Quantity: 1

Notes: Wide, flat serrated jaws with angled ring handles; No ratchets

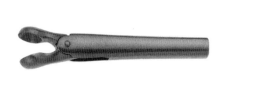

FIGURE 11-81

Watson-Williams polyp forceps

Size: 7.75"

Quantity: 1

Notes: Flat rounded jaws available in 9 mm or 6 mm diameter surface; No ratchets; Angled ring handles

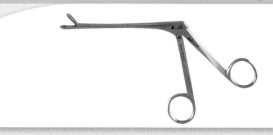

FIGURE 11-82

Lewis septum forceps

Size: 8.0"

Quantity: 1

Notes: Flat serrated jaws; Hinge situated along shanks for minimal opening; No ratchets; Angled ring handles

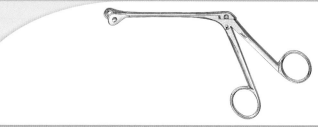

FIGURE 11-83

Rubin septal morselizer

Size: 8.0"

Quantity: 1

Notes: Flat heavily serrated jaws; Double-action hinges to minimize visual obstruction during firm grasping and crushing of tissue; Angled spring handles; Tip guard

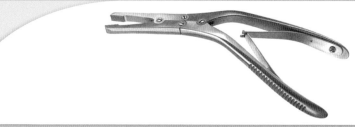

FIGURE 11-84

Ballenger tonsil forceps

Size: 8.5"

Quantity: 1

Notes: Curved jaws with 3 × 3 teeth; One open ring with ratchet locks

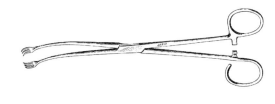

FIGURE 11-85

Intranasal and Pharyngeal Instrumentation – GRASPING FORCEPS *continued*

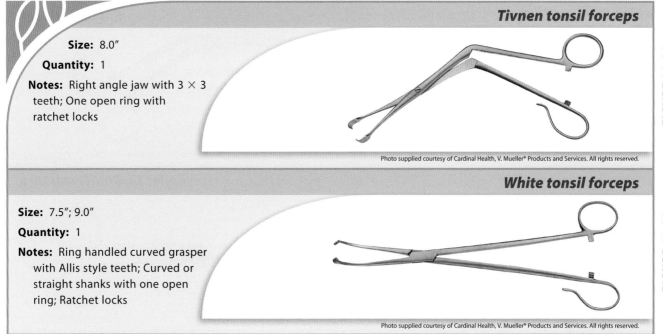

Tivnen tonsil forceps

Size: 8.0″

Quantity: 1

Notes: Right angle jaw with 3 × 3 teeth; One open ring with ratchet locks

FIGURE 11-86

White tonsil forceps

Size: 7.5″; 9.0″

Quantity: 1

Notes: Ring handled curved grasper with Allis style teeth; Curved or straight shanks with one open ring; Ratchet locks

FIGURE 11-87

Intranasal and Pharyngeal Instrumentation – DISSECTION INSTRUMENTS

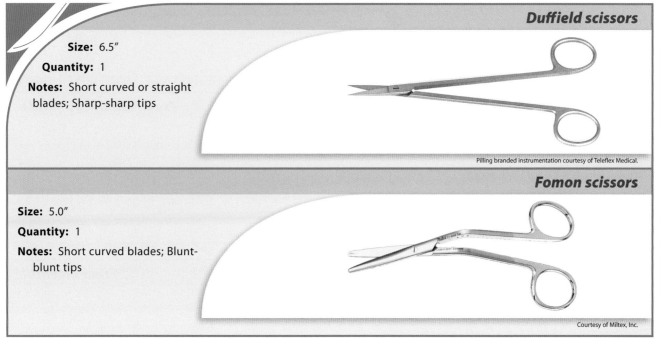

Duffield scissors

Size: 6.5″

Quantity: 1

Notes: Short curved or straight blades; Sharp-sharp tips

FIGURE 11-88

Fomon scissors

Size: 5.0″

Quantity: 1

Notes: Short curved blades; Blunt-blunt tips

FIGURE 11-89

continues

Intranasal and Pharyngeal Instrumentation – DISSECTION INSTRUMENTS *continued*

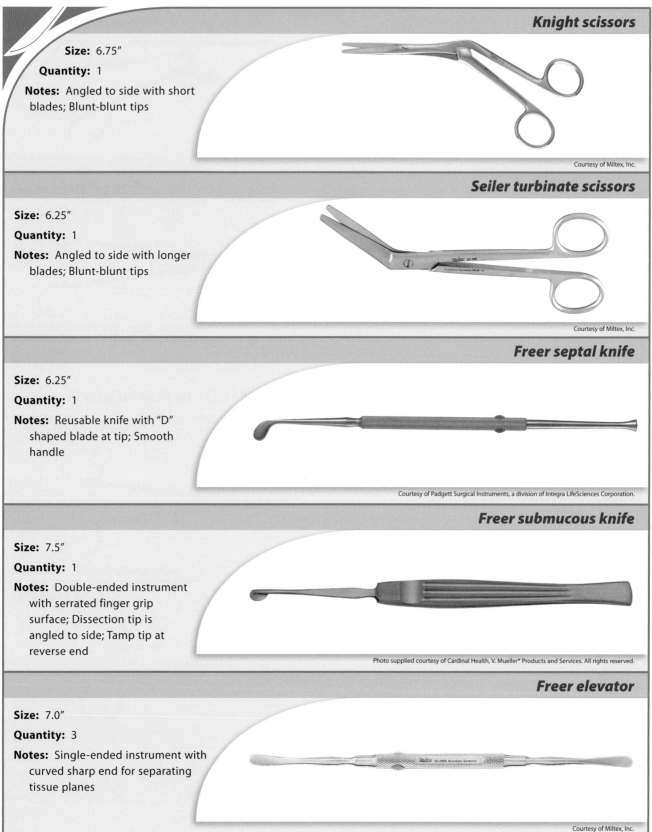

Knight scissors

Size: 6.75"

Quantity: 1

Notes: Angled to side with short blades; Blunt-blunt tips

Courtesy of Miltex, Inc.

FIGURE 11-90

Seiler turbinate scissors

Size: 6.25"

Quantity: 1

Notes: Angled to side with longer blades; Blunt-blunt tips

Courtesy of Miltex, Inc.

FIGURE 11-91

Freer septal knife

Size: 6.25"

Quantity: 1

Notes: Reusable knife with "D" shaped blade at tip; Smooth handle

Courtesy of Padgett Surgical Instruments, a division of Integra LifeSciences Corporation.

FIGURE 11-92

Freer submucous knife

Size: 7.5"

Quantity: 1

Notes: Double-ended instrument with serrated finger grip surface; Dissection tip is angled to side; Tamp tip at reverse end

Photo supplied courtesy of Cardinal Health, V. Mueller® Products and Services. All rights reserved.

FIGURE 11-93

Freer elevator

Size: 7.0"

Quantity: 3

Notes: Single-ended instrument with curved sharp end for separating tissue planes

Courtesy of Miltex, Inc.

FIGURE 11-94

Intranasal and Pharyngeal Instrumentation – DISSECTION INSTRUMENTS *continued*

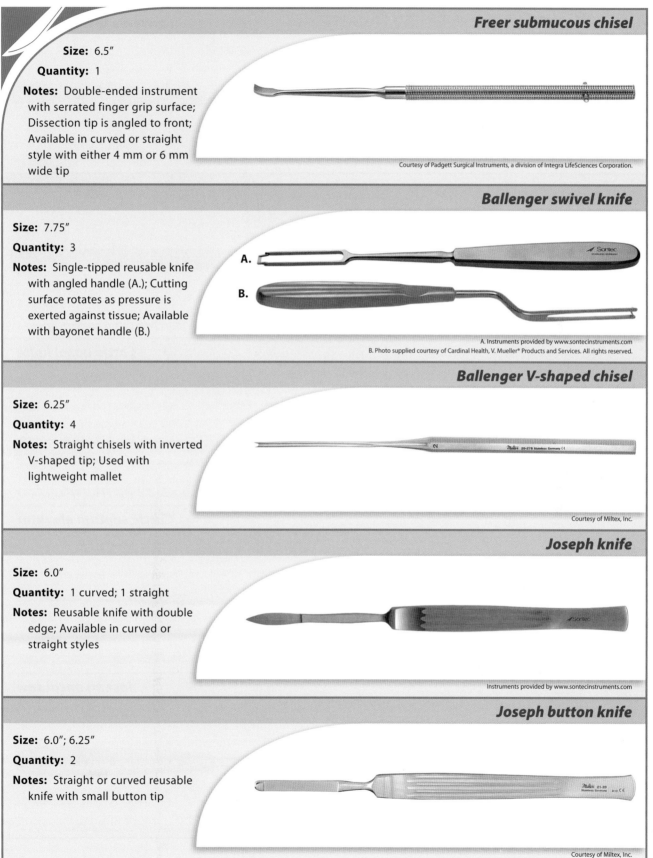

Freer submucous chisel

Size: 6.5"

Quantity: 1

Notes: Double-ended instrument with serrated finger grip surface; Dissection tip is angled to front; Available in curved or straight style with either 4 mm or 6 mm wide tip

Courtesy of Padgett Surgical Instruments, a division of Integra LifeSciences Corporation.

FIGURE 11-95

Ballenger swivel knife

Size: 7.75"

Quantity: 3

Notes: Single-tipped reusable knife with angled handle (A.); Cutting surface rotates as pressure is exerted against tissue; Available with bayonet handle (B.)

A.

B.

A. Instruments provided by www.sontecinstruments.com
B. Photo supplied courtesy of Cardinal Health, V. Mueller® Products and Services. All rights reserved.

FIGURE 11-96

Ballenger V-shaped chisel

Size: 6.25"

Quantity: 4

Notes: Straight chisels with inverted V-shaped tip; Used with lightweight mallet

Courtesy of Miltex, Inc.

FIGURE 11-97

Joseph knife

Size: 6.0"

Quantity: 1 curved; 1 straight

Notes: Reusable knife with double edge; Available in curved or straight styles

Instruments provided by www.sontecinstruments.com

FIGURE 11-98

Joseph button knife

Size: 6.0"; 6.25"

Quantity: 2

Notes: Straight or curved reusable knife with small button tip

Courtesy of Miltex, Inc.

FIGURE 11-99

continues

Intranasal and Pharyngeal Instrumentation – DISSECTION INSTRUMENTS *continued*

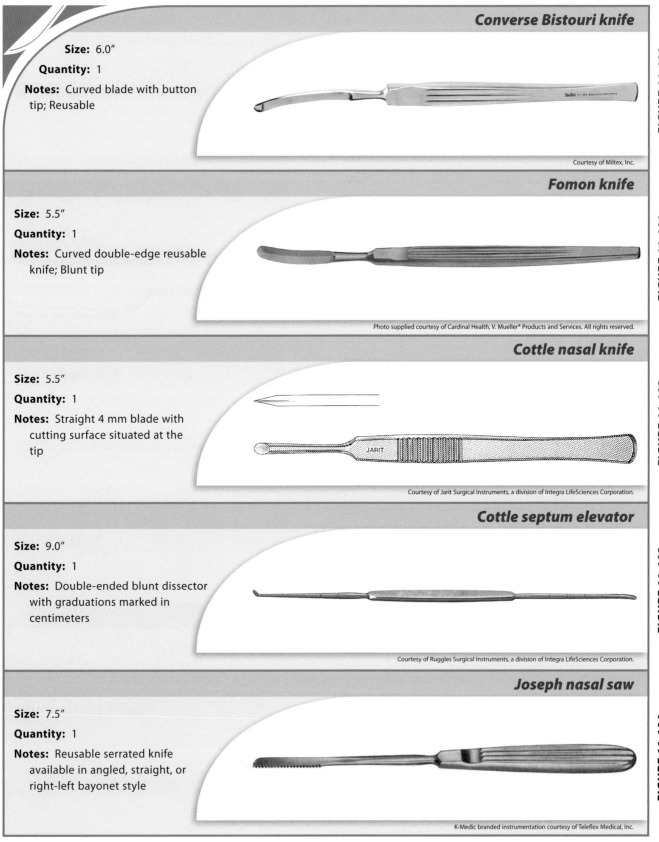

Converse Bistouri knife

Size: 6.0"

Quantity: 1

Notes: Curved blade with button tip; Reusable

FIGURE 11-100

Fomon knife

Size: 5.5"

Quantity: 1

Notes: Curved double-edge reusable knife; Blunt tip

FIGURE 11-101

Cottle nasal knife

Size: 5.5"

Quantity: 1

Notes: Straight 4 mm blade with cutting surface situated at the tip

FIGURE 11-102

Cottle septum elevator

Size: 9.0"

Quantity: 1

Notes: Double-ended blunt dissector with graduations marked in centimeters

FIGURE 11-103

Joseph nasal saw

Size: 7.5"

Quantity: 1

Notes: Reusable serrated knife available in angled, straight, or right-left bayonet style

FIGURE 11-104

Intranasal and Pharyngeal Instrumentation – DISSECTION INSTRUMENTS *continued*

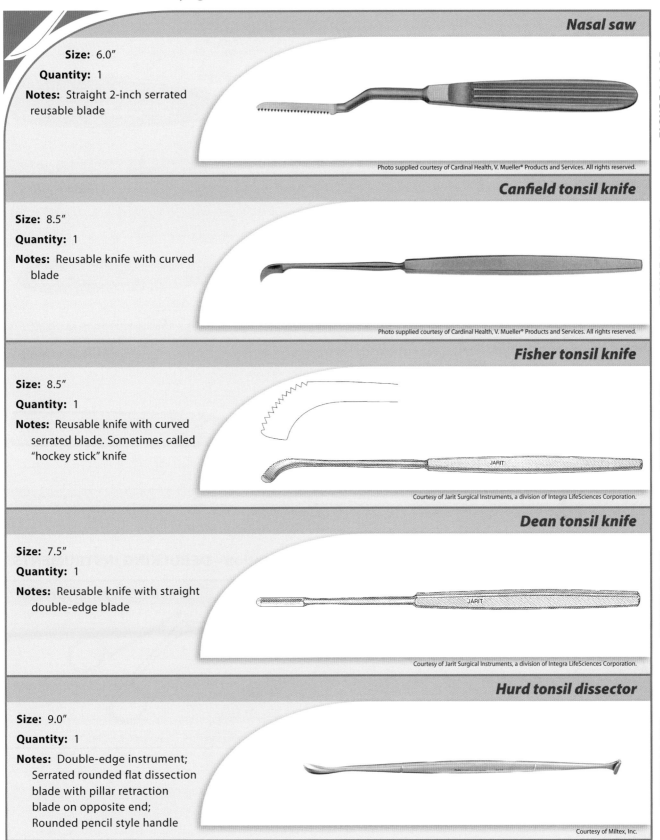

Nasal saw

Size: 6.0"

Quantity: 1

Notes: Straight 2-inch serrated reusable blade

FIGURE 11-105

Canfield tonsil knife

Size: 8.5"

Quantity: 1

Notes: Reusable knife with curved blade

FIGURE 11-106

Fisher tonsil knife

Size: 8.5"

Quantity: 1

Notes: Reusable knife with curved serrated blade. Sometimes called "hockey stick" knife

FIGURE 11-107

Dean tonsil knife

Size: 7.5"

Quantity: 1

Notes: Reusable knife with straight double-edge blade

FIGURE 11-108

Hurd tonsil dissector

Size: 9.0"

Quantity: 1

Notes: Double-edge instrument; Serrated rounded flat dissection blade with pillar retraction blade on opposite end; Rounded pencil style handle

FIGURE 11-109

continues

Intranasal and Pharyngeal Instrumentation – DISSECTION INSTRUMENTS *continued*

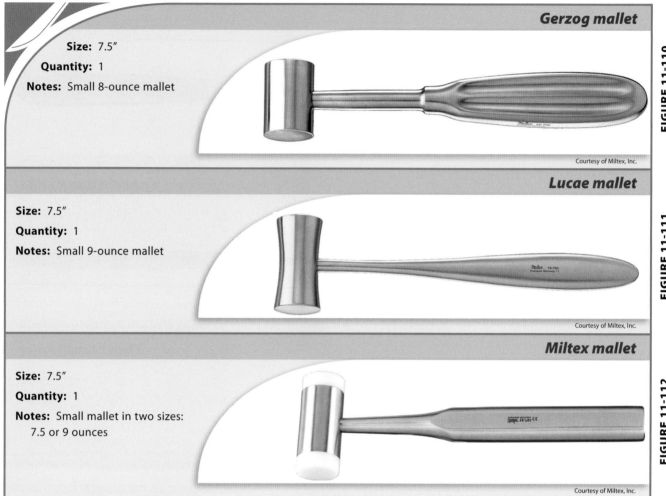

Gerzog mallet

Size: 7.5″

Quantity: 1

Notes: Small 8-ounce mallet

Courtesy of Miltex, Inc.

FIGURE 11-110

Lucae mallet

Size: 7.5″

Quantity: 1

Notes: Small 9-ounce mallet

Courtesy of Miltex, Inc.

FIGURE 11-111

Miltex mallet

Size: 7.5″

Quantity: 1

Notes: Small mallet in two sizes: 7.5 or 9 ounces

Courtesy of Miltex, Inc.

FIGURE 11-112

Intranasal and Pharyngeal Instrumentation – DEBULKING INSTRUMENTS

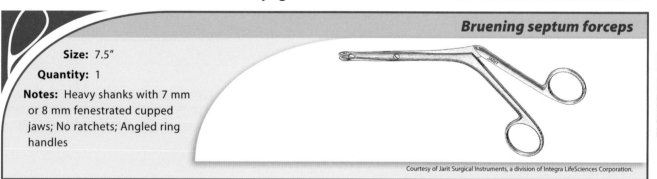

Bruening septum forceps

Size: 7.5″

Quantity: 1

Notes: Heavy shanks with 7 mm or 8 mm fenestrated cupped jaws; No ratchets; Angled ring handles

Courtesy of Jarit Surgical Instruments, a division of Integra LifeSciences Corporation.

FIGURE 11-113

Intranasal and Pharyngeal Instrumentation – DEBULKING INSTRUMENTS *continued*

Jansen-Middleton forceps

Size: 7.5″

Quantity: 2

Notes: Double-action angled spring handles; Spoon-shaped jaws or flat oval cutting jaws

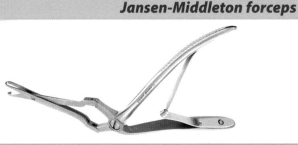

FIGURE 11-114

Takahashi ethmoid forceps

Size: 4.5″

Quantity: 1

Notes: Angled ring handles; No ratchets; Elongated cup jaws

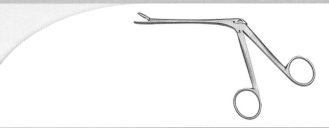

FIGURE 11-115

Wilde (Blakesley) ethmoid forceps

Size: 5.0″

Quantity: 4

Notes: Angled ring handles; No ratchets; Pointed fenestrated cutting jaws available in four sizes

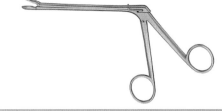

FIGURE 11-116

Gruenwald nasal forceps

Size: 4.5″

Quantity: 3

Notes: Angled ring handles; No ratchets; Sharp cutting oval jaws available in three sizes

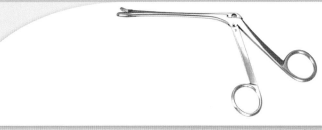

FIGURE 11-117

Struyken turbinate forceps

Size: 4.5″

Quantity: 1

Notes: Angled ring handles; No ratchets; Sharp cutting narrow oval jaws

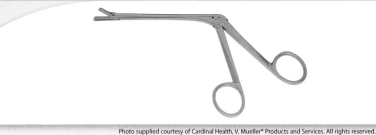

FIGURE 11-118

continues

Intranasal and Pharyngeal Instrumentation – DEBULKING INSTRUMENTS *continued*

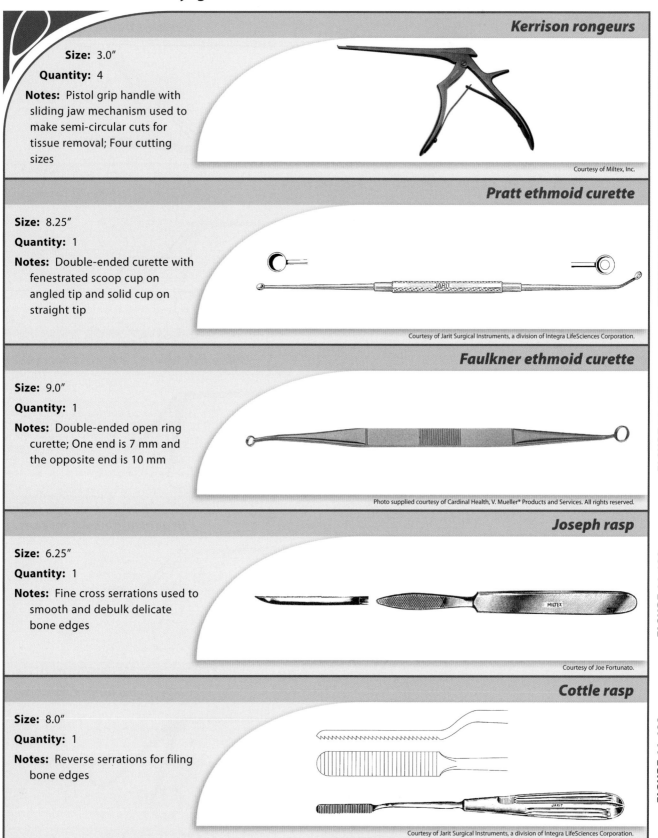

Kerrison rongeurs

Size: 3.0″

Quantity: 4

Notes: Pistol grip handle with sliding jaw mechanism used to make semi-circular cuts for tissue removal; Four cutting sizes

Courtesy of Miltex, Inc.

FIGURE 11-119

Pratt ethmoid curette

Size: 8.25″

Quantity: 1

Notes: Double-ended curette with fenestrated scoop cup on angled tip and solid cup on straight tip

Courtesy of Jarit Surgical Instruments, a division of Integra LifeSciences Corporation.

FIGURE 11-120

Faulkner ethmoid curette

Size: 9.0″

Quantity: 1

Notes: Double-ended open ring curette; One end is 7 mm and the opposite end is 10 mm

Photo supplied courtesy of Cardinal Health, V. Mueller® Products and Services. All rights reserved.

FIGURE 11-121

Joseph rasp

Size: 6.25″

Quantity: 1

Notes: Fine cross serrations used to smooth and debulk delicate bone edges

Courtesy of Joe Fortunato.

FIGURE 11-122

Cottle rasp

Size: 8.0″

Quantity: 1

Notes: Reverse serrations for filing bone edges

Courtesy of Jarit Surgical Instruments, a division of Integra LifeSciences Corporation.

FIGURE 11-123

Intranasal and Pharyngeal Instrumentation – DEBULKING INSTRUMENTS *continued*

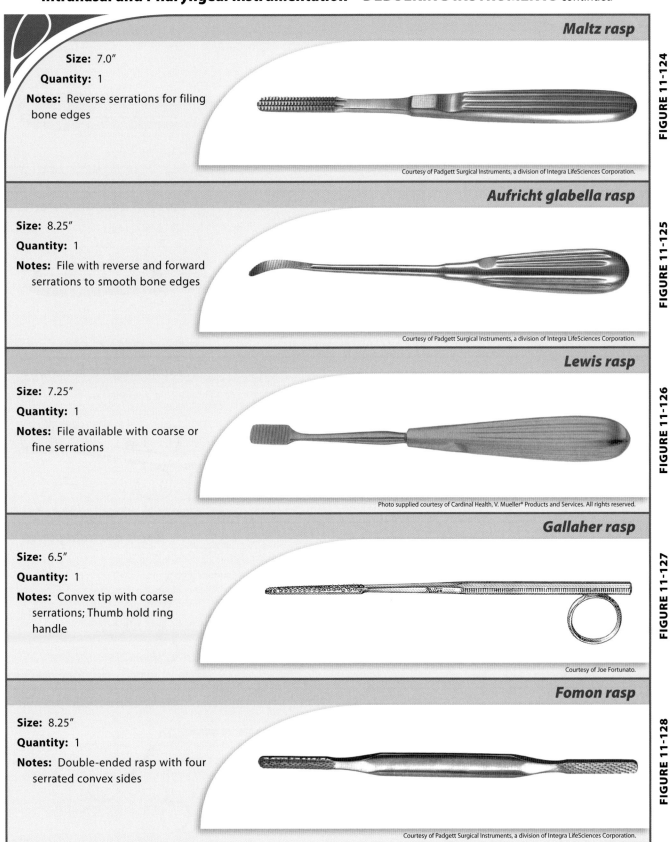

Maltz rasp

FIGURE 11-124

Size: 7.0″

Quantity: 1

Notes: Reverse serrations for filing bone edges

Courtesy of Padgett Surgical Instruments, a division of Integra LifeSciences Corporation.

Aufricht glabella rasp

FIGURE 11-125

Size: 8.25″

Quantity: 1

Notes: File with reverse and forward serrations to smooth bone edges

Courtesy of Padgett Surgical Instruments, a division of Integra LifeSciences Corporation.

Lewis rasp

FIGURE 11-126

Size: 7.25″

Quantity: 1

Notes: File available with coarse or fine serrations

Photo supplied courtesy of Cardinal Health, V. Mueller® Products and Services. All rights reserved.

Gallaher rasp

FIGURE 11-127

Size: 6.5″

Quantity: 1

Notes: Convex tip with coarse serrations; Thumb hold ring handle

Courtesy of Joe Fortunato.

Fomon rasp

FIGURE 11-128

Size: 8.25″

Quantity: 1

Notes: Double-ended rasp with four serrated convex sides

Courtesy of Padgett Surgical Instruments, a division of Integra LifeSciences Corporation.

continues

Intranasal and Pharyngeal Instrumentation – DEBULKING INSTRUMENTS *continued*

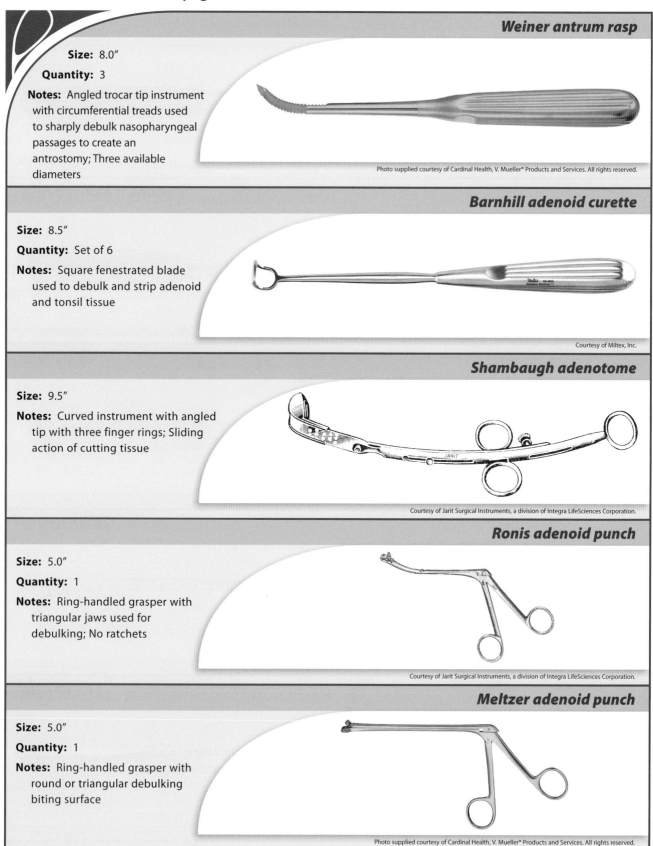

Weiner antrum rasp

Size: 8.0"

Quantity: 3

Notes: Angled trocar tip instrument with circumferential treads used to sharply debulk nasopharyngeal passages to create an antrostomy; Three available diameters

FIGURE 11-129

Barnhill adenoid curette

Size: 8.5"

Quantity: Set of 6

Notes: Square fenestrated blade used to debulk and strip adenoid and tonsil tissue

FIGURE 11-130

Shambaugh adenotome

Size: 9.5"

Notes: Curved instrument with angled tip with three finger rings; Sliding action of cutting tissue

FIGURE 11-131

Ronis adenoid punch

Size: 5.0"

Quantity: 1

Notes: Ring-handled grasper with triangular jaws used for debulking; No ratchets

FIGURE 11-132

Meltzer adenoid punch

Size: 5.0"

Quantity: 1

Notes: Ring-handled grasper with round or triangular debulking biting surface

FIGURE 11-133

Intranasal and Pharyngeal Instrumentation – PROBES AND DILATORS

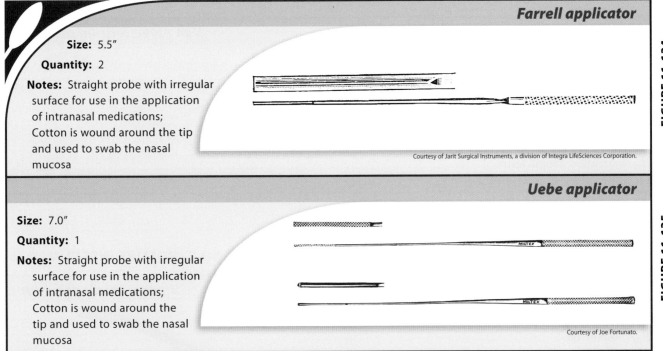

Farrell applicator

Size: 5.5″

Quantity: 2

Notes: Straight probe with irregular surface for use in the application of intranasal medications; Cotton is wound around the tip and used to swab the nasal mucosa

Courtesy of Jarit Surgical Instruments, a division of Integra LifeSciences Corporation.

FIGURE 11-134

Uebe applicator

Size: 7.0″

Quantity: 1

Notes: Straight probe with irregular surface for use in the application of intranasal medications; Cotton is wound around the tip and used to swab the nasal mucosa

Courtesy of Joe Fortunato.

FIGURE 11-135

Intranasal and Pharyngeal Instrumentation – EVACUATION AND INSTILLATION INSTRUMENTS

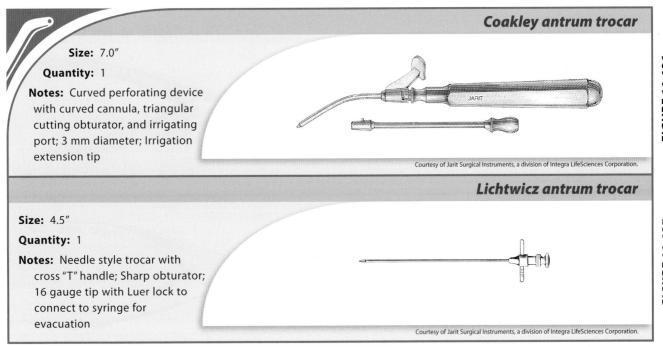

Coakley antrum trocar

Size: 7.0″

Quantity: 1

Notes: Curved perforating device with curved cannula, triangular cutting obturator, and irrigating port; 3 mm diameter; Irrigation extension tip

Courtesy of Jarit Surgical Instruments, a division of Integra LifeSciences Corporation.

FIGURE 11-136

Lichtwicz antrum trocar

Size: 4.5″

Quantity: 1

Notes: Needle style trocar with cross "T" handle; Sharp obturator; 16 gauge tip with Luer lock to connect to syringe for evacuation

Courtesy of Jarit Surgical Instruments, a division of Integra LifeSciences Corporation.

FIGURE 11-137

continues

Intranasal and Pharyngeal Instrumentation –
EVACUATION AND INSTILLATION INSTRUMENTS *continued*

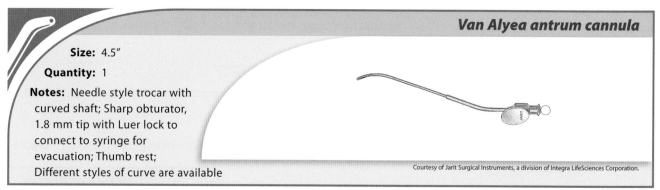

Van Alyea antrum cannula

Size: 4.5″

Quantity: 1

Notes: Needle style trocar with curved shaft; Sharp obturator, 1.8 mm tip with Luer lock to connect to syringe for evacuation; Thumb rest; Different styles of curve are available

Courtesy of Jarit Surgical Instruments, a division of Integra LifeSciences Corporation.

FIGURE 11-138

Intranasal and Pharyngeal Instrumentation – RETRACTION AND EXPOSURE INSTRUMENTS

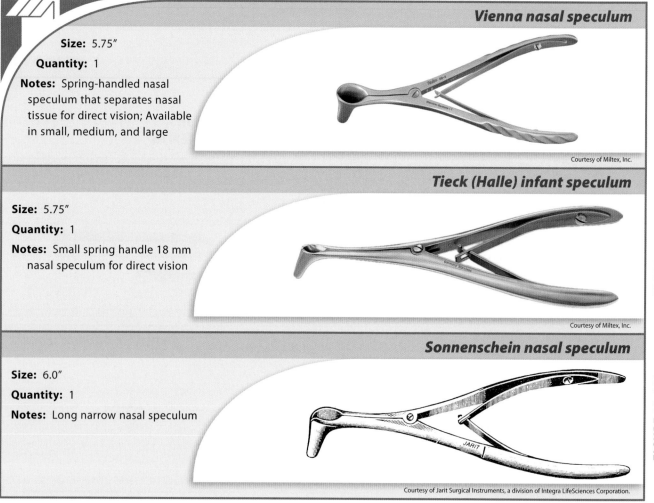

Vienna nasal speculum

Size: 5.75″

Quantity: 1

Notes: Spring-handled nasal speculum that separates nasal tissue for direct vision; Available in small, medium, and large

Courtesy of Miltex, Inc.

FIGURE 11-139

Tieck (Halle) infant speculum

Size: 5.75″

Quantity: 1

Notes: Small spring handle 18 mm nasal speculum for direct vision

Courtesy of Miltex, Inc.

FIGURE 11-140

Sonnenschein nasal speculum

Size: 6.0″

Quantity: 1

Notes: Long narrow nasal speculum

Courtesy of Jarit Surgical Instruments, a division of Integra LifeSciences Corporation.

FIGURE 11-141

Intranasal and Pharyngeal Instrumentation –
RETRACTION AND EXPOSURE INSTRUMENTS *continued*

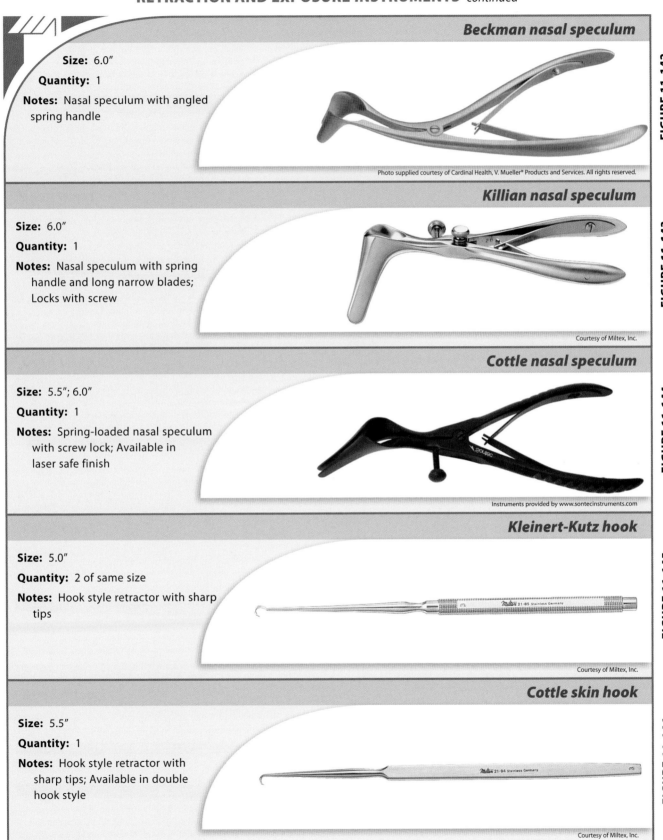

Beckman nasal speculum

Size: 6.0″

Quantity: 1

Notes: Nasal speculum with angled spring handle

FIGURE 11-142

Killian nasal speculum

Size: 6.0″

Quantity: 1

Notes: Nasal speculum with spring handle and long narrow blades; Locks with screw

FIGURE 11-143

Cottle nasal speculum

Size: 5.5″; 6.0″

Quantity: 1

Notes: Spring-loaded nasal speculum with screw lock; Available in laser safe finish

FIGURE 11-144

Kleinert-Kutz hook

Size: 5.0″

Quantity: 2 of same size

Notes: Hook style retractor with sharp tips

FIGURE 11-145

Cottle skin hook

Size: 5.5″

Quantity: 1

Notes: Hook style retractor with sharp tips; Available in double hook style

FIGURE 11-146

continues

Intranasal and Pharyngeal Instrumentation –
RETRACTION AND EXPOSURE INSTRUMENTS *continued*

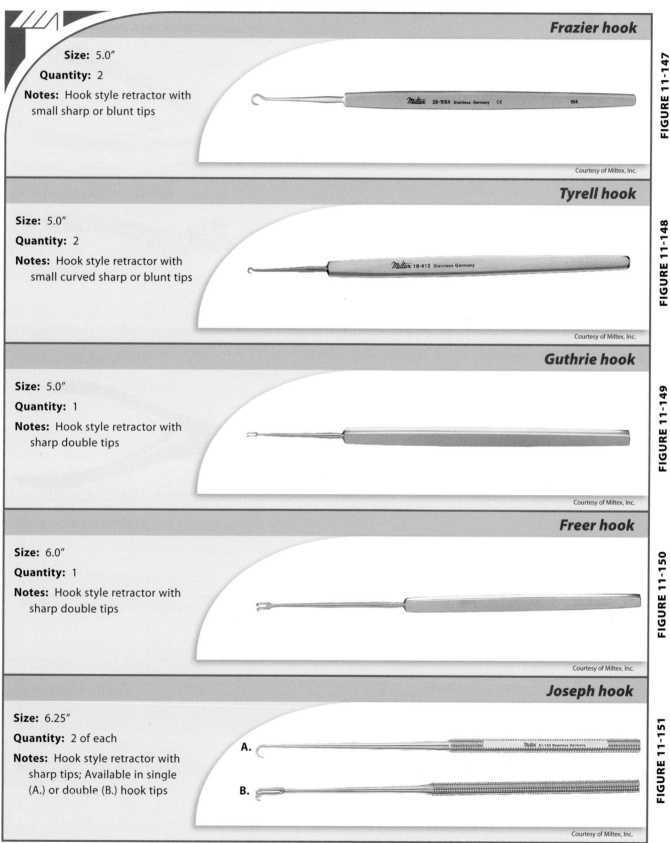

Frazier hook

Size: 5.0"

Quantity: 2

Notes: Hook style retractor with small sharp or blunt tips

Courtesy of Miltex, Inc.

FIGURE 11-147

Tyrell hook

Size: 5.0"

Quantity: 2

Notes: Hook style retractor with small curved sharp or blunt tips

Courtesy of Miltex, Inc.

FIGURE 11-148

Guthrie hook

Size: 5.0"

Quantity: 1

Notes: Hook style retractor with sharp double tips

Courtesy of Miltex, Inc.

FIGURE 11-149

Freer hook

Size: 6.0"

Quantity: 1

Notes: Hook style retractor with sharp double tips

Courtesy of Miltex, Inc.

FIGURE 11-150

Joseph hook

Size: 6.25"

Quantity: 2 of each

Notes: Hook style retractor with sharp tips; Available in single (A.) or double (B.) hook tips

A.

B.

Courtesy of Miltex, Inc.

FIGURE 11-151

Intranasal and Pharyngeal Instrumentation –
RETRACTION AND EXPOSURE INSTRUMENTS *continued*

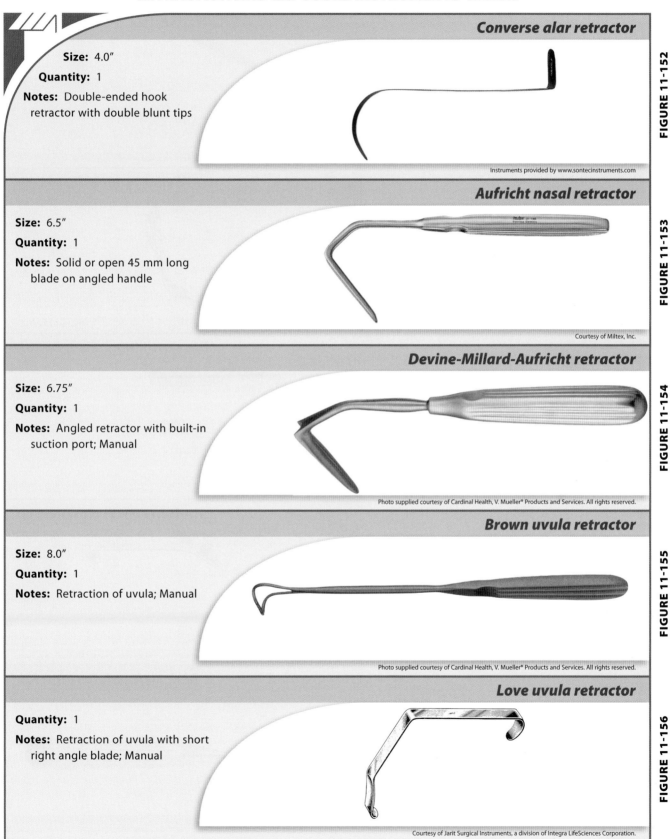

Converse alar retractor

Size: 4.0″

Quantity: 1

Notes: Double-ended hook retractor with double blunt tips

Instruments provided by www.sontecinstruments.com

FIGURE 11-152

Aufricht nasal retractor

Size: 6.5″

Quantity: 1

Notes: Solid or open 45 mm long blade on angled handle

Courtesy of Miltex, Inc.

FIGURE 11-153

Devine-Millard-Aufricht retractor

Size: 6.75″

Quantity: 1

Notes: Angled retractor with built-in suction port; Manual

Photo supplied courtesy of Cardinal Health, V. Mueller® Products and Services. All rights reserved.

FIGURE 11-154

Brown uvula retractor

Size: 8.0″

Quantity: 1

Notes: Retraction of uvula; Manual

Photo supplied courtesy of Cardinal Health, V. Mueller® Products and Services. All rights reserved.

FIGURE 11-155

Love uvula retractor

Quantity: 1

Notes: Retraction of uvula with short right angle blade; Manual

Courtesy of Jarit Surgical Instruments, a division of Integra LifeSciences Corporation.

FIGURE 11-156

continues

Intranasal and Pharyngeal Instrumentation –
RETRACTION AND EXPOSURE INSTRUMENTS *continued*

Yankauer pharyngeal speculum

Quantity: 1

Notes: Tubular speculum for direct vision of the pharynx; Manual

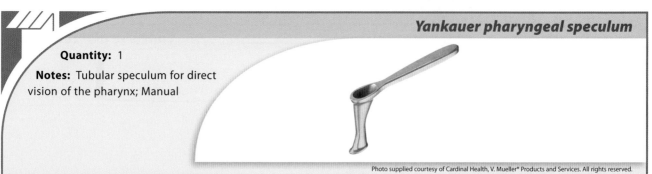

FIGURE 11-157

Wieder tongue depressor

Size: 28 mm; 36 mm

Quantity: 1

Notes: Manual right angle tongue retractor; Contact surface is cover leaf shaped with traction serrations

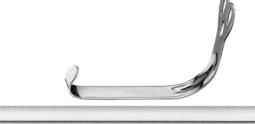

FIGURE 11-158

Bosworth tongue depressor

Size: 25 mm

Quantity: 1

Notes: Manual right angle retractor with fenestrated blade; Smooth surface

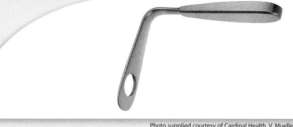

FIGURE 11-159

Andrews tongue depressor

Size: 21 mm

Quantity: 1

Notes: Manual right angle tongue retractor

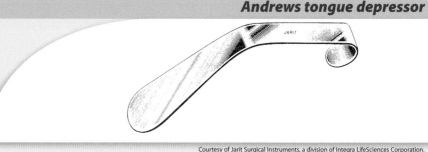

FIGURE 11-160

Blair cleft palate retractor

Size: 7.75"; 8.0"

Quantity: 1

Notes: Manual right angle blunt retractor

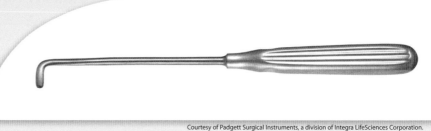

FIGURE 11-161

Intranasal and Pharyngeal Instrumentation –
RETRACTION AND EXPOSURE INSTRUMENTS *continued*

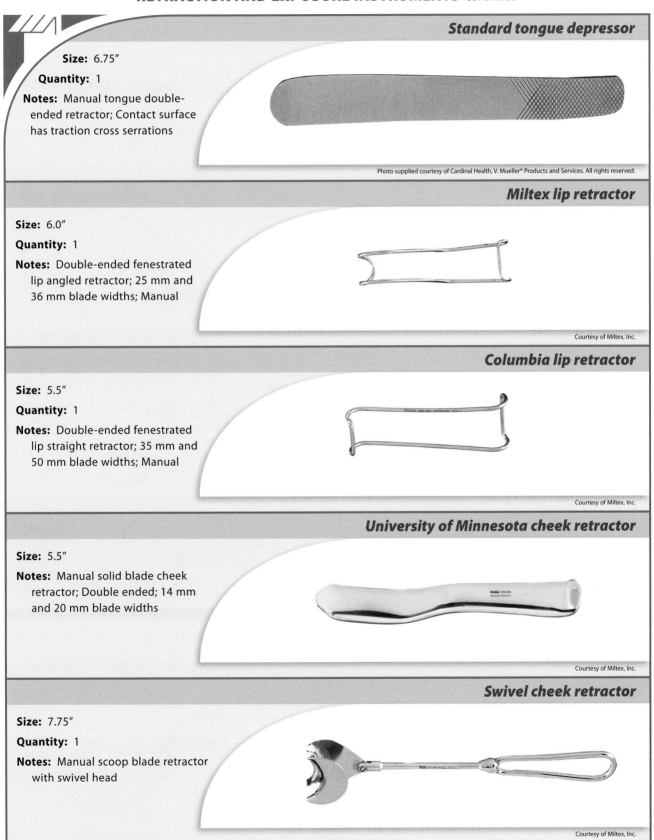

Standard tongue depressor

Size: 6.75"

Quantity: 1

Notes: Manual tongue double-ended retractor; Contact surface has traction cross serrations

FIGURE 11-162

Miltex lip retractor

Size: 6.0"

Quantity: 1

Notes: Double-ended fenestrated lip angled retractor; 25 mm and 36 mm blade widths; Manual

FIGURE 11-163

Columbia lip retractor

Size: 5.5"

Quantity: 1

Notes: Double-ended fenestrated lip straight retractor; 35 mm and 50 mm blade widths; Manual

FIGURE 11-164

University of Minnesota cheek retractor

Size: 5.5"

Notes: Manual solid blade cheek retractor; Double ended; 14 mm and 20 mm blade widths

FIGURE 11-165

Swivel cheek retractor

Size: 7.75"

Quantity: 1

Notes: Manual scoop blade retractor with swivel head

FIGURE 11-166

continues

Intranasal and Pharyngeal Instrumentation –
RETRACTION AND EXPOSURE INSTRUMENTS *continued*

FIGURE 11-167

Colver tonsil retractor

Size: 8.0"

Quantity: 1

Notes: Right angle tip with long slender handle

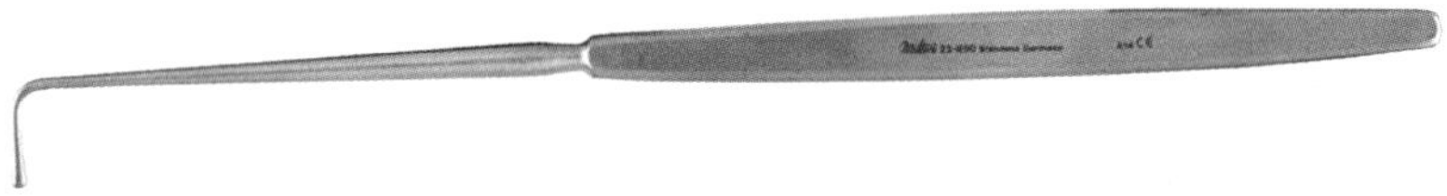

Courtesy of Miltex, Inc.

FIGURE 11-168

Davis mouth gag

Size: 6.25"

Quantity: 1

Notes: Self-retaining mouth retractor with built-in suction port; Side opening; Available in right or left models; Ratchet locks on vertical plane

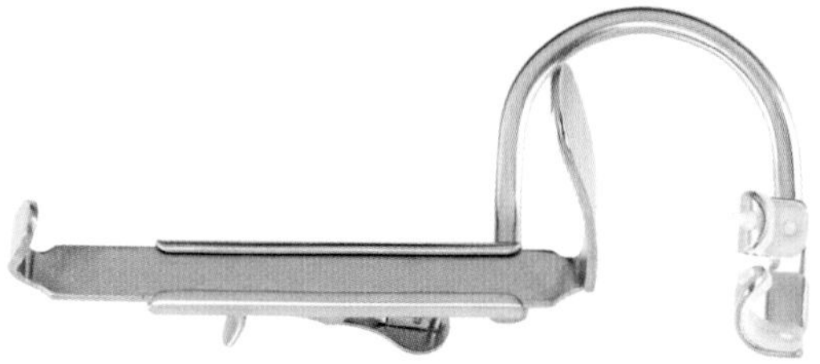

Courtesy of Miltex, Inc.

FIGURE 11-169

Sluder-Jansen mouth gag

Size: 5.5"

Quantity: 1

Notes: Self-retaining mouth retractor with ratchets

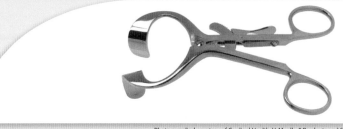

Photo supplied courtesy of Cardinal Health, V. Mueller® Products and Services. All rights reserved.

FIGURE 11-170

McIvor mouth gag

Size: 5.75"

Quantity: 1

Notes: Self-retaining mouth retractor; Ratchet locks on vertical plane

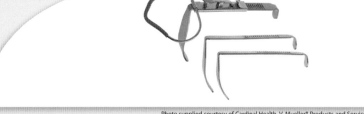

Photo supplied courtesy of Cardinal Health, V. Mueller® Products and Services. All rights reserved.

FIGURE 11-171

Jennings mouth gag

Size: 6.0"; 4.75"; 3.75"

Quantity: 1

Notes: Self-retaining mouth retractor with side ratchets; Reversible for right or left locking

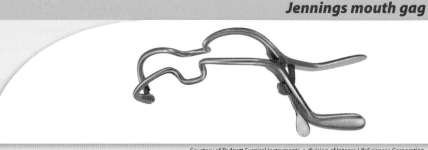

Courtesy of Padgett Surgical Instruments, a division of Integra LifeSciences Corporation.

Intranasal and Pharyngeal Instrumentation –
RETRACTION AND EXPOSURE INSTRUMENTS *continued*

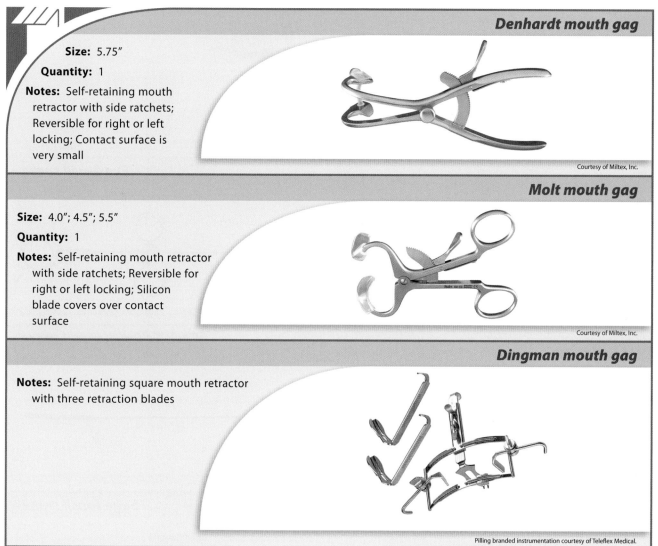

Denhardt mouth gag

Size: 5.75″

Quantity: 1

Notes: Self-retaining mouth retractor with side ratchets; Reversible for right or left locking; Contact surface is very small

Courtesy of Miltex, Inc.

FIGURE 11-172

Molt mouth gag

Size: 4.0″; 4.5″; 5.5″

Quantity: 1

Notes: Self-retaining mouth retractor with side ratchets; Reversible for right or left locking; Silicon blade covers over contact surface

Courtesy of Miltex, Inc.

FIGURE 11-173

Dingman mouth gag

Notes: Self-retaining square mouth retractor with three retraction blades

Pilling branded instrumentation courtesy of Teleflex Medical.

FIGURE 11-174

Intranasal and Pharyngeal Instrumentation – SPECIALTY SPECIFIC INSTRUMENTS

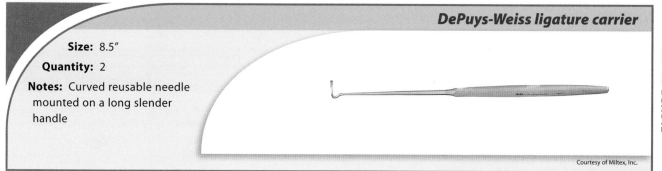

DePuys-Weiss ligature carrier

Size: 8.5″

Quantity: 2

Notes: Curved reusable needle mounted on a long slender handle

Courtesy of Miltex, Inc.

FIGURE 11-175

continues

Intranasal and Pharyngeal Instrumentation – SPECIALTY SPECIFIC INSTRUMENTS *continued*

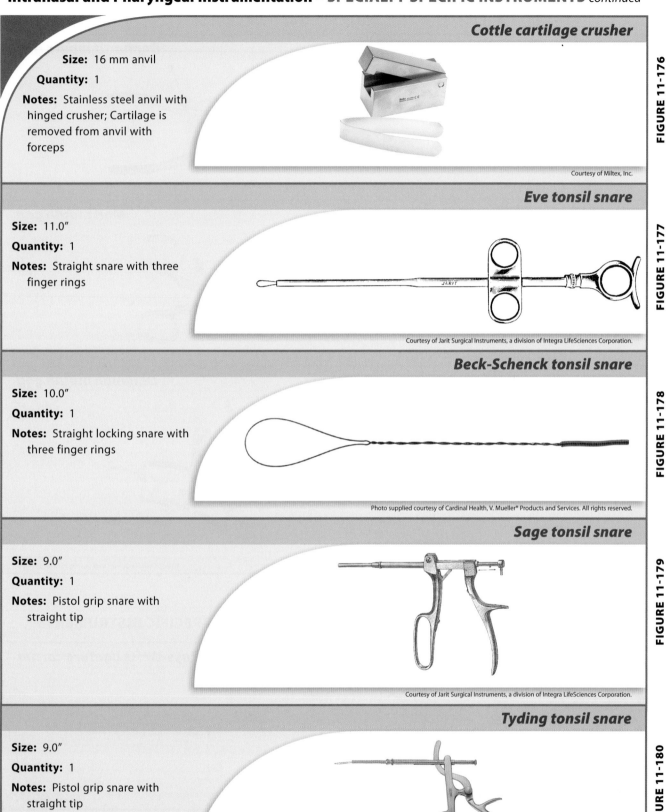

Cottle cartilage crusher

Size: 16 mm anvil

Quantity: 1

Notes: Stainless steel anvil with hinged crusher; Cartilage is removed from anvil with forceps

Courtesy of Miltex, Inc.

FIGURE 11-176

Eve tonsil snare

Size: 11.0"

Quantity: 1

Notes: Straight snare with three finger rings

Courtesy of Jarit Surgical Instruments, a division of Integra LifeSciences Corporation.

FIGURE 11-177

Beck-Schenck tonsil snare

Size: 10.0"

Quantity: 1

Notes: Straight locking snare with three finger rings

Photo supplied courtesy of Cardinal Health, V. Mueller® Products and Services. All rights reserved.

FIGURE 11-178

Sage tonsil snare

Size: 9.0"

Quantity: 1

Notes: Pistol grip snare with straight tip

Courtesy of Jarit Surgical Instruments, a division of Integra LifeSciences Corporation.

FIGURE 11-179

Tyding tonsil snare

Size: 9.0"

Quantity: 1

Notes: Pistol grip snare with straight tip

Courtesy of Miltex, Inc.

FIGURE 11-180

Intranasal and Pharyngeal Instrumentation – SPECIALTY SPECIFIC INSTRUMENTS continued

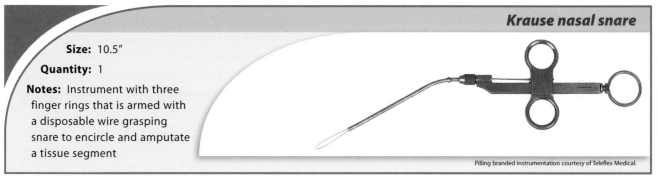

Krause nasal snare

Size: 10.5″

Quantity: 1

Notes: Instrument with three finger rings that is armed with a disposable wire grasping snare to encircle and amputate a tissue segment

Pilling branded instrumentation courtesy of Teleflex Medical.

FIGURE 11-181

ANTERIOR NECK INSTRUMENTATION

Anterior neck instrumentation is used for surface and subcutaneous structures associated with glandular, digestive, endocrine, and airway components. Neck dissection can be very tedious and time consuming because of the neck's complex vascular and neuro-logic structures. The short and medium foundation instrument sets are commonly used; however, the long foundation set could be required for deep esophageal dissection. Anterior neck procedures are primarily soft tissue dissection. Few additional specialty instruments are needed for dissection and exposure.

Thyroidectomy and Neck Dissection Instrumentation

Thyroidectomy and Neck Dissection Instrumentation – PROBES AND DILATORS

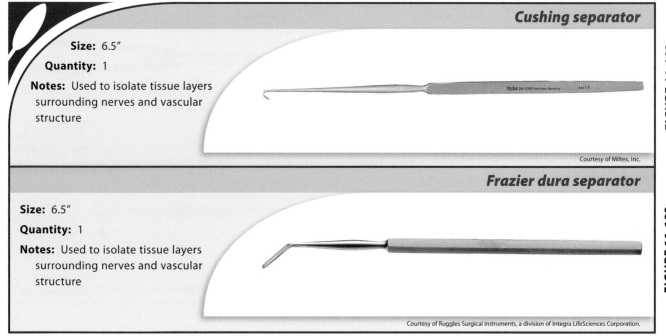

Cushing separator

Size: 6.5″

Quantity: 1

Notes: Used to isolate tissue layers surrounding nerves and vascular structure

Courtesy of Miltex, Inc.

FIGURE 11-182

Frazier dura separator

Size: 6.5″

Quantity: 1

Notes: Used to isolate tissue layers surrounding nerves and vascular structure

Courtesy of Ruggles Surgical Instruments, a division of Integra LifeSciences Corporation.

FIGURE 11-183

continues

Thyroidectomy and Neck Dissection Instrumentation – PROBES AND DILATORS *continued*

Dandy nerve hook

Size: 9.0″

Quantity: 1

Notes: Used to isolate tissue layers surrounding nerves and vascular structure

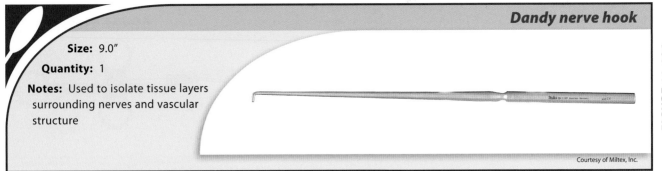

Courtesy of Miltex, Inc.

FIGURE 11-184

Thyroidectomy and Neck Dissection Instrumentation –
RETRACTION AND EXPOSURE INSTRUMENTS

Lahey retractor

Size: 7.75″

Quantity: 2

Notes: Right angle retractor with solid blade; Manual

Courtesy of Miltex, Inc.

FIGURE 11-185

Green retractor

Size: 8.5″

Quantity: 2

Notes: Right angle retractor with curved open blade; Manual

Courtesy of Miltex, Inc.

FIGURE 11-186

Senn retractor

Size: 6.25″

Quantity: 2

Notes: Double-ended retractor with a solid right angle blade at one end and a sharp or blunt rake on the opposite end; Manual

Courtesy of Miltex, Inc.

FIGURE 11-187

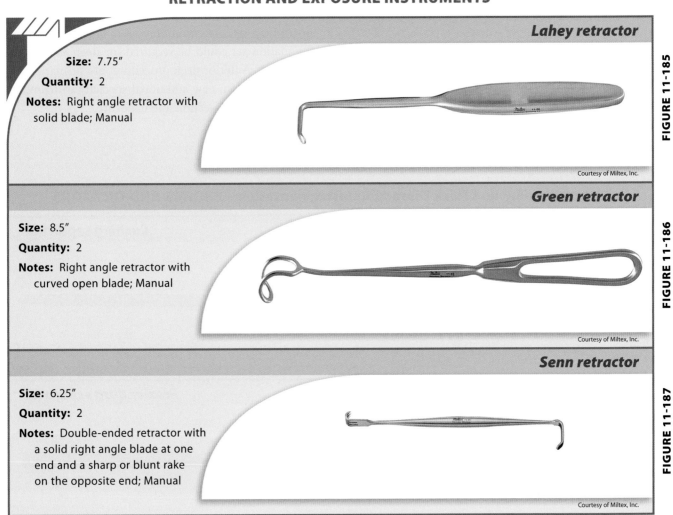

Thyroidectomy and Neck Dissection Instrumentation –
RETRACTION AND EXPOSURE INSTRUMENTS *continued*

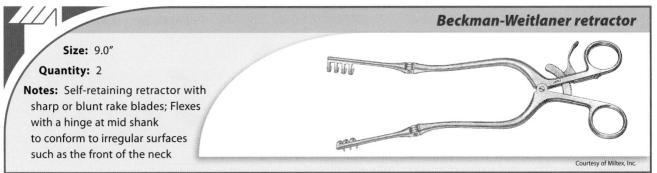

Beckman-Weitlaner retractor

Size: 9.0″

Quantity: 2

Notes: Self-retaining retractor with sharp or blunt rake blades; Flexes with a hinge at mid shank to conform to irregular surfaces such as the front of the neck

Courtesy of Miltex, Inc.

FIGURE 11-188

Tracheostomy-Tracheotomy Instrumentation

The short foundation set contains sufficient instruments for a tracheotomy. Additional exposure and airway maintenance instruments as listed in this collection are required.

Tracheostomy-Tracheotomy Instrumentation – PROBES AND DILATORS

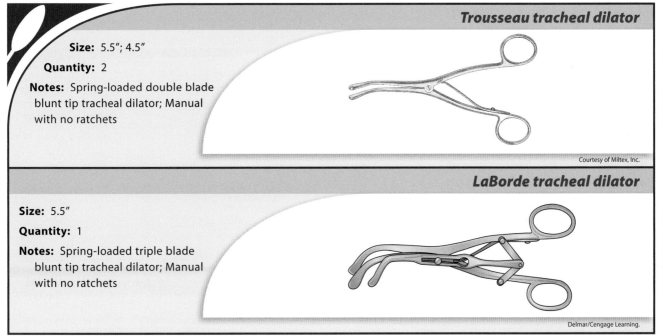

Trousseau tracheal dilator

Size: 5.5″; 4.5″

Quantity: 2

Notes: Spring-loaded double blade blunt tip tracheal dilator; Manual with no ratchets

Courtesy of Miltex, Inc.

FIGURE 11-189

LaBorde tracheal dilator

Size: 5.5″

Quantity: 1

Notes: Spring-loaded triple blade blunt tip tracheal dilator; Manual with no ratchets

Delmar/Cengage Learning.

FIGURE 11-190

Tracheostomy-Tracheotomy Instrumentation –
EVACUATION AND INSTILLATION INSTRUMENTS

Lewis laryngectomy tube

Size: Individually sized for each patient

Quantity: Assorted sizes

Notes: Reusable three-part cannula system for prolonged percutaneous airway support after laryngectomy; Wide diameter; Components are the sleeve, inner cannula, and insertion obturator made of sterling silver

FIGURE 11-191

Tracheostomy-Tracheotomy Instrumentation –
RETRACTION AND EXPOSURE INSTRUMENTS

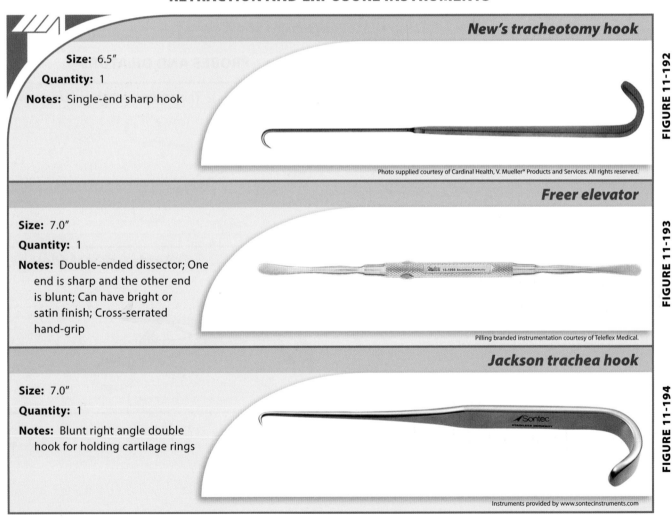

New's tracheotomy hook

Size: 6.5″

Quantity: 1

Notes: Single-end sharp hook

FIGURE 11-192

Freer elevator

Size: 7.0″

Quantity: 1

Notes: Double-ended dissector; One end is sharp and the other end is blunt; Can have bright or satin finish; Cross-serrated hand-grip

FIGURE 11-193

Jackson trachea hook

Size: 7.0″

Quantity: 1

Notes: Blunt right angle double hook for holding cartilage rings

FIGURE 11-194

Tracheostomy-Tracheotomy Instrumentation –
RETRACTION AND EXPOSURE INSTRUMENTS *continued*

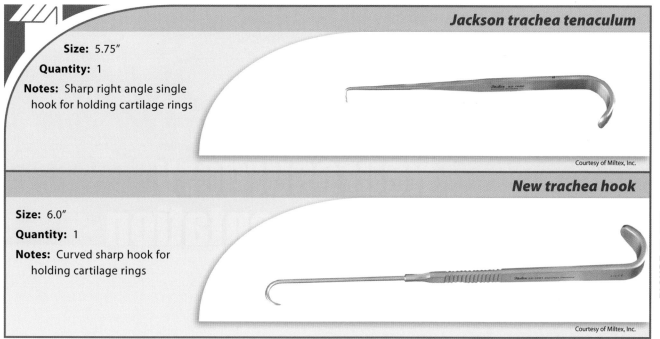

Jackson trachea tenaculum

Size: 5.75"

Quantity: 1

Notes: Sharp right angle single hook for holding cartilage rings

Courtesy of Miltex, Inc.

FIGURE 11-195

New trachea hook

Size: 6.0"

Quantity: 1

Notes: Curved sharp hook for holding cartilage rings

Courtesy of Miltex, Inc.

FIGURE 11-196

SUMMARY

Surgery of the mouth and anterior neck commonly include exposing structural components of the upper airway. Safety considerations include avoiding the use of electrosurgery pencils in the presence of oxygen. An ignition spark could cause an upper airway fire that is disastrous and potentially fatal for the patient.

Most procedures of the anterior neck can be performed with the medium foundation set instrumentation with the addition of minimal clamps, hooks, and dilation instrumentation used around and in the trachea.

Intraoral instrumentation will be longer, curved, or bayonet-styled, and have smaller jaws to enhance visualization while manipulating tissue within the confined space of the mouth and throat.

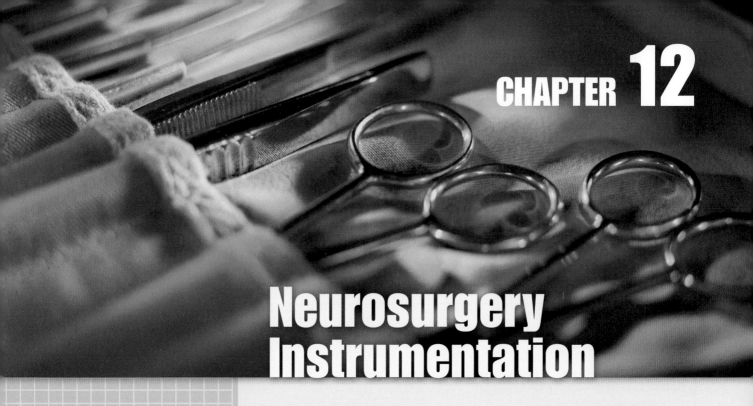

Neurosurgery Instrumentation

INTRODUCTION

Neurosurgery is unique because it involves working with every form of tissue and instrumentation from every category. Neurologic procedures can be performed on any body part ranging from head-to-toe, literally. Soft tissue dissection for peripheral nerves in the superficial regions of the body can be performed using short or medium foundation sets with the addition of assorted nerve hooks and dissectors.

The sections in this chapter include intracranial, spinal, and cervical instrumentation used in combination with medium and long foundation sets.

INTRACRANIAL INSTRUMENTATION

Intracranial procedures require the use of instrumentation for several types of tissue. A medium foundation set is used to open and close the soft tissues of the scalp. The scalp edges are handled with care because injury to hair follicles or follicular blood supply may cause baldness in the area of the vascular distribution. Temporary occlusion scalp clips are applied around the edges of the incision for hemostasis and are removed at the end of the procedure. This preserves the blood supply, yet keeps the field of vision clear during the surgical procedure without harming the blood supply.

Instrumentation for intracranial surgery includes drills, saws, burrs, and rongeurs for entering the skull and elevators for blunt dissection of the adherent layers of periosteum and dura mater. Fine soft tissue is dissected with delicate specialty devices and microscopic instrumentation. Instruments used with microscopes are described in Chapter 14.

Intracranial Instrumentation – CLAMPS

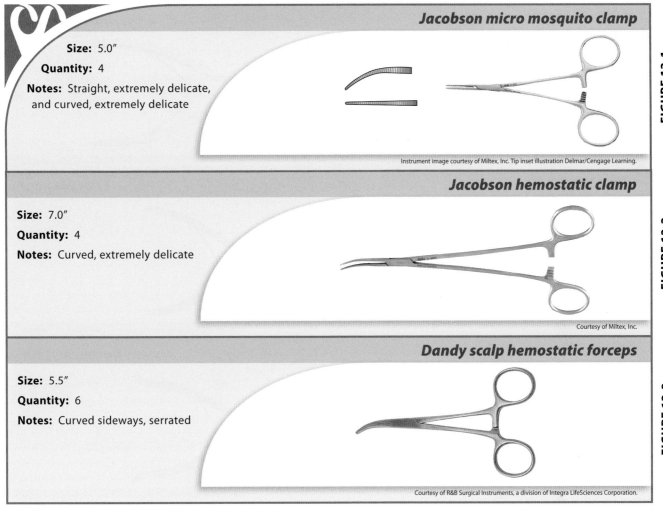

Jacobson micro mosquito clamp

Size: 5.0″

Quantity: 4

Notes: Straight, extremely delicate, and curved, extremely delicate

Instrument image courtesy of Miltex, Inc. Tip inset illustration Delmar/Cengage Learning.

FIGURE 12-1

Jacobson hemostatic clamp

Size: 7.0″

Quantity: 4

Notes: Curved, extremely delicate

Courtesy of Miltex, Inc.

FIGURE 12-2

Dandy scalp hemostatic forceps

Size: 5.5″

Quantity: 6

Notes: Curved sideways, serrated

Courtesy of R&B Surgical Instruments, a division of Integra LifeSciences Corporation.

FIGURE 12-3

Intracranial Instrumentation – GRASPING FORCEPS

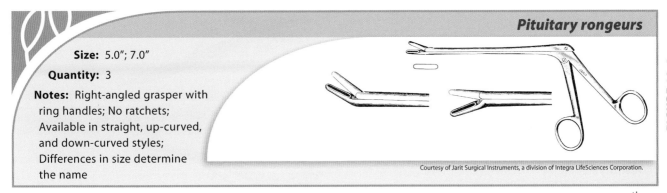

Pituitary rongeurs

Size: 5.0″; 7.0″

Quantity: 3

Notes: Right-angled grasper with ring handles; No ratchets; Available in straight, up-curved, and down-curved styles; Differences in size determine the name

Courtesy of Jarit Surgical Instruments, a division of Integra LifeSciences Corporation.

FIGURE 12-4

continues

Intracranial Instrumentation – GRASPING FORCEPS *continued*

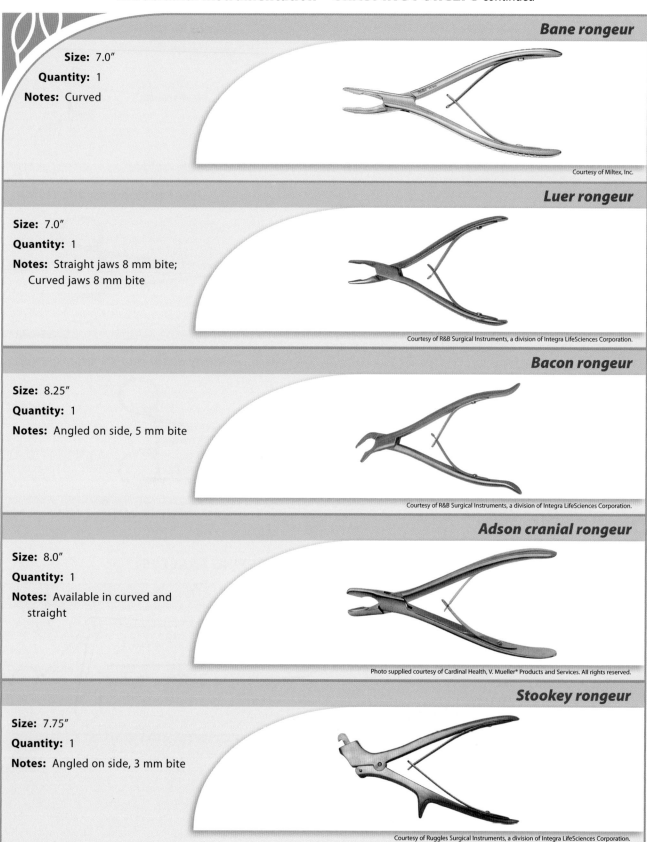

Bane rongeur

Size: 7.0"

Quantity: 1

Notes: Curved

Courtesy of Miltex, Inc.

FIGURE 12-5

Luer rongeur

Size: 7.0"

Quantity: 1

Notes: Straight jaws 8 mm bite;
Curved jaws 8 mm bite

Courtesy of R&B Surgical Instruments, a division of Integra LifeSciences Corporation.

FIGURE 12-6

Bacon rongeur

Size: 8.25"

Quantity: 1

Notes: Angled on side, 5 mm bite

Courtesy of R&B Surgical Instruments, a division of Integra LifeSciences Corporation.

FIGURE 12-7

Adson cranial rongeur

Size: 8.0"

Quantity: 1

Notes: Available in curved and
straight

Photo supplied courtesy of Cardinal Health, V. Mueller® Products and Services. All rights reserved.

FIGURE 12-8

Stookey rongeur

Size: 7.75"

Quantity: 1

Notes: Angled on side, 3 mm bite

Courtesy of Ruggles Surgical Instruments, a division of Integra LifeSciences Corporation.

FIGURE 12-9

Intracranial Instrumentation – GRASPING FORCEPS *continued*

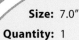

Zaufel-Jansen rongeur

Size: 7.0″

Quantity: 1

Notes: Slightly curved jaws 5 mm wide

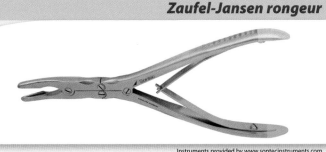

FIGURE 12-10

Beyer rongeur

Size: 7.0″

Quantity: 1

Notes: Slightly curved jaws 3.5 mm wide

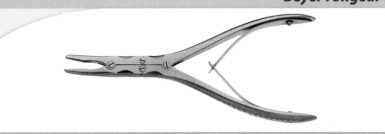

FIGURE 12-11

Stille-Luer rongeur

Size: 8.75″; 9.0″

Quantity: 1 of each

Notes: Straight jaws, 9 × 15 mm; Curved jaws, 9 × 15 mm; Duckbill rongeur, angled on side jaws, 6 × 12 mm

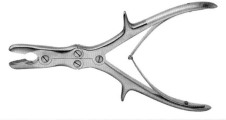

FIGURE 12-12

DeVilbiss cranial rongeur

Size: 8.25″

Quantity: 1

Notes: Two blades

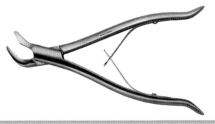

FIGURE 12-13

Oldberg pituitary rongeur

Size: 7.0″

Notes: Round cup jaws 6 mm

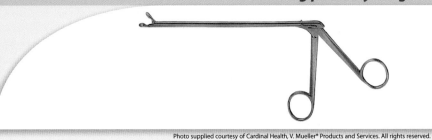

FIGURE 12-14

continues

Intracranial Instrumentation – GRASPING FORCEPS *continued*

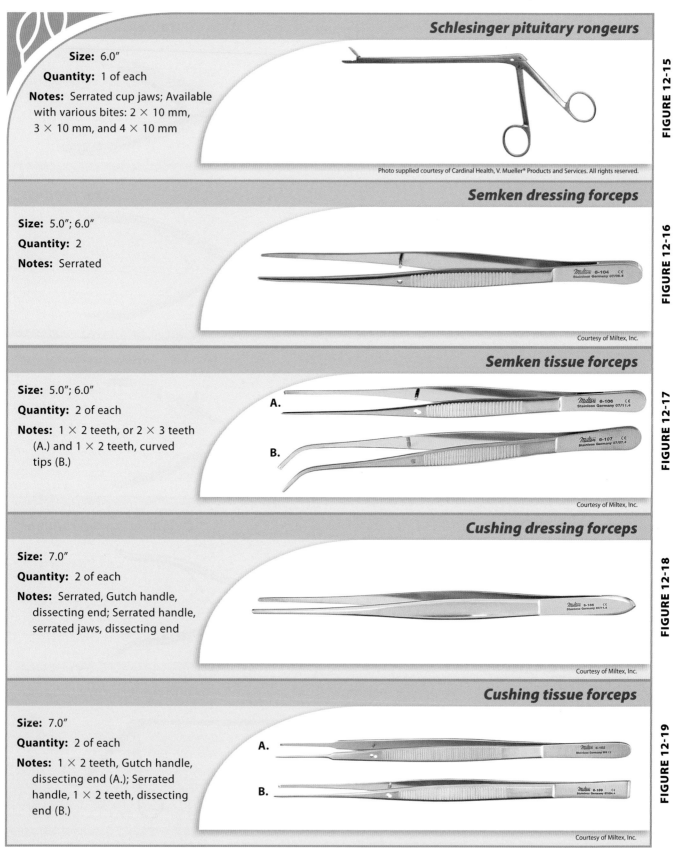

Schlesinger pituitary rongeurs

Size: 6.0"

Quantity: 1 of each

Notes: Serrated cup jaws; Available with various bites: 2 × 10 mm, 3 × 10 mm, and 4 × 10 mm

FIGURE 12-15

Semken dressing forceps

Size: 5.0"; 6.0"

Quantity: 2

Notes: Serrated

FIGURE 12-16

Semken tissue forceps

Size: 5.0"; 6.0"

Quantity: 2 of each

Notes: 1 × 2 teeth, or 2 × 3 teeth (A.) and 1 × 2 teeth, curved tips (B.)

A.

B.

FIGURE 12-17

Cushing dressing forceps

Size: 7.0"

Quantity: 2 of each

Notes: Serrated, Gutch handle, dissecting end; Serrated handle, serrated jaws, dissecting end

FIGURE 12-18

Cushing tissue forceps

Size: 7.0"

Quantity: 2 of each

Notes: 1 × 2 teeth, Gutch handle, dissecting end (A.); Serrated handle, 1 × 2 teeth, dissecting end (B.)

A.

B.

FIGURE 12-19

Intracranial Instrumentation – GRASPING FORCEPS *continued*

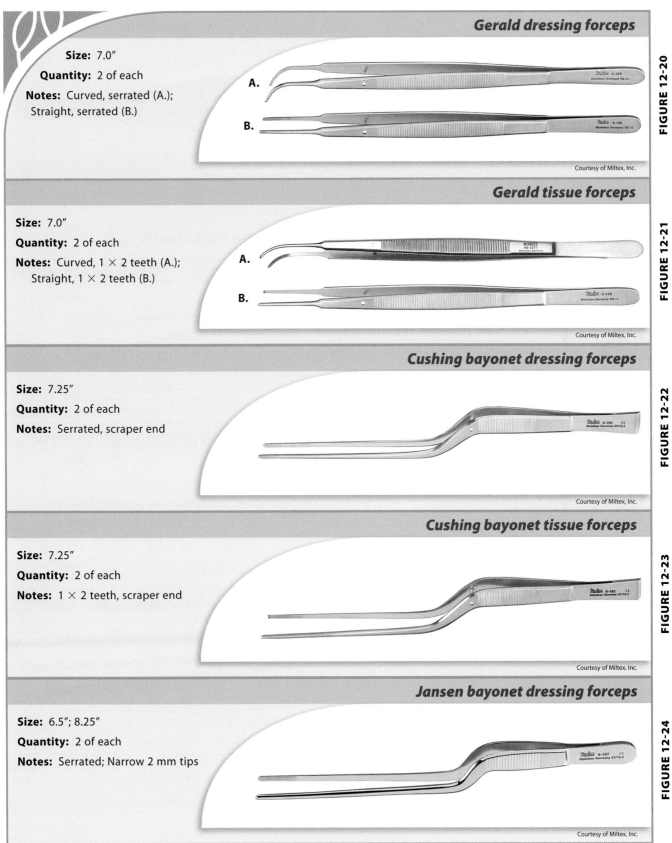

Gerald dressing forceps

Size: 7.0"

Quantity: 2 of each

Notes: Curved, serrated (A.); Straight, serrated (B.)

A.

B.

Courtesy of Miltex, Inc.

FIGURE 12-20

Gerald tissue forceps

Size: 7.0"

Quantity: 2 of each

Notes: Curved, 1 × 2 teeth (A.); Straight, 1 × 2 teeth (B.)

A.

B.

Courtesy of Miltex, Inc.

FIGURE 12-21

Cushing bayonet dressing forceps

Size: 7.25"

Quantity: 2 of each

Notes: Serrated, scraper end

Courtesy of Miltex, Inc.

FIGURE 12-22

Cushing bayonet tissue forceps

Size: 7.25"

Quantity: 2 of each

Notes: 1 × 2 teeth, scraper end

Courtesy of Miltex, Inc.

FIGURE 12-23

Jansen bayonet dressing forceps

Size: 6.5"; 8.25"

Quantity: 2 of each

Notes: Serrated; Narrow 2 mm tips

Courtesy of Miltex, Inc.

FIGURE 12-24

continues

Intracranial Instrumentation – GRASPING FORCEPS *continued*

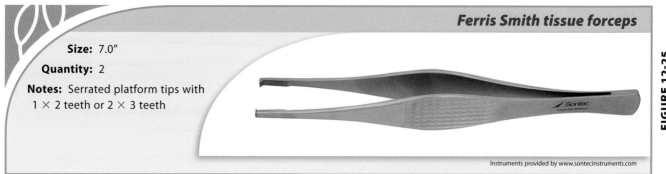

Ferris Smith tissue forceps

Size: 7.0″

Quantity: 2

Notes: Serrated platform tips with 1 × 2 teeth or 2 × 3 teeth

Instruments provided by www.sontecinstruments.com

FIGURE 12-25

Intracranial Instrumentation – DISSECTION INSTRUMENTS

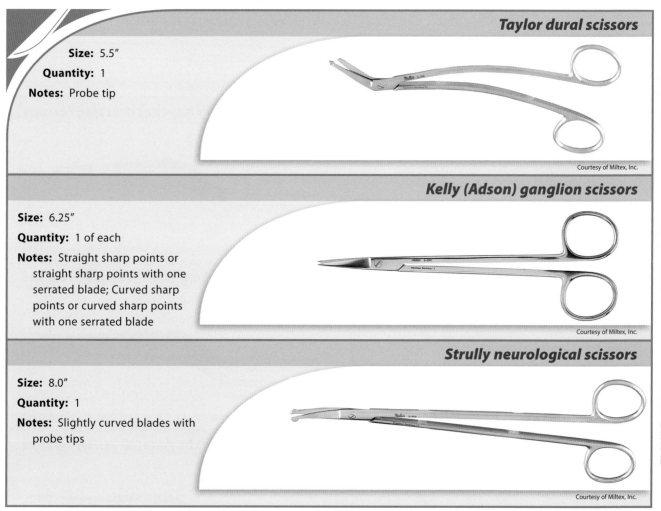

Taylor dural scissors

Size: 5.5″

Quantity: 1

Notes: Probe tip

Courtesy of Miltex, Inc.

FIGURE 12-26

Kelly (Adson) ganglion scissors

Size: 6.25″

Quantity: 1 of each

Notes: Straight sharp points or straight sharp points with one serrated blade; Curved sharp points or curved sharp points with one serrated blade

Courtesy of Miltex, Inc.

FIGURE 12-27

Strully neurological scissors

Size: 8.0″

Quantity: 1

Notes: Slightly curved blades with probe tips

Courtesy of Miltex, Inc.

FIGURE 12-28

Intracranial Instrumentation – DISSECTION INSTRUMENTS *continued*

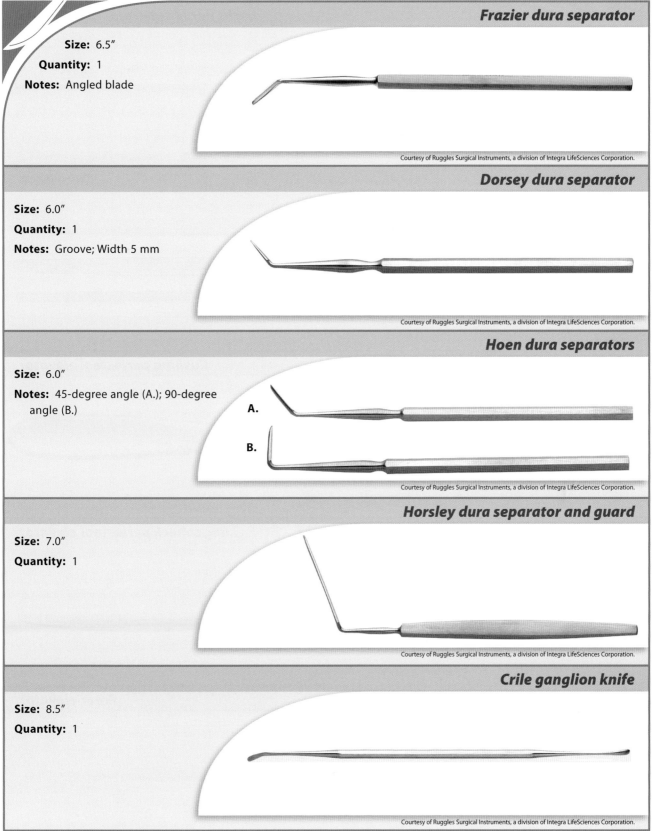

Frazier dura separator

Size: 6.5″
Quantity: 1
Notes: Angled blade

Courtesy of Ruggles Surgical Instruments, a division of Integra LifeSciences Corporation.

FIGURE 12-29

Dorsey dura separator

Size: 6.0″
Quantity: 1
Notes: Groove; Width 5 mm

Courtesy of Ruggles Surgical Instruments, a division of Integra LifeSciences Corporation.

FIGURE 12-30

Hoen dura separators

Size: 6.0″
Notes: 45-degree angle (A.); 90-degree angle (B.)

A.

B.

Courtesy of Ruggles Surgical Instruments, a division of Integra LifeSciences Corporation.

FIGURE 12-31

Horsley dura separator and guard

Size: 7.0″
Quantity: 1

Courtesy of Ruggles Surgical Instruments, a division of Integra LifeSciences Corporation.

FIGURE 12-32

Crile ganglion knife

Size: 8.5″
Quantity: 1

Courtesy of Ruggles Surgical Instruments, a division of Integra LifeSciences Corporation.

FIGURE 12-33

continues

Intracranial Instrumentation – DISSECTION INSTRUMENTS *continued*

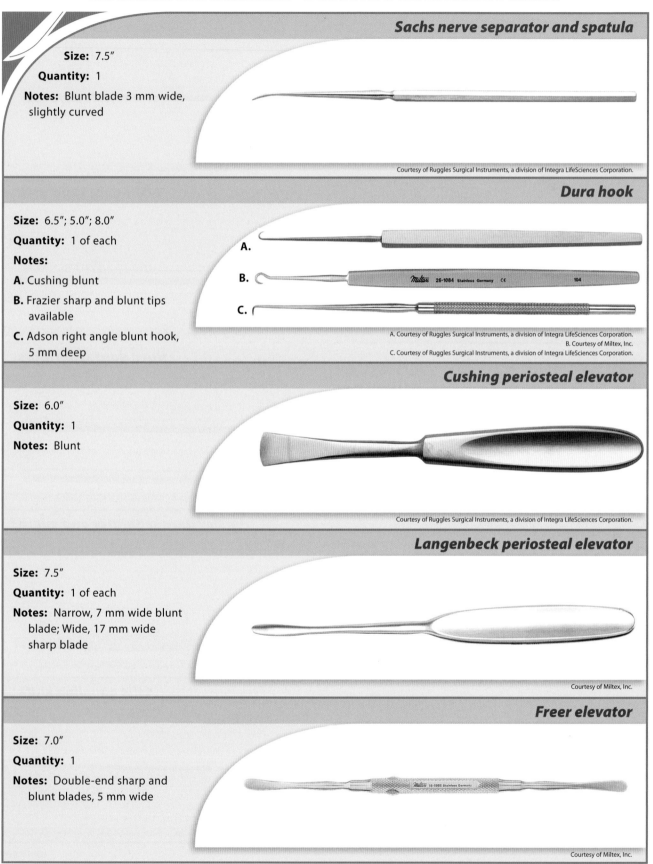

Sachs nerve separator and spatula

Size: 7.5″

Quantity: 1

Notes: Blunt blade 3 mm wide, slightly curved

FIGURE 12-34

Courtesy of Ruggles Surgical Instruments, a division of Integra LifeSciences Corporation.

Dura hook

Size: 6.5″; 5.0″; 8.0″

Quantity: 1 of each

Notes:

A. Cushing blunt

B. Frazier sharp and blunt tips available

C. Adson right angle blunt hook, 5 mm deep

A.

B.

C.

FIGURE 12-35

A. Courtesy of Ruggles Surgical Instruments, a division of Integra LifeSciences Corporation.
B. Courtesy of Miltex, Inc.
C. Courtesy of Ruggles Surgical Instruments, a division of Integra LifeSciences Corporation.

Cushing periosteal elevator

Size: 6.0″

Quantity: 1

Notes: Blunt

FIGURE 12-36

Courtesy of Ruggles Surgical Instruments, a division of Integra LifeSciences Corporation.

Langenbeck periosteal elevator

Size: 7.5″

Quantity: 1 of each

Notes: Narrow, 7 mm wide blunt blade; Wide, 17 mm wide sharp blade

FIGURE 12-37

Courtesy of Miltex, Inc.

Freer elevator

Size: 7.0″

Quantity: 1

Notes: Double-end sharp and blunt blades, 5 mm wide

FIGURE 12-38

Courtesy of Miltex, Inc.

Intracranial Instrumentation – DISSECTION INSTRUMENTS *continued*

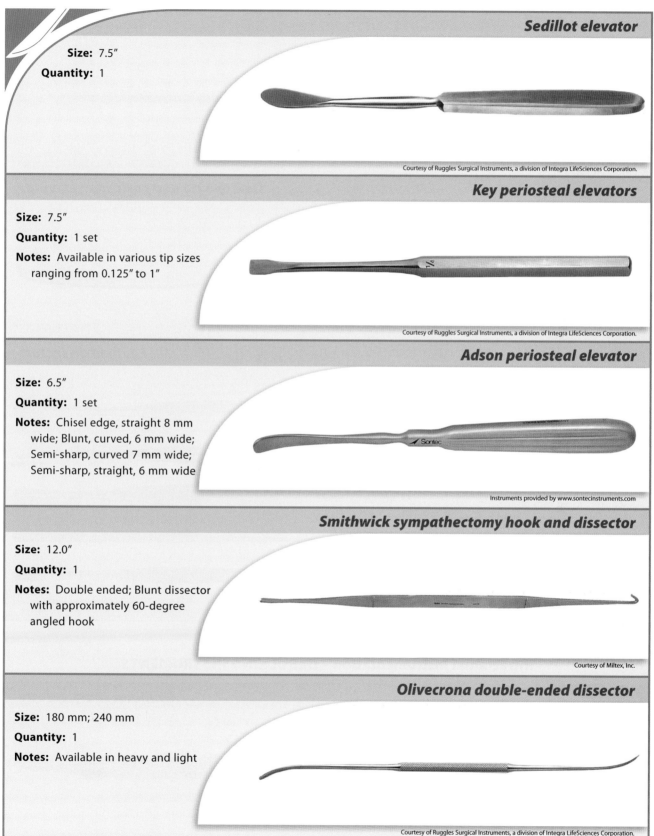

Sedillot elevator

Size: 7.5"
Quantity: 1

Courtesy of Ruggles Surgical Instruments, a division of Integra LifeSciences Corporation.

FIGURE 12-39

Key periosteal elevators

Size: 7.5"
Quantity: 1 set
Notes: Available in various tip sizes ranging from 0.125" to 1"

Courtesy of Ruggles Surgical Instruments, a division of Integra LifeSciences Corporation.

FIGURE 12-40

Adson periosteal elevator

Size: 6.5"
Quantity: 1 set
Notes: Chisel edge, straight 8 mm wide; Blunt, curved, 6 mm wide; Semi-sharp, curved 7 mm wide; Semi-sharp, straight, 6 mm wide

Instruments provided by www.sontecinstruments.com

FIGURE 12-41

Smithwick sympathectomy hook and dissector

Size: 12.0"
Quantity: 1
Notes: Double ended; Blunt dissector with approximately 60-degree angled hook

Courtesy of Miltex, Inc.

FIGURE 12-42

Olivecrona double-ended dissector

Size: 180 mm; 240 mm
Quantity: 1
Notes: Available in heavy and light

Courtesy of Ruggles Surgical Instruments, a division of Integra LifeSciences Corporation.

FIGURE 12-43

continues

Intracranial Instrumentation – DISSECTION INSTRUMENTS *continued*

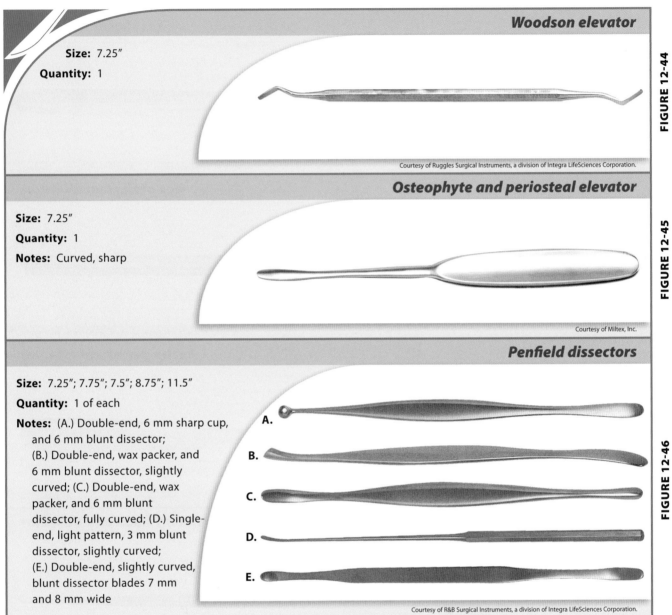

Woodson elevator

Size: 7.25″

Quantity: 1

FIGURE 12-44

Osteophyte and periosteal elevator

Size: 7.25″

Quantity: 1

Notes: Curved, sharp

FIGURE 12-45

Penfield dissectors

Size: 7.25″; 7.75″; 7.5″; 8.75″; 11.5″

Quantity: 1 of each

Notes: (A.) Double-end, 6 mm sharp cup, and 6 mm blunt dissector; (B.) Double-end, wax packer, and 6 mm blunt dissector, slightly curved; (C.) Double-end, wax packer, and 6 mm blunt dissector, fully curved; (D.) Single-end, light pattern, 3 mm blunt dissector, slightly curved; (E.) Double-end, slightly curved, blunt dissector blades 7 mm and 8 mm wide

A.

B.

C.

D.

E.

FIGURE 12-46

Intracranial Instrumentation – DEBULKING INSTRUMENTS

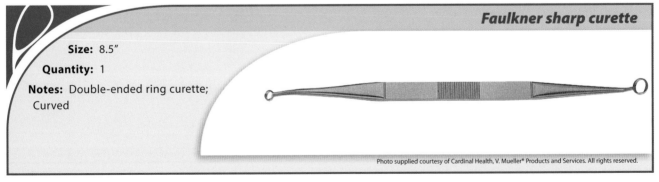

Faulkner sharp curette

Size: 8.5″

Quantity: 1

Notes: Double-ended ring curette; Curved

FIGURE 12-47

Intracranial Instrumentation – DEBULKING INSTRUMENTS *continued*

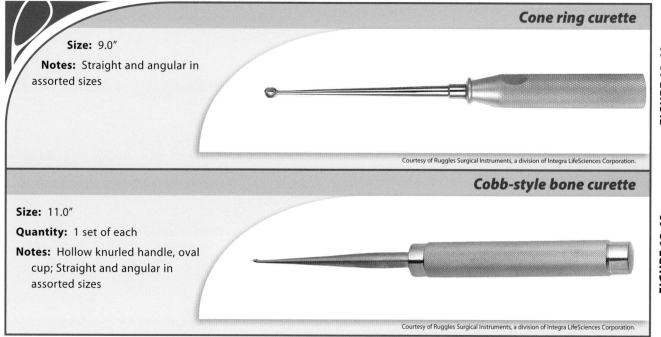

Cone ring curette

Size: 9.0″

Notes: Straight and angular in assorted sizes

Courtesy of Ruggles Surgical Instruments, a division of Integra LifeSciences Corporation.

FIGURE 12-48

Cobb-style bone curette

Size: 11.0″

Quantity: 1 set of each

Notes: Hollow knurled handle, oval cup; Straight and angular in assorted sizes

Courtesy of Ruggles Surgical Instruments, a division of Integra LifeSciences Corporation.

FIGURE 12-49

Intracranial Instrumentation – PROBES AND DILATORS

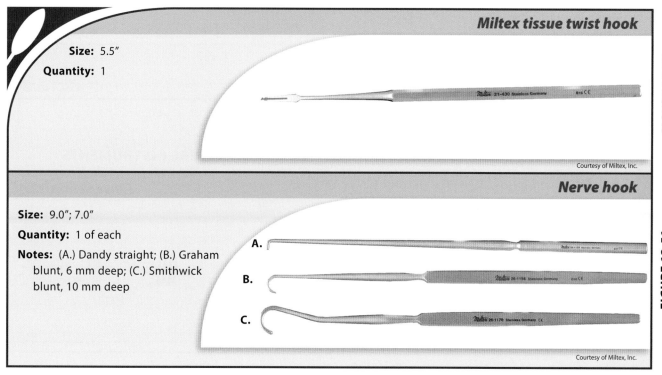

Miltex tissue twist hook

Size: 5.5″

Quantity: 1

Courtesy of Miltex, Inc.

FIGURE 12-50

Nerve hook

Size: 9.0″; 7.0″

Quantity: 1 of each

Notes: (A.) Dandy straight; (B.) Graham blunt, 6 mm deep; (C.) Smithwick blunt, 10 mm deep

A.

B.

C.

Courtesy of Miltex, Inc.

FIGURE 12-51

Intracranial Instrumentation – EVACUATION AND INSTILLATION INSTRUMENTS

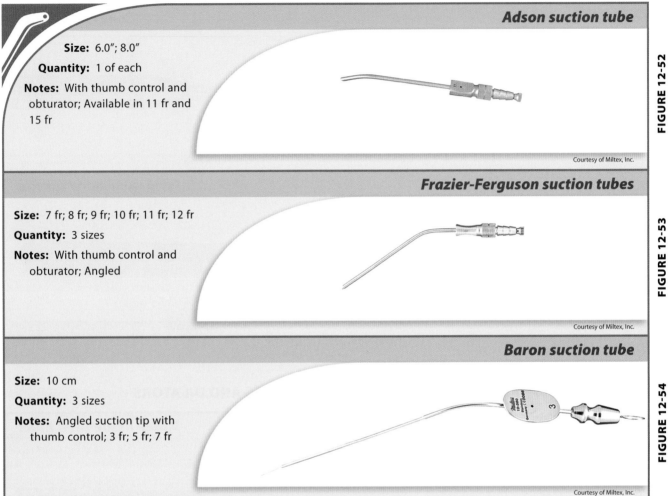

Adson suction tube

Size: 6.0"; 8.0"

Quantity: 1 of each

Notes: With thumb control and obturator; Available in 11 fr and 15 fr

Courtesy of Miltex, Inc.

FIGURE 12-52

Frazier-Ferguson suction tubes

Size: 7 fr; 8 fr; 9 fr; 10 fr; 11 fr; 12 fr

Quantity: 3 sizes

Notes: With thumb control and obturator; Angled

Courtesy of Miltex, Inc.

FIGURE 12-53

Baron suction tube

Size: 10 cm

Quantity: 3 sizes

Notes: Angled suction tip with thumb control; 3 fr; 5 fr; 7 fr

Courtesy of Miltex, Inc.

FIGURE 12-54

Intracranial Instrumentation – RETRACTION AND EXPOSURE INSTRUMENTS

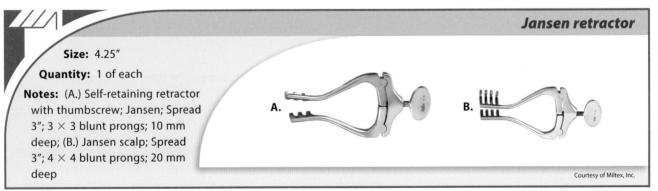

Jansen retractor

Size: 4.25"

Quantity: 1 of each

Notes: (A.) Self-retaining retractor with thumbscrew; Jansen; Spread 3"; 3 × 3 blunt prongs; 10 mm deep; (B.) Jansen scalp; Spread 3"; 4 × 4 blunt prongs; 20 mm deep

A.

B.

Courtesy of Miltex, Inc.

FIGURE 12-55

Intracranial Instrumentation – RETRACTION AND EXPOSURE INSTRUMENTS *continued*

Scalp contour retractor

Size: 5.5"

Quantity: 1

Notes: 3 × 4 prongs; Can be sharp or blunt

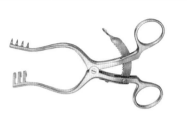

K-Medic branded instrumentation courtesy of Teleflex Medical, Inc.

FIGURE 12-56

Beckman-Weitlaner retractors

Size: 5.5"; 6.5"; 9.0"

Quantity: 1

Notes: Hinged blades, 3 × 4 teeth; Available with sharp or blunt prongs

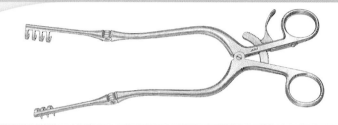

Courtesy of Jarit Surgical Instruments, a division of Integra LifeSciences Corporation.

FIGURE 12-57

LEYLA self-retaining brain retractor set

Size: Universal

Quantity: 1 set

Notes: Flexible self-locking retractor base attaches to side rail of surgical table; Assembles in two pieces that can hold up to five flexible arms; Ball joint adjustment

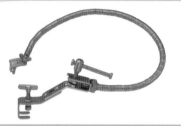

Photo supplied courtesy of Cardinal Health, V. Mueller® Products and Services. All rights reserved.

FIGURE 12-58

Yasargil brain retractor

Notes: Flexible self-locking retractor base that attaches to overhead bar on surgical bed. Available in titanium

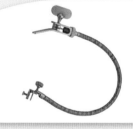
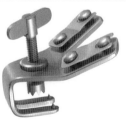

Courtesy of Joe Fortunato.

FIGURE 12-59

continues

Intracranial Instrumentation – RETRACTION AND EXPOSURE INSTRUMENTS *continued*

Fukushima retraction system

Notes: Adjustable table mounted brain retractor system compatible with Mayfield skull pin fixation

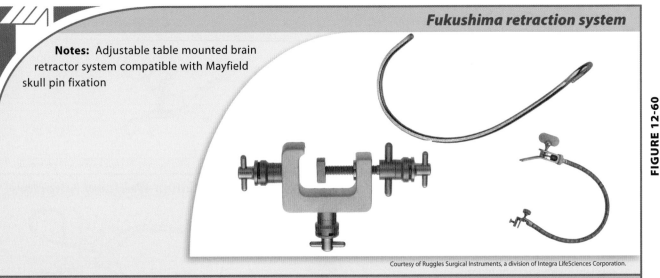

Courtesy of Ruggles Surgical Instruments, a division of Integra LifeSciences Corporation.

FIGURE 12-60

Fukushima brain spatulas

Size: 225 mm

Quantity: 1 of each size

Notes: Malleable brain spatula for use with self-retaining system; Ebonized for use with laser

A. Small tip 2.2 mm
B. Medium tip 3.8 mm
C. Large tip 5.8 mm
D. Extra large tip 7.0 mm

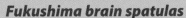

Courtesy of Ruggles Surgical Instruments, a division of Integra LifeSciences Corporation.

FIGURE 12-61

Fukushima dura spatula

Size: 205 mm

Quantity: 1 of each size

Notes: Rigid dura spatula

A. Small tip 60-degree curved end
B. Small tip 2.2 mm
C. Medium tip 3.8 mm
D. Large tip 5.8 mm

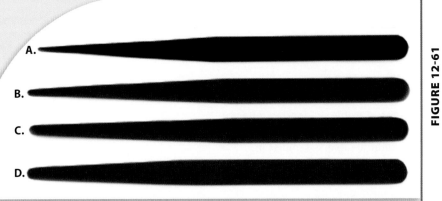

Courtesy of Ruggles Surgical Instruments, a division of Integra LifeSciences Corporation.

FIGURE 12-62

Intracranial Instrumentation – RETRACTION AND EXPOSURE INSTRUMENTS *continued*

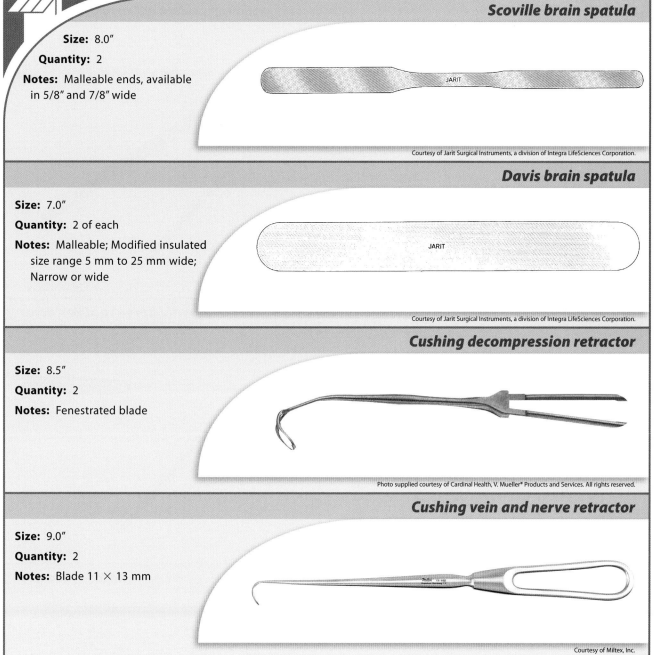

Scoville brain spatula

Size: 8.0"

Quantity: 2

Notes: Malleable ends, available in 5/8" and 7/8" wide

FIGURE 12-63

Courtesy of Jarit Surgical Instruments, a division of Integra LifeSciences Corporation.

Davis brain spatula

Size: 7.0"

Quantity: 2 of each

Notes: Malleable; Modified insulated size range 5 mm to 25 mm wide; Narrow or wide

FIGURE 12-64

Courtesy of Jarit Surgical Instruments, a division of Integra LifeSciences Corporation.

Cushing decompression retractor

Size: 8.5"

Quantity: 2

Notes: Fenestrated blade

FIGURE 12-65

Photo supplied courtesy of Cardinal Health, V. Mueller® Products and Services. All rights reserved.

Cushing vein and nerve retractor

Size: 9.0"

Quantity: 2

Notes: Blade 11 × 13 mm

FIGURE 12-66

Courtesy of Miltex, Inc.

continues

Intracranial Instrumentation – RETRACTION AND EXPOSURE INSTRUMENTS *continued*

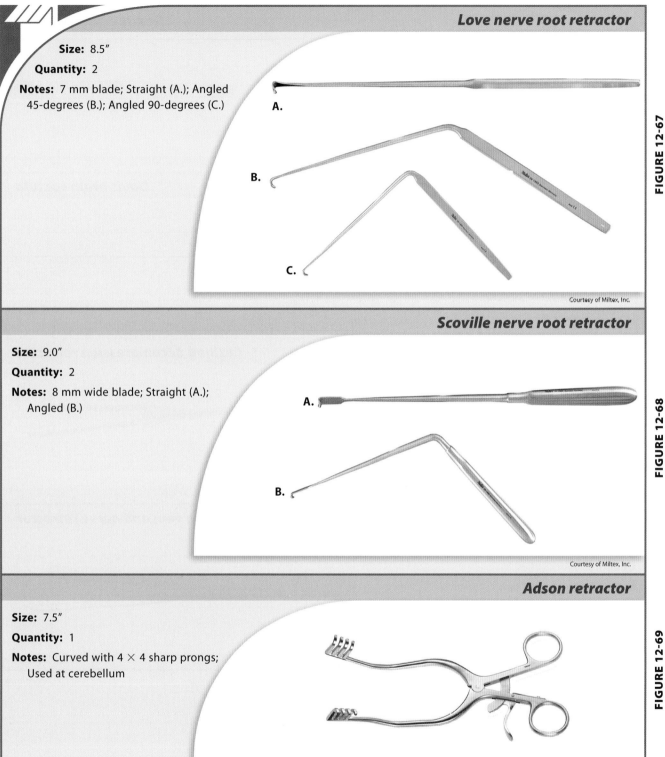

Love nerve root retractor

Size: 8.5″

Quantity: 2

Notes: 7 mm blade; Straight (A.); Angled 45-degrees (B.); Angled 90-degrees (C.)

A.

B.

C.

Courtesy of Miltex, Inc.

FIGURE 12-67

Scoville nerve root retractor

Size: 9.0″

Quantity: 2

Notes: 8 mm wide blade; Straight (A.); Angled (B.)

A.

B.

Courtesy of Miltex, Inc.

FIGURE 12-68

Adson retractor

Size: 7.5″

Quantity: 1

Notes: Curved with 4 × 4 sharp prongs; Used at cerebellum

Courtesy of Ruggles Surgical Instruments, a division of Integra LifeSciences Corporation.

FIGURE 12-69

Intracranial Instrumentation – APPROXIMATION AND CLOSURE INSTRUMENTS

Adson aneurysm needle

Size: 9.0"

Quantity: 1

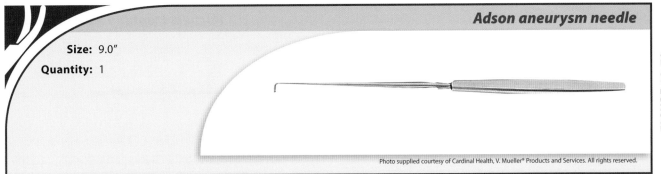

FIGURE 12-70

Intracranial Instrumentation – SPECIALTY SPECIFIC INSTRUMENTS

Gigli saw handle

Quantity: 2

Notes: Gigli saw handles are used in pairs; The flexible blade attaches to hooks at the base of the handle; The surgeon pulls the blade back and forth in alternating motions to cut the bone

Courtesy of Miltex, Inc.

FIGURE 12-71

Gigli saw blade

Size: 12.0"; 20.0"; 30.0"

Quantity: 1

Notes: Universal blade connections for gigli handles; Take care with serrated edge; Disposable styles are preferred

Courtesy of Miltex, Inc.

FIGURE 12-72

Bailey gigli saw guide

Size: 12.0"

Quantity: 1

Notes: Flexible; Permits placement of gigli saw without tissue damage

Courtesy of Joe Fortunato.

FIGURE 12-73

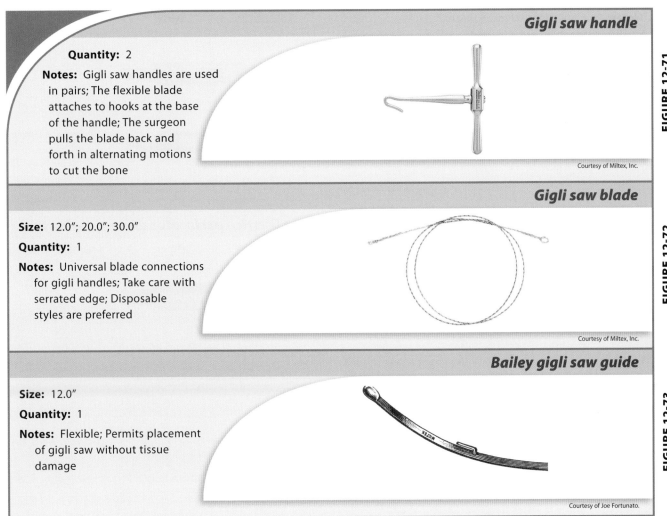

continues

Intracranial Instrumentation – SPECIALTY SPECIFIC INSTRUMENTS *continued*

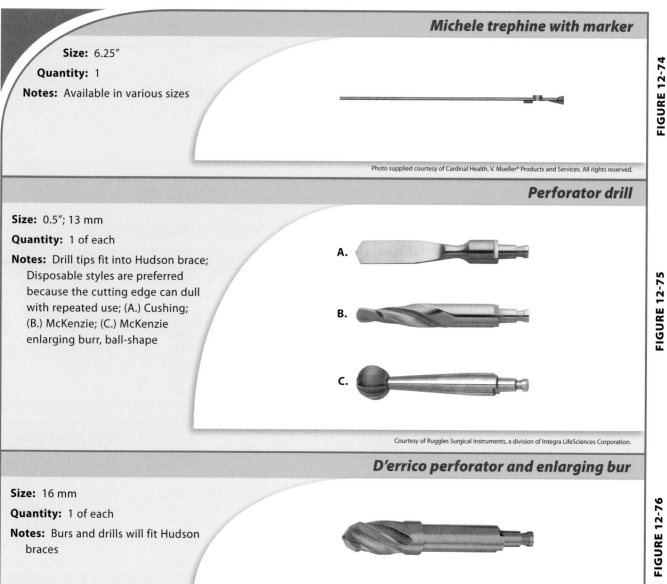

Michele trephine with marker

Size: 6.25″

Quantity: 1

Notes: Available in various sizes

FIGURE 12-74

Perforator drill

Size: 0.5″; 13 mm

Quantity: 1 of each

Notes: Drill tips fit into Hudson brace; Disposable styles are preferred because the cutting edge can dull with repeated use; (A.) Cushing; (B.) McKenzie; (C.) McKenzie enlarging burr, ball-shape

A.

B.

C.

FIGURE 12-75

D'errico perforator and enlarging bur

Size: 16 mm

Quantity: 1 of each

Notes: Burs and drills will fit Hudson braces

FIGURE 12-76

Intracranial Instrumentation – SPECIALTY SPECIFIC INSTRUMENTS *continued*

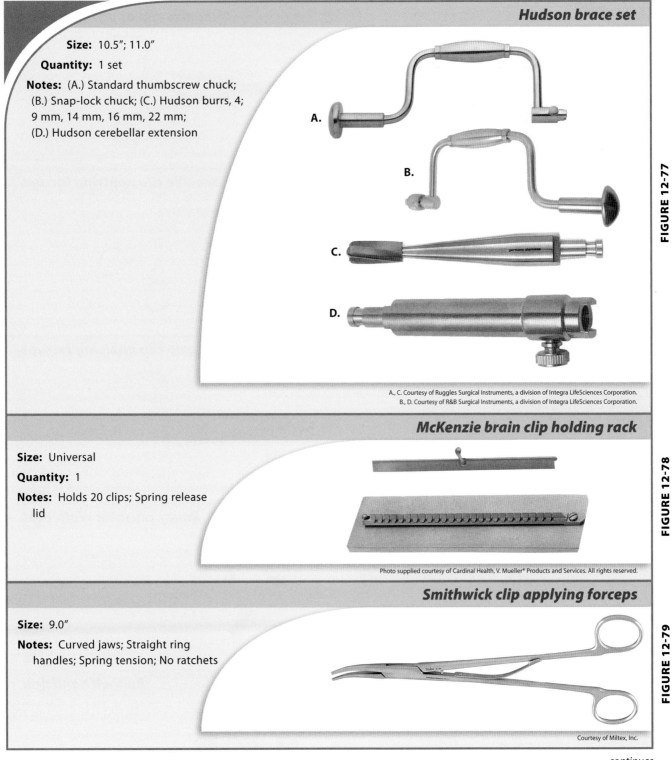

Hudson brace set

Size: 10.5″; 11.0″

Quantity: 1 set

Notes: (A.) Standard thumbscrew chuck;
(B.) Snap-lock chuck; (C.) Hudson burrs, 4;
9 mm, 14 mm, 16 mm, 22 mm;
(D.) Hudson cerebellar extension

A.

B.

C.

D.

A., C. Courtesy of Ruggles Surgical Instruments, a division of Integra LifeSciences Corporation.
B., D. Courtesy of R&B Surgical Instruments, a division of Integra LifeSciences Corporation.

FIGURE 12-77

McKenzie brain clip holding rack

Size: Universal

Quantity: 1

Notes: Holds 20 clips; Spring release
lid

Photo supplied courtesy of Cardinal Health, V. Mueller® Products and Services. All rights reserved.

FIGURE 12-78

Smithwick clip applying forceps

Size: 9.0″

Notes: Curved jaws; Straight ring
handles; Spring tension; No ratchets

Courtesy of Miltex, Inc.

FIGURE 12-79

continues

Intracranial Instrumentation – SPECIALTY SPECIFIC INSTRUMENTS *continued*

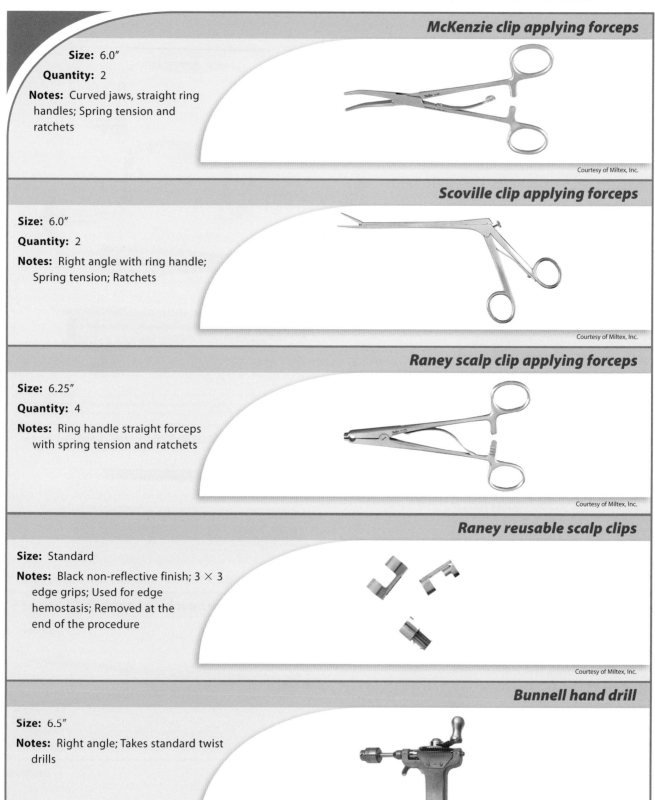

McKenzie clip applying forceps

Size: 6.0"

Quantity: 2

Notes: Curved jaws, straight ring handles; Spring tension and ratchets

Courtesy of Miltex, Inc.

FIGURE 12-80

Scoville clip applying forceps

Size: 6.0"

Quantity: 2

Notes: Right angle with ring handle; Spring tension; Ratchets

Courtesy of Miltex, Inc.

FIGURE 12-81

Raney scalp clip applying forceps

Size: 6.25"

Quantity: 4

Notes: Ring handle straight forceps with spring tension and ratchets

Courtesy of Miltex, Inc.

FIGURE 12-82

Raney reusable scalp clips

Size: Standard

Notes: Black non-reflective finish; 3 × 3 edge grips; Used for edge hemostasis; Removed at the end of the procedure

Courtesy of Miltex, Inc.

FIGURE 12-83

Bunnell hand drill

Size: 6.5"

Notes: Right angle; Takes standard twist drills

Courtesy of Ruggles Surgical Instruments, a division of Integra LifeSciences Corporation.

FIGURE 12-84

SPINE INSTRUMENTATION

Spinal surgery involves soft and compact tissue handling. Although neurologic tissue is commonly the arena of the neurosurgeon, orthopaedic surgeons perform spinal procedures. Both disciplines take precautionary measures to preserve delicate tissues.

A medium or long foundation set is used to enter the surgical site, and compact tissue instrumentation is used for bone and fibrous disc material. Instrumentation in this group is commonly used for vertebrae between the thorax and sacrum. Implants can be placed during procedures for stabilization or deformity correction.

Spine Instrumentation – DISSECTION AND DEBULKING INSTRUMENTS

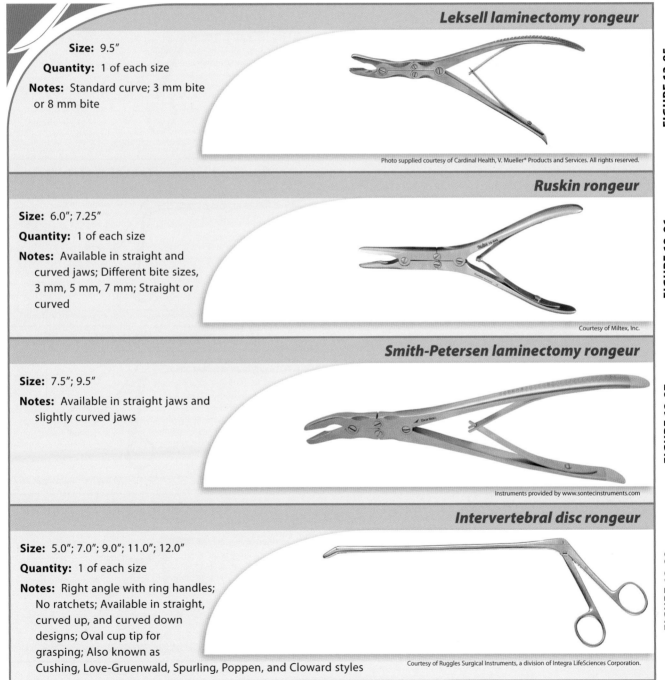

Leksell laminectomy rongeur

Size: 9.5"

Quantity: 1 of each size

Notes: Standard curve; 3 mm bite or 8 mm bite

FIGURE 12-85

Ruskin rongeur

Size: 6.0"; 7.25"

Quantity: 1 of each size

Notes: Available in straight and curved jaws; Different bite sizes, 3 mm, 5 mm, 7 mm; Straight or curved

FIGURE 12-86

Smith-Petersen laminectomy rongeur

Size: 7.5"; 9.5"

Notes: Available in straight jaws and slightly curved jaws

FIGURE 12-87

Intervertebral disc rongeur

Size: 5.0"; 7.0"; 9.0"; 11.0"; 12.0"

Quantity: 1 of each size

Notes: Right angle with ring handles; No ratchets; Available in straight, curved up, and curved down designs; Oval cup tip for grasping; Also known as Cushing, Love-Gruenwald, Spurling, Poppen, and Cloward styles

FIGURE 12-88

continues

Spine Instrumentation – DISSECTION AND DEBULKING INSTRUMENTS *continued*

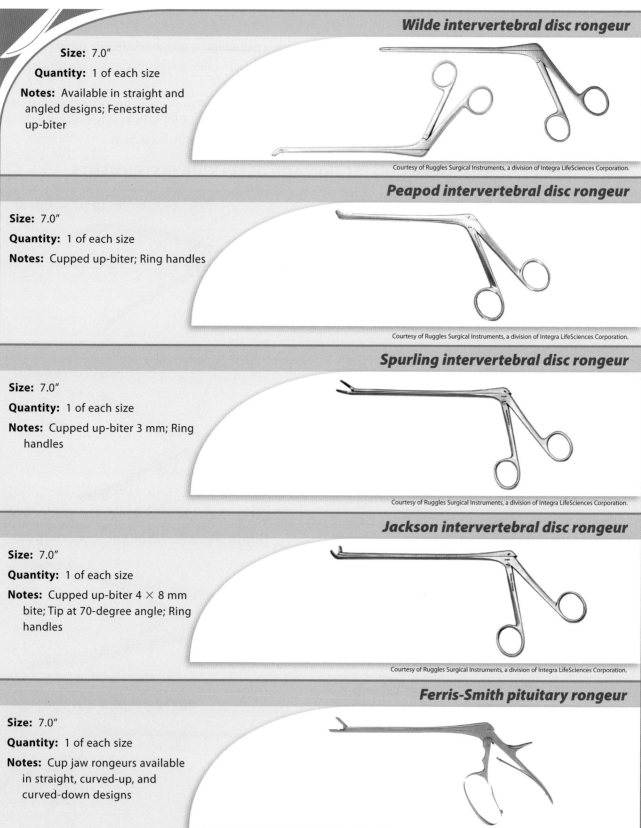

Wilde intervertebral disc rongeur

Size: 7.0″

Quantity: 1 of each size

Notes: Available in straight and angled designs; Fenestrated up-biter

FIGURE 12-89

Peapod intervertebral disc rongeur

Size: 7.0″

Quantity: 1 of each size

Notes: Cupped up-biter; Ring handles

FIGURE 12-90

Spurling intervertebral disc rongeur

Size: 7.0″

Quantity: 1 of each size

Notes: Cupped up-biter 3 mm; Ring handles

FIGURE 12-91

Jackson intervertebral disc rongeur

Size: 7.0″

Quantity: 1 of each size

Notes: Cupped up-biter 4 × 8 mm bite; Tip at 70-degree angle; Ring handles

FIGURE 12-92

Ferris-Smith pituitary rongeur

Size: 7.0″

Quantity: 1 of each size

Notes: Cup jaw rongeurs available in straight, curved-up, and curved-down designs

FIGURE 12-93

Spine Instrumentation – DISSECTION AND DEBULKING INSTRUMENTS *continued*

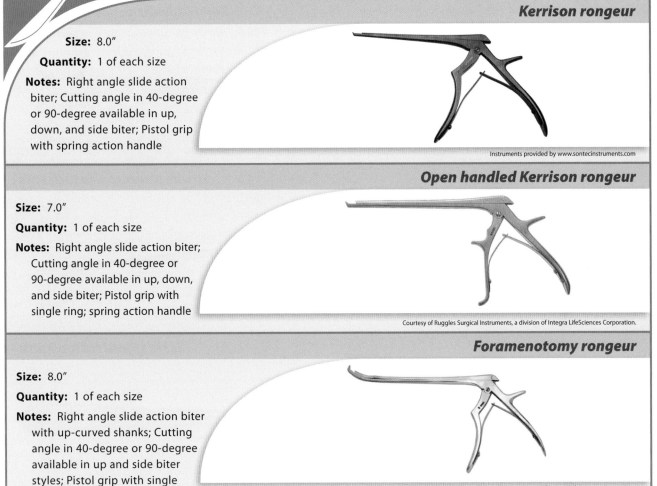

Kerrison rongeur

Size: 8.0"

Quantity: 1 of each size

Notes: Right angle slide action biter; Cutting angle in 40-degree or 90-degree available in up, down, and side biter; Pistol grip with spring action handle

Instruments provided by www.sontecinstruments.com

FIGURE 12-94

Open handled Kerrison rongeur

Size: 7.0"

Quantity: 1 of each size

Notes: Right angle slide action biter; Cutting angle in 40-degree or 90-degree available in up, down, and side biter; Pistol grip with single ring; spring action handle

Courtesy of Ruggles Surgical Instruments, a division of Integra LifeSciences Corporation.

FIGURE 12-95

Foramenotomy rongeur

Size: 8.0"

Quantity: 1 of each size

Notes: Right angle slide action biter with up-curved shanks; Cutting angle in 40-degree or 90-degree available in up and side biter styles; Pistol grip with single ring spring action handle

Courtesy of Ruggles Surgical Instruments, a division of Integra LifeSciences Corporation.

FIGURE 12-96

Spine Instrumentation – DISSECTION INSTRUMENTS

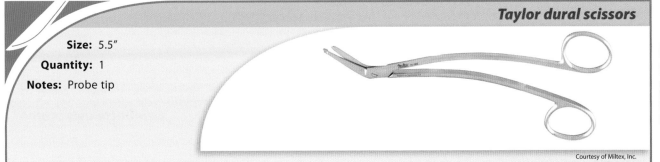

Taylor dural scissors

Size: 5.5"

Quantity: 1

Notes: Probe tip

Courtesy of Miltex, Inc.

FIGURE 12-97

continues

Spine Instrumentation – DISSECTION INSTRUMENTS *continued*

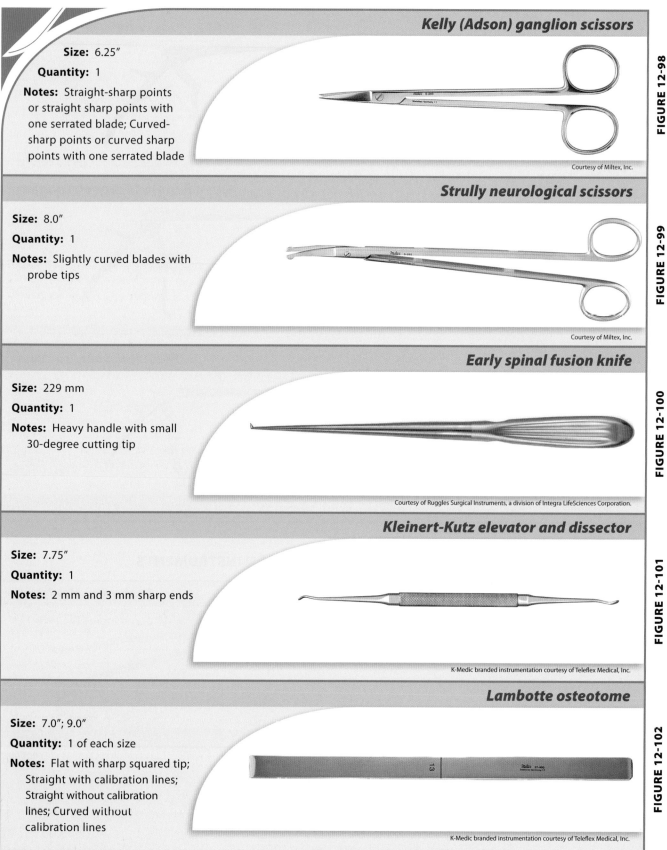

Kelly (Adson) ganglion scissors

Size: 6.25"

Quantity: 1

Notes: Straight-sharp points or straight sharp points with one serrated blade; Curved-sharp points or curved sharp points with one serrated blade

Courtesy of Miltex, Inc.

FIGURE 12-98

Strully neurological scissors

Size: 8.0"

Quantity: 1

Notes: Slightly curved blades with probe tips

Courtesy of Miltex, Inc.

FIGURE 12-99

Early spinal fusion knife

Size: 229 mm

Quantity: 1

Notes: Heavy handle with small 30-degree cutting tip

Courtesy of Ruggles Surgical Instruments, a division of Integra LifeSciences Corporation.

FIGURE 12-100

Kleinert-Kutz elevator and dissector

Size: 7.75"

Quantity: 1

Notes: 2 mm and 3 mm sharp ends

K-Medic branded instrumentation courtesy of Teleflex Medical, Inc.

FIGURE 12-101

Lambotte osteotome

Size: 7.0"; 9.0"

Quantity: 1 of each size

Notes: Flat with sharp squared tip; Straight with calibration lines; Straight without calibration lines; Curved without calibration lines

K-Medic branded instrumentation courtesy of Teleflex Medical, Inc.

FIGURE 12-102

Spine Instrumentation – DISSECTION INSTRUMENTS *continued*

Hibbs osteotome

Size: 9.0"

Quantity: 1 of each size

Notes: Curved or straight sharp tip; Hexagonal handle; 0.25"; 0.38"; 0.5"; 0.63"; 0.75"; 0.88"; 1.0"; 1.13"; 1.25"; 1.5"

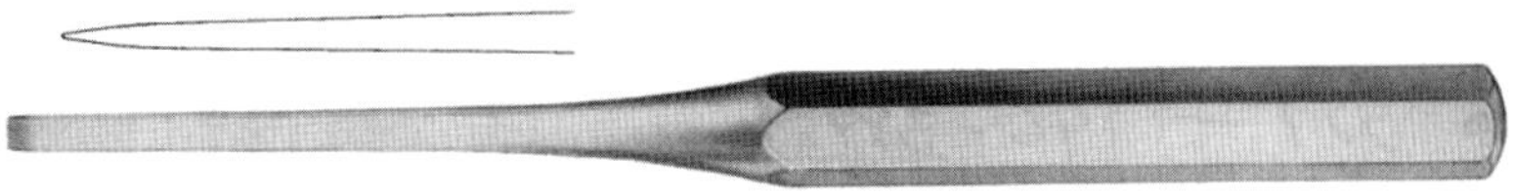

K-Medic branded instrumentation courtesy of Teleflex Medical, Inc.

FIGURE 12-103

Smith-Peterson gouge

Size: 8.0"

Quantity: 1 of each size

Notes: Rounded handle with flat end for mallet use; Straight; Curved

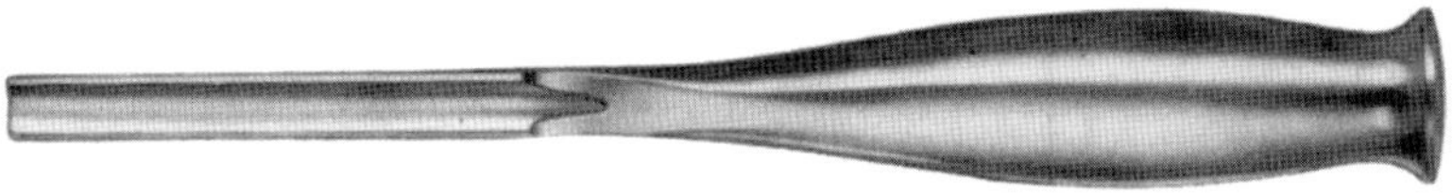

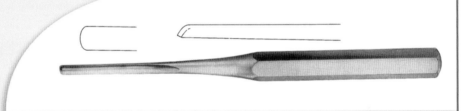

K-Medic branded instrumentation courtesy of Teleflex Medical, Inc.

FIGURE 12-104

Hibbs gouge

Size: 9.0"

Quantity: 1 of each size

Notes: Straight; Curved

K-Medic branded instrumentation courtesy of Teleflex Medical, Inc.

FIGURE 12-105

Cobb-type spinal gouge

Size: 11.0"

Notes: Rounded head; 7 mm blade width; Straight; Medium curve; Strong curve; Reverse curve

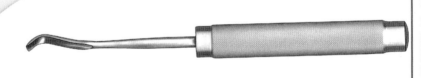

K-Medic branded instrumentation courtesy of Teleflex Medical, Inc.

FIGURE 12-106

Liston bone cutting forceps

Size: 5.5"; 6.75"; 7.5"; 8.5"

Quantity: 1 of each size

Notes: Straight; Angled on flat

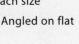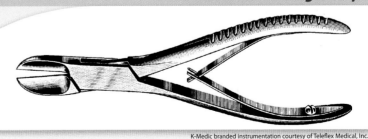

K-Medic branded instrumentation courtesy of Teleflex Medical, Inc.

FIGURE 12-107

continues

Spine Instrumentation – DISSECTION INSTRUMENTS *continued*

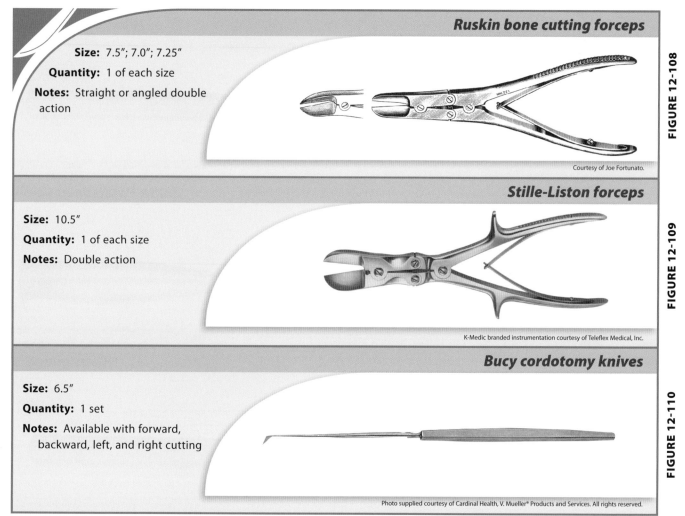

Ruskin bone cutting forceps

Size: 7.5"; 7.0"; 7.25"

Quantity: 1 of each size

Notes: Straight or angled double action

FIGURE 12-108

Stille-Liston forceps

Size: 10.5"

Quantity: 1 of each size

Notes: Double action

FIGURE 12-109

Bucy cordotomy knives

Size: 6.5"

Quantity: 1 set

Notes: Available with forward, backward, left, and right cutting

FIGURE 12-110

Spine Instrumentation – DEBULKING INSTRUMENTS

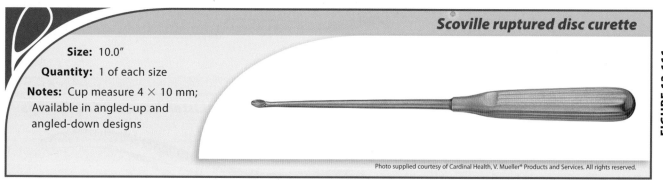

Scoville ruptured disc curette

Size: 10.0"

Quantity: 1 of each size

Notes: Cup measure 4 × 10 mm; Available in angled-up and angled-down designs

FIGURE 12-111

Spine Instrumentation – DEBULKING INSTRUMENTS *continued*

Spratt (Brun) bone curettes

Size: 6.5"

Quantity: 1 of each size

Notes: Oval cups; Available in various sizes ranging from a size 5/0 to a size 6

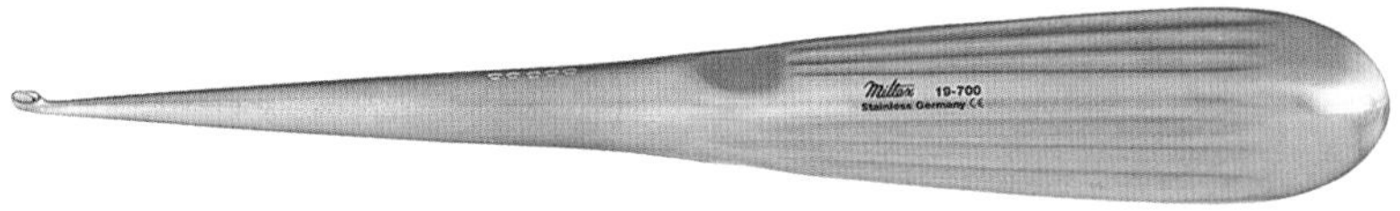

Courtesy of Miltex, Inc.

FIGURE 12-112

Brun bone curettes

Size: 6.75"

Quantity: 1 of each size

Notes: Round cups; Available in various sizes ranging from 7 mm to 14 mm

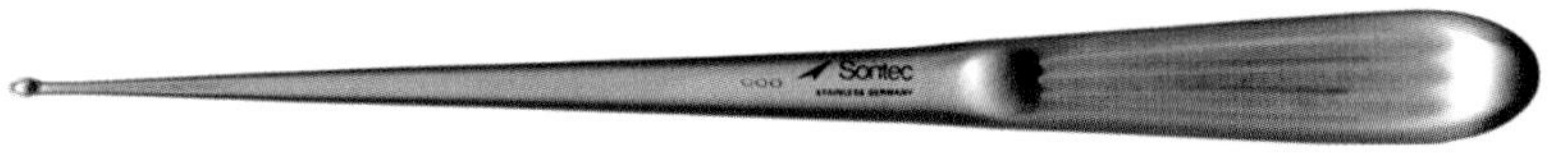

Instruments provided by www.sontecinstruments.com

FIGURE 12-113

Ruggles flatback spinal fusion curette

Size: 9"

Quantity: 1 of each size

Notes: Straight; Angled 40-degree; Angled 90-degree; Reversed angle

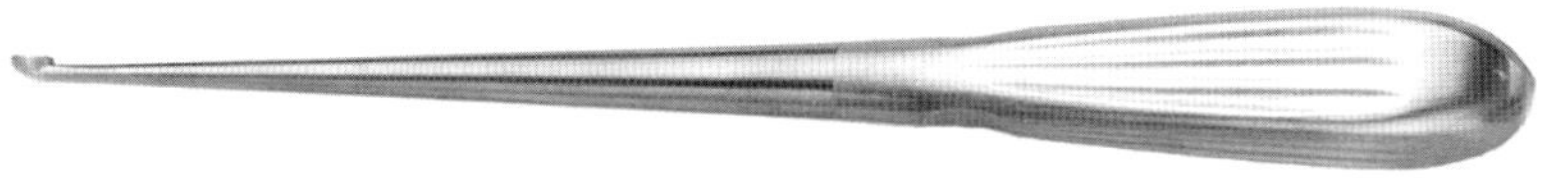

Courtesy of Ruggles Surgical Instruments, a division of Integra LifeSciences Corporation.

FIGURE 12-114

Sisco bayonet spinal fusion curette

Size: 9"

Notes: Reverse angle up; Angle 90-degree; Straight; Reverse angle down; Angle 40-degree

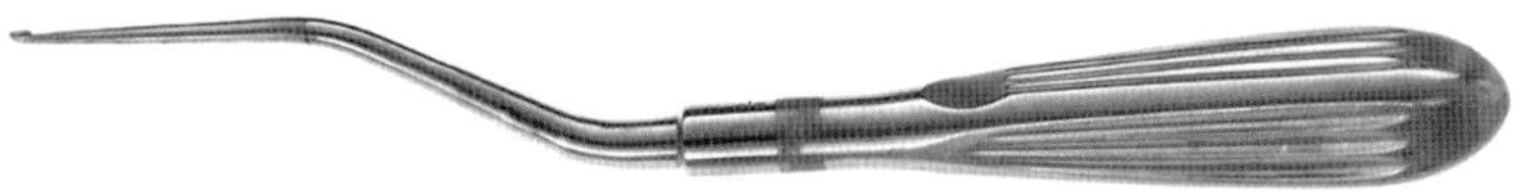

Courtesy of Ruggles Surgical Instruments, a division of Integra LifeSciences Corporation.

FIGURE 12-115

Ruggles lumbar axial curettes

Size: 260 mm; 276 mm

Quantity: 1 of each size

Notes: Reverse angled up; Reverse angled down; Angled up; Angled down; Straight up; Straight down

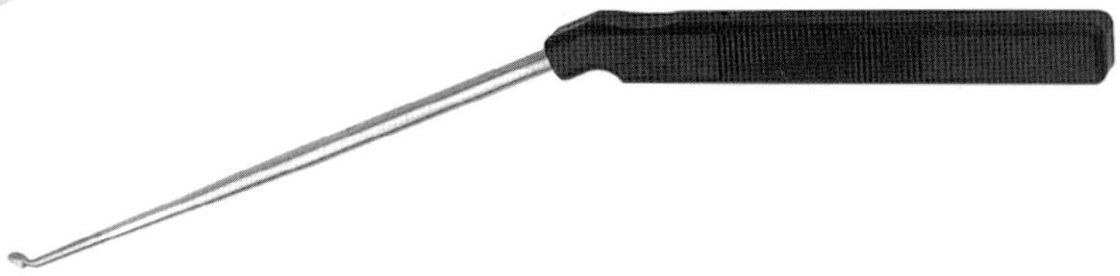

Courtesy of Ruggles Surgical Instruments, a division of Integra LifeSciences Corporation.

FIGURE 12-116

Spine Instrumentation – PROBES AND DILATORS

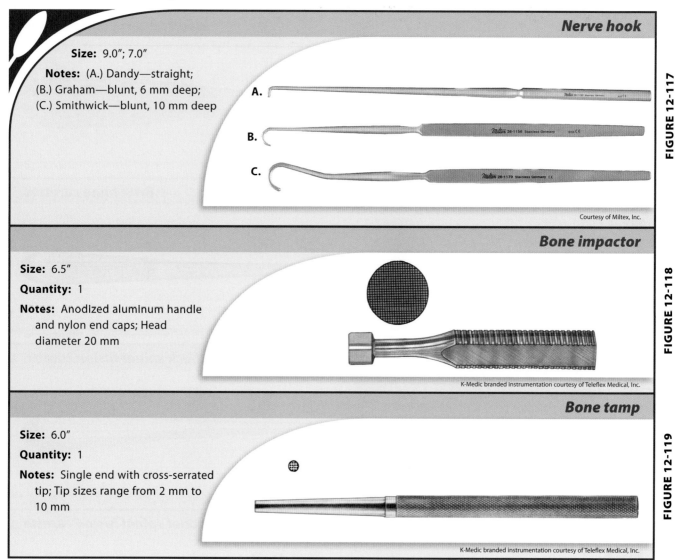

Nerve hook

Size: 9.0"; 7.0"

Notes: (A.) Dandy—straight;
(B.) Graham—blunt, 6 mm deep;
(C.) Smithwick—blunt, 10 mm deep

A.

B.

C.

Courtesy of Miltex, Inc.

FIGURE 12-117

Bone impactor

Size: 6.5"

Quantity: 1

Notes: Anodized aluminum handle and nylon end caps; Head diameter 20 mm

K-Medic branded instrumentation courtesy of Teleflex Medical, Inc.

FIGURE 12-118

Bone tamp

Size: 6.0"

Quantity: 1

Notes: Single end with cross-serrated tip; Tip sizes range from 2 mm to 10 mm

K-Medic branded instrumentation courtesy of Teleflex Medical, Inc.

FIGURE 12-119

Spine Instrumentation – RETRACTION AND EXPOSURE INSTRUMENTS

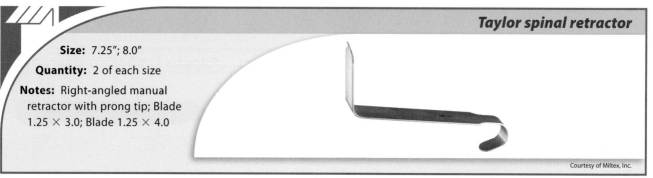

Taylor spinal retractor

Size: 7.25"; 8.0"

Quantity: 2 of each size

Notes: Right-angled manual retractor with prong tip; Blade 1.25 × 3.0; Blade 1.25 × 4.0

Courtesy of Miltex, Inc.

FIGURE 12-120

Spine Instrumentation – RETRACTION AND EXPOSURE INSTRUMENTS *continued*

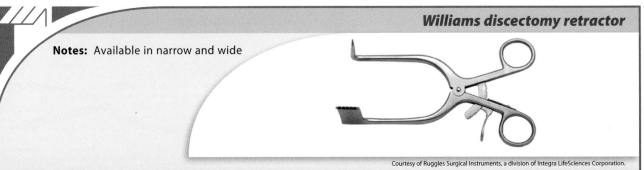

Williams discectomy retractor

Notes: Available in narrow and wide

FIGURE 12-121

Tuffier retractor

Size: 6.5″

Quantity: 2

Notes: Grooved blades, 6.5″ spread

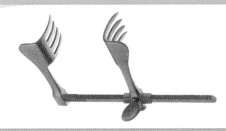

FIGURE 12-122

Meyerding laminectomy retractor

Size: 9.5″

Quantity: 4

Notes: Right angle manual retractor with toothed traction edge; Large blade 3.5 × 2.0; Medium blade 3.0 × 1.0; Small blade 2.0 × 5/8

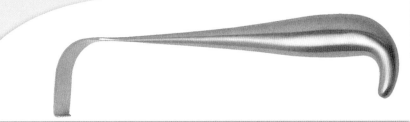

FIGURE 12-123

Beckman-Weitlaner retractor

Size: 5.5″; 6.5″; 9.0″

Quantity: 2 sizes

Notes: Ring handle self-retaining retractor; Hinged with 3 × 4 teeth; Sharp or blunt

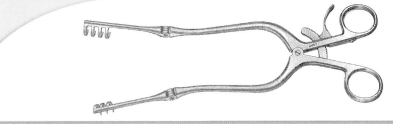

FIGURE 12-124

Beckman-Adson laminectomy retractor

Size: 12.5″

Quantity: 2

Notes: Ring handle with ratchets; Hinged, sharp 4 × 4 teeth

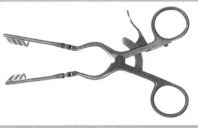

FIGURE 12-125

continues

Spine Instrumentation – RETRACTION AND EXPOSURE INSTRUMENTS *continued*

Beckman-Eaton laminectomy retractor

Size: 12.75"

Quantity: 2

Notes: Ring handle with ratchets; Hinged, sharp 7 × 7 teeth

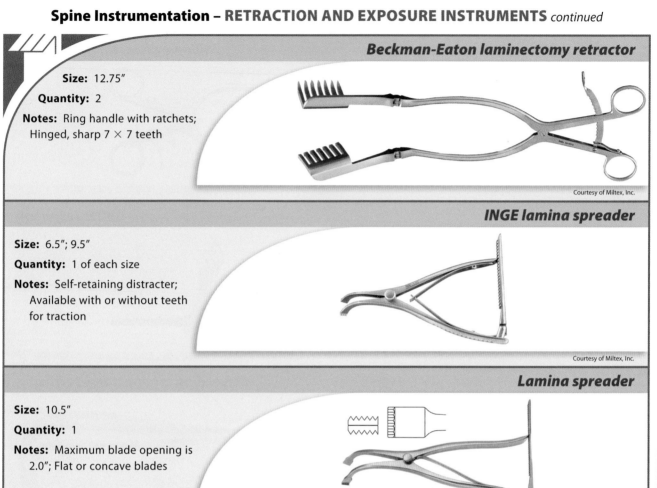

Courtesy of Miltex, Inc.

FIGURE 12-126

INGE lamina spreader

Size: 6.5"; 9.5"

Quantity: 1 of each size

Notes: Self-retaining distracter; Available with or without teeth for traction

Courtesy of Miltex, Inc.

FIGURE 12-127

Lamina spreader

Size: 10.5"

Quantity: 1

Notes: Maximum blade opening is 2.0"; Flat or concave blades

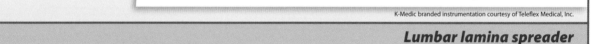

K-Medic branded instrumentation courtesy of Teleflex Medical, Inc.

FIGURE 12-128

Lumbar lamina spreader

Size: 3.5"; 4.24"

Quantity: 1 of each size

Notes: Spring handle locking distraction bone separator

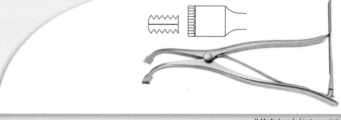

K-Medic branded instrumentation courtesy of Teleflex Medical, Inc.

FIGURE 12-129

Vertebra spreader

Size: 5.0"

Quantity: 1

Notes: Small self-retaining bone distractor with ratchet

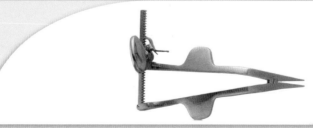

Courtesy of Ruggles Surgical Instruments, a division of Integra LifeSciences Corporation.

FIGURE 12-130

Spine Instrumentation – RETRACTION AND EXPOSURE INSTRUMENTS continued

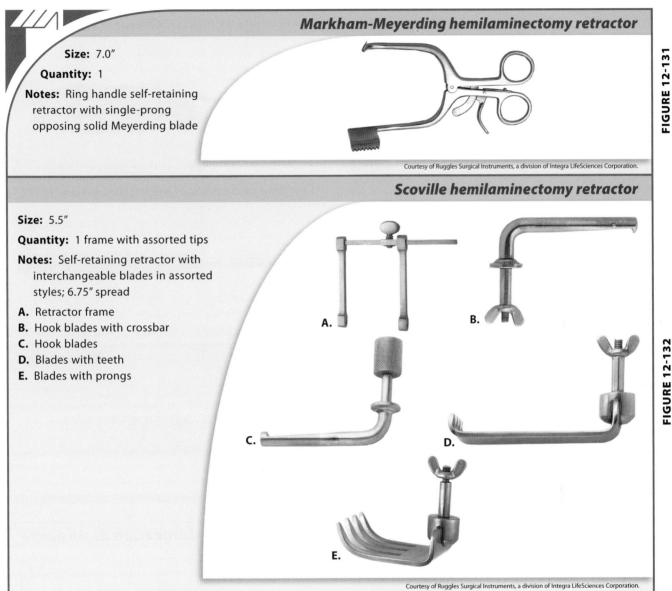

Markham-Meyerding hemilaminectomy retractor

Size: 7.0″

Quantity: 1

Notes: Ring handle self-retaining retractor with single-prong opposing solid Meyerding blade

Courtesy of Ruggles Surgical Instruments, a division of Integra LifeSciences Corporation.

FIGURE 12-131

Scoville hemilaminectomy retractor

Size: 5.5″

Quantity: 1 frame with assorted tips

Notes: Self-retaining retractor with interchangeable blades in assorted styles; 6.75″ spread

A. Retractor frame
B. Hook blades with crossbar
C. Hook blades
D. Blades with teeth
E. Blades with prongs

Courtesy of Ruggles Surgical Instruments, a division of Integra LifeSciences Corporation.

FIGURE 12-132

Spine Instrumentation – SPECIALTY SPECIFIC INSTRUMENTS

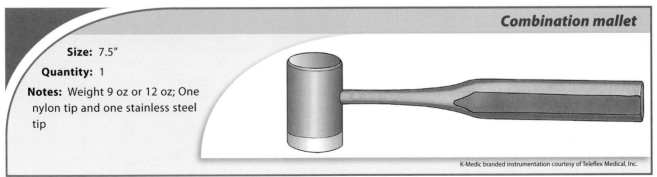

Combination mallet

Size: 7.5″

Quantity: 1

Notes: Weight 9 oz or 12 oz; One nylon tip and one stainless steel tip

K-Medic branded instrumentation courtesy of Teleflex Medical, Inc.

FIGURE 12-133

continues

Spine Instrumentation – SPECIALTY SPECIFIC INSTRUMENTS *continued*

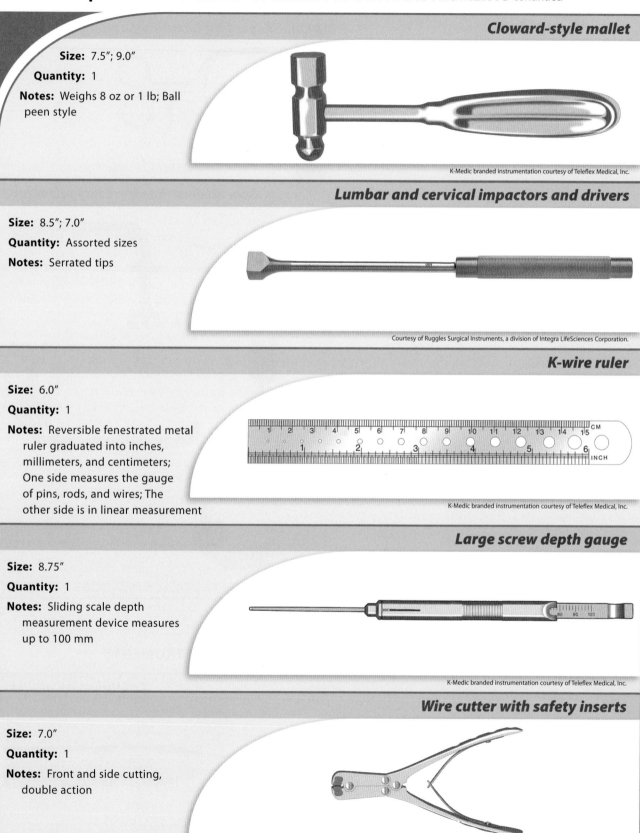

Cloward-style mallet

Size: 7.5"; 9.0"

Quantity: 1

Notes: Weighs 8 oz or 1 lb; Ball peen style

K-Medic branded instrumentation courtesy of Teleflex Medical, Inc.

FIGURE 12-134

Lumbar and cervical impactors and drivers

Size: 8.5"; 7.0"

Quantity: Assorted sizes

Notes: Serrated tips

Courtesy of Ruggles Surgical Instruments, a division of Integra LifeSciences Corporation.

FIGURE 12-135

K-wire ruler

Size: 6.0"

Quantity: 1

Notes: Reversible fenestrated metal ruler graduated into inches, millimeters, and centimeters; One side measures the gauge of pins, rods, and wires; The other side is in linear measurement

K-Medic branded instrumentation courtesy of Teleflex Medical, Inc.

FIGURE 12-136

Large screw depth gauge

Size: 8.75"

Quantity: 1

Notes: Sliding scale depth measurement device measures up to 100 mm

K-Medic branded instrumentation courtesy of Teleflex Medical, Inc.

FIGURE 12-137

Wire cutter with safety inserts

Size: 7.0"

Quantity: 1

Notes: Front and side cutting, double action

K-Medic branded instrumentation courtesy of Teleflex Medical, Inc.

FIGURE 12-138

Spine Instrumentation – SPECIALTY SPECIFIC INSTRUMENTS *continued*

Loute wire tightener

Size: 8.5″

Quantity: 1

Notes: Used for deep cerclage; Screw knobs

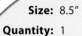
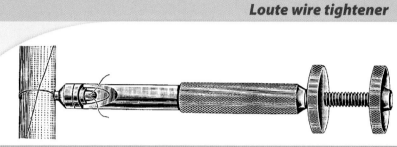

K-Medic branded instrumentation courtesy of Teleflex Medical, Inc.

FIGURE 12-139

Jet wire twister

Size: 11.0″

Quantity: 1

Notes: Used for cerclage of soft wire; Ratchet locks; Cross-serrated jaws

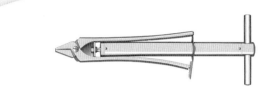

K-Medic branded instrumentation courtesy of Teleflex Medical, Inc.

FIGURE 12-140

Universal rod bender

Size: 11.0″

Quantity: 1

Notes: Bends rods up to 7 mm; Adjustable dial head and recessed hand grips

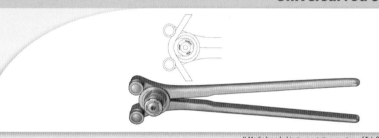

K-Medic branded instrumentation courtesy of Teleflex Medical, Inc.

FIGURE 12-141

Bone compass

Size: 8.0″

Quantity: 1

Notes: Set screw-locking caliper

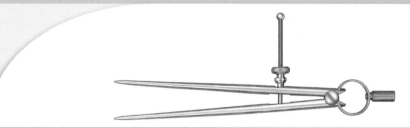

K-Medic branded instrumentation courtesy of Teleflex Medical, Inc.

FIGURE 12-142

Castroviejo caliper

Size: 6.5″

Quantity: 1

Notes: Set screw-locking measurement up to 40 mm

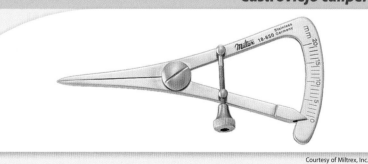

Courtesy of Miltrex, Inc.

FIGURE 12-143

continues

Spine Instrumentation – SPECIALTY SPECIFIC INSTRUMENTS *continued*

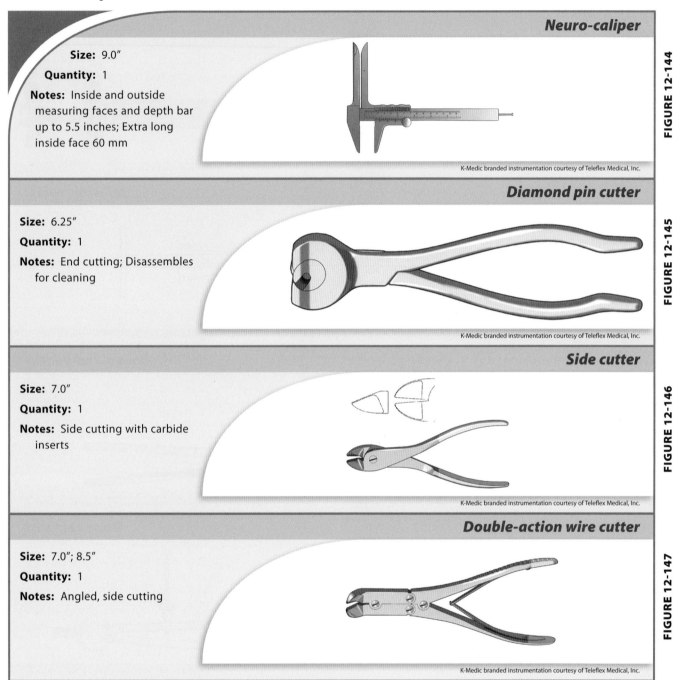

Neuro-caliper

Size: 9.0"

Quantity: 1

Notes: Inside and outside measuring faces and depth bar up to 5.5 inches; Extra long inside face 60 mm

K-Medic branded instrumentation courtesy of Teleflex Medical, Inc.

FIGURE 12-144

Diamond pin cutter

Size: 6.25"

Quantity: 1

Notes: End cutting; Disassembles for cleaning

K-Medic branded instrumentation courtesy of Teleflex Medical, Inc.

FIGURE 12-145

Side cutter

Size: 7.0"

Quantity: 1

Notes: Side cutting with carbide inserts

K-Medic branded instrumentation courtesy of Teleflex Medical, Inc.

FIGURE 12-146

Double-action wire cutter

Size: 7.0"; 8.5"

Quantity: 1

Notes: Angled, side cutting

K-Medic branded instrumentation courtesy of Teleflex Medical, Inc.

FIGURE 12-147

CERVICAL SPINE INSTRUMENTATION

Cervical spine procedures may use many of the typical lower spine instruments in addition to many of the instruments in the next group. Tissue depth will vary according to the approach used to enter the surgical site. The surgical methods involve prevention of injury to adjacent tissues such as anterior throat structures.

Cervical Spine Instrumentation – GRASPING FORCEPS

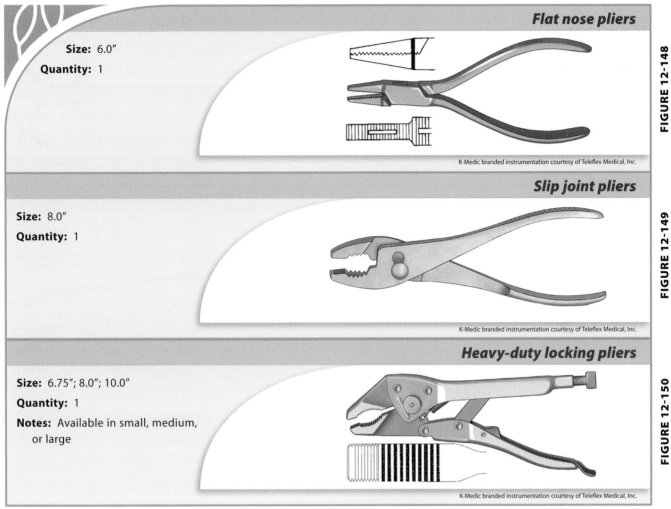

Flat nose pliers

Size: 6.0"

Quantity: 1

K-Medic branded instrumentation courtesy of Teleflex Medical, Inc.

FIGURE 12-148

Slip joint pliers

Size: 8.0"

Quantity: 1

K-Medic branded instrumentation courtesy of Teleflex Medical, Inc.

FIGURE 12-149

Heavy-duty locking pliers

Size: 6.75"; 8.0"; 10.0"

Quantity: 1

Notes: Available in small, medium, or large

K-Medic branded instrumentation courtesy of Teleflex Medical, Inc.

FIGURE 12-150

Cervical Spine Instrumentation – DISSECTION INSTRUMENTS

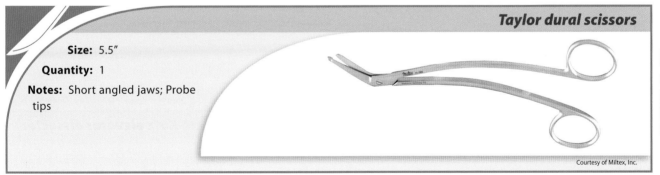

Taylor dural scissors

Size: 5.5"

Quantity: 1

Notes: Short angled jaws; Probe tips

Courtesy of Miltex, Inc.

FIGURE 12-151

continues

Cervical Spine Instrumentation – DISSECTION INSTRUMENTS *continued*

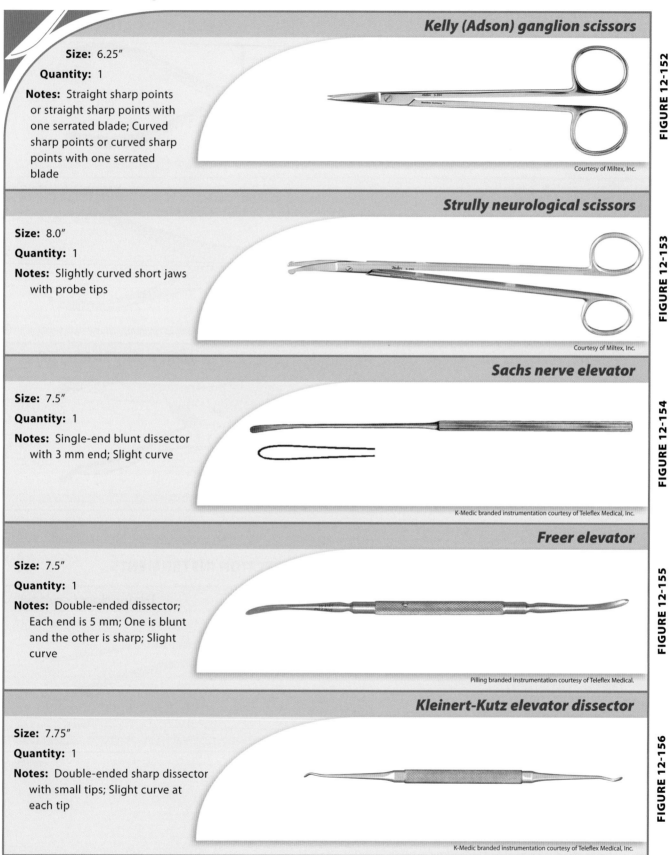

Kelly (Adson) ganglion scissors

Size: 6.25″

Quantity: 1

Notes: Straight sharp points or straight sharp points with one serrated blade; Curved sharp points or curved sharp points with one serrated blade

Courtesy of Miltex, Inc.

FIGURE 12-152

Strully neurological scissors

Size: 8.0″

Quantity: 1

Notes: Slightly curved short jaws with probe tips

Courtesy of Miltex, Inc.

FIGURE 12-153

Sachs nerve elevator

Size: 7.5″

Quantity: 1

Notes: Single-end blunt dissector with 3 mm end; Slight curve

K-Medic branded instrumentation courtesy of Teleflex Medical, Inc.

FIGURE 12-154

Freer elevator

Size: 7.5″

Quantity: 1

Notes: Double-ended dissector; Each end is 5 mm; One is blunt and the other is sharp; Slight curve

Pilling branded instrumentation courtesy of Teleflex Medical.

FIGURE 12-155

Kleinert-Kutz elevator dissector

Size: 7.75″

Quantity: 1

Notes: Double-ended sharp dissector with small tips; Slight curve at each tip

K-Medic branded instrumentation courtesy of Teleflex Medical, Inc.

FIGURE 12-156

Cervical Spine Instrumentation – DISSECTION INSTRUMENTS *continued*

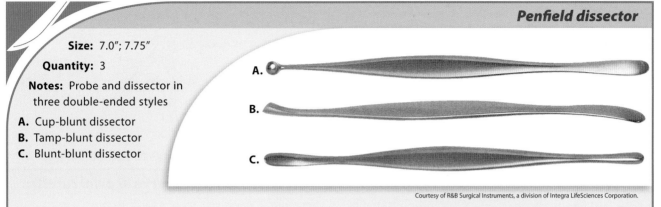

Penfield dissector

Size: 7.0″; 7.75″

Quantity: 3

Notes: Probe and dissector in three double-ended styles

A. Cup-blunt dissector
B. Tamp-blunt dissector
C. Blunt-blunt dissector

FIGURE 12-157

Cervical Spine Instrumentation – DEBULKING INSTRUMENTS

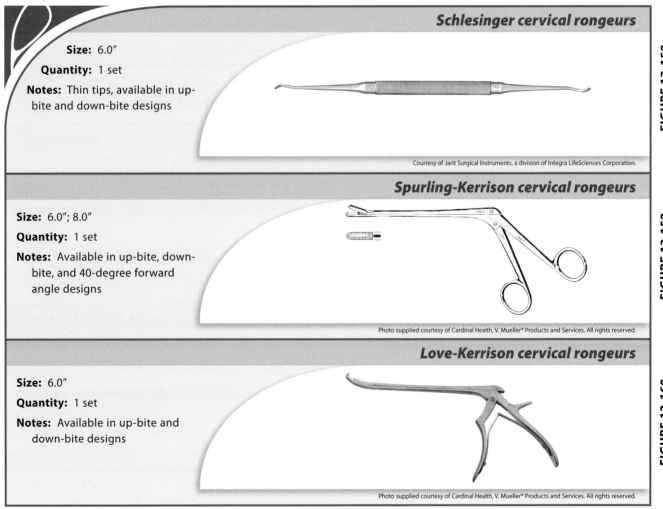

Schlesinger cervical rongeurs

Size: 6.0″

Quantity: 1 set

Notes: Thin tips, available in up-bite and down-bite designs

FIGURE 12-158

Spurling-Kerrison cervical rongeurs

Size: 6.0″; 8.0″

Quantity: 1 set

Notes: Available in up-bite, down-bite, and 40-degree forward angle designs

FIGURE 12-159

Love-Kerrison cervical rongeurs

Size: 6.0″

Quantity: 1 set

Notes: Available in up-bite and down-bite designs

FIGURE 12-160

continues

Cervical Spine Instrumentation – DEBULKING INSTRUMENTS *continued*

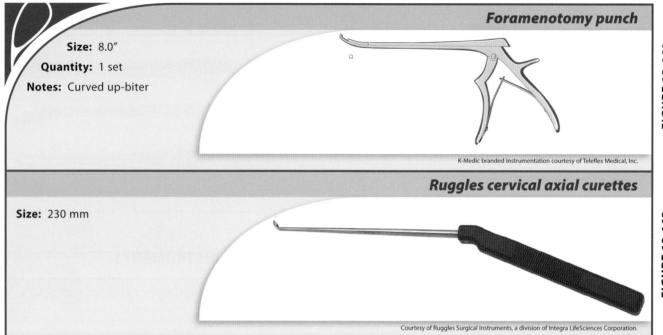

Foramenotomy punch

Size: 8.0″

Quantity: 1 set

Notes: Curved up-biter

K-Medic branded instrumentation courtesy of Teleflex Medical, Inc.

FIGURE 12-161

Ruggles cervical axial curettes

Size: 230 mm

Courtesy of Ruggles Surgical Instruments, a division of Integra LifeSciences Corporation.

FIGURE 12-162

Cervical Spine Instrumentation – PROBES AND DILATORS

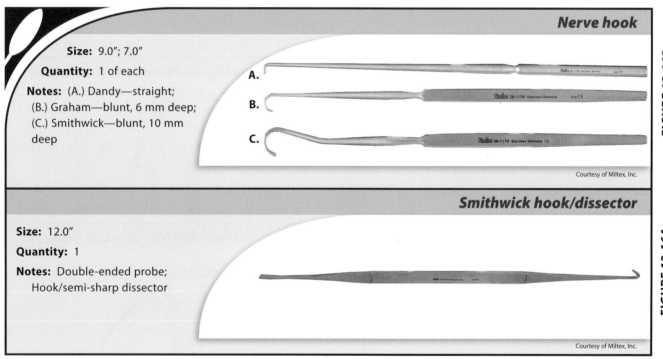

Nerve hook

Size: 9.0″; 7.0″

Quantity: 1 of each

Notes: (A.) Dandy—straight;
(B.) Graham—blunt, 6 mm deep;
(C.) Smithwick—blunt, 10 mm
deep

A.

B.

C.

Courtesy of Miltex, Inc.

FIGURE 12-163

Smithwick hook/dissector

Size: 12.0″

Quantity: 1

Notes: Double-ended probe;
Hook/semi-sharp dissector

Courtesy of Miltex, Inc.

FIGURE 12-164

Cervical Spine Instrumentation – RETRACTION AND EXPOSURE INSTRUMENTS

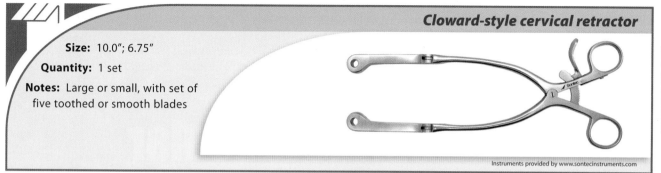

Cloward-style cervical retractor

Size: 10.0"; 6.75"

Quantity: 1 set

Notes: Large or small, with set of five toothed or smooth blades

Instruments provided by www.sontecinstruments.com

FIGURE 12-165

Cervical Spine Instrumentation – SPECIALTY SPECIFIC INSTRUMENTS

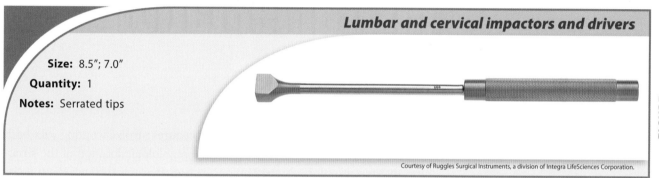

Lumbar and cervical impactors and drivers

Size: 8.5"; 7.0"

Quantity: 1

Notes: Serrated tips

Courtesy of Ruggles Surgical Instruments, a division of Integra LifeSciences Corporation.

FIGURE 12-166

SUMMARY

Neurologic surgical procedures can involve all types of tissues. Procedures may involve very delicate instrumentation used under a microscope or heavy instrumentation used to debulk bone.

Regardless of the type of surrounding tissue involved with the surgical procedure, consideration must be given to the focus of the dissection—the nerves and nervous tissue. Nervous tissue is very delicate and easily injured by inadvertent pressure or forceful displacement with retractors. Regeneration, or healing of injured nervous tissue, is not consistent and may result in permanent damage not only to the nerve itself, but to structures innervated distally, such as blood vessels and muscles.

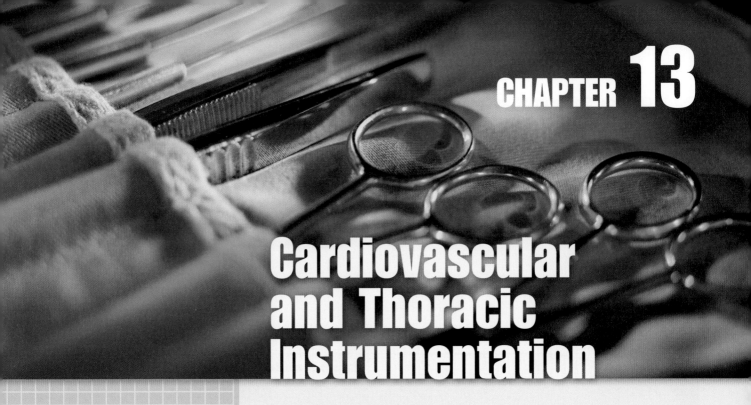

CHAPTER 13

Cardiovascular and Thoracic Instrumentation

INTRODUCTION

Cardiac, vascular, and thoracic surgical procedures involve working with both soft and compact tissues depending on the physiologic location of the structures that require surgical intervention. Incisional access through the soft tissues of skin is accomplished by the use of one of the foundation sets depending on the depth of the target tissues. After the skin and outer tissues are incised the main part of the procedure will require additional instrumentation.

CARDIOVASCULAR INSTRUMENTATION

Most cardiovascular procedures are performed using similar instruments of varying lengths and weight. Some of the instrumentation has unusual curves, angles, or jaws designated right or left. Some of the curves are designed to fit the circumference of the vessel. The size and weight of the vascular instruments will be determined according to the texture and condition of the tissues. Some clamps will have jaw covers, referred to as *shods,* to cushion the hold and prevent slippage. Small segments of tubular silicone referred to as *suture boots* can be slipped onto the jaws of tiny hemostats for snug traction when holding suture. Clamps such as the Fogarty style have small holes along the jaws for snapping on special jaw liners. Shods, suture boots, and jaw liners are counted items and are closely contained.

If the facility does not have shods or suture boots on hand, the scrub person can fashion shods for the jaws of clamps from sterile Robinson red rubber catheters sized 10 fr to 16 fr and suture boots from 3 fr to 5 fr infant feeding tubes. IV tubing is not used because only the inner lumen is sterile and the exterior is not. The size is selected according to the clamp jaw width. The scrub person cuts the tubing on the sterile field and reports the number of cut segments to the circulator for addition to the surgical counts. The wide connecting ends are discarded. Care is taken to determine if the patient is latex sensitive before selecting tubing to cut on the field.

Cardiovascular Instrumentation – CLAMPS

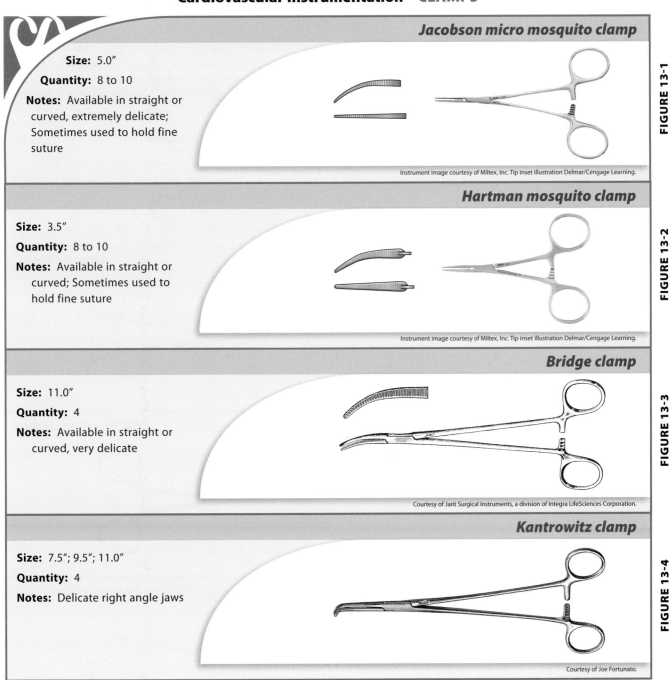

Jacobson micro mosquito clamp

Size: 5.0"

Quantity: 8 to 10

Notes: Available in straight or curved, extremely delicate; Sometimes used to hold fine suture

Instrument image courtesy of Miltex, Inc. Tip inset illustration Delmar/Cengage Learning.

FIGURE 13-1

Hartman mosquito clamp

Size: 3.5"

Quantity: 8 to 10

Notes: Available in straight or curved; Sometimes used to hold fine suture

Instrument image courtesy of Miltex, Inc. Tip inset illustration Delmar/Cengage Learning.

FIGURE 13-2

Bridge clamp

Size: 11.0"

Quantity: 4

Notes: Available in straight or curved, very delicate

Courtesy of Jarit Surgical Instruments, a division of Integra LifeSciences Corporation.

FIGURE 13-3

Kantrowitz clamp

Size: 7.5"; 9.5"; 11.0"

Quantity: 4

Notes: Delicate right angle jaws

Courtesy of Joe Fortunato.

FIGURE 13-4

continues

Cardiovascular Instrumentation – CLAMPS *continued*

Finochietto clamp

Size: 9.0″

Quantity: 4

Notes: Slightly curved jaws

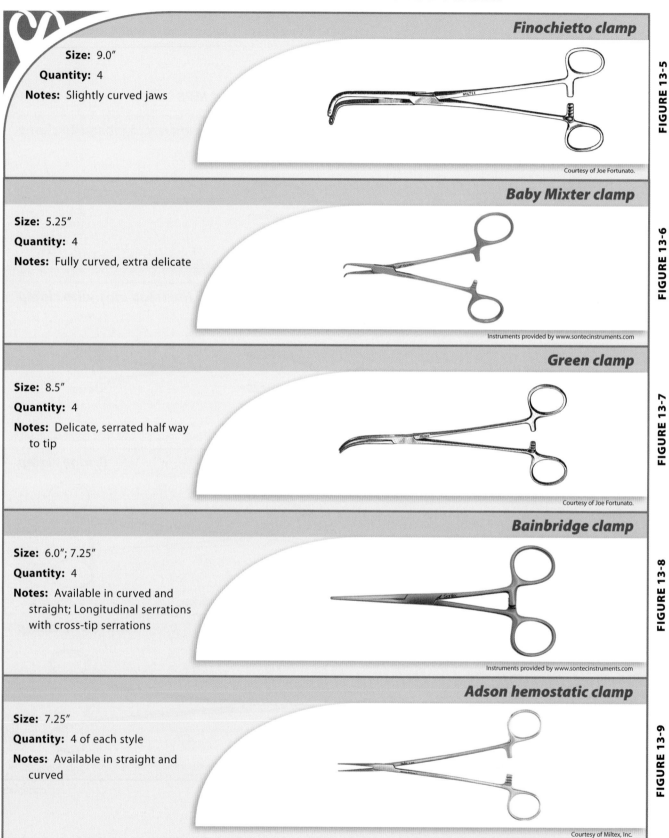

Courtesy of Joe Fortunato.

FIGURE 13-5

Baby Mixter clamp

Size: 5.25″

Quantity: 4

Notes: Fully curved, extra delicate

Instruments provided by www.sontecinstruments.com

FIGURE 13-6

Green clamp

Size: 8.5″

Quantity: 4

Notes: Delicate, serrated half way to tip

Courtesy of Joe Fortunato.

FIGURE 13-7

Bainbridge clamp

Size: 6.0″; 7.25″

Quantity: 4

Notes: Available in curved and straight; Longitudinal serrations with cross-tip serrations

Instruments provided by www.sontecinstruments.com

FIGURE 13-8

Adson hemostatic clamp

Size: 7.25″

Quantity: 4 of each style

Notes: Available in straight and curved

Courtesy of Miltex, Inc.

FIGURE 13-9

Cardiovascular Instrumentation – CLAMPS *continued*

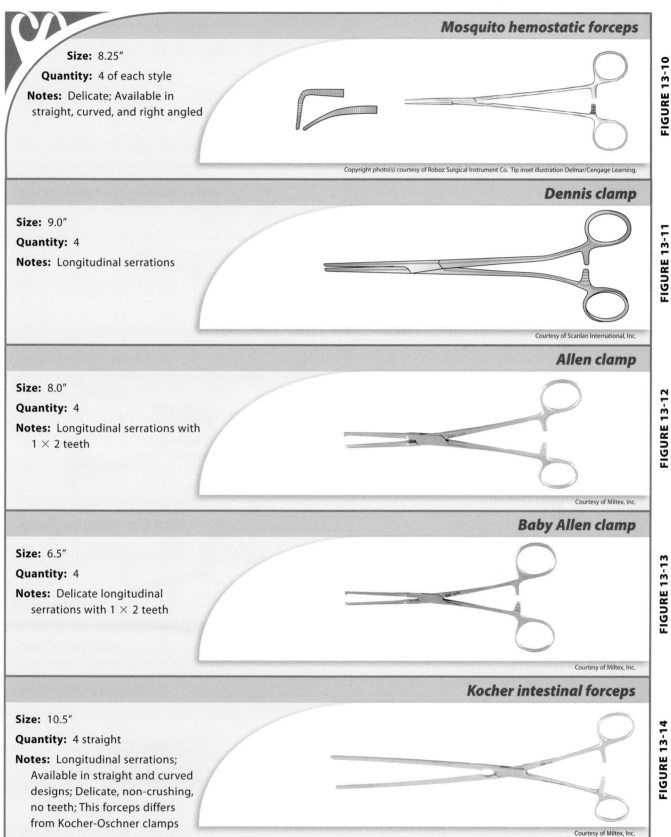

Mosquito hemostatic forceps

Size: 8.25"

Quantity: 4 of each style

Notes: Delicate; Available in straight, curved, and right angled

Copyright photo(s) courtesy of Roboz Surgical Instrument Co. Tip inset illustration Delmar/Cengage Learning.

FIGURE 13-10

Dennis clamp

Size: 9.0"

Quantity: 4

Notes: Longitudinal serrations

Courtesy of Scanlan International, Inc.

FIGURE 13-11

Allen clamp

Size: 8.0"

Quantity: 4

Notes: Longitudinal serrations with 1 × 2 teeth

Courtesy of Miltex, Inc.

FIGURE 13-12

Baby Allen clamp

Size: 6.5"

Quantity: 4

Notes: Delicate longitudinal serrations with 1 × 2 teeth

Courtesy of Miltex, Inc.

FIGURE 13-13

Kocher intestinal forceps

Size: 10.5"

Quantity: 4 straight

Notes: Longitudinal serrations; Available in straight and curved designs; Delicate, non-crushing, no teeth; This forceps differs from Kocher-Oschner clamps

Courtesy of Miltex, Inc.

FIGURE 13-14

continues

Cardiovascular Instrumentation – CLAMPS *continued*

Gemini-Mixter forceps

Size: 5.25″

Quantity: 4

Notes: Delicate, fully curved jaws

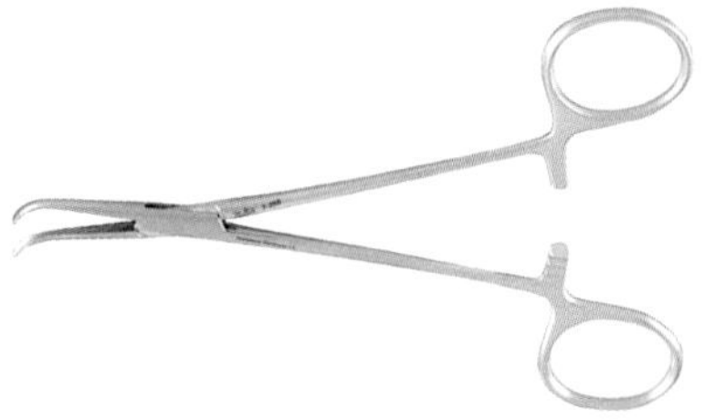

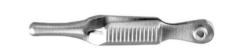

Courtesy of Miltex, Inc.

FIGURE 13-15

Johns Hopkins bulldog clamp

Size: 1.25″; 2.0″; 2.5″; 3.0″; 3.5″

Quantity: Assorted sizes

Notes: Available in straight or curved designs

Courtesy of Miltex, Inc.

FIGURE 13-16

Glover bulldog clamps

Size: 7.0″; 8.0″; 9.0″; 11.0″

Quantity: Assorted sizes

Notes: Spring tension adjusting screw; Available in straight or curved designs

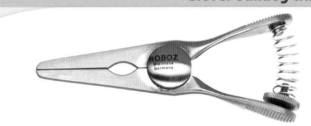

Copyright photo(s) courtesy of Roboz Surgical Instrument Co.

FIGURE 13-17

DeBakey bulldog clamp

Size: 7.5″; 8.5″; 10.5″; 12.0″

Quantity: Assorted sizes

Notes: Cross action; Available in straight or curved designs

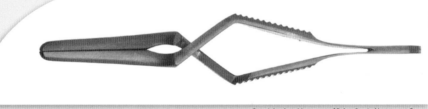

Copyright photo(s) courtesy of Roboz Surgical Instrument Co.

FIGURE 13-18

Dieffenbach serrefine

Size: 2.25″

Quantity: 4

Notes: Available in straight or curved designs

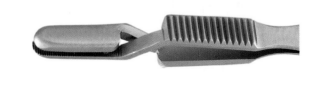

Copyright photo(s) courtesy of Roboz Surgical Instrument Co.

FIGURE 13-19

Cardiovascular Instrumentation – CLAMPS *continued*

Dietrich micro bulldog clamp

Size: 1.88"; 1.75"

Quantity: 4

Notes: Straight or angled jaws with 8 × 1.2 mm

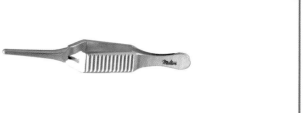

Courtesy of Miltex, Inc.

FIGURE 13-20

DeBakey ring-handled bulldog clamp

Size: 5.0"; 4.75"; 4.0"; 4.88"; 4.75"

Quantity: 1 of each

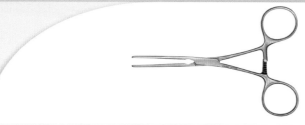

Copyright photo(s) courtesy of Roboz Surgical Instrument Co.

FIGURE 13-21

Lee right angle bronchus and general purpose vascular clamp

Size: 9.0"

Quantity: 2

Notes: Used for vascular and thoracic applications

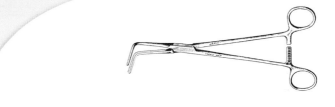

Courtesy of Jarit Surgical Instruments, a division of Integra LifeSciences Corporation.

FIGURE 13-22

Glover patent ductus clamp

Size: 8.0"

Quantity: 2

Notes: 3 cm jaws; Available in straight or angular

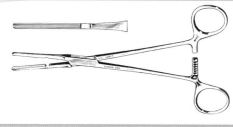

Courtesy of Jarit Surgical Instruments, a division of Integra LifeSciences Corporation.

FIGURE 13-23

DeBakey vascular clamp for aortic aneurism

Size: 10.0"; 10.5"; 12.25"; 12.75"

Quantity: 4

Notes: Slightly curved jaws and strongly curved jaws

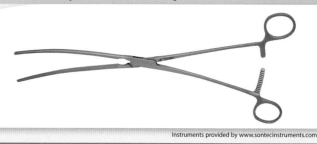

Instruments provided by www.sontecinstruments.com

FIGURE 13-24

continues

Cardiovascular Instrumentation – CLAMPS *continued*

DeBakey multipurpose clamps

Size: A. 9.5"; 8.25"; 9.5"; 12.0"
B. 9.0"; 8.0"; 10.5"

Quantity: 2 of each size

Notes: (A.) Obtuse angle 60-degree;
(B.) Right angle 90-degree

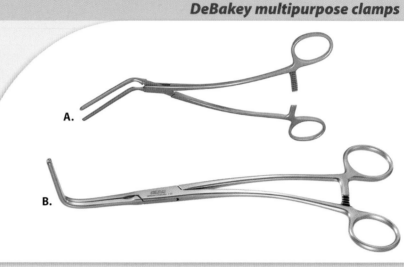

FIGURE 13-25

DeBakey tangential occlusion clamp

Size: 8.0"; 10.0"; 10.25"; 10.5"; 11.0"

Quantity: 2 each of at least three sizes

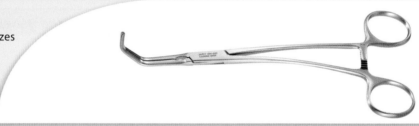

FIGURE 13-26

Satinsky-DeBakey vascular clamp for vena cava

Size: 9.75"

Quantity: 2

Notes: Available in small, medium,
and large

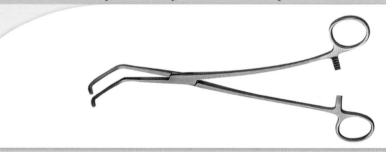

FIGURE 13-27

Cooley pediatric vascular clamp for anastomosis

Size: 6.5"

Quantity: 2

Notes: 5 mm graduations on jaws

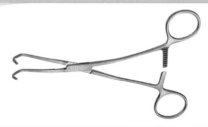

FIGURE 13-28

Cardiovascular Instrumentation – CLAMPS *continued*

DeBakey pediatric multipurpose clamp

Size: 6.5"; 6.0"; 5.5"

Quantity: 2 of each size and angle

Notes: Available in 30-degree, 60-degree, and 90-degree angles

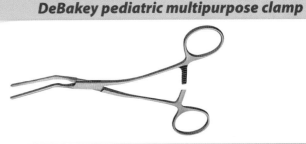

FIGURE 13-29

DeBakey-Derra vascular clamp for anastomosis

Size: 6.25"; 6.75"; 7.0"

Quantity: 2 of each

Notes: Available with small, medium, or large jaws

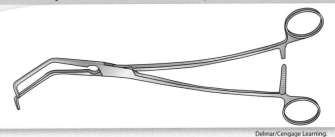

FIGURE 13-30

Cooley pediatric vascular clamps

Size: 5.5"

Quantity: 2 of each

Notes: Jaws 25 mm; Straight or angled jaws; Straight or angled handles

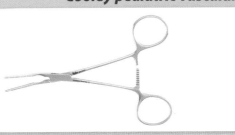

FIGURE 13-31

Cooley clamps pediatric vascular clamps

Size: 4.75"

Quantity: 2 of each

Notes: 5 mm calibrations on outer sides of jaws; Right angle, straight handles

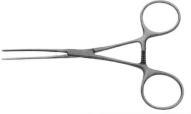

FIGURE 13-32

Cooley-Satinsky clamp

Size: 5.5"

Quantity: 2

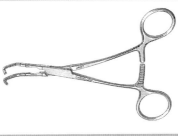

FIGURE 13-33

continues

Cardiovascular Instrumentation – CLAMPS *continued*

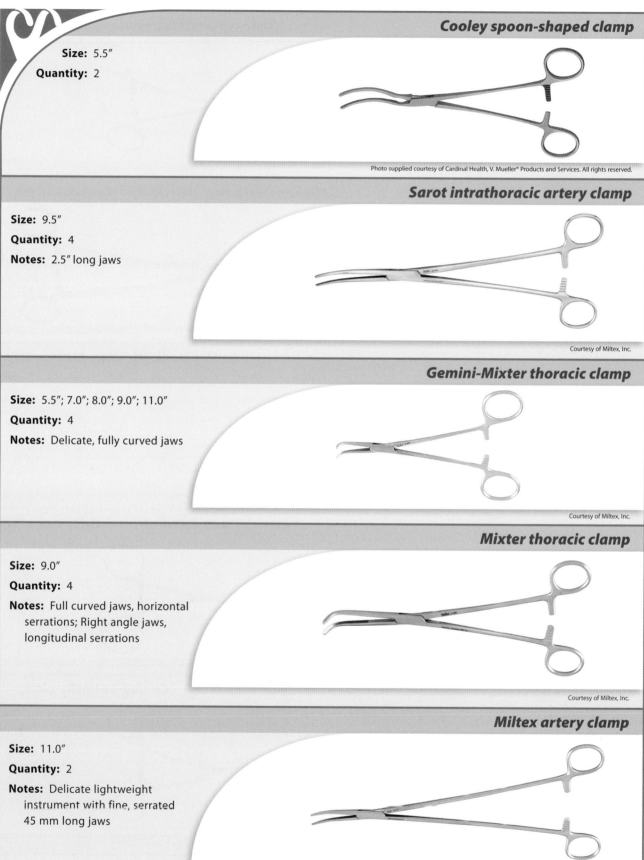

Cooley spoon-shaped clamp

Size: 5.5"

Quantity: 2

FIGURE 13-34

Sarot intrathoracic artery clamp

Size: 9.5"

Quantity: 4

Notes: 2.5" long jaws

FIGURE 13-35

Gemini-Mixter thoracic clamp

Size: 5.5"; 7.0"; 8.0"; 9.0"; 11.0"

Quantity: 4

Notes: Delicate, fully curved jaws

FIGURE 13-36

Mixter thoracic clamp

Size: 9.0"

Quantity: 4

Notes: Full curved jaws, horizontal serrations; Right angle jaws, longitudinal serrations

FIGURE 13-37

Miltex artery clamp

Size: 11.0"

Quantity: 2

Notes: Delicate lightweight instrument with fine, serrated 45 mm long jaws

FIGURE 13-38

Cardiovascular Instrumentation – CLAMPS *continued*

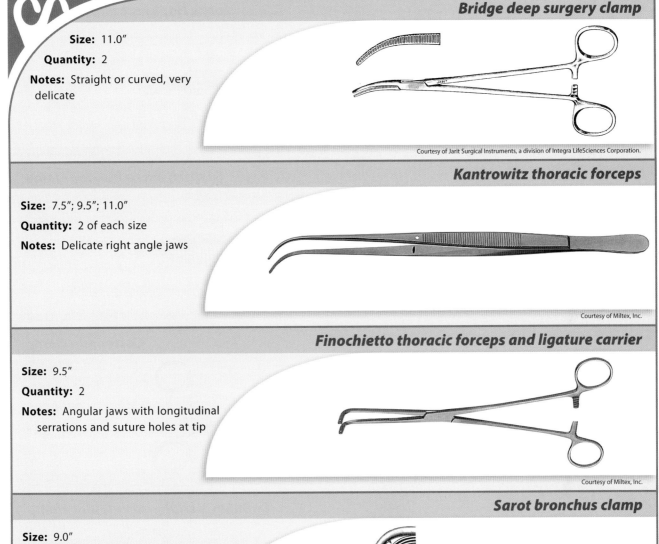

Bridge deep surgery clamp

Size: 11.0"

Quantity: 2

Notes: Straight or curved, very delicate

Courtesy of Jarit Surgical Instruments, a division of Integra LifeSciences Corporation.

FIGURE 13-39

Kantrowitz thoracic forceps

Size: 7.5"; 9.5"; 11.0"

Quantity: 2 of each size

Notes: Delicate right angle jaws

Courtesy of Miltex, Inc.

FIGURE 13-40

Finochietto thoracic forceps and ligature carrier

Size: 9.5"

Quantity: 2

Notes: Angular jaws with longitudinal serrations and suture holes at tip

Courtesy of Miltex, Inc.

FIGURE 13-41

Sarot bronchus clamp

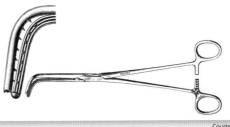

Size: 9.0"

Quantity: 2

Notes: Left and right clamps with interdigitating teeth full length of 35 mm jaws

Courtesy of Joe Fortunato.

FIGURE 13-42

Crawford coarctation clamp

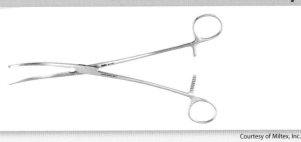

Size: 9.5"

Quantity: 2

Notes: Slightly curved jaws 65 mm with longitudinal serrations

Courtesy of Miltex, Inc.

FIGURE 13-43

continues

Cardiovascular Instrumentation – CLAMPS *continued*

Johns Hopkins bulldog clamps

Size: 1.5"; 2.0"; 2.5"; 3.0"; 3.5"

Quantity: Assorted sizes, 2 of each

Notes: Available straight or curved

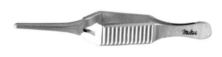

Courtesy of Miltex, Inc.

FIGURE 13-44

Dietrich micro bulldog clamp

Size: 1.88"

Quantity: 1 of each size

Notes: Straight or angled jaws,
8 × 1.2 mm

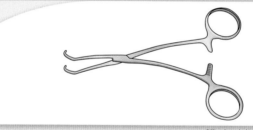

Courtesy of Miltex, Inc.

FIGURE 13-45

Castaneda clamp

Size: 6.0"

Quantity: 4

Notes: Long, slightly curved
handles, long curved jaw; Used
in neonates

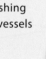

Pilling branded instrumentation courtesy of Teleflex Medical.

FIGURE 13-46

DeBakey peripheral vascular clamp

Size: 7.25"

Quantity: 2

Notes: Occluding noncrushing
clamps used on larger vessels

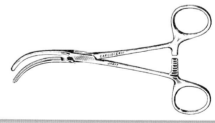

Courtesy of Jarit Surgical Instruments, a division of Integra LifeSciences Corporation.

FIGURE 13-47

Cleveland Clinic baby renal clamp

Size: 5.75"

Quantity: 2 right; 2 left

Notes: Delicate DeBakey style
clamps with right angle jaws;
Available in right or left angles

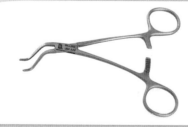

Pilling branded instrumentation courtesy of Teleflex Medical.

FIGURE 13-48

Cardiovascular Instrumentation – CLAMPS *continued*

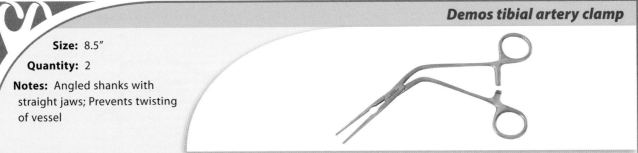

Demos tibial artery clamp

Size: 8.5"

Quantity: 2

Notes: Angled shanks with straight jaws; Prevents twisting of vessel

Pilling branded instrumentation courtesy of Teleflex Medical.

FIGURE 13-49

Cooley vascular clamp

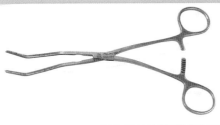

Size: 7.25"; 11.75"; 8.5"

Quantity: 4

Notes: Long, slender clamp; Curved shafts, angled jaws; Available in vessel, renal, iliac, curved, down angle

Pilling branded instrumentation courtesy of Teleflex Medical.

FIGURE 13-50

Gerbode patent ductus clamp

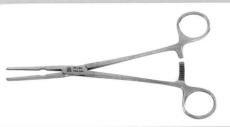

Size: 8.0"

Quantity: 2

Notes: Long straight jaw with open crest at box lock

Pilling branded instrumentation courtesy of Teleflex Medical.

FIGURE 13-51

Hufnagel clamp

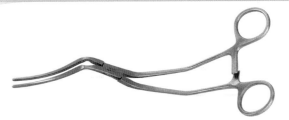

Size: 9.5"

Quantity: 2

Notes: Used for grasping and occluding the ascending aorta; Angled shanks with down angled jaws

Pilling branded instrumentation courtesy of Teleflex Medical.

FIGURE 13-52

Crawford coarctation clamp

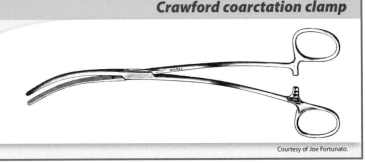

Size: 8.0"; 13.0"

Quantity: 2 of each

Notes: Angled shanks and curved jaws with longitudinal serrations full length of jaw

Courtesy of Joe Fortunato.

FIGURE 13-53

continues

Cardiovascular Instrumentation – CLAMPS *continued*

Stoney aortic clamp

Size: 6.88"; 9.0"

Quantity: 2

Notes: Sharp angled jaws

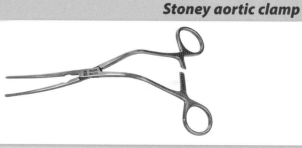

Pilling branded instrumentation courtesy of Teleflex Medical.

FIGURE 13-54

Grant aortic aneurysm clamp

Size: 10.5"; 9.25"

Quantity: 2

Notes: Multi-angled shanks and jaws; Used for the aorta of thin patients; Also referred to as "Texas twister"

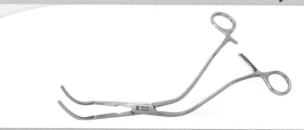

Pilling branded instrumentation courtesy of Teleflex Medical.

FIGURE 13-55

Lambert abdominal aorta clamp

Size: 8.75"

Quantity: 2

Notes: Handles angled upward

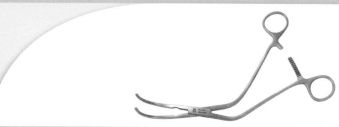

Pilling branded instrumentation courtesy of Teleflex Medical.

FIGURE 13-56

Strong aorta clamps

Size: 8.0"

Quantity: 2

Notes: Down-angled shanks with up-curved platform jaws

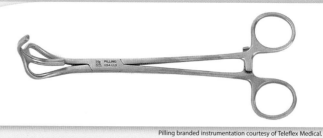

Pilling branded instrumentation courtesy of Teleflex Medical.

FIGURE 13-57

Cardiovascular Instrumentation – GRASPING FORCEPS

DeBakey thoracic tissue forceps

Size: 6.0"; 7.5"; 9.5"; 12.0"

Quantity: 2 of each size

Notes: Lightweight forceps; 2.5 mm wide tips

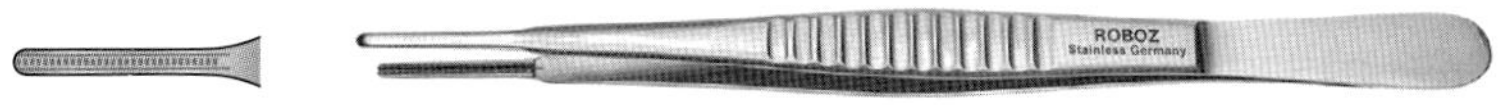

Copyright photo(s) courtesy of Roboz Surgical Instrument Co. Tip inset illustration Delmar/Cengage Learning.

FIGURE 13-58

DeBakey vascular tissue forceps

Size: 6.0"; 7.5"; 7.75"; 9.5"

Quantity: 2 of each size

Notes: 1.5 mm wide tips; Available in lightweight fenestrated handle design

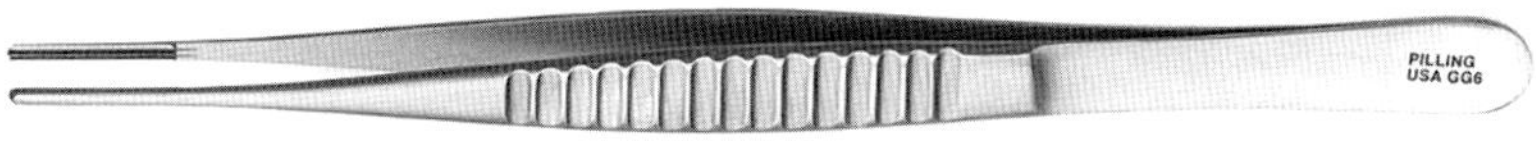

Pilling branded instrumentation courtesy of Teleflex Medical.

FIGURE 13-59

Cooley vascular tissue forceps

Size: 6.0"; 8.0"

Quantity: 2

Notes: Tips 2 mm wide

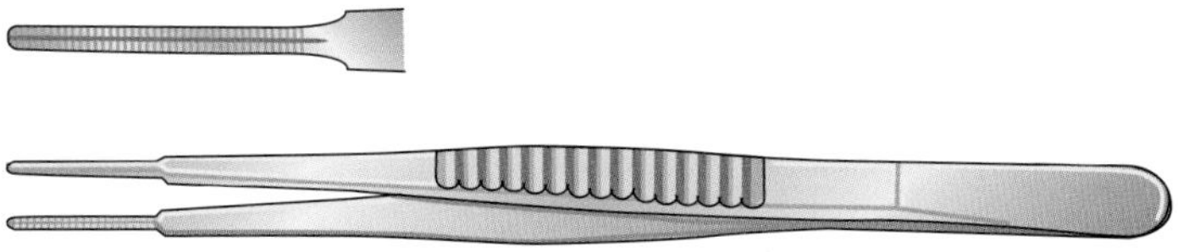

Delmar/Cengage Learning.

FIGURE 13-60

Kelly tissue forceps

Size: 9.0"

Quantity: 2

Notes: Slotted Gutch handle; Available with 1 × 2 teeth, 2 × 3 teeth, or 3 × 4 teeth

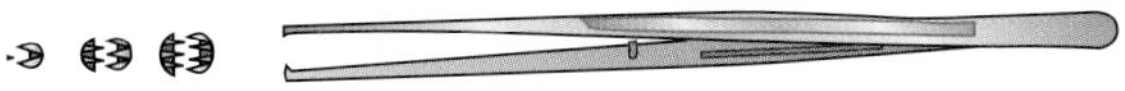

Delmar/Cengage Learning.

FIGURE 13-61

Mayo-Russian tissue forceps

Size: 9.0"

Quantity: 2

Notes: Fenestrated jaws, slotted groove handles

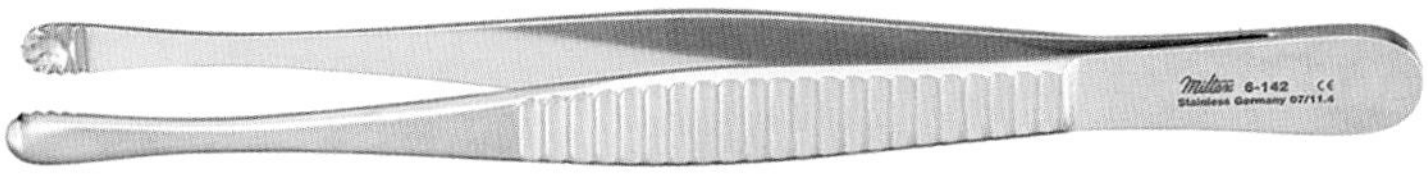

Courtesy of Miltrex, Inc.

FIGURE 13-62

continues

Cardiovascular Instrumentation – GRASPING FORCEPS *continued*

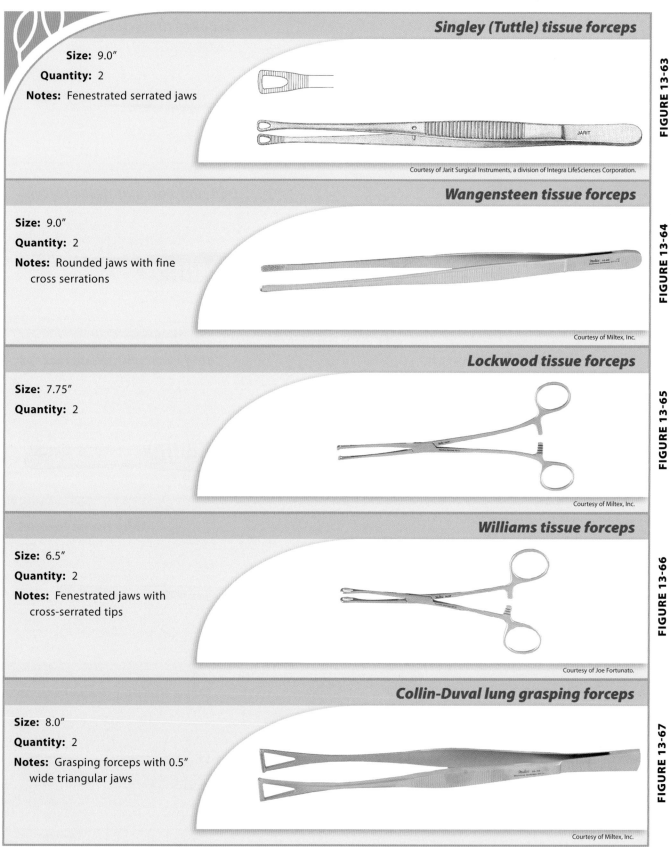

Singley (Tuttle) tissue forceps

Size: 9.0″

Quantity: 2

Notes: Fenestrated serrated jaws

Courtesy of Jarit Surgical Instruments, a division of Integra LifeSciences Corporation.

FIGURE 13-63

Wangensteen tissue forceps

Size: 9.0″

Quantity: 2

Notes: Rounded jaws with fine cross serrations

Courtesy of Miltex, Inc.

FIGURE 13-64

Lockwood tissue forceps

Size: 7.75″

Quantity: 2

Courtesy of Miltex, Inc.

FIGURE 13-65

Williams tissue forceps

Size: 6.5″

Quantity: 2

Notes: Fenestrated jaws with cross-serrated tips

Courtesy of Joe Fortunato.

FIGURE 13-66

Collin-Duval lung grasping forceps

Size: 8.0″

Quantity: 2

Notes: Grasping forceps with 0.5″ wide triangular jaws

Courtesy of Miltex, Inc.

FIGURE 13-67

Cardiovascular Instrumentation – GRASPING FORCEPS *continued*

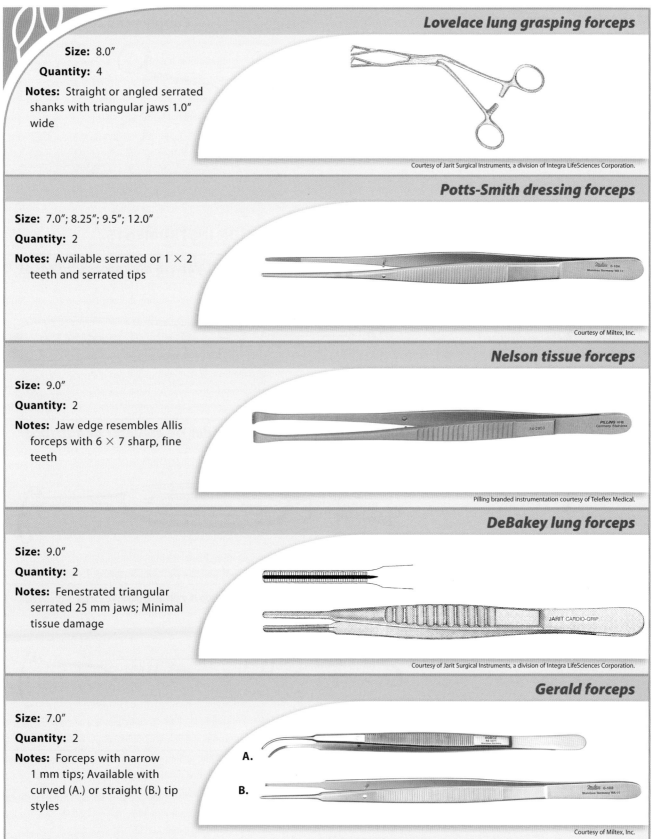

Lovelace lung grasping forceps

Size: 8.0"

Quantity: 4

Notes: Straight or angled serrated shanks with triangular jaws 1.0" wide

Courtesy of Jarit Surgical Instruments, a division of Integra LifeSciences Corporation.

FIGURE 13-68

Potts-Smith dressing forceps

Size: 7.0"; 8.25"; 9.5"; 12.0"

Quantity: 2

Notes: Available serrated or 1 × 2 teeth and serrated tips

Courtesy of Miltex, Inc.

FIGURE 13-69

Nelson tissue forceps

Size: 9.0"

Quantity: 2

Notes: Jaw edge resembles Allis forceps with 6 × 7 sharp, fine teeth

Pilling branded instrumentation courtesy of Teleflex Medical.

FIGURE 13-70

DeBakey lung forceps

Size: 9.0"

Quantity: 2

Notes: Fenestrated triangular serrated 25 mm jaws; Minimal tissue damage

Courtesy of Jarit Surgical Instruments, a division of Integra LifeSciences Corporation.

FIGURE 13-71

Gerald forceps

Size: 7.0"

Quantity: 2

Notes: Forceps with narrow 1 mm tips; Available with curved (A.) or straight (B.) tip styles

A.

B.

Courtesy of Miltex, Inc.

FIGURE 13-72

continues

Cardiovascular Instrumentation – GRASPING FORCEPS *continued*

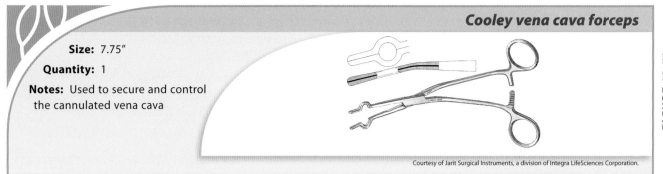

Cooley vena cava forceps

Size: 7.75″

Quantity: 1

Notes: Used to secure and control the cannulated vena cava

Courtesy of Jarit Surgical Instruments, a division of Integra LifeSciences Corporation.

FIGURE 13-73

Cardiovascular Instrumentation – DISSECTION INSTRUMENTS

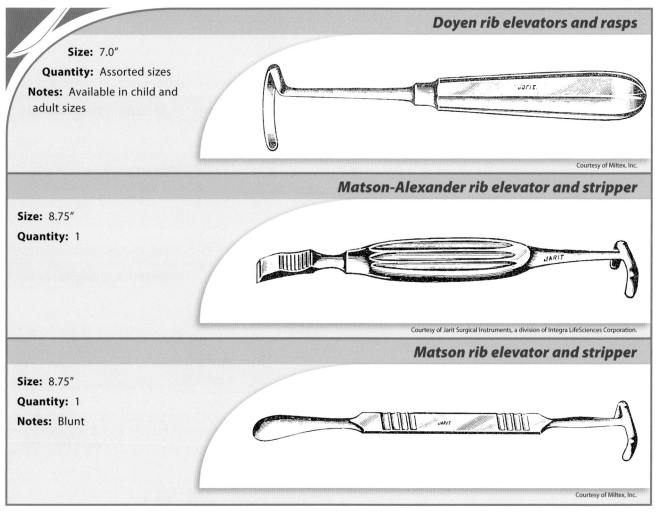

Doyen rib elevators and rasps

Size: 7.0″

Quantity: Assorted sizes

Notes: Available in child and adult sizes

Courtesy of Miltex, Inc.

FIGURE 13-74

Matson-Alexander rib elevator and stripper

Size: 8.75″

Quantity: 1

Courtesy of Jarit Surgical Instruments, a division of Integra LifeSciences Corporation.

FIGURE 13-75

Matson rib elevator and stripper

Size: 8.75″

Quantity: 1

Notes: Blunt

Courtesy of Miltex, Inc.

FIGURE 13-76

Cardiovascular Instrumentation – DISSECTION INSTRUMENTS *continued*

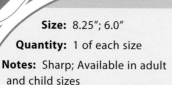

Alexander-Farabeuf periosteotome

Size: 8.25"; 6.0"

Quantity: 1 of each size

Notes: Sharp; Available in adult and child sizes

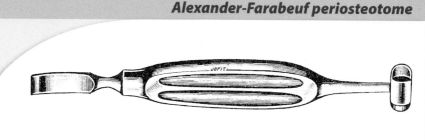

Courtesy of Jarit Surgical Instruments, a division of Integra LifeSciences Corporation.

FIGURE 13-77

Sedillot periosteal elevator

Size: 7.5"

Quantity: 1

Notes: Blade 17 mm wide, blunt

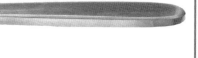

Courtesy of Miltex, Inc.

FIGURE 13-78

Bethune rib shears

Size: 13.75"

Quantity: 1

Notes: Double curved handles

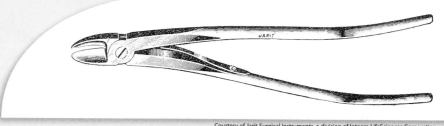

Courtesy of Jarit Surgical Instruments, a division of Integra LifeSciences Corporation.

FIGURE 13-79

Gluck rib shears

Size: 8.5"

Quantity: 1

Notes: Used to cut ribs

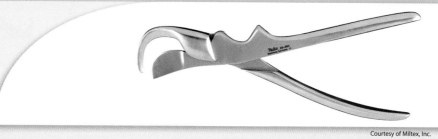

Courtesy of Miltex, Inc.

FIGURE 13-80

Stille pattern rib shears

Size: 8.5"

Quantity: 1

Notes: Used to cut ribs

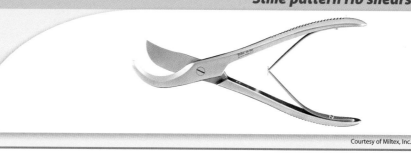

Courtesy of Miltex, Inc.

FIGURE 13-81

continues

Cardiovascular Instrumentation – DISSECTION INSTRUMENTS *continued*

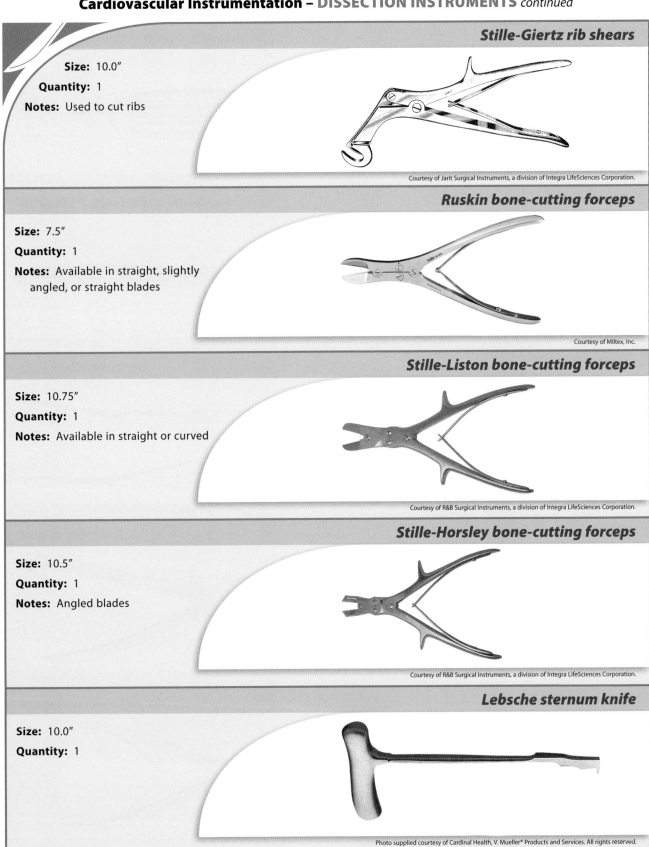

Stille-Giertz rib shears

Size: 10.0"

Quantity: 1

Notes: Used to cut ribs

Courtesy of Jarit Surgical Instruments, a division of Integra LifeSciences Corporation.

FIGURE 13-82

Ruskin bone-cutting forceps

Size: 7.5"

Quantity: 1

Notes: Available in straight, slightly angled, or straight blades

Courtesy of Miltex, Inc.

FIGURE 13-83

Stille-Liston bone-cutting forceps

Size: 10.75"

Quantity: 1

Notes: Available in straight or curved

Courtesy of R&B Surgical Instruments, a division of Integra LifeSciences Corporation.

FIGURE 13-84

Stille-Horsley bone-cutting forceps

Size: 10.5"

Quantity: 1

Notes: Angled blades

Courtesy of R&B Surgical Instruments, a division of Integra LifeSciences Corporation.

FIGURE 13-85

Lebsche sternum knife

Size: 10.0"

Quantity: 1

Photo supplied courtesy of Cardinal Health, V. Mueller® Products and Services. All rights reserved.

FIGURE 13-86

Cardiovascular Instrumentation – DISSECTION INSTRUMENTS *continued*

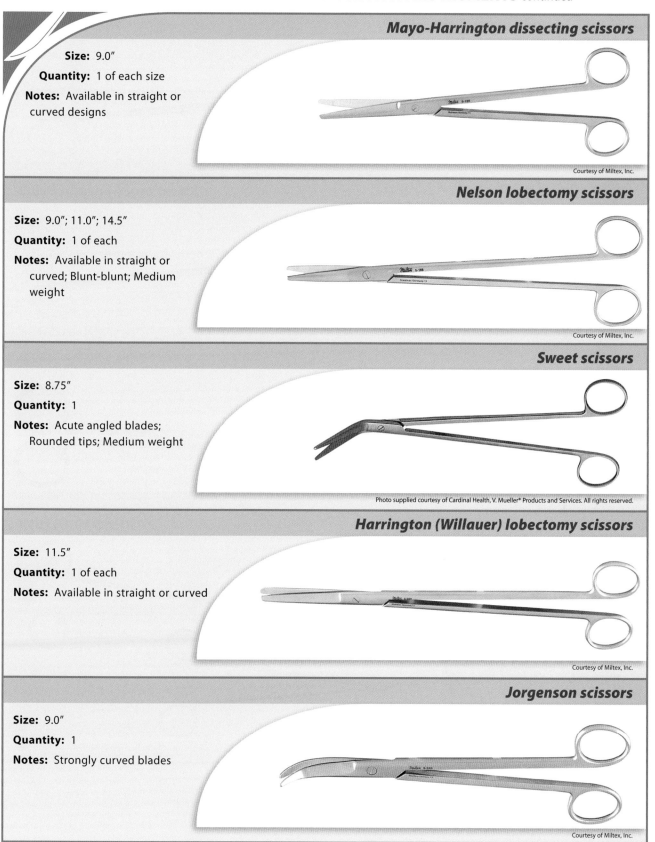

Mayo-Harrington dissecting scissors

Size: 9.0"

Quantity: 1 of each size

Notes: Available in straight or curved designs

Courtesy of Miltex, Inc.

FIGURE 13-87

Nelson lobectomy scissors

Size: 9.0"; 11.0"; 14.5"

Quantity: 1 of each

Notes: Available in straight or curved; Blunt-blunt; Medium weight

Courtesy of Miltex, Inc.

FIGURE 13-88

Sweet scissors

Size: 8.75"

Quantity: 1

Notes: Acute angled blades; Rounded tips; Medium weight

Photo supplied courtesy of Cardinal Health, V. Mueller® Products and Services. All rights reserved.

FIGURE 13-89

Harrington (Willauer) lobectomy scissors

Size: 11.5"

Quantity: 1 of each

Notes: Available in straight or curved

Courtesy of Miltex, Inc.

FIGURE 13-90

Jorgenson scissors

Size: 9.0"

Quantity: 1

Notes: Strongly curved blades

Courtesy of Miltex, Inc.

FIGURE 13-91

continues

Cardiovascular Instrumentation – DISSECTION INSTRUMENTS *continued*

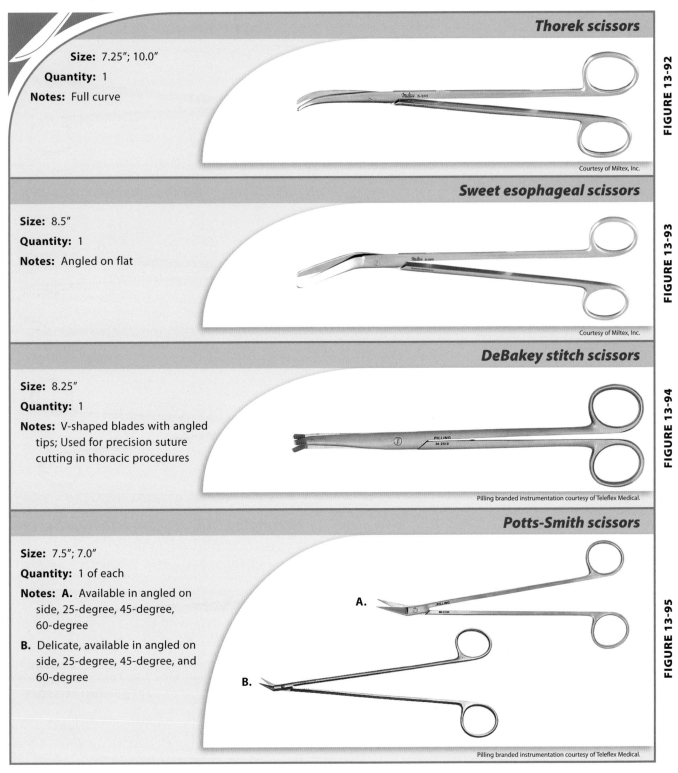

Thorek scissors

Size: 7.25"; 10.0"

Quantity: 1

Notes: Full curve

Courtesy of Miltex, Inc.

FIGURE 13-92

Sweet esophageal scissors

Size: 8.5"

Quantity: 1

Notes: Angled on flat

Courtesy of Miltex, Inc.

FIGURE 13-93

DeBakey stitch scissors

Size: 8.25"

Quantity: 1

Notes: V-shaped blades with angled tips; Used for precision suture cutting in thoracic procedures

Pilling branded instrumentation courtesy of Teleflex Medical.

FIGURE 13-94

Potts-Smith scissors

Size: 7.5"; 7.0"

Quantity: 1 of each

Notes: A. Available in angled on side, 25-degree, 45-degree, 60-degree

B. Delicate, available in angled on side, 25-degree, 45-degree, and 60-degree

Pilling branded instrumentation courtesy of Teleflex Medical.

FIGURE 13-95

Cardiovascular Instrumentation – DISSECTION INSTRUMENTS *continued*

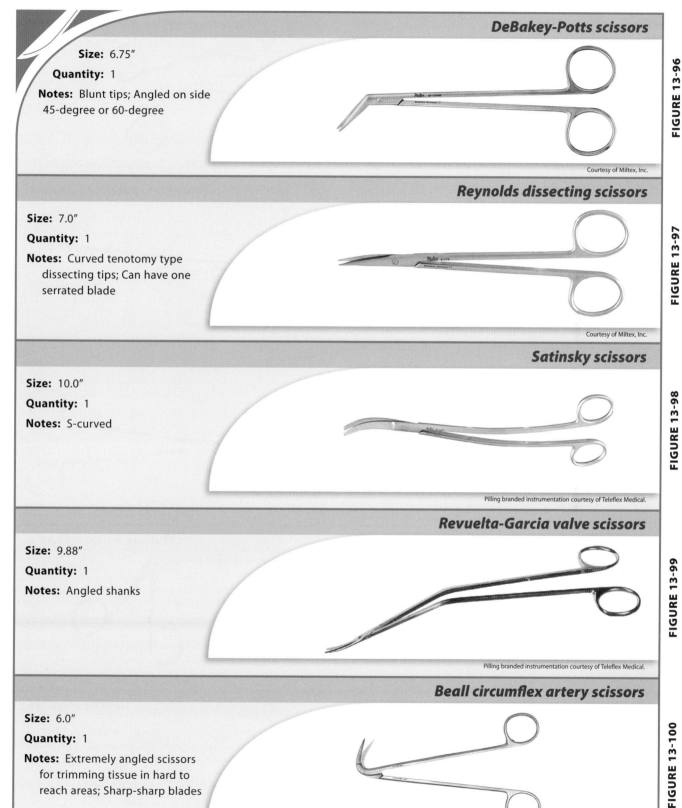

DeBakey-Potts scissors

Size: 6.75"

Quantity: 1

Notes: Blunt tips; Angled on side 45-degree or 60-degree

Courtesy of Miltex, Inc.

FIGURE 13-96

Reynolds dissecting scissors

Size: 7.0"

Quantity: 1

Notes: Curved tenotomy type dissecting tips; Can have one serrated blade

Courtesy of Miltex, Inc.

FIGURE 13-97

Satinsky scissors

Size: 10.0"

Quantity: 1

Notes: S-curved

Pilling branded instrumentation courtesy of Teleflex Medical.

FIGURE 13-98

Revuelta-Garcia valve scissors

Size: 9.88"

Quantity: 1

Notes: Angled shanks

Pilling branded instrumentation courtesy of Teleflex Medical.

FIGURE 13-99

Beall circumflex artery scissors

Size: 6.0"

Quantity: 1

Notes: Extremely angled scissors for trimming tissue in hard to reach areas; Sharp-sharp blades

Pilling branded instrumentation courtesy of Teleflex Medical.

FIGURE 13-100

continues

Cardiovascular Instrumentation – DISSECTION INSTRUMENTS *continued*

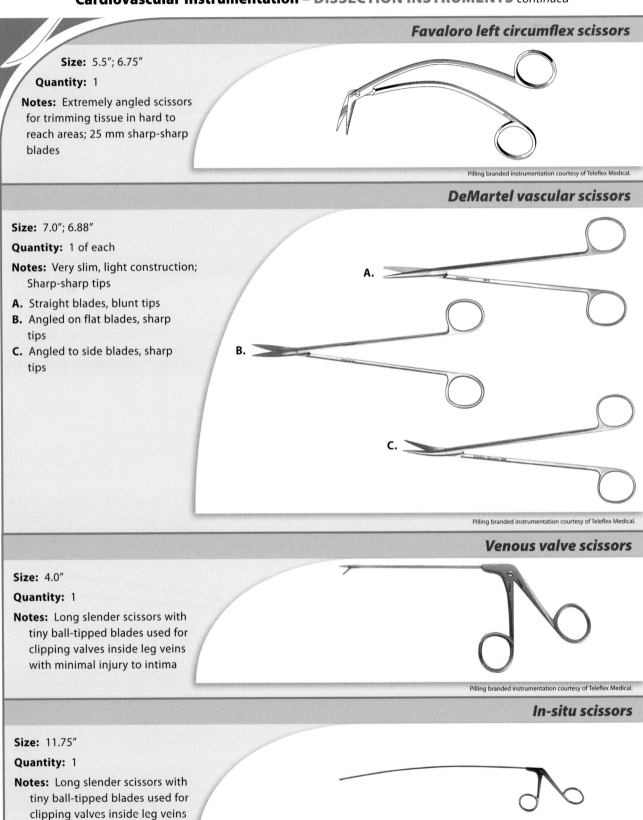

Favaloro left circumflex scissors

Size: 5.5"; 6.75"

Quantity: 1

Notes: Extremely angled scissors for trimming tissue in hard to reach areas; 25 mm sharp-sharp blades

Pilling branded instrumentation courtesy of Teleflex Medical.

FIGURE 13-101

DeMartel vascular scissors

Size: 7.0"; 6.88"

Quantity: 1 of each

Notes: Very slim, light construction; Sharp-sharp tips

A. Straight blades, blunt tips

B. Angled on flat blades, sharp tips

C. Angled to side blades, sharp tips

Pilling branded instrumentation courtesy of Teleflex Medical.

FIGURE 13-102

Venous valve scissors

Size: 4.0"

Quantity: 1

Notes: Long slender scissors with tiny ball-tipped blades used for clipping valves inside leg veins with minimal injury to intima

Pilling branded instrumentation courtesy of Teleflex Medical.

FIGURE 13-103

In-situ scissors

Size: 11.75"

Quantity: 1

Notes: Long slender scissors with tiny ball-tipped blades used for clipping valves inside leg veins with minimal injury to intima

Pilling branded instrumentation courtesy of Teleflex Medical.

FIGURE 13-104

Cardiovascular Instrumentation – DISSECTION INSTRUMENTS *continued*

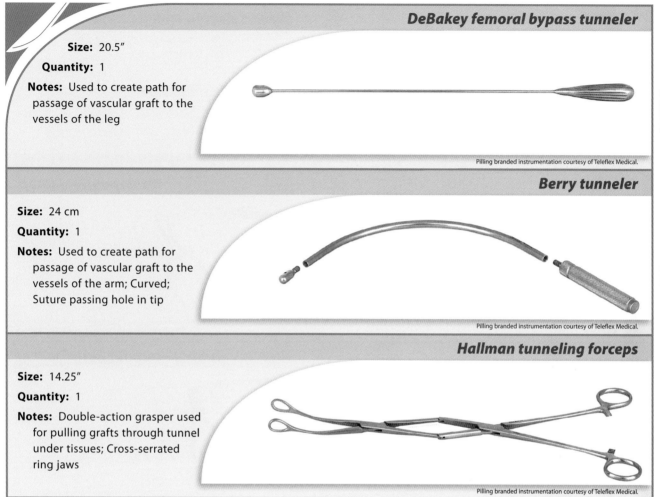

DeBakey femoral bypass tunneler

Size: 20.5″

Quantity: 1

Notes: Used to create path for passage of vascular graft to the vessels of the leg

Pilling branded instrumentation courtesy of Teleflex Medical.

FIGURE 13-105

Berry tunneler

Size: 24 cm

Quantity: 1

Notes: Used to create path for passage of vascular graft to the vessels of the arm; Curved; Suture passing hole in tip

Pilling branded instrumentation courtesy of Teleflex Medical.

FIGURE 13-106

Hallman tunneling forceps

Size: 14.25″

Quantity: 1

Notes: Double-action grasper used for pulling grafts through tunnel under tissues; Cross-serrated ring jaws

Pilling branded instrumentation courtesy of Teleflex Medical.

FIGURE 13-107

Cardiovascular Instrumentation – PROBES AND DILATORS

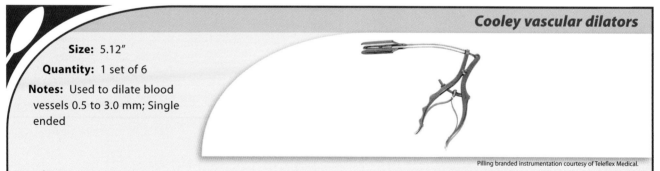

Cooley vascular dilators

Size: 5.12″

Quantity: 1 set of 6

Notes: Used to dilate blood vessels 0.5 to 3.0 mm; Single ended

Pilling branded instrumentation courtesy of Teleflex Medical.

FIGURE 13-108

continues

Cardiovascular Instrumentation – PROBES AND DILATORS *continued*

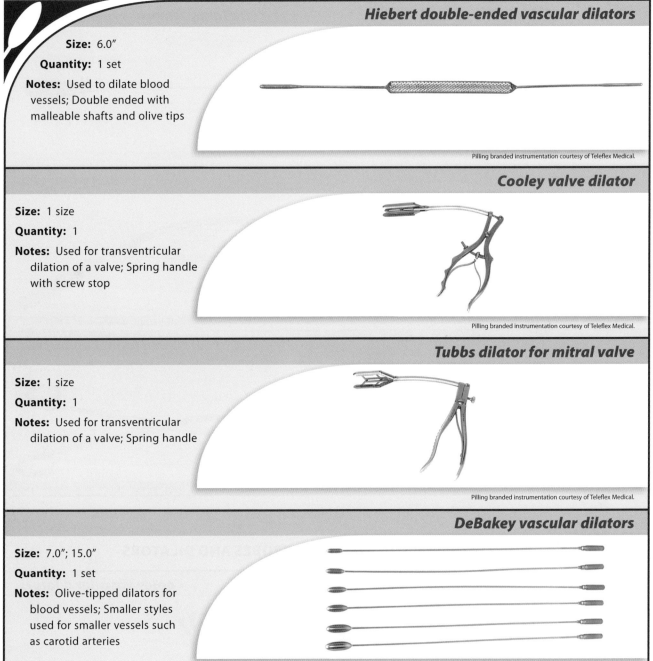

Hiebert double-ended vascular dilators

Size: 6.0″

Quantity: 1 set

Notes: Used to dilate blood vessels; Double ended with malleable shafts and olive tips

Pilling branded instrumentation courtesy of Teleflex Medical.

FIGURE 13-109

Cooley valve dilator

Size: 1 size

Quantity: 1

Notes: Used for transventricular dilation of a valve; Spring handle with screw stop

Pilling branded instrumentation courtesy of Teleflex Medical.

FIGURE 13-110

Tubbs dilator for mitral valve

Size: 1 size

Quantity: 1

Notes: Used for transventricular dilation of a valve; Spring handle

Pilling branded instrumentation courtesy of Teleflex Medical.

FIGURE 13-111

DeBakey vascular dilators

Size: 7.0″; 15.0″

Quantity: 1 set

Notes: Olive-tipped dilators for blood vessels; Smaller styles used for smaller vessels such as carotid arteries

Pilling branded instrumentation courtesy of Teleflex Medical.

FIGURE 13-112

Cardiovascular Instrumentation – EVACUATION AND INSTILLATION INSTRUMENTS

Heparin cannulae with Luer lock

Size: 1.88"; 2.5"; 2.31"; 2.13"; 5.94"; 4.31"; 4.75"; 3.38"; 3.25"

Quantity: 1 of each size

Notes: Applications include peripheral vascular, cardiac, general, orthopedic, urology, and neurosurgery; Used to irrigate, flush, and inject solutions into lumens; Reusable

A. Stoney heparin injector, 1.88" length

B. Zanger heparin cannula, 2.5" length

C. Horsley heparin cannula, 2.31" length

D. DeBakey heparin cannula, malleable, 5.94" length

E. Garrett heparin injector 4.31" length

F. Samson heparin injector, malleable, 3.38" length

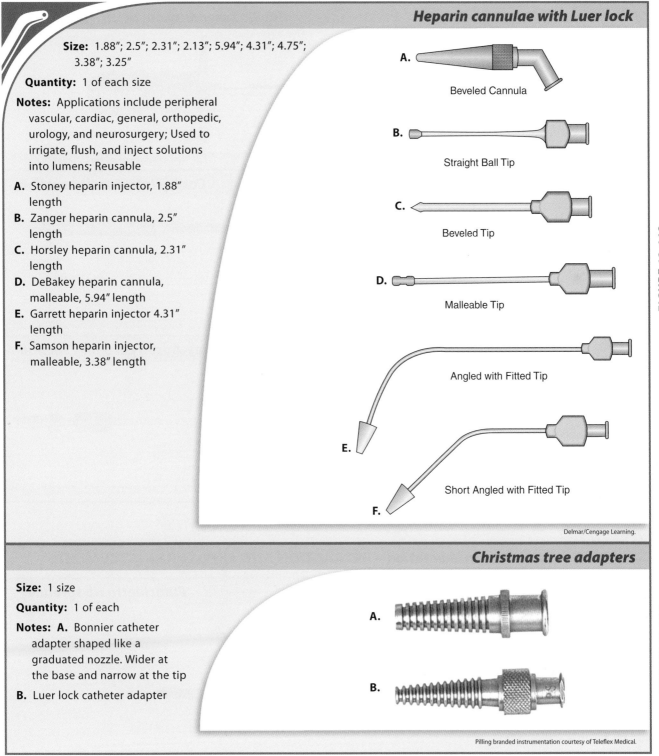

A. Beveled Cannula

B. Straight Ball Tip

C. Beveled Tip

D. Malleable Tip

Angled with Fitted Tip

E.

Short Angled with Fitted Tip

F.

Delmar/Cengage Learning.

FIGURE 13-113

Christmas tree adapters

Size: 1 size

Quantity: 1 of each

Notes: **A.** Bonnier catheter adapter shaped like a graduated nozzle. Wider at the base and narrow at the tip

B. Luer lock catheter adapter

A.

B.

Pilling branded instrumentation courtesy of Teleflex Medical.

FIGURE 13-114

continues

Cardiovascular Instrumentation – EVACUATION AND INSTILLATION INSTRUMENTS *continued*

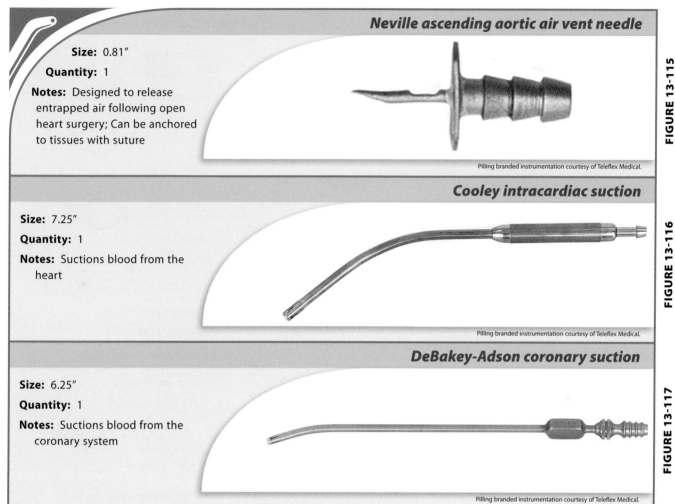

Neville ascending aortic air vent needle

Size: 0.81"

Quantity: 1

Notes: Designed to release entrapped air following open heart surgery; Can be anchored to tissues with suture

Pilling branded instrumentation courtesy of Teleflex Medical.

FIGURE 13-115

Cooley intracardiac suction

Size: 7.25"

Quantity: 1

Notes: Suctions blood from the heart

Pilling branded instrumentation courtesy of Teleflex Medical.

FIGURE 13-116

DeBakey-Adson coronary suction

Size: 6.25"

Quantity: 1

Notes: Suctions blood from the coronary system

Pilling branded instrumentation courtesy of Teleflex Medical.

FIGURE 13-117

Cardiovascular Instrumentation – RETRACTION AND EXPOSURE INSTRUMENTS

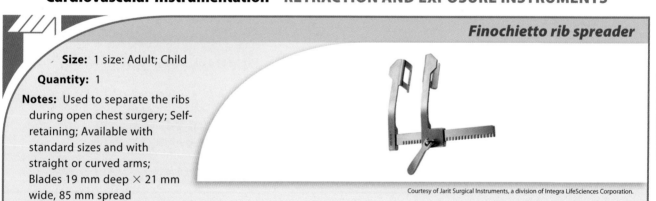

Finochietto rib spreader

Size: 1 size: Adult; Child

Quantity: 1

Notes: Used to separate the ribs during open chest surgery; Self-retaining; Available with standard sizes and with straight or curved arms; Blades 19 mm deep × 21 mm wide, 85 mm spread

Courtesy of Jarit Surgical Instruments, a division of Integra LifeSciences Corporation.

FIGURE 13-118

Cardiovascular Instrumentation – RETRACTION AND EXPOSURE INSTRUMENTS *continued*

Burford-Finochietto rib spreader

Size: 1 size

Quantity: 1 set

Notes: Self-retaining retractor; 8.0", 10.0", or 12.0" spread

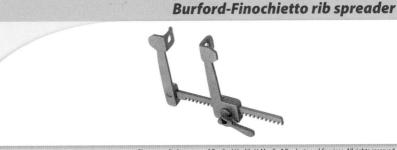

FIGURE 13-119

Harken rib spreaders and scapula retractors

Size: 1 size

Quantity: 1

Notes: 8.0" or 10.0" spread

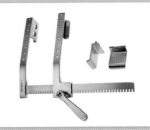

FIGURE 13-120

Tuffier rib spreader

Size: 1 size

Quantity: 1

Notes: 2.0 × 1.75, grooved blades, 6.5" spread

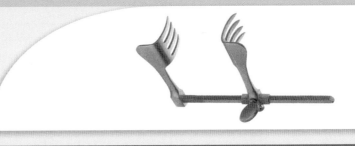

FIGURE 13-121

Israel retractor

Size: 9.0"

Quantity: 2

Notes: Blunt, either 4 or 6 prongs

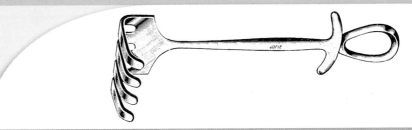

FIGURE 13-122

Allison lung retractor

Size: 12.75"

Quantity: 2

Notes: 2.0" wide blade

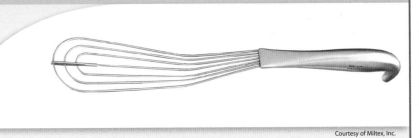

FIGURE 13-123

continues

Cardiovascular Instrumentation – RETRACTION AND EXPOSURE INSTRUMENTS *continued*

Davidson scapula retractor

Size: 8.5"

Quantity: 2

Notes: Blade 3.5" wide and 3.25" deep

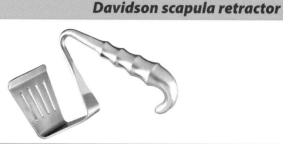

Courtesy of Miltex, Inc.

Favaloro self-retaining retractor

Size: 1 size

Quantity: 1 set

Notes: Table-mounted self-retaining retractor used during internal mammary artery retractor; Available with sharp or blunt rake style retractor blades

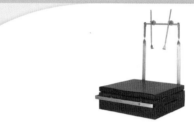

Pilling branded instrumentation courtesy of Teleflex Medical.

Harrington splanchnik retractor

Size: 12.0"; 9.5"

Quantity: 2

Notes: Available with large, small, or extra small blades

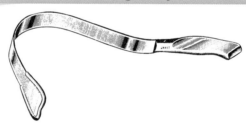

Courtesy of Jarit Surgical Instruments, a division of Integra LifeSciences Corporation.

Cheanvechai-Favaloro retractor

Size: 1 size

Quantity: 1 set

Notes: Table-mounted self-retaining retractor used during internal mammary artery retractor; Available with sharp or blunt rake style retractor blades; Adjusts with ratchets

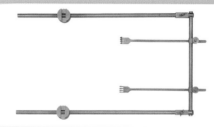

Photo supplied courtesy of Cardinal Health, V. Mueller® Products and Services. All rights reserved.

Strong T-bar retractor

Size: 1 size

Quantity: 1 set

Notes: Adjustable table-mounted self-retaining retractor with one central upright "T" mount and a cross bar for the retractor blades

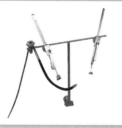

Pilling branded instrumentation courtesy of Teleflex Medical.

Cardiovascular Instrumentation – RETRACTION AND EXPOSURE INSTRUMENTS *continued*

Wilcox pediatric cardiac retractors

Size: 1 size

Quantity: 1 set

Notes: Self-retaining retractor for pediatric cardiac surgery

A. Retractor

B. Assorted pediatric retractor blades

C. Pediatric Allison retractor

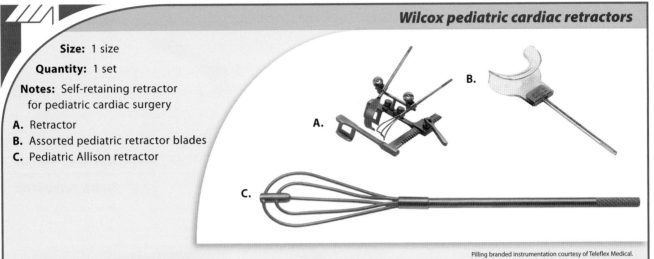

Pilling branded instrumentation courtesy of Teleflex Medical.

FIGURE 13-129

Amato retractor

Size: 1 size

Quantity: 1 set

Notes: Self-retaining sternal retractor

A. 4-blade, small, max spread 2.38"

B. 6-blade, large, max spread 2.75"

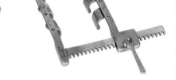

Pilling branded instrumentation courtesy of Teleflex Medical.

FIGURE 13-130

Holman lung retractors

Size: 14.88"; 15.75"

Quantity: 2

Notes: Manual retractor available in small and medium; Distal paddle-shaped blade easily reshaped by hand

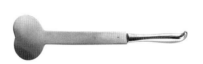

Pilling branded instrumentation courtesy of Teleflex Medical.

FIGURE 13-131

Parsonnet epicardial retractor

Size: 1.88"

Quantity: 1

Notes: Self-retaining retractor designed to retract the epicardial fat during coronary bypass procedures

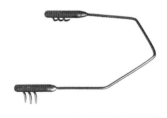

Pilling branded instrumentation courtesy of Teleflex Medical.

FIGURE 13-132

continues

Cardiovascular Instrumentation – RETRACTION AND EXPOSURE INSTRUMENTS *continued*

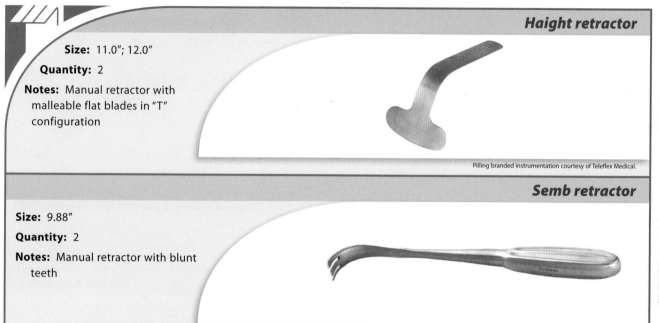

Haight retractor

Size: 11.0"; 12.0"

Quantity: 2

Notes: Manual retractor with malleable flat blades in "T" configuration

Pilling branded instrumentation courtesy of Teleflex Medical.

FIGURE 13-133

Semb retractor

Size: 9.88"

Quantity: 2

Notes: Manual retractor with blunt teeth

Pilling branded instrumentation courtesy of Teleflex Medical.

FIGURE 13-134

Cardiovascular Instrumentation – APPROXIMATION AND CLOSURE INSTRUMENTS

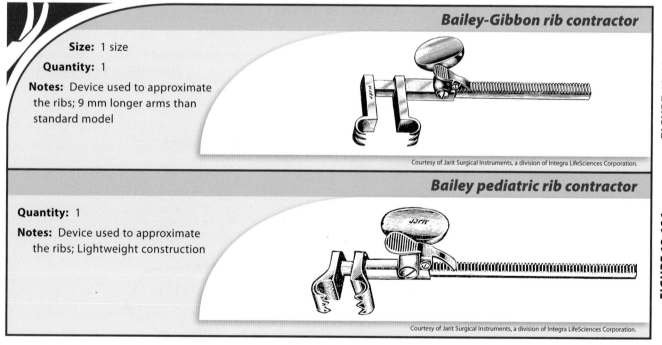

Bailey-Gibbon rib contractor

Size: 1 size

Quantity: 1

Notes: Device used to approximate the ribs; 9 mm longer arms than standard model

Courtesy of Jarit Surgical Instruments, a division of Integra LifeSciences Corporation.

FIGURE 13-135

Bailey pediatric rib contractor

Quantity: 1

Notes: Device used to approximate the ribs; Lightweight construction

Courtesy of Jarit Surgical Instruments, a division of Integra LifeSciences Corporation.

FIGURE 13-136

Cardiovascular Instrumentation – APPROXIMATION AND CLOSURE INSTRUMENTS *continued*

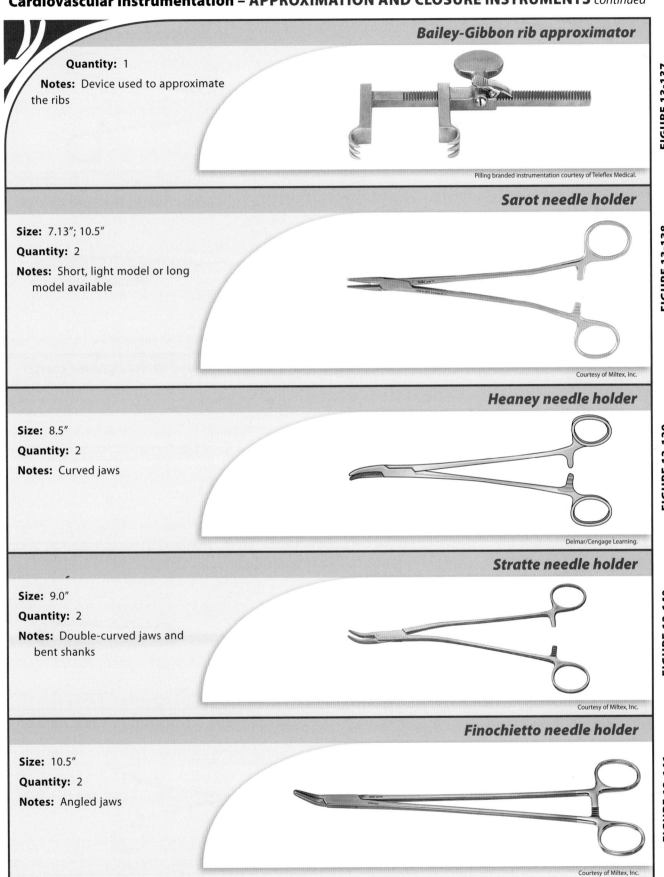

Bailey-Gibbon rib approximator

Quantity: 1

Notes: Device used to approximate the ribs

Pilling branded instrumentation courtesy of Teleflex Medical.

FIGURE 13-137

Sarot needle holder

Size: 7.13"; 10.5"

Quantity: 2

Notes: Short, light model or long model available

Courtesy of Miltex, Inc.

FIGURE 13-138

Heaney needle holder

Size: 8.5"

Quantity: 2

Notes: Curved jaws

Delmar/Cengage Learning.

FIGURE 13-139

Stratte needle holder

Size: 9.0"

Quantity: 2

Notes: Double-curved jaws and bent shanks

Courtesy of Miltex, Inc.

FIGURE 13-140

Finochietto needle holder

Size: 10.5"

Quantity: 2

Notes: Angled jaws

Courtesy of Miltex, Inc.

FIGURE 13-141

continues

Cardiovascular Instrumentation – APPROXIMATION AND CLOSURE INSTRUMENTS *continued*

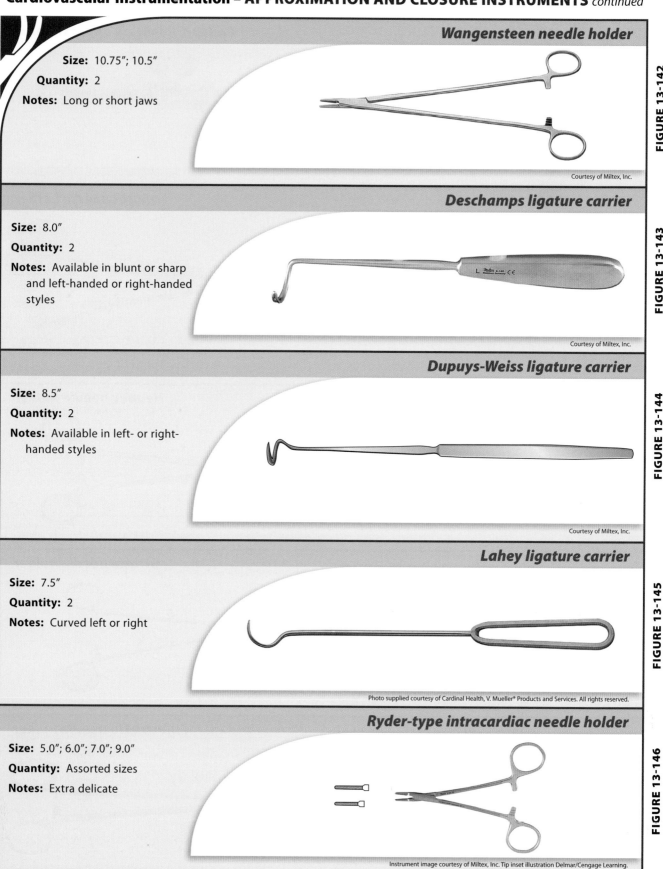

Wangensteen needle holder

Size: 10.75"; 10.5"

Quantity: 2

Notes: Long or short jaws

Courtesy of Miltex, Inc.

FIGURE 13-142

Deschamps ligature carrier

Size: 8.0"

Quantity: 2

Notes: Available in blunt or sharp and left-handed or right-handed styles

Courtesy of Miltex, Inc.

FIGURE 13-143

Dupuys-Weiss ligature carrier

Size: 8.5"

Quantity: 2

Notes: Available in left- or right-handed styles

Courtesy of Miltex, Inc.

FIGURE 13-144

Lahey ligature carrier

Size: 7.5"

Quantity: 2

Notes: Curved left or right

Photo supplied courtesy of Cardinal Health, V. Mueller® Products and Services. All rights reserved.

FIGURE 13-145

Ryder-type intracardiac needle holder

Size: 5.0"; 6.0"; 7.0"; 9.0"

Quantity: Assorted sizes

Notes: Extra delicate

Instrument image courtesy of Miltex, Inc. Tip inset illustration Delmar/Cengage Learning.

FIGURE 13-146

Cardiovascular Instrumentation – APPROXIMATION AND CLOSURE INSTRUMENTS *continued*

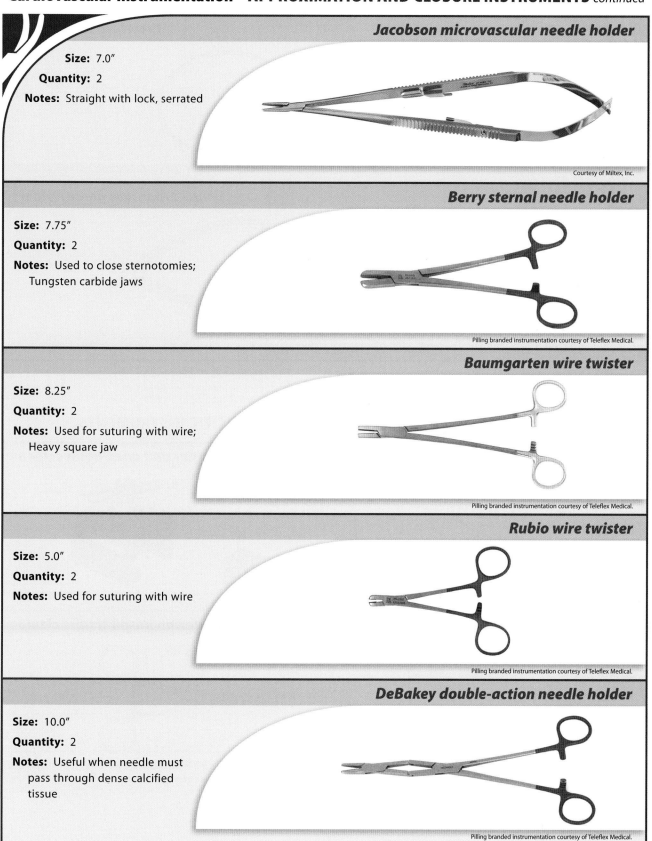

Jacobson microvascular needle holder

Size: 7.0″

Quantity: 2

Notes: Straight with lock, serrated

Courtesy of Miltex, Inc.

FIGURE 13-147

Berry sternal needle holder

Size: 7.75″

Quantity: 2

Notes: Used to close sternotomies; Tungsten carbide jaws

Pilling branded instrumentation courtesy of Teleflex Medical.

FIGURE 13-148

Baumgarten wire twister

Size: 8.25″

Quantity: 2

Notes: Used for suturing with wire; Heavy square jaw

Pilling branded instrumentation courtesy of Teleflex Medical.

FIGURE 13-149

Rubio wire twister

Size: 5.0″

Quantity: 2

Notes: Used for suturing with wire

Pilling branded instrumentation courtesy of Teleflex Medical.

FIGURE 13-150

DeBakey double-action needle holder

Size: 10.0″

Quantity: 2

Notes: Useful when needle must pass through dense calcified tissue

Pilling branded instrumentation courtesy of Teleflex Medical.

FIGURE 13-151

continues

Cardiovascular Instrumentation – **APPROXIMATION AND CLOSURE INSTRUMENTS** *continued*

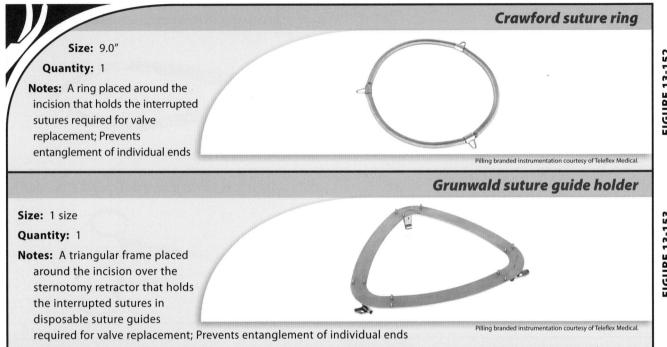

Crawford suture ring

Size: 9.0″

Quantity: 1

Notes: A ring placed around the incision that holds the interrupted sutures required for valve replacement; Prevents entanglement of individual ends

Pilling branded instrumentation courtesy of Teleflex Medical.

FIGURE 13-152

Grunwald suture guide holder

Size: 1 size

Quantity: 1

Notes: A triangular frame placed around the incision over the sternotomy retractor that holds the interrupted sutures in disposable suture guides required for valve replacement; Prevents entanglement of individual ends

Pilling branded instrumentation courtesy of Teleflex Medical.

FIGURE 13-153

Cardiovascular Instrumentation – **SPECIALTY SPECIFIC INSTRUMENTS**

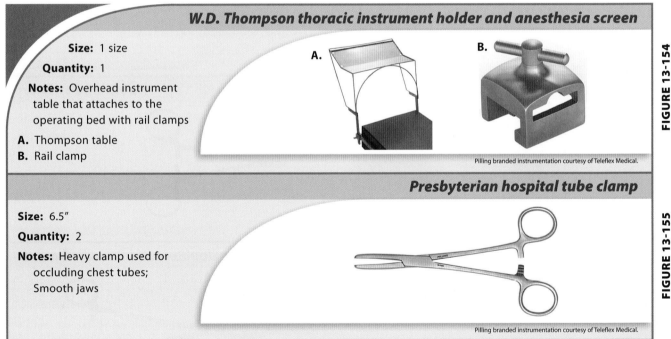

W.D. Thompson thoracic instrument holder and anesthesia screen

Size: 1 size

Quantity: 1

Notes: Overhead instrument table that attaches to the operating bed with rail clamps

A. Thompson table
B. Rail clamp

A.

B.

Pilling branded instrumentation courtesy of Teleflex Medical.

FIGURE 13-154

Presbyterian hospital tube clamp

Size: 6.5″

Quantity: 2

Notes: Heavy clamp used for occluding chest tubes; Smooth jaws

Pilling branded instrumentation courtesy of Teleflex Medical.

FIGURE 13-155

Cardiovascular Instrumentation – SPECIALTY SPECIFIC INSTRUMENTS continued

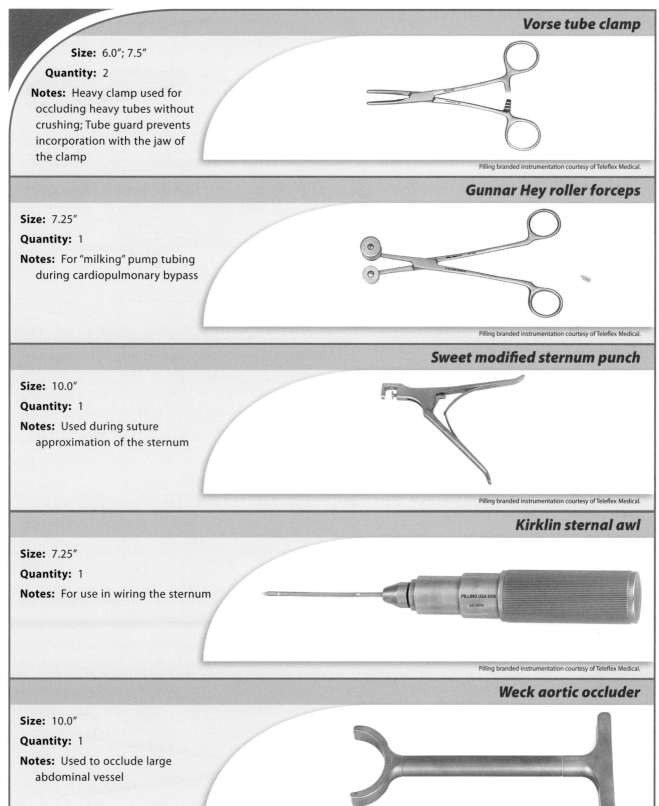

Vorse tube clamp

Size: 6.0"; 7.5"

Quantity: 2

Notes: Heavy clamp used for occluding heavy tubes without crushing; Tube guard prevents incorporation with the jaw of the clamp

Pilling branded instrumentation courtesy of Teleflex Medical.

FIGURE 13-156

Gunnar Hey roller forceps

Size: 7.25"

Quantity: 1

Notes: For "milking" pump tubing during cardiopulmonary bypass

Pilling branded instrumentation courtesy of Teleflex Medical.

FIGURE 13-157

Sweet modified sternum punch

Size: 10.0"

Quantity: 1

Notes: Used during suture approximation of the sternum

Pilling branded instrumentation courtesy of Teleflex Medical.

FIGURE 13-158

Kirklin sternal awl

Size: 7.25"

Quantity: 1

Notes: For use in wiring the sternum

Pilling branded instrumentation courtesy of Teleflex Medical.

FIGURE 13-159

Weck aortic occluder

Size: 10.0"

Quantity: 1

Notes: Used to occlude large abdominal vessel

Pilling branded instrumentation courtesy of Teleflex Medical.

FIGURE 13-160

continues

Cardiovascular Instrumentation – SPECIALTY SPECIFIC INSTRUMENTS *continued*

Riahi coronary compressor

Size: 9.35"

Quantity: 1

Notes: Compresses coronary artery without the use of a clamp

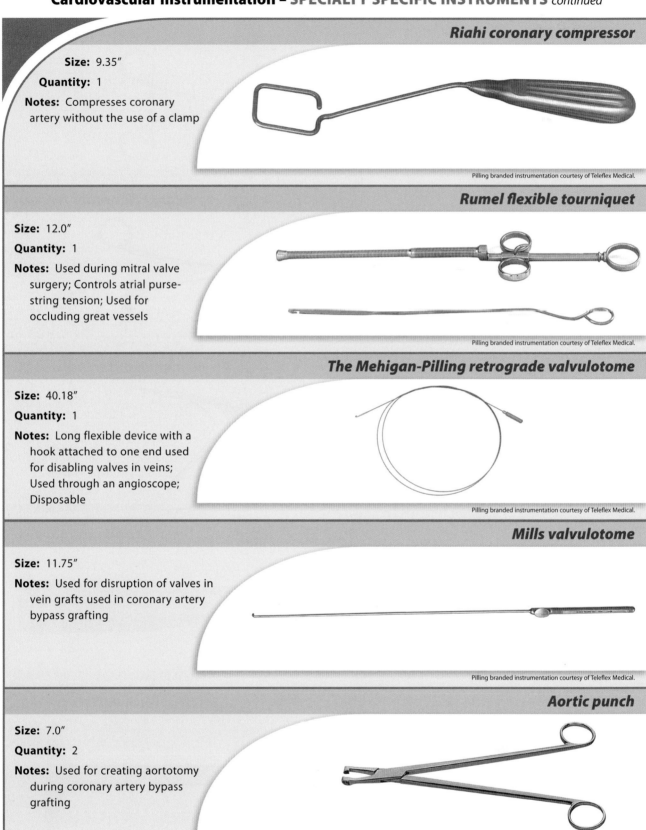

FIGURE 13-161

Rumel flexible tourniquet

Size: 12.0"

Quantity: 1

Notes: Used during mitral valve surgery; Controls atrial purse-string tension; Used for occluding great vessels

FIGURE 13-162

The Mehigan-Pilling retrograde valvulotome

Size: 40.18"

Quantity: 1

Notes: Long flexible device with a hook attached to one end used for disabling valves in veins; Used through an angioscope; Disposable

FIGURE 13-163

Mills valvulotome

Size: 11.75"

Notes: Used for disruption of valves in vein grafts used in coronary artery bypass grafting

FIGURE 13-164

Aortic punch

Size: 7.0"

Quantity: 2

Notes: Used for creating aortotomy during coronary artery bypass grafting

FIGURE 13-165

Cardiovascular Instrumentation – SPECIALTY SPECIFIC INSTRUMENTS *continued*

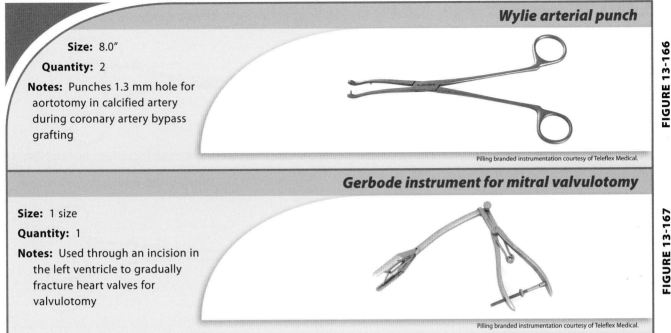

Wylie arterial punch

Size: 8.0"

Quantity: 2

Notes: Punches 1.3 mm hole for aortotomy in calcified artery during coronary artery bypass grafting

FIGURE 13-166

Pilling branded instrumentation courtesy of Teleflex Medical.

Gerbode instrument for mitral valvulotomy

Size: 1 size

Quantity: 1

Notes: Used through an incision in the left ventricle to gradually fracture heart valves for valvulotomy

FIGURE 13-167

Pilling branded instrumentation courtesy of Teleflex Medical.

CAROTID INSTRUMENTATION

Soft tissue foundation instrumentation is used to incise the tissues over and around the carotid arteries. The main instruments used in the endarterectomy portion of the procedure are clamps and dissectors. Some surgeons prefer to shunt the artery rather than simply occlude the blood flow with a clamp. The degree of plaque formation and volume of calcification are the determining factors as to which instrumentation is used. It is important to have an assortment of artery clamps and shunt clamps on hand. The shunts are disposable.

Carotid Instrumentation – CLAMPS

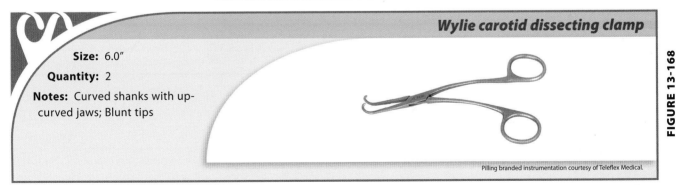

Wylie carotid dissecting clamp

Size: 6.0"

Quantity: 2

Notes: Curved shanks with up-curved jaws; Blunt tips

FIGURE 13-168

Pilling branded instrumentation courtesy of Teleflex Medical.

continues

Carotid Instrumentation – CLAMPS *continued*

Wylie external carotid clamp

Size: 3.0"; 8.0"

Quantity: 2

Notes: Angled occlusion clamp designed to clamp the external carotid

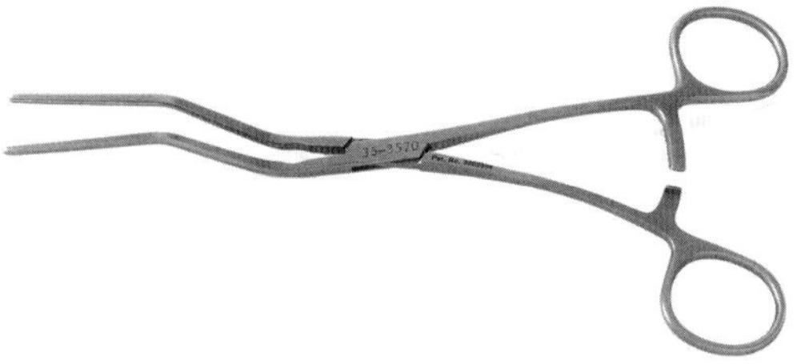

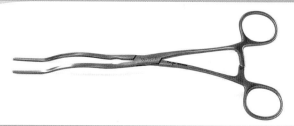

Pilling branded instrumentation courtesy of Teleflex Medical.

FIGURE 13-169

Wylie internal carotid clamp

Size: 3.0"; 8.25"

Quantity: 2

Notes: Angled occlusion clamp designed to clamp the internal carotid

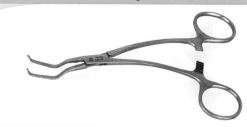

Pilling branded instrumentation courtesy of Teleflex Medical.

FIGURE 13-170

Thompson carotid closure clamp

Size: 6.25"

Quantity: 2

Notes: Curved shanks with angled jaws

Pilling branded instrumentation courtesy of Teleflex Medical.

FIGURE 13-171

Cooley carotid, subclavian, and renal clamp

Size: 7.25"

Quantity: 2

Notes: Curved shanks with angled jaws; Graduated markings on jaws

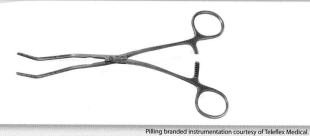

Pilling branded instrumentation courtesy of Teleflex Medical.

FIGURE 13-172

Carotid Instrumentation – CLAMPS *continued*

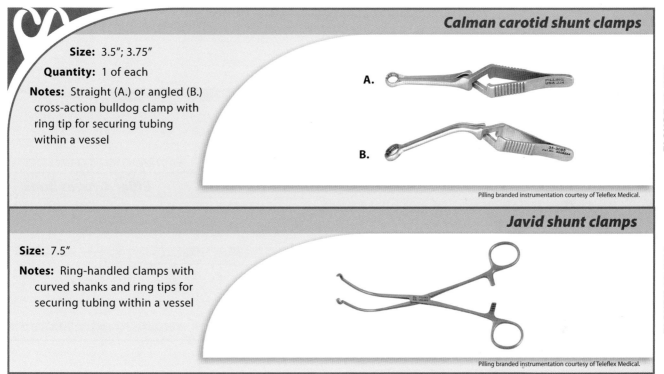

Calman carotid shunt clamps

Size: 3.5"; 3.75"

Quantity: 1 of each

Notes: Straight (A.) or angled (B.) cross-action bulldog clamp with ring tip for securing tubing within a vessel

A.

B.

Pilling branded instrumentation courtesy of Teleflex Medical.

FIGURE 13-173

Javid shunt clamps

Size: 7.5"

Notes: Ring-handled clamps with curved shanks and ring tips for securing tubing within a vessel

Pilling branded instrumentation courtesy of Teleflex Medical.

FIGURE 13-174

Carotid Instrumentation – DISSECTION INSTRUMENTS

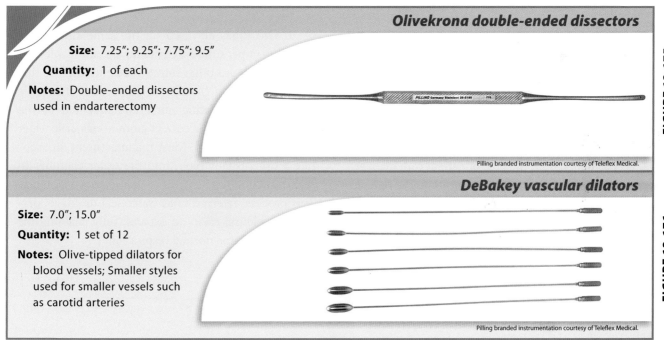

Olivekrona double-ended dissectors

Size: 7.25"; 9.25"; 7.75"; 9.5"

Quantity: 1 of each

Notes: Double-ended dissectors used in endarterectomy

Pilling branded instrumentation courtesy of Teleflex Medical.

FIGURE 13-175

DeBakey vascular dilators

Size: 7.0"; 15.0"

Quantity: 1 set of 12

Notes: Olive-tipped dilators for blood vessels; Smaller styles used for smaller vessels such as carotid arteries

Pilling branded instrumentation courtesy of Teleflex Medical.

FIGURE 13-176

continues

Carotid Instrumentation – DISSECTION INSTRUMENTS *continued*

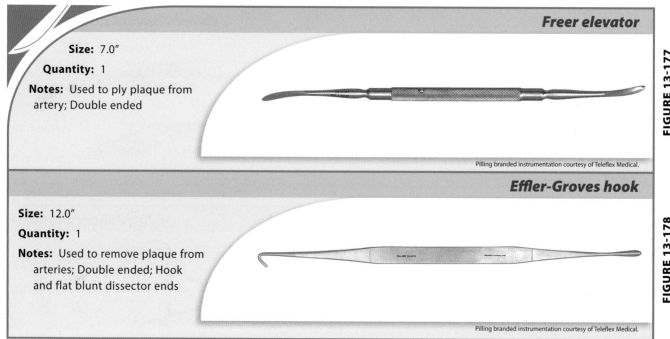

Freer elevator

Size: 7.0″

Quantity: 1

Notes: Used to ply plaque from artery; Double ended

Pilling branded instrumentation courtesy of Teleflex Medical.

FIGURE 13-177

Effler-Groves hook

Size: 12.0″

Quantity: 1

Notes: Used to remove plaque from arteries; Double ended; Hook and flat blunt dissector ends

Pilling branded instrumentation courtesy of Teleflex Medical.

FIGURE 13-178

SUMMARY

Cardiothoracic surgery is performed on patients who are compromised with several conditions, such as inadequate circulation, diabetes, obesity, or other comorbidity. Entering the chest of any patient interrupts the integrity of the mediastinum and interferes with the performance of the lungs, regardless of the surgical procedure performed.

Postoperatively, the goal of patient care management is the restoration of the intrathoracic vacuum required for respiration. As the patient's chest is closed, one or two large bore drainage tubes are inserted into the chest either through the lateral chest wall or through the median sternotomy incision.

If two tubes are used on the same side of the chest, the upper tube evacuates air and the lower tube drains blood and other intrathoracic fluids. The disposable collection chamber is delivered to the sterile field by the circulating nurse and prepared by the scrub person with the correct amount of sterile water to create a water seal. Most manufacturers incorporate a tint (usually blue) into the water chamber to make the fluid level easy to visualize from a distance. This process, referred to as water seal drainage, permits the pleural cavity to expand, fully enabling the patient to resume normal respiration.

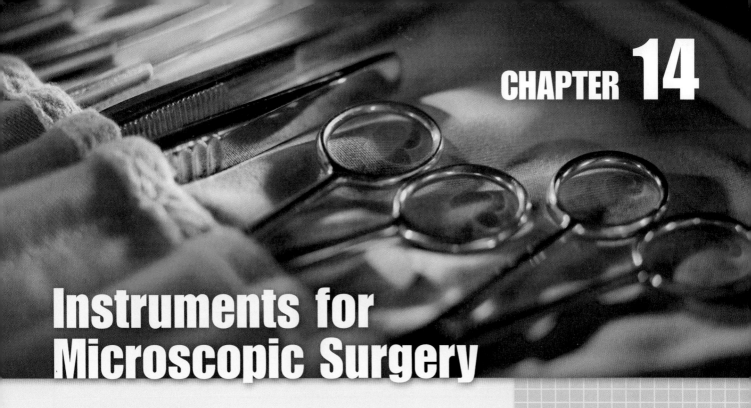

CHAPTER **14**

Instruments for Microscopic Surgery

INTRODUCTION

Microscopic surgery is an application that can be extended to most surgical specialties. All tissues can be surgically dissected using microscopic techniques. Performing microscopic procedures requires the operator to have a steady hand and a high level of concentration. The scrub person is critical to this process because the surgeon will need to maintain accommodation of vision through the microscopic lens and trust that the correct instrument oriented in the correct position will be placed in his or her extended hand. If the surgeon has to look away from the microscope each time the instrumentation is passed, the visual adjustment can cause misjudgment of distance or instrument placement during tissue manipulation. Manual dexterity is critical for a safe and effective microscopic procedure.

MULTIPURPOSE MICROSURGERY INSTRUMENTATION

Surgical procedures using a microscope require instruments with extremely fine tips and handles that do not obscure the user's vision during the procedure. Sutures and devices manipulated by micro instrumentation are equally fine and delicate and cannot be handled with conventional instrumentation without causing damage to the structure. The instrumentation described in this section is selected according to the particular target tissue being manipulated under microscopy.

The microscopic part of the procedure takes place after the outer tissues have been incised. Opening the skin and gross dissection requires the use of the appropriate foundation set. The most commonly used sets for intraabdominal procedures are the medium and long foundation sets. Examples of microscopic procedures within the abdomen include vascular attachments of transplantation and salpingoplasty.

Multipurpose Microsurgery Instrumentation – CLAMPS

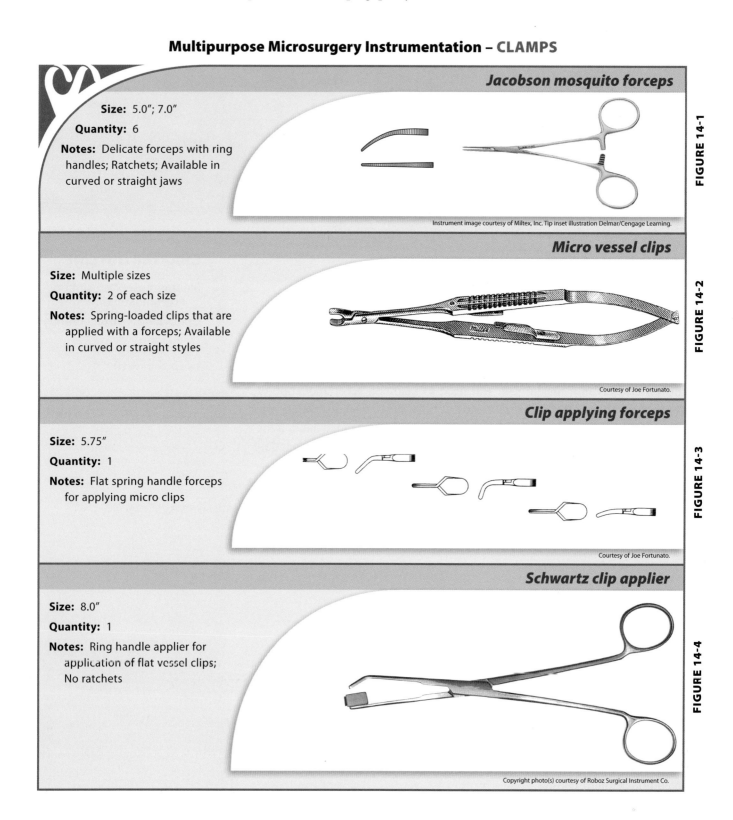

Jacobson mosquito forceps

Size: 5.0"; 7.0"

Quantity: 6

Notes: Delicate forceps with ring handles; Ratchets; Available in curved or straight jaws

Instrument image courtesy of Miltex, Inc. Tip inset illustration Delmar/Cengage Learning.

FIGURE 14-1

Micro vessel clips

Size: Multiple sizes

Quantity: 2 of each size

Notes: Spring-loaded clips that are applied with a forceps; Available in curved or straight styles

Courtesy of Joe Fortunato.

FIGURE 14-2

Clip applying forceps

Size: 5.75"

Quantity: 1

Notes: Flat spring handle forceps for applying micro clips

Courtesy of Joe Fortunato.

FIGURE 14-3

Schwartz clip applier

Size: 8.0"

Quantity: 1

Notes: Ring handle applier for application of flat vessel clips; No ratchets

Copyright photo(s) courtesy of Roboz Surgical Instrument Co.

FIGURE 14-4

Multipurpose Microsurgery Instrumentation – GRASPING FORCEPS

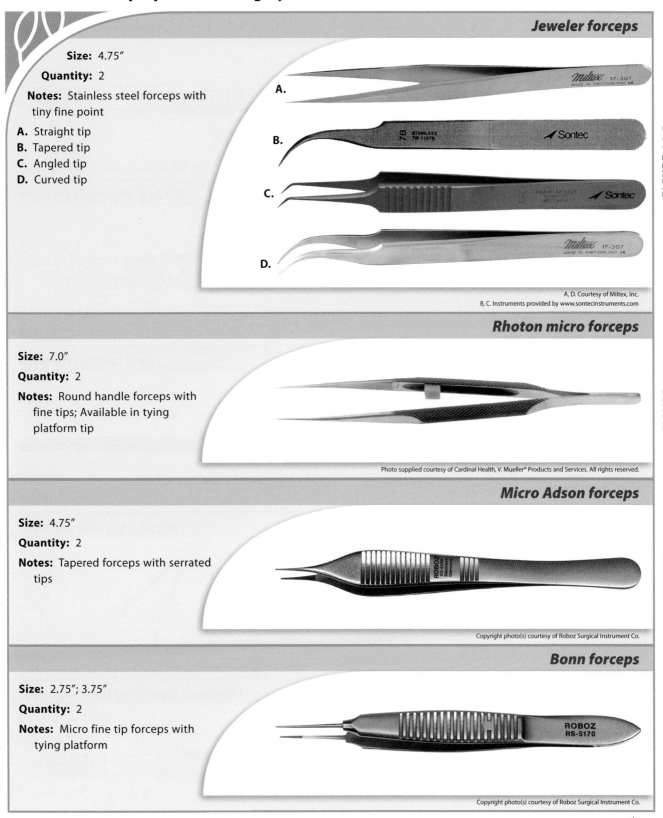

Jeweler forceps

Size: 4.75″

Quantity: 2

Notes: Stainless steel forceps with tiny fine point

A. Straight tip
B. Tapered tip
C. Angled tip
D. Curved tip

A.
B.
C.
D.

A, D. Courtesy of Miltex, Inc.
B, C. Instruments provided by www.sontecinstruments.com

FIGURE 14-5

Rhoton micro forceps

Size: 7.0″

Quantity: 2

Notes: Round handle forceps with fine tips; Available in tying platform tip

Photo supplied courtesy of Cardinal Health, V. Mueller® Products and Services. All rights reserved.

FIGURE 14-6

Micro Adson forceps

Size: 4.75″

Quantity: 2

Notes: Tapered forceps with serrated tips

Copyright photo(s) courtesy of Roboz Surgical Instrument Co.

FIGURE 14-7

Bonn forceps

Size: 2.75″; 3.75″

Quantity: 2

Notes: Micro fine tip forceps with tying platform

Copyright photo(s) courtesy of Roboz Surgical Instrument Co.

FIGURE 14-8

continues

Multipurpose Microsurgery Instrumentation – GRASPING FORCEPS *continued*

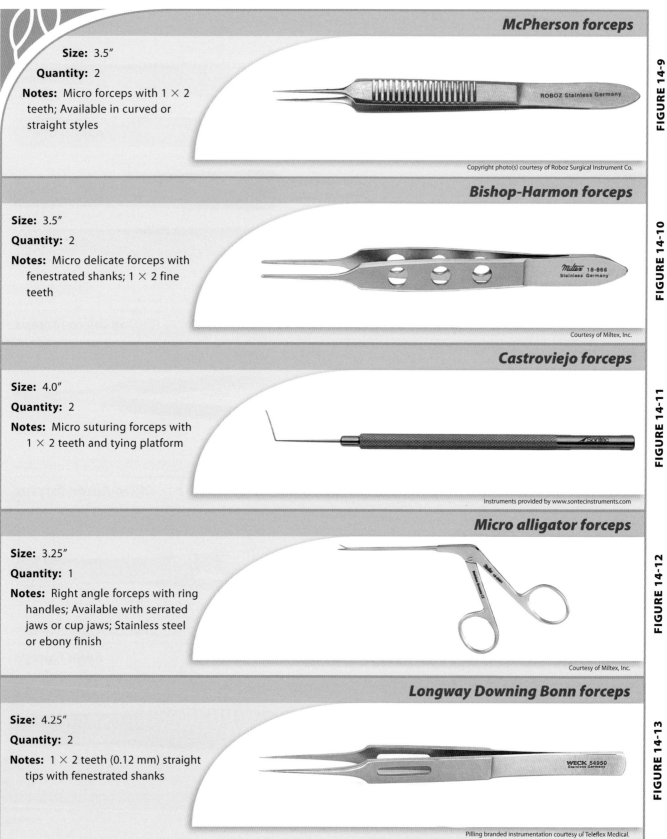

McPherson forceps

Size: 3.5"

Quantity: 2

Notes: Micro forceps with 1 × 2 teeth; Available in curved or straight styles

Copyright photo(s) courtesy of Roboz Surgical Instrument Co.

FIGURE 14-9

Bishop-Harmon forceps

Size: 3.5"

Quantity: 2

Notes: Micro delicate forceps with fenestrated shanks; 1 × 2 fine teeth

Courtesy of Miltex, Inc.

FIGURE 14-10

Castroviejo forceps

Size: 4.0"

Quantity: 2

Notes: Micro suturing forceps with 1 × 2 teeth and tying platform

Instruments provided by www.sontecinstruments.com

FIGURE 14-11

Micro alligator forceps

Size: 3.25"

Quantity: 1

Notes: Right angle forceps with ring handles; Available with serrated jaws or cup jaws; Stainless steel or ebony finish

Courtesy of Miltex, Inc.

FIGURE 14-12

Longway Downing Bonn forceps

Size: 4.25"

Quantity: 2

Notes: 1 × 2 teeth (0.12 mm) straight tips with fenestrated shanks

Pilling branded instrumentation courtesy of Teleflex Medical.

FIGURE 14-13

Multipurpose Microsurgery Instrumentation – GRASPING FORCEPS *continued*

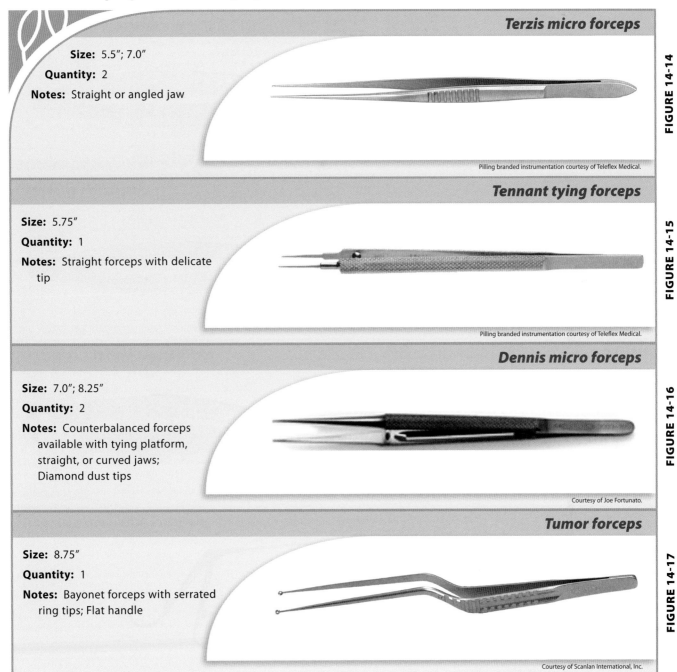

Terzis micro forceps

Size: 5.5"; 7.0"

Quantity: 2

Notes: Straight or angled jaw

Pilling branded instrumentation courtesy of Teleflex Medical.

FIGURE 14-14

Tennant tying forceps

Size: 5.75"

Quantity: 1

Notes: Straight forceps with delicate tip

Pilling branded instrumentation courtesy of Teleflex Medical.

FIGURE 14-15

Dennis micro forceps

Size: 7.0"; 8.25"

Quantity: 2

Notes: Counterbalanced forceps available with tying platform, straight, or curved jaws; Diamond dust tips

Courtesy of Joe Fortunato.

FIGURE 14-16

Tumor forceps

Size: 8.75"

Quantity: 1

Notes: Bayonet forceps with serrated ring tips; Flat handle

Courtesy of Scanlan International, Inc.

FIGURE 14-17

Multipurpose Microsurgery Instrumentation – DISSECTION INSTRUMENTS

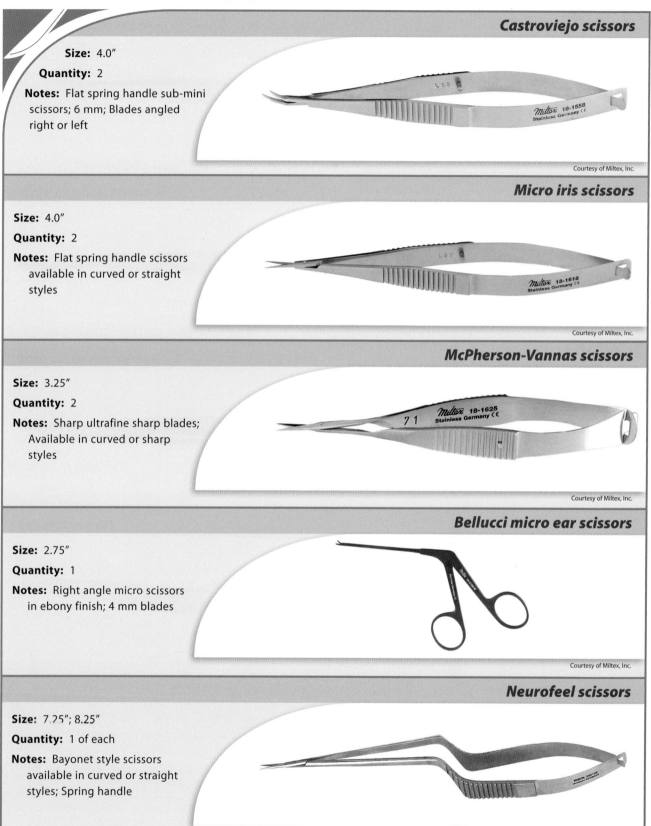

Castroviejo scissors

Size: 4.0"

Quantity: 2

Notes: Flat spring handle sub-mini scissors; 6 mm; Blades angled right or left

Courtesy of Miltex, Inc.

FIGURE 14-18

Micro iris scissors

Size: 4.0"

Quantity: 2

Notes: Flat spring handle scissors available in curved or straight styles

Courtesy of Miltex, Inc.

FIGURE 14-19

McPherson-Vannas scissors

Size: 3.25"

Quantity: 2

Notes: Sharp ultrafine sharp blades; Available in curved or sharp styles

Courtesy of Miltex, Inc.

FIGURE 14-20

Bellucci micro ear scissors

Size: 2.75"

Quantity: 1

Notes: Right angle micro scissors in ebony finish; 4 mm blades

Courtesy of Miltex, Inc.

FIGURE 14-21

Neurofeel scissors

Size: 7.25"; 8.25"

Quantity: 1 of each

Notes: Bayonet style scissors available in curved or straight styles; Spring handle

Pilling branded instrumentation courtesy of Teleflex Medical.

FIGURE 14-22

Multipurpose Microsurgery Instrumentation – DISSECTION INSTRUMENTS *continued*

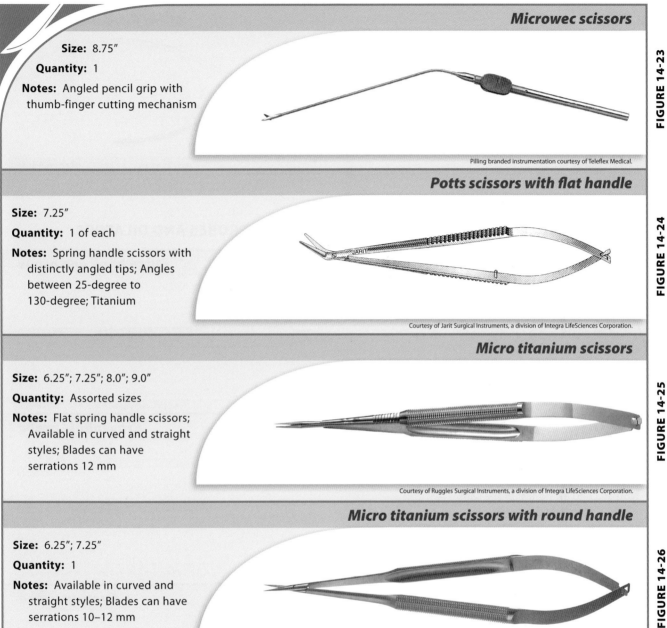

Microwec scissors

Size: 8.75″

Quantity: 1

Notes: Angled pencil grip with thumb-finger cutting mechanism

FIGURE 14-23

Pilling branded instrumentation courtesy of Teleflex Medical.

Potts scissors with flat handle

Size: 7.25″

Quantity: 1 of each

Notes: Spring handle scissors with distinctly angled tips; Angles between 25-degree to 130-degree; Titanium

FIGURE 14-24

Courtesy of Jarit Surgical Instruments, a division of Integra LifeSciences Corporation.

Micro titanium scissors

Size: 6.25″; 7.25″; 8.0″; 9.0″

Quantity: Assorted sizes

Notes: Flat spring handle scissors; Available in curved and straight styles; Blades can have serrations 12 mm

FIGURE 14-25

Courtesy of Ruggles Surgical Instruments, a division of Integra LifeSciences Corporation.

Micro titanium scissors with round handle

Size: 6.25″; 7.25″

Quantity: 1

Notes: Available in curved and straight styles; Blades can have serrations 10–12 mm

FIGURE 14-26

Courtesy of Padgett Surgical Instruments, a division of Integra LifeSciences Corporation.

Multipurpose Microsurgery Instrumentation – DEBULKING INSTRUMENTS

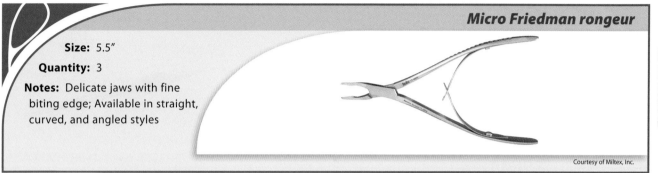

Micro Friedman rongeur

Size: 5.5"

Quantity: 3

Notes: Delicate jaws with fine biting edge; Available in straight, curved, and angled styles

Courtesy of Miltex, Inc.

FIGURE 14-27

Multipurpose Microsurgery Instrumentation – PROBES AND DILATORS

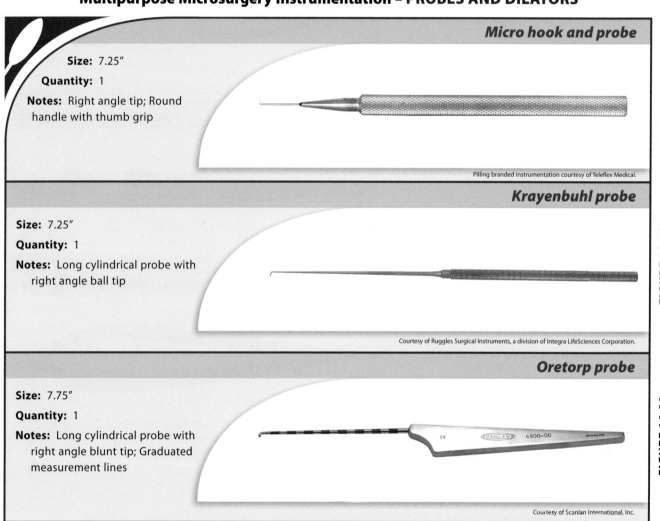

Micro hook and probe

Size: 7.25"

Quantity: 1

Notes: Right angle tip; Round handle with thumb grip

Pilling branded instrumentation courtesy of Teleflex Medical.

FIGURE 14-28

Krayenbuhl probe

Size: 7.25"

Quantity: 1

Notes: Long cylindrical probe with right angle ball tip

Courtesy of Ruggles Surgical Instruments, a division of Integra LifeSciences Corporation.

FIGURE 14-29

Oretorp probe

Size: 7.75"

Quantity: 1

Notes: Long cylindrical probe with right angle blunt tip; Graduated measurement lines

Courtesy of Scanlan International, Inc.

FIGURE 14-30

Multipurpose Microsurgery Instrumentation –
EVACUATION AND INSTILLATION INSTRUMENTS

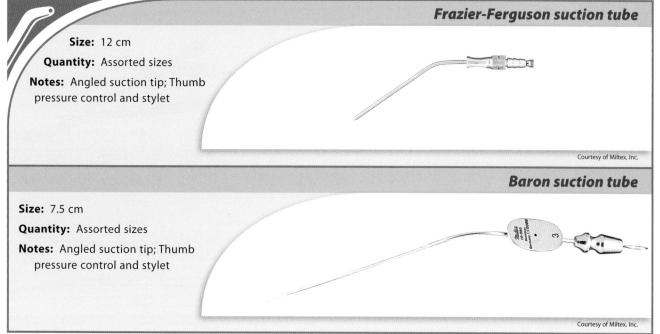

Frazier-Ferguson suction tube

Size: 12 cm

Quantity: Assorted sizes

Notes: Angled suction tip; Thumb pressure control and stylet

Courtesy of Miltex, Inc.

FIGURE 14-31

Baron suction tube

Size: 7.5 cm

Quantity: Assorted sizes

Notes: Angled suction tip; Thumb pressure control and stylet

Courtesy of Miltex, Inc.

FIGURE 14-32

Multipurpose Microsurgery Instrumentation –
APPROXIMATION AND CLOSURE INSTRUMENTS

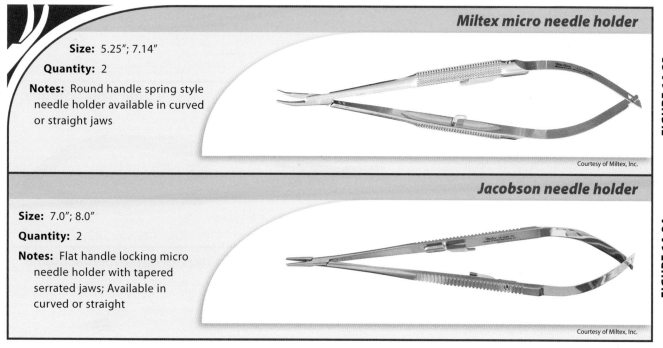

Miltex micro needle holder

Size: 5.25"; 7.14"

Quantity: 2

Notes: Round handle spring style needle holder available in curved or straight jaws

Courtesy of Miltex, Inc.

FIGURE 14-33

Jacobson needle holder

Size: 7.0"; 8.0"

Quantity: 2

Notes: Flat handle locking micro needle holder with tapered serrated jaws; Available in curved or straight

Courtesy of Miltex, Inc.

FIGURE 14-34

continues

Multipurpose Microsurgery Instrumentation –
APPROXIMATION AND CLOSURE INSTRUMENTS *continued*

Kalt needle holder

Size: 5.25"

Quantity: 2

Notes: Flat handle needle holder with spring action and thumb release; Delicate cross-serrated jaws

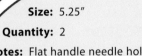
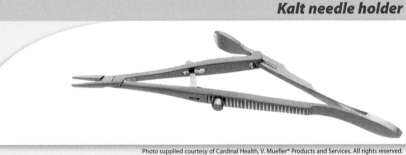

FIGURE 14-35

Green needle holder

Size: 4.25"

Quantity: 2

Notes: Spring handle needle holder for suturing and tying

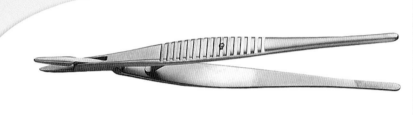

FIGURE 14-36

Castroviejo needle holder

Size: 5.5"

Quantity: 2

Notes: Spring flat handle needle holder; Available as locking or non-locking; Extra fine tip in curved or straight styles; Titanium

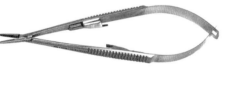

FIGURE 14-37

Paton needle holder

Size: 4.5"

Quantity: 1

Notes: Spring handle needle holder; Non-locking

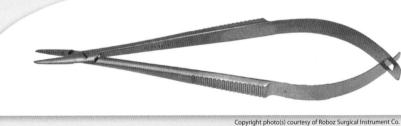

FIGURE 14-38

McPherson micro needle holder

Size: 4.0"

Quantity: 1

Notes: Spring handle with smooth notched jaws; Curved; Locking

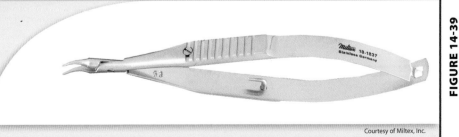

FIGURE 14-39

Multipurpose Microsurgery Instrumentation –
APPROXIMATION AND CLOSURE INSTRUMENTS *continued*

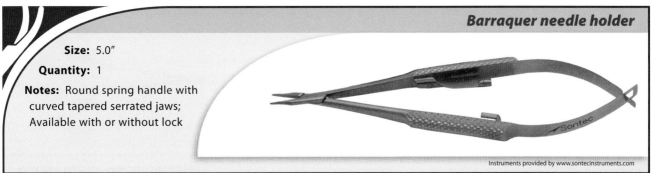

Barraquer needle holder

Size: 5.0″

Quantity: 1

Notes: Round spring handle with curved tapered serrated jaws; Available with or without lock

FIGURE 14-40

OPHTHALMIC INSTRUMENTATION

Ophthalmic surgeons use many of the basic micro instruments listed in the microscopic basic instrumentation list. The eye has many structures that require the use of highly specialized instruments for handling the lens, the cornea, the sclera, and conjunctiva. The lacrimal structures and musculature are commonly included in the realm of ophthalmic surgery and employ many probes and hooks. This collection of instruments would not be assembled as a set. Procedure-specific instruments would be packaged together as appropriate sets. Foundation sets would not be included unless skin incisions are performed.

Ophthalmic Instrumentation – CLAMPS

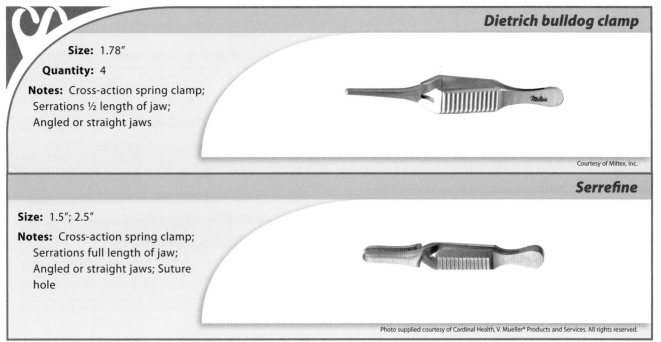

Dietrich bulldog clamp

Size: 1.78″

Quantity: 4

Notes: Cross-action spring clamp; Serrations ½ length of jaw; Angled or straight jaws

FIGURE 14-41

Serrefine

Size: 1.5″; 2.5″

Notes: Cross-action spring clamp; Serrations full length of jaw; Angled or straight jaws; Suture hole

FIGURE 14-42

continues

Ophthalmic Instrumentation – CLAMPS *continued*

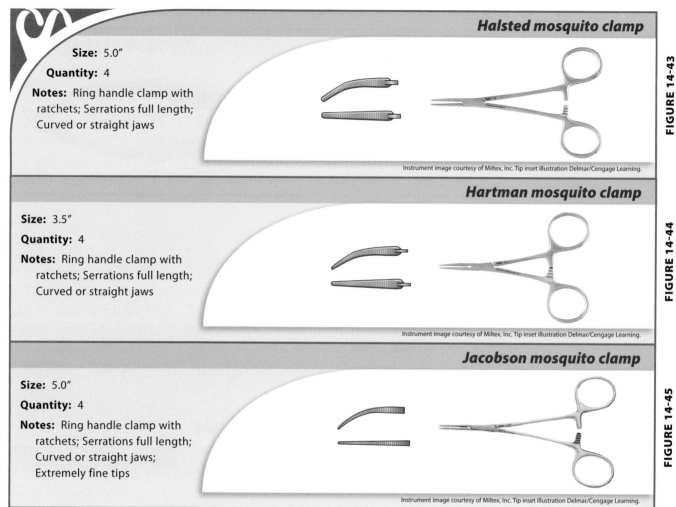

Halsted mosquito clamp

Size: 5.0″

Quantity: 4

Notes: Ring handle clamp with ratchets; Serrations full length; Curved or straight jaws

Instrument image courtesy of Miltex, Inc. Tip inset illustration Delmar/Cengage Learning.

FIGURE 14-43

Hartman mosquito clamp

Size: 3.5″

Quantity: 4

Notes: Ring handle clamp with ratchets; Serrations full length; Curved or straight jaws

Instrument image courtesy of Miltex, Inc. Tip inset illustration Delmar/Cengage Learning.

FIGURE 14-44

Jacobson mosquito clamp

Size: 5.0″

Quantity: 4

Notes: Ring handle clamp with ratchets; Serrations full length; Curved or straight jaws; Extremely fine tips

Instrument image courtesy of Miltex, Inc. Tip inset illustration Delmar/Cengage Learning.

FIGURE 14-45

Ophthalmic Instrumentation – GRASPING FORCEPS

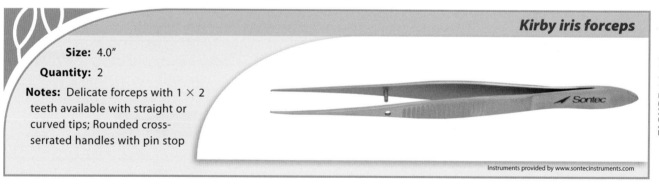

Kirby iris forceps

Size: 4.0″

Quantity: 2

Notes: Delicate forceps with 1 × 2 teeth available with straight or curved tips; Rounded cross-serrated handles with pin stop

Instruments provided by www.sontecinstruments.com

FIGURE 14-46

Ophthalmic Instrumentation – GRASPING FORCEPS *continued*

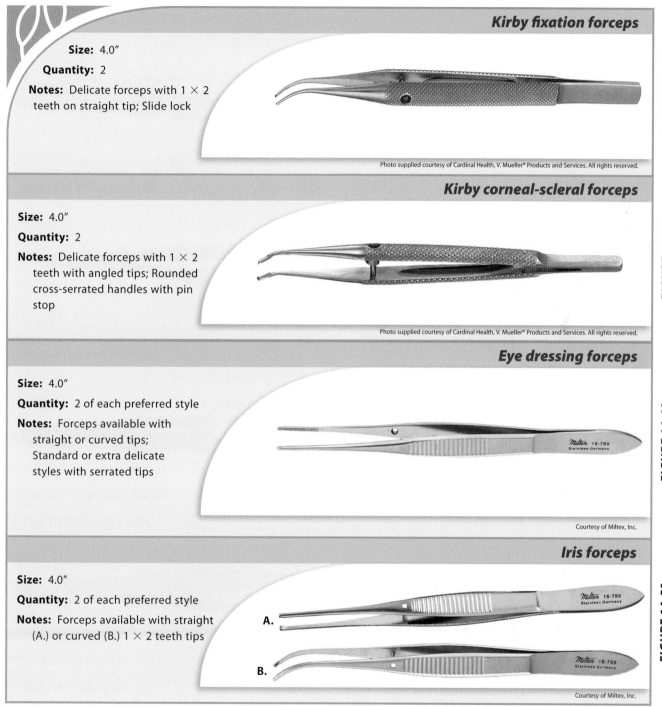

Kirby fixation forceps

Size: 4.0″

Quantity: 2

Notes: Delicate forceps with 1 × 2 teeth on straight tip; Slide lock

FIGURE 14-47

Kirby corneal-scleral forceps

Size: 4.0″

Quantity: 2

Notes: Delicate forceps with 1 × 2 teeth with angled tips; Rounded cross-serrated handles with pin stop

FIGURE 14-48

Eye dressing forceps

Size: 4.0″

Quantity: 2 of each preferred style

Notes: Forceps available with straight or curved tips; Standard or extra delicate styles with serrated tips

FIGURE 14-49

Iris forceps

Size: 4.0″

Quantity: 2 of each preferred style

Notes: Forceps available with straight (A.) or curved (B.) 1 × 2 teeth tips

A.

B.

FIGURE 14-50

continues

Ophthalmic Instrumentation – GRASPING FORCEPS *continued*

O'Connor iris forceps

Size: 3.75″

Quantity: 2

Notes: Forceps with angled jaws; 1 × 2 teeth

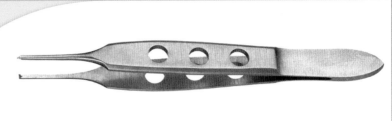

FIGURE 14-51

Bracken iris forceps

Size: 4.0″

Quantity: 2

Notes: Forceps with slightly curved jaws; Fine cross-serrated tips

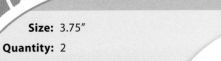

FIGURE 14-52

Foerster eye forceps

Size: 3.75″

Quantity: 2

Notes: Forceps with fenestrated octagonal handles; Available in curved or straight tips with smooth or 1 × 2 teeth

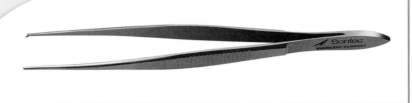

FIGURE 14-53

Stevens iris forceps

Size: 4.0″

Quantity: 2

Notes: Straight forceps with 1 × 2 teeth; Narrow 1 mm tips

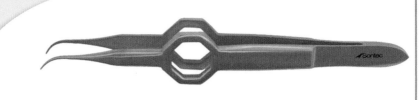

FIGURE 14-54

Graefe iris forceps

Size: 2.75″

Quantity: Assorted sizes of choice

Notes: Forceps available with 1 × 2 toothed curved or straight tips

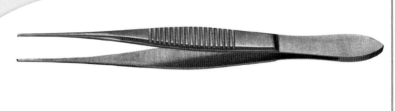
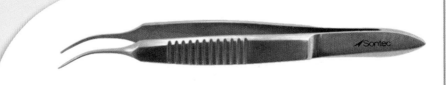

FIGURE 14-55

Ophthalmic Instrumentation – GRASPING FORCEPS *continued*

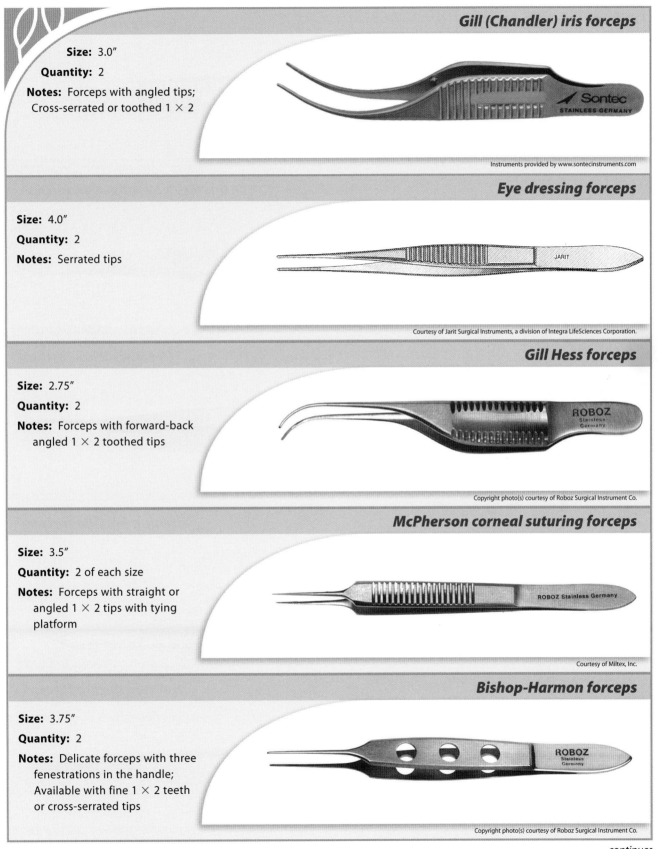

Gill (Chandler) iris forceps

Size: 3.0″

Quantity: 2

Notes: Forceps with angled tips; Cross-serrated or toothed 1 × 2

Instruments provided by www.sontecinstruments.com

FIGURE 14-56

Eye dressing forceps

Size: 4.0″

Quantity: 2

Notes: Serrated tips

Courtesy of Jarit Surgical Instruments, a division of Integra LifeSciences Corporation.

FIGURE 14-57

Gill Hess forceps

Size: 2.75″

Quantity: 2

Notes: Forceps with forward-back angled 1 × 2 toothed tips

Copyright photo(s) courtesy of Roboz Surgical Instrument Co.

FIGURE 14-58

McPherson corneal suturing forceps

Size: 3.5″

Quantity: 2 of each size

Notes: Forceps with straight or angled 1 × 2 tips with tying platform

Courtesy of Miltex, Inc.

FIGURE 14-59

Bishop-Harmon forceps

Size: 3.75″

Quantity: 2

Notes: Delicate forceps with three fenestrations in the handle; Available with fine 1 × 2 teeth or cross-serrated tips

Copyright photo(s) courtesy of Roboz Surgical Instrument Co.

FIGURE 14-60

continues

Ophthalmic Instrumentation – GRASPING FORCEPS *continued*

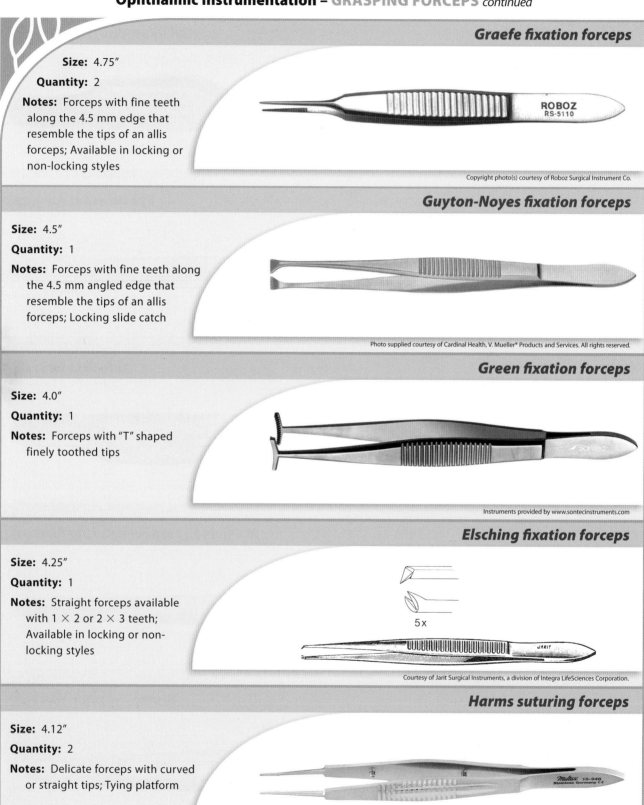

Graefe fixation forceps

Size: 4.75"

Quantity: 2

Notes: Forceps with fine teeth along the 4.5 mm edge that resemble the tips of an allis forceps; Available in locking or non-locking styles

FIGURE 14-61

Guyton-Noyes fixation forceps

Size: 4.5"

Quantity: 1

Notes: Forceps with fine teeth along the 4.5 mm angled edge that resemble the tips of an allis forceps; Locking slide catch

FIGURE 14-62

Green fixation forceps

Size: 4.0"

Quantity: 1

Notes: Forceps with "T" shaped finely toothed tips

FIGURE 14-63

Elsching fixation forceps

Size: 4.25"

Quantity: 1

Notes: Straight forceps available with 1 × 2 or 2 × 3 teeth; Available in locking or non-locking styles

5 x

FIGURE 14-64

Harms suturing forceps

Size: 4.12"

Quantity: 2

Notes: Delicate forceps with curved or straight tips; Tying platform

FIGURE 14-65

Ophthalmic Instrumentation – GRASPING FORCEPS *continued*

Nugent forceps

Size: 4.25"

Quantity: 1

Notes: Forceps with angled cross-serrated tips

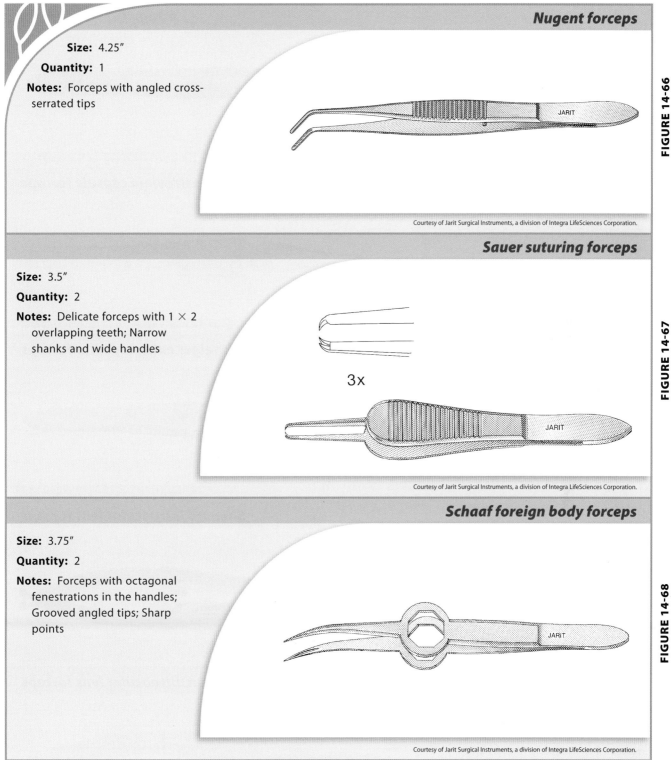

Courtesy of Jarit Surgical Instruments, a division of Integra LifeSciences Corporation.

FIGURE 14-66

Sauer suturing forceps

Size: 3.5"

Quantity: 2

Notes: Delicate forceps with 1 × 2 overlapping teeth; Narrow shanks and wide handles

3x

Courtesy of Jarit Surgical Instruments, a division of Integra LifeSciences Corporation.

FIGURE 14-67

Schaaf foreign body forceps

Size: 3.75"

Quantity: 2

Notes: Forceps with octagonal fenestrations in the handles; Grooved angled tips; Sharp points

Courtesy of Jarit Surgical Instruments, a division of Integra LifeSciences Corporation.

FIGURE 14-68

continues

Ophthalmic Instrumentation – GRASPING FORCEPS *continued*

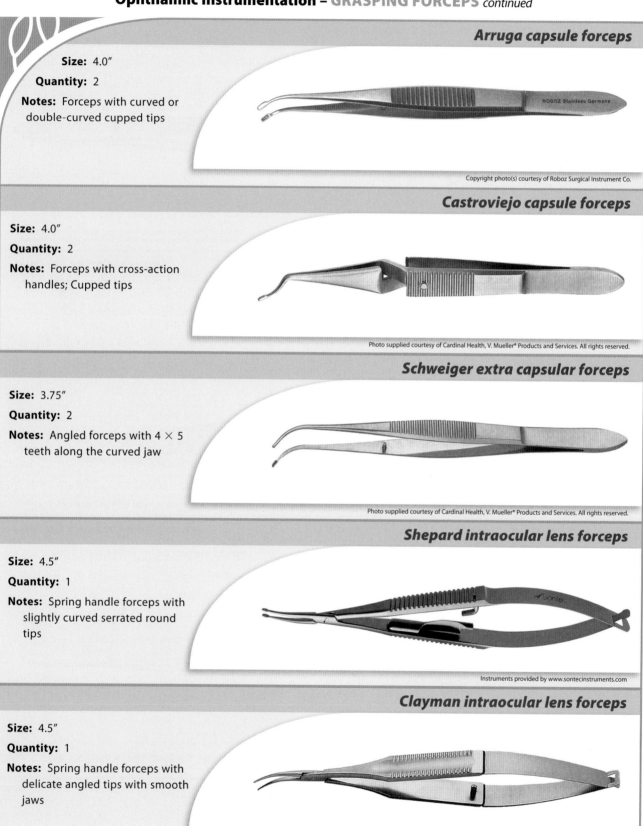

Arruga capsule forceps

Size: 4.0″

Quantity: 2

Notes: Forceps with curved or double-curved cupped tips

FIGURE 14-69

Castroviejo capsule forceps

Size: 4.0″

Quantity: 2

Notes: Forceps with cross-action handles; Cupped tips

FIGURE 14-70

Schweiger extra capsular forceps

Size: 3.75″

Quantity: 2

Notes: Angled forceps with 4 × 5 teeth along the curved jaw

FIGURE 14-71

Shepard intraocular lens forceps

Size: 4.5″

Quantity: 1

Notes: Spring handle forceps with slightly curved serrated round tips

FIGURE 14-72

Clayman intraocular lens forceps

Size: 4.5″

Quantity: 1

Notes: Spring handle forceps with delicate angled tips with smooth jaws

FIGURE 14-73

Ophthalmic Instrumentation – GRASPING FORCEPS *continued*

Littauer cilia forceps

Size: 3.5"

Quantity: 1

Notes: Forceps with 4 mm wide jaws and fine horizontal serrations

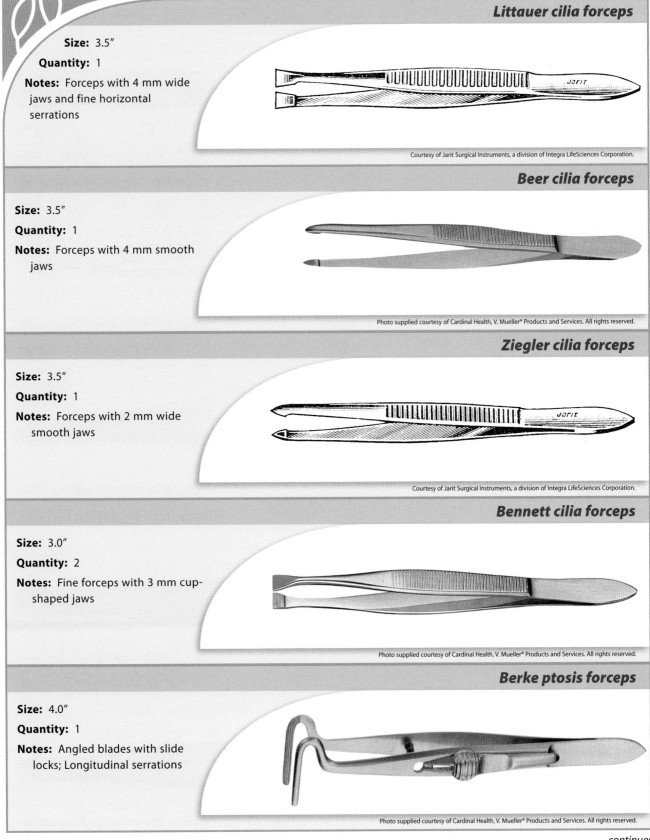

FIGURE 14-74

Beer cilia forceps

Size: 3.5"

Quantity: 1

Notes: Forceps with 4 mm smooth jaws

FIGURE 14-75

Ziegler cilia forceps

Size: 3.5"

Quantity: 1

Notes: Forceps with 2 mm wide smooth jaws

FIGURE 14-76

Bennett cilia forceps

Size: 3.0"

Quantity: 2

Notes: Fine forceps with 3 mm cup-shaped jaws

FIGURE 14-77

Berke ptosis forceps

Size: 4.0"

Quantity: 1

Notes: Angled blades with slide locks; Longitudinal serrations

FIGURE 14-78

continues

Ophthalmic Instrumentation – GRASPING FORCEPS *continued*

Erhardt lid forceps

Size: 3.5"

Quantity: 1

Notes: Flat lid plate with fine serrations and slide lock on fine toothed edge

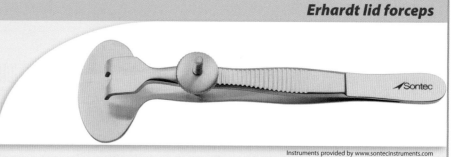

FIGURE 14-79

Lambert chalazion forceps

Size: 3.5"

Quantity: 1

Notes: Forceps with one solid plate and one round fenestrated ring; Screw lock

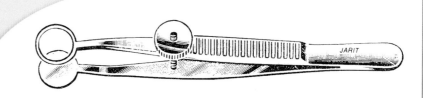

FIGURE 14-80

Wies chalazion forceps

Size: 4.0"

Quantity: 1

Notes: Forceps with one solid plate and one round fenestrated ring; Top angle of ring is flat; Screw lock

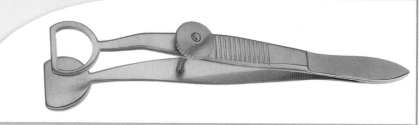

FIGURE 14-81

Desmarres chalazion forceps

Size: 3.5"

Quantity: 1

Notes: Forceps with one solid plate and one ovoid fenestrated ring; Screw lock

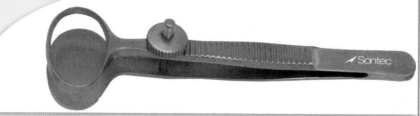

FIGURE 14-82

Prince trachoma forceps

Size: 3.5"

Quantity: 1

Notes: Forceps with two 8 × 10 mm fenestrated ovoid rings; No lock

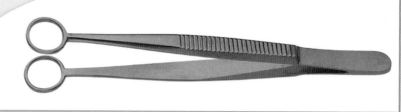

FIGURE 14-83

Ophthalmic Instrumentation – GRASPING FORCEPS *continued*

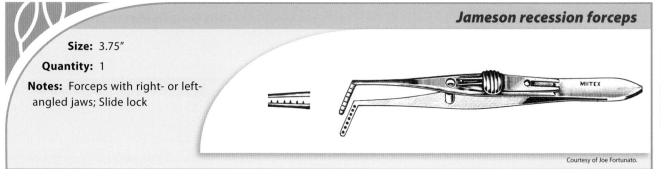

Jameson recession forceps

Size: 3.75″

Quantity: 1

Notes: Forceps with right- or left-angled jaws; Slide lock

FIGURE 14-84

Ophthalmic Instrumentation – DISSECTION INSTRUMENTS

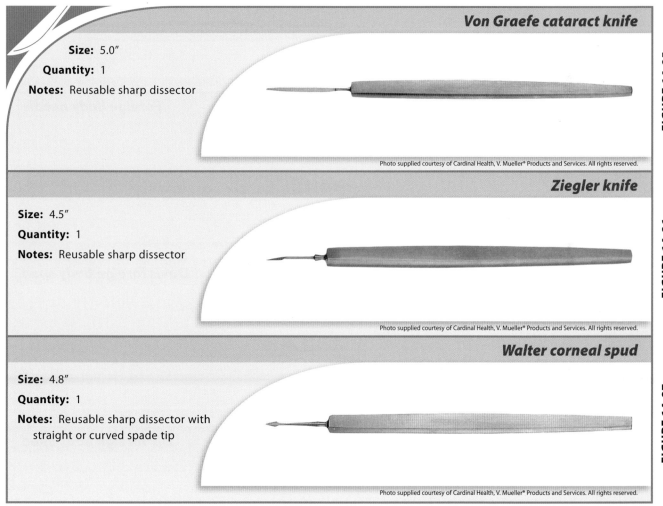

Von Graefe cataract knife

Size: 5.0″

Quantity: 1

Notes: Reusable sharp dissector

FIGURE 14-85

Ziegler knife

Size: 4.5″

Quantity: 1

Notes: Reusable sharp dissector

FIGURE 14-86

Walter corneal spud

Size: 4.8″

Quantity: 1

Notes: Reusable sharp dissector with straight or curved spade tip

FIGURE 14-87

continues

Ophthalmic Instrumentation – DISSECTION INSTRUMENTS *continued*

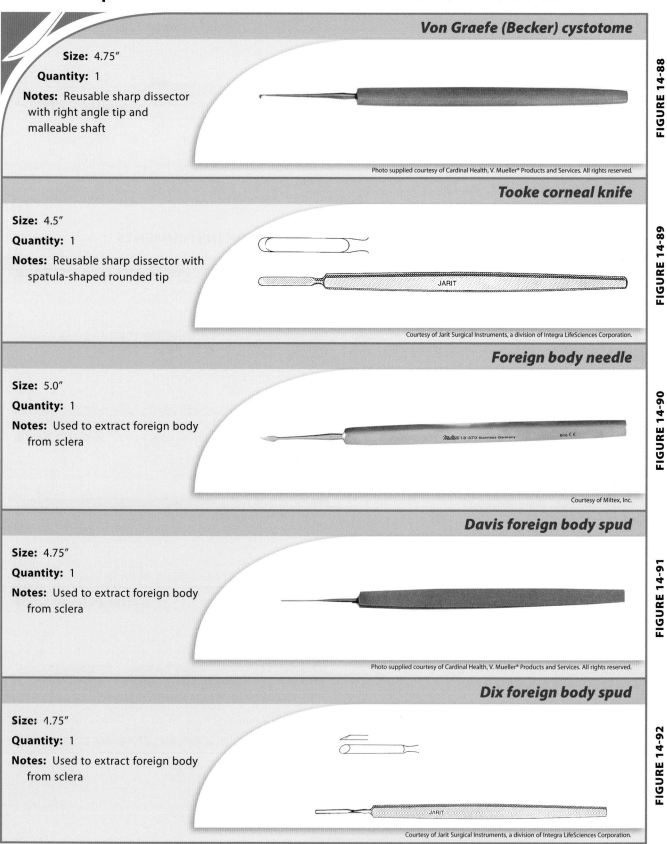

Von Graefe (Becker) cystotome

Size: 4.75″

Quantity: 1

Notes: Reusable sharp dissector with right angle tip and malleable shaft

FIGURE 14-88

Tooke corneal knife

Size: 4.5″

Quantity: 1

Notes: Reusable sharp dissector with spatula-shaped rounded tip

FIGURE 14-89

Foreign body needle

Size: 5.0″

Quantity: 1

Notes: Used to extract foreign body from sclera

FIGURE 14-90

Davis foreign body spud

Size: 4.75″

Quantity: 1

Notes: Used to extract foreign body from sclera

FIGURE 14-91

Dix foreign body spud

Size: 4.75″

Quantity: 1

Notes: Used to extract foreign body from sclera

FIGURE 14-92

Ophthalmic Instrumentation – DISSECTION INSTRUMENTS *continued*

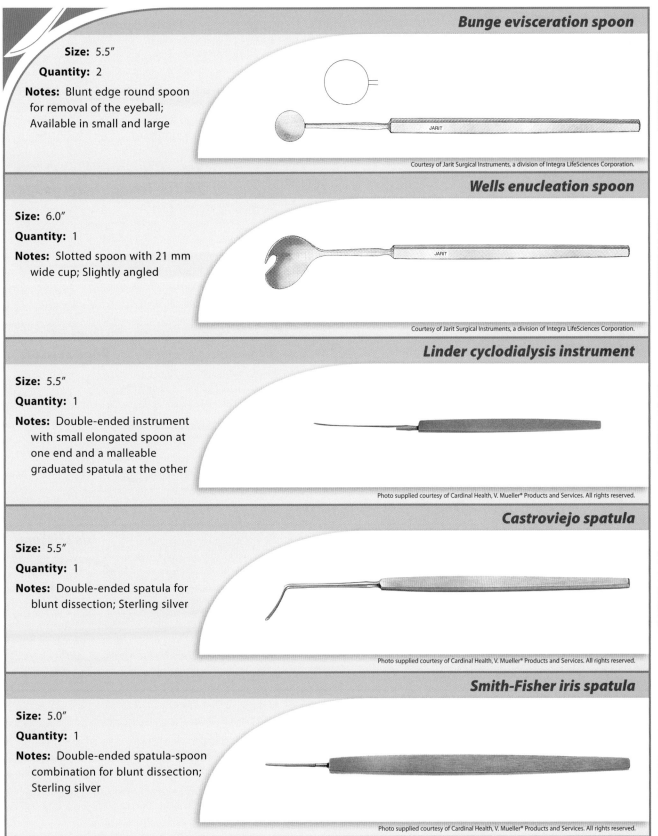

Bunge evisceration spoon

Size: 5.5″

Quantity: 2

Notes: Blunt edge round spoon for removal of the eyeball; Available in small and large

FIGURE 14-93

Wells enucleation spoon

Size: 6.0″

Quantity: 1

Notes: Slotted spoon with 21 mm wide cup; Slightly angled

FIGURE 14-94

Linder cyclodialysis instrument

Size: 5.5″

Quantity: 1

Notes: Double-ended instrument with small elongated spoon at one end and a malleable graduated spatula at the other

FIGURE 14-95

Castroviejo spatula

Size: 5.5″

Quantity: 1

Notes: Double-ended spatula for blunt dissection; Sterling silver

FIGURE 14-96

Smith-Fisher iris spatula

Size: 5.0″

Quantity: 1

Notes: Double-ended spatula-spoon combination for blunt dissection; Sterling silver

FIGURE 14-97

continues

Ophthalmic Instrumentation – DISSECTION INSTRUMENTS *continued*

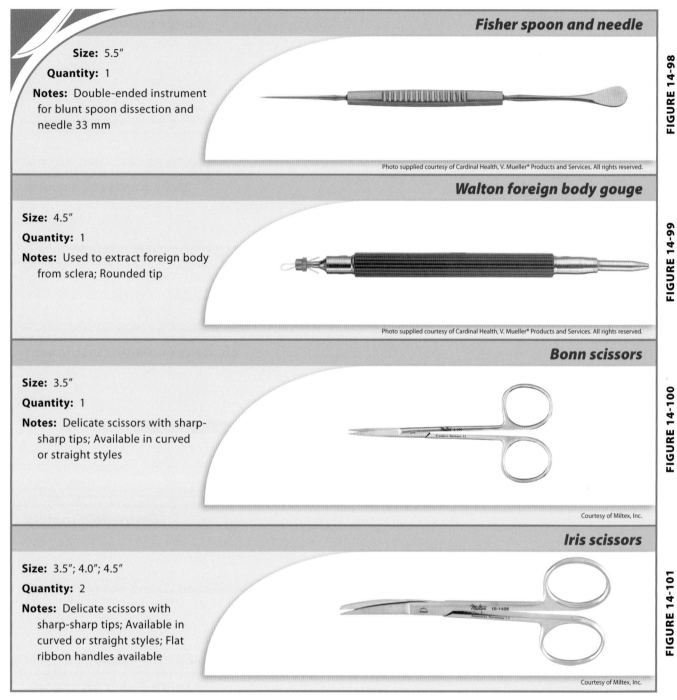

Fisher spoon and needle

Size: 5.5″

Quantity: 1

Notes: Double-ended instrument for blunt spoon dissection and needle 33 mm

FIGURE 14-98

Walton foreign body gouge

Size: 4.5″

Quantity: 1

Notes: Used to extract foreign body from sclera; Rounded tip

FIGURE 14-99

Bonn scissors

Size: 3.5″

Quantity: 1

Notes: Delicate scissors with sharp-sharp tips; Available in curved or straight styles

FIGURE 14-100

Iris scissors

Size: 3.5″; 4.0″; 4.5″

Quantity: 2

Notes: Delicate scissors with sharp-sharp tips; Available in curved or straight styles; Flat ribbon handles available

FIGURE 14-101

Ophthalmic Instrumentation – DISSECTION INSTRUMENTS *continued*

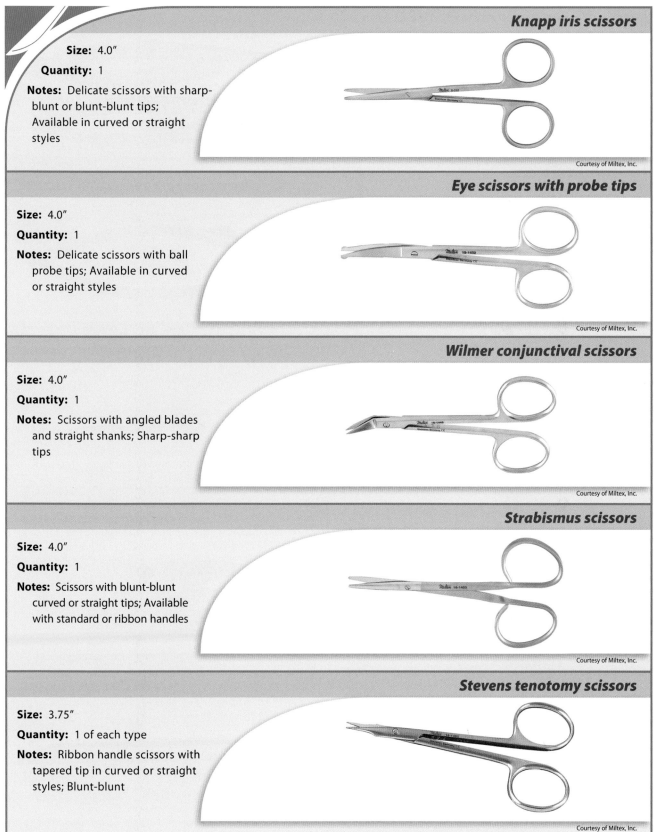

Knapp iris scissors

Size: 4.0"

Quantity: 1

Notes: Delicate scissors with sharp-blunt or blunt-blunt tips; Available in curved or straight styles

Courtesy of Miltex, Inc.

FIGURE 14-102

Eye scissors with probe tips

Size: 4.0"

Quantity: 1

Notes: Delicate scissors with ball probe tips; Available in curved or straight styles

Courtesy of Miltex, Inc.

FIGURE 14-103

Wilmer conjunctival scissors

Size: 4.0"

Quantity: 1

Notes: Scissors with angled blades and straight shanks; Sharp-sharp tips

Courtesy of Miltex, Inc.

FIGURE 14-104

Strabismus scissors

Size: 4.0"

Quantity: 1

Notes: Scissors with blunt-blunt curved or straight tips; Available with standard or ribbon handles

Courtesy of Miltex, Inc.

FIGURE 14-105

Stevens tenotomy scissors

Size: 3.75"

Quantity: 1 of each type

Notes: Ribbon handle scissors with tapered tip in curved or straight styles; Blunt-blunt

Courtesy of Miltex, Inc.

FIGURE 14-106

continues

Ophthalmic Instrumentation – DISSECTION INSTRUMENTS *continued*

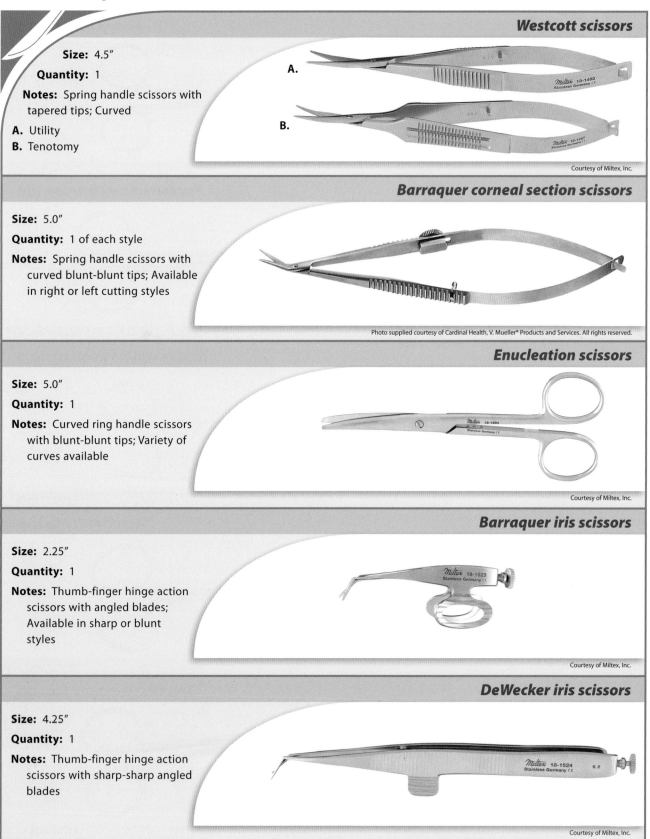

Westcott scissors

Size: 4.5"

Quantity: 1

Notes: Spring handle scissors with tapered tips; Curved

A. Utility

B. Tenotomy

Courtesy of Miltex, Inc.

FIGURE 14-107

Barraquer corneal section scissors

Size: 5.0"

Quantity: 1 of each style

Notes: Spring handle scissors with curved blunt-blunt tips; Available in right or left cutting styles

Photo supplied courtesy of Cardinal Health, V. Mueller® Products and Services. All rights reserved.

FIGURE 14-108

Enucleation scissors

Size: 5.0"

Quantity: 1

Notes: Curved ring handle scissors with blunt-blunt tips; Variety of curves available

Courtesy of Miltex, Inc.

FIGURE 14-109

Barraquer iris scissors

Size: 2.25"

Quantity: 1

Notes: Thumb-finger hinge action scissors with angled blades; Available in sharp or blunt styles

Courtesy of Miltex, Inc.

FIGURE 14-110

DeWecker iris scissors

Size: 4.25"

Quantity: 1

Notes: Thumb-finger hinge action scissors with sharp-sharp angled blades

Courtesy of Miltex, Inc.

FIGURE 14-111

Ophthalmic Instrumentation – DISSECTION INSTRUMENTS *continued*

Noyes iridectomy scissors

Size: 5.5″

Quantity: 1

Notes: Straight scissors with adapted spring handle; Sharp-sharp

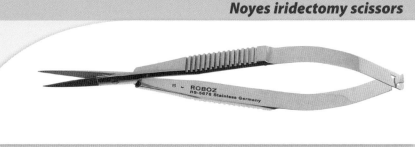

Copyright photo(s) courtesy of Roboz Surgical Instrument Co.

FIGURE 14-112

McClure iris scissors

Size: 3.75″

Quantity: 1

Notes: Spring handle scissors with side-angled sharp-sharp blades

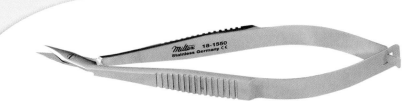

Courtesy of Miltex, Inc.

FIGURE 14-113

McGuire corneal scissors

Size: 4.12″

Quantity: 1

Notes: Ring handle scissors with double curve tips; Blunt-blunt; Available in right and left styles

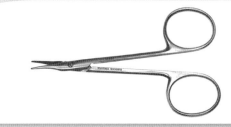

Copyright photo(s) courtesy of Roboz Surgical Instrument Co.

FIGURE 14-114

Aebli corneal scissors

Size: 4.0″

Quantity: 1

Notes: Ring handle scissors with side-angled tapered tips; Blunt-blunt; Available in right and left styles

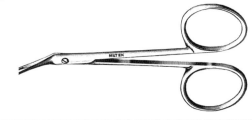

Courtesy of Joe Fortunato.

FIGURE 14-115

Vannas capsulotomy scissors

Size: 3.25″

Quantity: 1

Notes: Spring handle scissors with sharp-sharp tips; Available in curved or angled styles

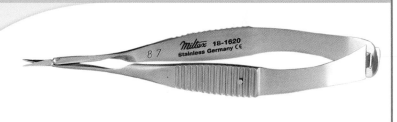

Courtesy of Miltex, Inc.

FIGURE 14-116

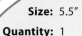

Ophthalmic Instrumentation – DEBULKING INSTRUMENTS

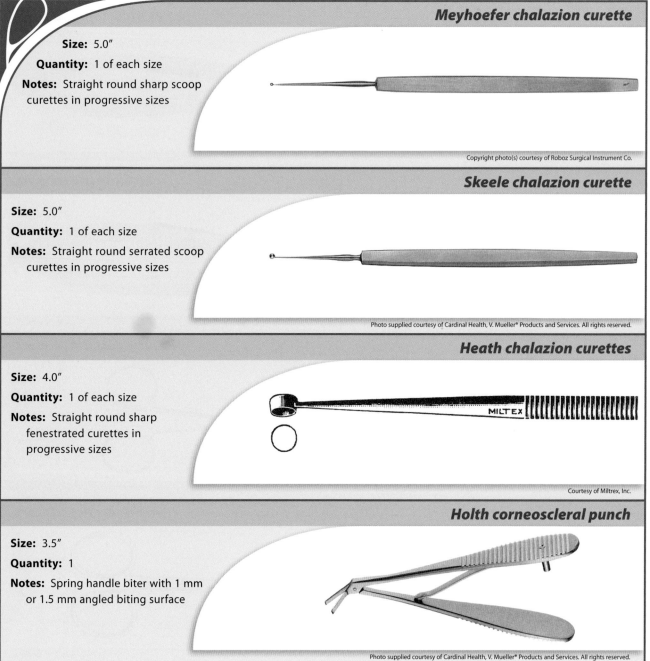

Meyhoefer chalazion curette

Size: 5.0"

Quantity: 1 of each size

Notes: Straight round sharp scoop curettes in progressive sizes

FIGURE 14-117

Skeele chalazion curette

Size: 5.0"

Quantity: 1 of each size

Notes: Straight round serrated scoop curettes in progressive sizes

FIGURE 14-118

Heath chalazion curettes

Size: 4.0"

Quantity: 1 of each size

Notes: Straight round sharp fenestrated curettes in progressive sizes

MILTEX

FIGURE 14-119

Holth corneoscleral punch

Size: 3.5"

Quantity: 1

Notes: Spring handle biter with 1 mm or 1.5 mm angled biting surface

FIGURE 14-120

Ophthalmic Instrumentation – HOOKS AND DILATORS

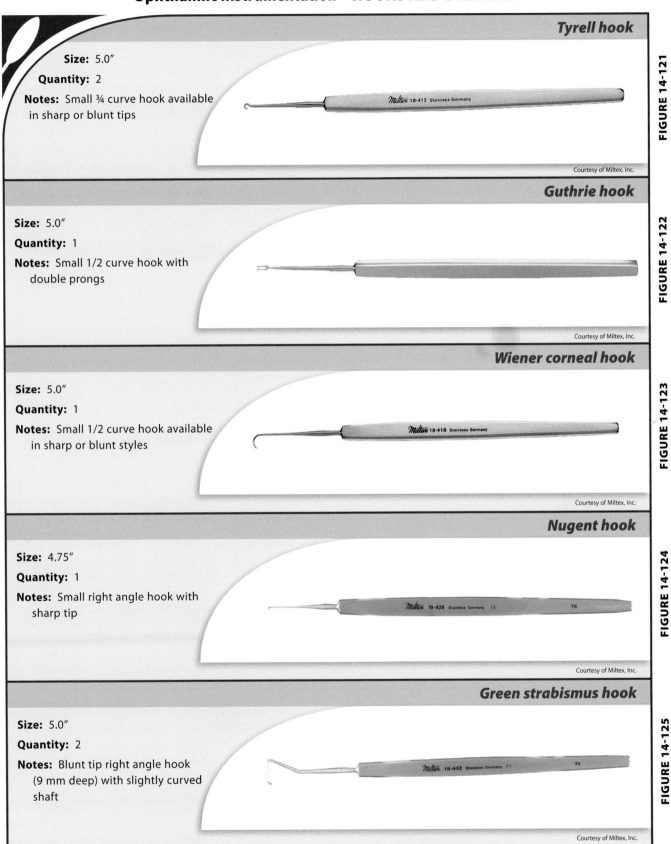

Tyrell hook

Size: 5.0"

Quantity: 2

Notes: Small ¾ curve hook available in sharp or blunt tips

Courtesy of Miltex, Inc.

FIGURE 14-121

Guthrie hook

Size: 5.0"

Quantity: 1

Notes: Small 1/2 curve hook with double prongs

Courtesy of Miltex, Inc.

FIGURE 14-122

Wiener corneal hook

Size: 5.0"

Quantity: 1

Notes: Small 1/2 curve hook available in sharp or blunt styles

Courtesy of Miltex, Inc.

FIGURE 14-123

Nugent hook

Size: 4.75"

Quantity: 1

Notes: Small right angle hook with sharp tip

Courtesy of Miltex, Inc.

FIGURE 14-124

Green strabismus hook

Size: 5.0"

Quantity: 2

Notes: Blunt tip right angle hook (9 mm deep) with slightly curved shaft

Courtesy of Miltex, Inc.

FIGURE 14-125

continues

Ophthalmic Instrumentation – HOOKS AND DILATORS *continued*

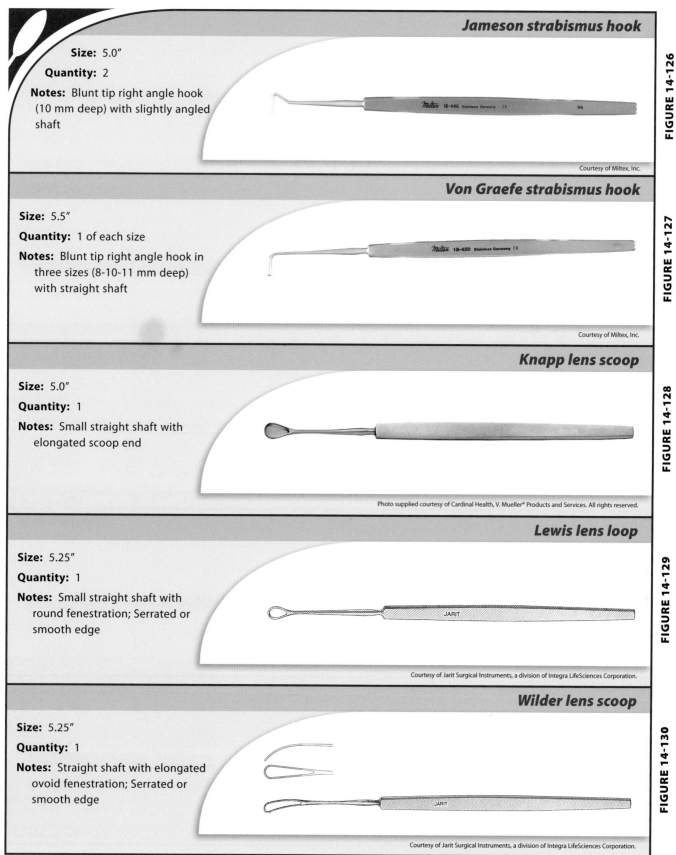

Jameson strabismus hook

Size: 5.0"

Quantity: 2

Notes: Blunt tip right angle hook (10 mm deep) with slightly angled shaft

Courtesy of Miltex, Inc.

FIGURE 14-126

Von Graefe strabismus hook

Size: 5.5"

Quantity: 1 of each size

Notes: Blunt tip right angle hook in three sizes (8-10-11 mm deep) with straight shaft

Courtesy of Miltex, Inc.

FIGURE 14-127

Knapp lens scoop

Size: 5.0"

Quantity: 1

Notes: Small straight shaft with elongated scoop end

Photo supplied courtesy of Cardinal Health, V. Mueller® Products and Services. All rights reserved.

FIGURE 14-128

Lewis lens loop

Size: 5.25"

Quantity: 1

Notes: Small straight shaft with round fenestration; Serrated or smooth edge

Courtesy of Jarit Surgical Instruments, a division of Integra LifeSciences Corporation.

FIGURE 14-129

Wilder lens scoop

Size: 5.25"

Quantity: 1

Notes: Straight shaft with elongated ovoid fenestration; Serrated or smooth edge

Courtesy of Jarit Surgical Instruments, a division of Integra LifeSciences Corporation.

FIGURE 14-130

Ophthalmic Instrumentation – HOOKS AND DILATORS *continued*

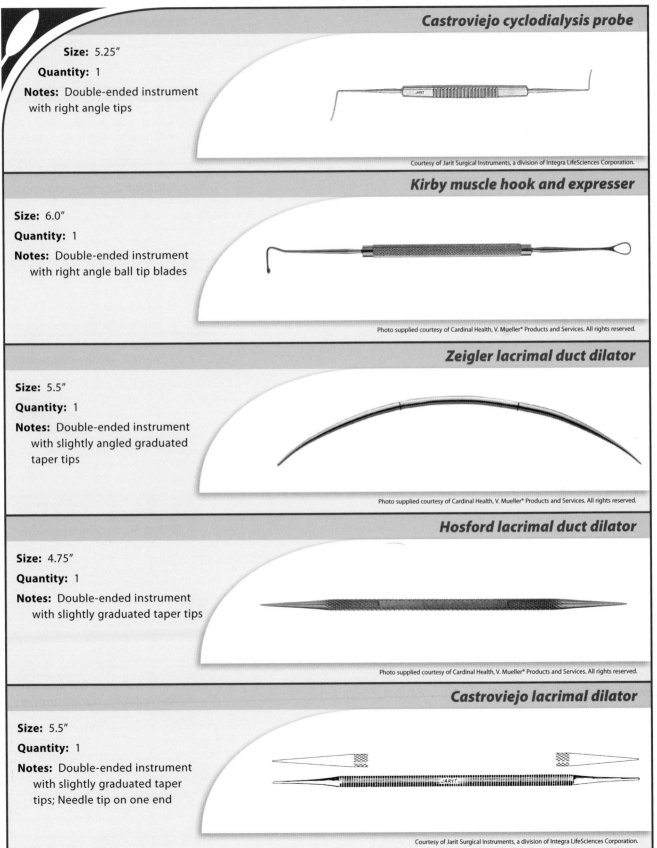

Castroviejo cyclodialysis probe

Size: 5.25″

Quantity: 1

Notes: Double-ended instrument with right angle tips

FIGURE 14-131

Kirby muscle hook and expresser

Size: 6.0″

Quantity: 1

Notes: Double-ended instrument with right angle ball tip blades

FIGURE 14-132

Zeigler lacrimal duct dilator

Size: 5.5″

Quantity: 1

Notes: Double-ended instrument with slightly angled graduated taper tips

FIGURE 14-133

Hosford lacrimal duct dilator

Size: 4.75″

Quantity: 1

Notes: Double-ended instrument with slightly graduated taper tips

FIGURE 14-134

Castroviejo lacrimal dilator

Size: 5.5″

Quantity: 1

Notes: Double-ended instrument with slightly graduated taper tips; Needle tip on one end

FIGURE 14-135

continues

Ophthalmic Instrumentation – HOOKS AND DILATORS *continued*

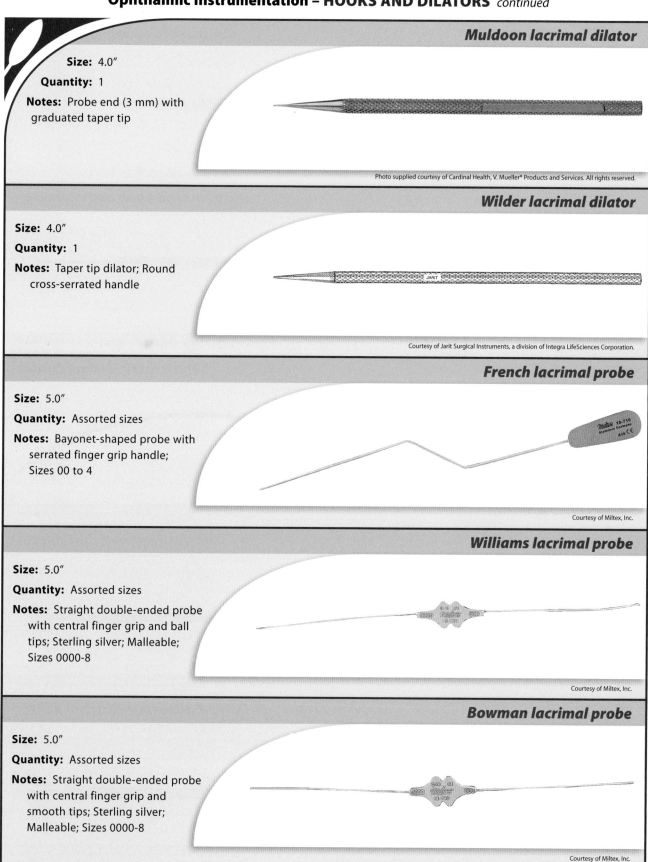

Muldoon lacrimal dilator

Size: 4.0"

Quantity: 1

Notes: Probe end (3 mm) with graduated taper tip

FIGURE 14-136

Wilder lacrimal dilator

Size: 4.0"

Quantity: 1

Notes: Taper tip dilator; Round cross-serrated handle

FIGURE 14-137

French lacrimal probe

Size: 5.0"

Quantity: Assorted sizes

Notes: Bayonet-shaped probe with serrated finger grip handle; Sizes 00 to 4

FIGURE 14-138

Williams lacrimal probe

Size: 5.0"

Quantity: Assorted sizes

Notes: Straight double-ended probe with central finger grip and ball tips; Sterling silver; Malleable; Sizes 0000-8

FIGURE 14-139

Bowman lacrimal probe

Size: 5.0"

Quantity: Assorted sizes

Notes: Straight double-ended probe with central finger grip and smooth tips; Sterling silver; Malleable; Sizes 0000-8

FIGURE 14-140

Ophthalmic Instrumentation – RETRACTION AND EXPOSURE INSTRUMENTS

Lancaster speculum

Size: 3.25″

Quantity: 1

Notes: Self-retaining spring retractor with screw lock and solid blades; Slightly angled

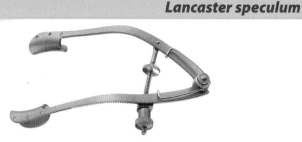

FIGURE 14-141

Knapp speculum

Size: 3.25″

Quantity: 1

Notes: Self-retaining spring retractor with screw lock and fenestrated blades; Slightly curved

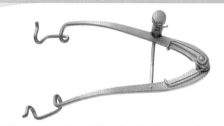

FIGURE 14-142

Castroviejo speculum

Size: 4.0″; 3.75″

Quantity: 1

Notes: Self-retaining retractor with screw-adjusted lock and fenestrated blades; Slightly angled; Available in small, medium, and large

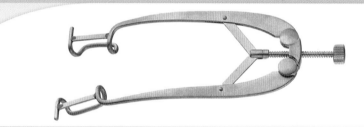

FIGURE 14-143

Lange speculum

Size: 3.75″

Quantity: 1

Notes: Self-retaining retractor with screw-adjusted lock and solid blades; Slightly angled

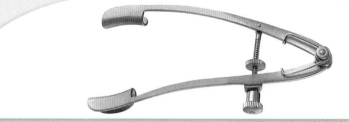

FIGURE 14-144

Williams speculum

Size: 3.25″; 2.75″

Quantity: 1

Notes: Self-retaining retractor with screw-adjusted lock and fenestrated blades; Slightly angled; Available in small and large

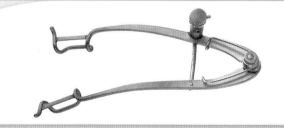

FIGURE 14-145

continues

Ophthalmic Instrumentation – RETRACTION AND EXPOSURE INSTRUMENTS *continued*

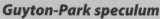

Guyton-Park speculum

Size: 3.5"

Quantity: 1

Notes: Self-retaining retractor with three solid or fenestrated blades and screw-adjusted lock; Slightly angled; Superior angle of blade has vertical suture posts for tying traction suture

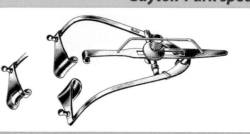

FIGURE 14-146

Maumee-Park speculum

Size: 3.5"

Quantity: 1

Notes: Self-retaining retractor with three solid blades and screw-adjusted lock; Slightly angled; Superior angle of blade has vertical suture posts for tying traction suture

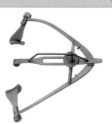

FIGURE 14-147

Barraquer speculum

Size: 1.75"

Quantity: 1

Notes: Spring style self-retaining retractor with simple wire blades; Available in small and large sizes

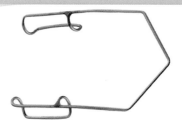

FIGURE 14-148

Sauer speculum

Size: 1.25"

Quantity: 1

Notes: Infant size self-retaining retractor with solid blades and ratchets

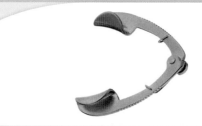

FIGURE 14-149

Murdock speculum

Size: 2.25"

Quantity: 1

Notes: Self-retaining retractor with fenestrated blades and slide lock

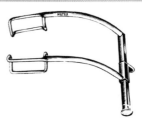

FIGURE 14-150

Ophthalmic Instrumentation – RETRACTION AND EXPOSURE INSTRUMENTS *continued*

McKinney speculum

Size: 2.12″

Quantity: 1

Notes: Self-retaining retractor with fenestrated blades and slide lock

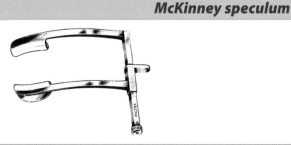

Courtesy of Joe Fortunato.

FIGURE 14-151

Cooke speculum

Size: 1.8″

Quantity: 1

Notes: Self-retaining retractor with fenestrated blades and slide screw lock; Infant and small child sized

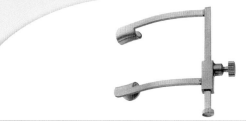

Photo supplied courtesy of Cardinal Health, V. Mueller® Products and Services. All rights reserved.

FIGURE 14-152

Mellinger speculum

Size: 2.75″

Quantity: 1

Notes: Self-retaining retractor with fenestrated or solid blades and slide ratchet lock

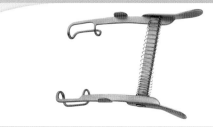

Photo supplied courtesy of Cardinal Health, V. Mueller® Products and Services. All rights reserved.

FIGURE 14-153

Agricola lacrimal retractor

Size: 1.5″

Quantity: 1

Notes: 3 × 3 pointed prongs on spring style self-retaining retractor

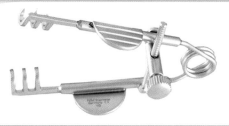

Courtesy of Miltex, Inc.

FIGURE 14-154

Meller lacrimal speculum

Size: 1.12″

Quantity: 1

Notes: 3 × 3 prongs; Spring style self-retaining retractor with screw lock

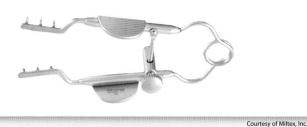

Courtesy of Miltex, Inc.

FIGURE 14-155

continues

Ophthalmic Instrumentation – RETRACTION AND EXPOSURE INSTRUMENTS *continued*

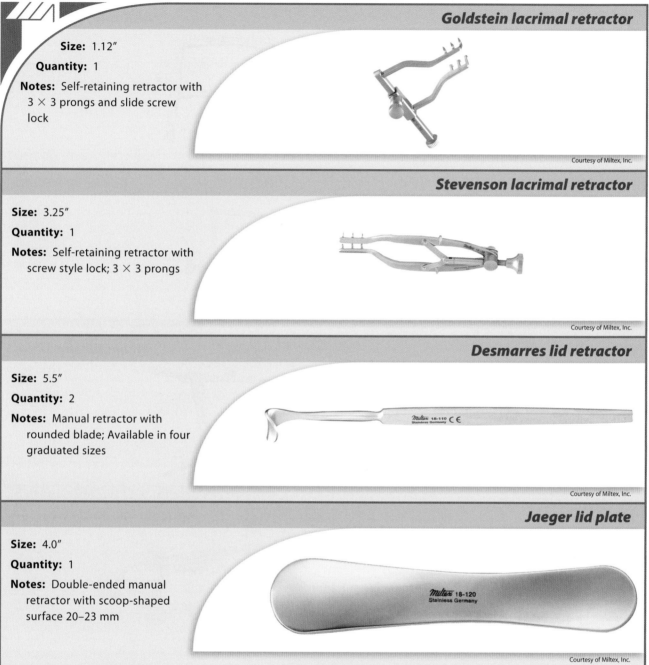

Goldstein lacrimal retractor

Size: 1.12"

Quantity: 1

Notes: Self-retaining retractor with 3 × 3 prongs and slide screw lock

Courtesy of Miltex, Inc.

FIGURE 14-156

Stevenson lacrimal retractor

Size: 3.25"

Quantity: 1

Notes: Self-retaining retractor with screw style lock; 3 × 3 prongs

Courtesy of Miltex, Inc.

FIGURE 14-157

Desmarres lid retractor

Size: 5.5"

Quantity: 2

Notes: Manual retractor with rounded blade; Available in four graduated sizes

Courtesy of Miltex, Inc.

FIGURE 14-158

Jaeger lid plate

Size: 4.0"

Quantity: 1

Notes: Double-ended manual retractor with scoop-shaped surface 20–23 mm

Courtesy of Miltex, Inc.

FIGURE 14-159

Ophthalmic Instrumentation – APPROXIMATION AND CLOSURE INSTRUMENTS

Kalt needle holder

Size: 5.25"

Quantity: 1

Notes: Adapted spring handle needle holder with one longer shank; Thumb pressure lock

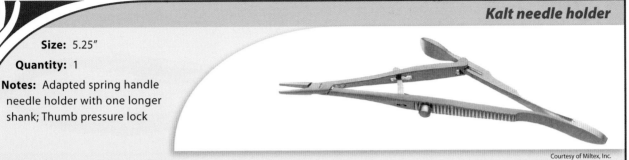

Courtesy of Miltex, Inc.

FIGURE 14-160

Green needle holder

Size: 4.25"

Quantity: 1

Notes: Spring handle needle holder with angled serrated jaws; No lock

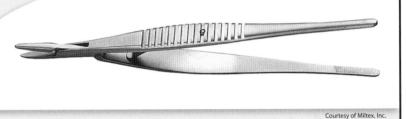

Courtesy of Miltex, Inc.

FIGURE 14-161

Castroviejo needle holder

Size: 5.5"

Quantity: Assorted sizes

Notes: Spring flat handle needle holder with curved delicate jaws; Available in curved or straight jaws; Locking or non-locking

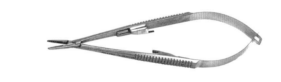

Courtesy of Miltex, Inc.

FIGURE 14-162

Paton needle holder

Size: 4.5"

Quantity: 1

Notes: Spring flat handle needle holder with straight jaws; No lock

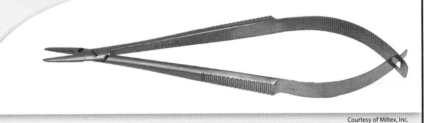

Courtesy of Miltex, Inc.

FIGURE 14-163

McPherson needle holder

Size: 4.0"

Quantity: 1

Notes: Spring flat handle needle holder with curved tapered jaws; Locking

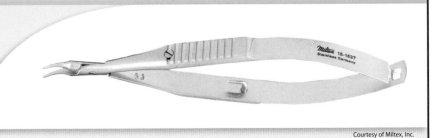

Courtesy of Miltex, Inc.

FIGURE 14-164

continues

Ophthalmic Instrumentation – APPROXIMATION AND CLOSURE INSTRUMENTS *continued*

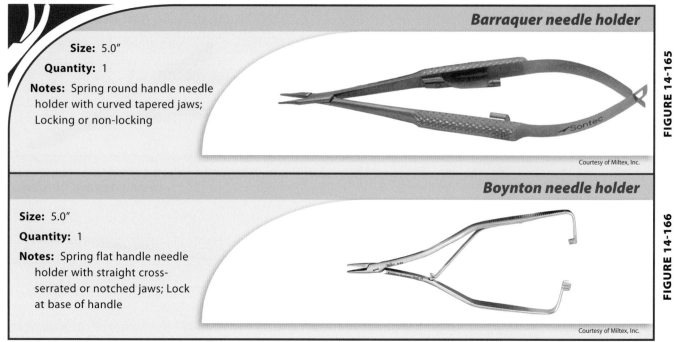

Barraquer needle holder

Size: 5.0"

Quantity: 1

Notes: Spring round handle needle holder with curved tapered jaws; Locking or non-locking

Courtesy of Miltex, Inc.

FIGURE 14-165

Boynton needle holder

Size: 5.0"

Quantity: 1

Notes: Spring flat handle needle holder with straight cross-serrated or notched jaws; Lock at base of handle

Courtesy of Miltex, Inc.

FIGURE 14-166

Ophthalmic Instrumentation – SPECIALTY SPECIFIC INSTRUMENTS

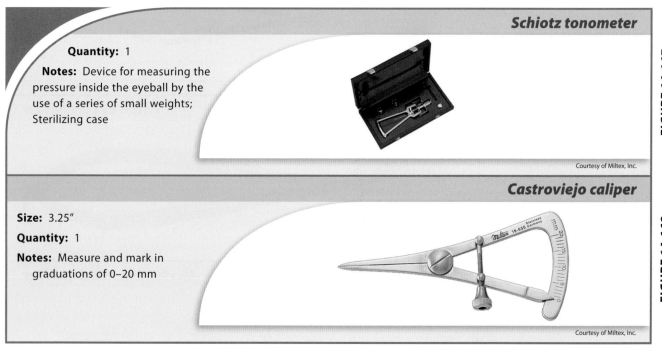

Schiotz tonometer

Quantity: 1

Notes: Device for measuring the pressure inside the eyeball by the use of a series of small weights; Sterilizing case

Courtesy of Miltex, Inc.

FIGURE 14-167

Castroviejo caliper

Size: 3.25"

Quantity: 1

Notes: Measure and mark in graduations of 0–20 mm

Courtesy of Miltex, Inc.

FIGURE 14-168

Ophthalmic Instrumentation – SPECIALTY SPECIFIC INSTRUMENTS *continued*

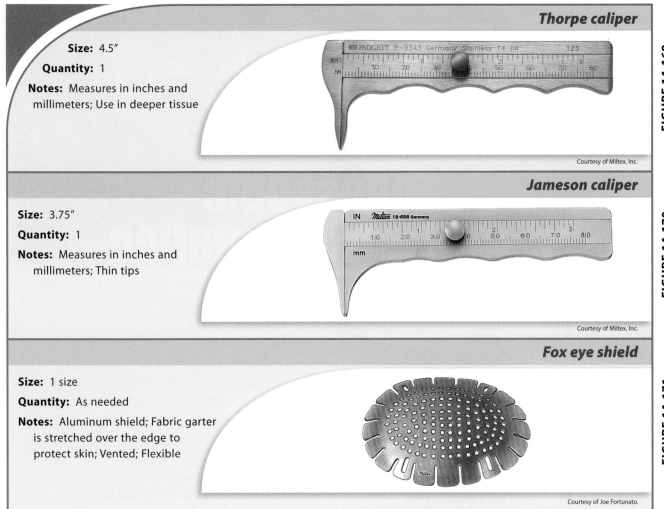

Thorpe caliper

Size: 4.5″

Quantity: 1

Notes: Measures in inches and millimeters; Use in deeper tissue

Courtesy of Miltex, Inc.

FIGURE 14-169

Jameson caliper

Size: 3.75″

Quantity: 1

Notes: Measures in inches and millimeters; Thin tips

Courtesy of Miltex, Inc.

FIGURE 14-170

Fox eye shield

Size: 1 size

Quantity: As needed

Notes: Aluminum shield; Fabric garter is stretched over the edge to protect skin; Vented; Flexible

Courtesy of Joe Fortunato.

FIGURE 14-171

SUMMARY

Many surgical procedures can be performed microscopically. Each procedure has its own inherent intricacies and complexities. Microscopic surgery requires high levels of experience and anatomic knowledge in the scrub person. The eye-hand coordination and dexterity necessary for the scrub person to develop takes many months or sometimes years to master.

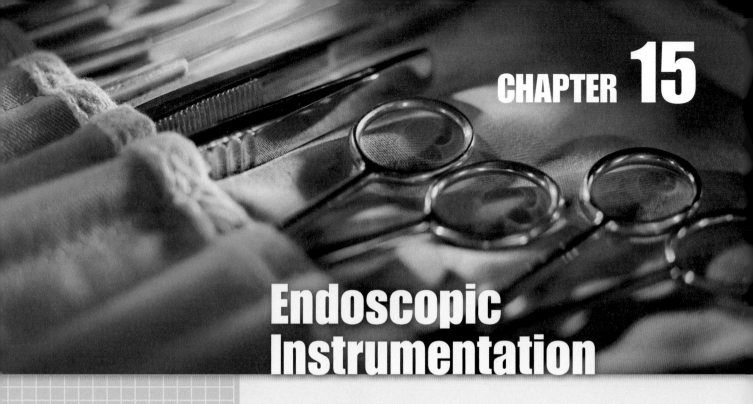

CHAPTER **15**

Endoscopic Instrumentation

INTRODUCTION

All endoscopy, regardless of whether entering the body through the skin or natural orifice, has several common practices that enable the surgeon to successfully perform the procedure. The absence of any one of these activities causes an alteration in the surgical endoscopic process that prevents successful completion. Failure to meet each endoscopic process criterion can result in the need for conversion to an open conventional procedure. This is not always easy to accomplish in an efficient manner because the instrumentation for an open procedure is significantly different and the set-up requires different equipment and supplies. The patient may need to be repositioned, reprepped, and redraped. Patient safety is a serious issue because the dispersive electrode can shift, causing electrical injury and lost instrumentation or sponges. In addition, the haste of the process may create an increased margin of error which is well documented in the literature concerning retained surgical instruments. Great care is taken to prevent injury to the patient and personnel.

METHODS OF ENDOSCOPIC ACCESS

Endoscopy can be performed through a percutaneous puncture through the skin or by a non-puncture method through a natural body orifice. Both methods employ an expansion medium to create a working space, instruments for manipulation and capture, evacuation of the expansion medium, and closure of the surgical site.

Percutaneous Endoscopy Procedures

Percutaneous endoscopic procedures require the use of a soft tissue foundation set to open the outer layers of skin for the introduction of the Veress needle and trocars and the closure of the tissue layers at the completion of the procedure.

The procedural process involves having several sizes of trocars inserted percutaneously through the skin to allow for placement of telescopes and other working instruments. The trocar is a two-part instrument that incorporates an outer sleeve and inner obturator that can be sharp or blunt. After placement of the trocar instrument, the inner obturator is removed and placed on the Mayo stand and the outer sleeve remains in place to form a channel for insertion of various endoscopic viewing and working instruments.

Non-Puncture Endoscopy

Non-puncture endoscopy requires the use of a viewing instrument with an incorporated working channel for graspers and dissectors. In colon resection open and percutaneous procedures, the surgeon may use an additional non-puncture sigmoidoscope inserted through the rectum to assess the anastomosis.

CREATION AND EVACUATION OF A WORKING SPACE

Endoscopic procedures require a proportionate working space wherein to accomplish the surgical tasks. Percutaneous punctures of the abdomen create a working space with insufflated carbon dioxide with a spring-loaded Luer lock Veress needle. This procedure is referred to as laparoscopy. The surgeon will use a scalpel with a small #15 or #11 blade to make an incision of 0.5 cm to place the Veress needle. The Veress needle is a sharp beveled cannula with a blunt retractable obturator that cuts through tissue layers as the surgeon presses it through the tissues. The obturator projects after each tissue layer is passed to prevent a sharps injury to non-target tissue. The insufflation tubing is attached to the Luer lock on the Veress needle and gas is infused to expand the peritoneal cavity.

The carbon dioxide is not harmful in a chemical sense because the body is well equipped to diffuse the gas across the peritoneal membrane and dispose of it through the lungs. Pressures of the insufflated gas are monitored by special sensors in the insufflation machine to prevent overdistention of the peritoneal cavity. If a disturbance of the gas flow occurs, the machine will alarm to alert the circulating nurse to adjust the pressure or troubleshoot the cause.

The gas is turned off briefly when the space is sufficiently expanded. The surgeon will slightly enlarge the incision with the scalpel and introduce the trocar assembly into the patient's abdomen. The gas tubing is disconnected from the Veress needle and attached to the trocar inflow port. The gas is restarted and flows sufficiently enough to maintain the desired volume of expansion for creation of the working space. The gas should be evacuated through the suction port at the end of the case. The carbon dioxide is considered a biologic contaminant and should not be released into the room air. Aerosolization could cause biologic material to come in contact with the skin or mucous membranes of the team.

Percutaneous puncture endoscopy through a joint capsule such as in arthroscopy requires the creation of a working space with infused fluid. The fluid is evacuated through an exit portal on the trocar to prevent overdistention of the capsule.

Endoscopy through a natural body orifice requires a working space as well. The oropharyngeal, nasal, aural, and bronchotracheal cavities are framed in native cartilaginous scaffolds and do not require an additional substrate or gas to create room to work. Other entrance areas such as the esophagus or rectum require the surgeon to use an insufflation bulb to separate collapsible tissue walls. This creates a working space by pumping in small amounts of ambient air, which is readily removed by suction.

Intrauterine and bladder working space is created by the instillation of solution. Exit portals permit the constant controlled evacuation of the expanded cavity to prevent overdistention or abnormal absorption. Volume instillation and evacuation ratios are continuously measured and recorded by the circulating nurse. Rectal endoscopy uses room air delivered by bulb hand pumps or an insufflation-suction machine to create the working space by separating the walls of the bowel. Size-appropriate rigid or flexible working instrumentation are passed through channels in the body of the scope for manipulation of tissue.

ILLUMINATION AND VISUALIZATION

When the endoscopic access and working space are established, the surgeon will need to illuminate the expanded cavity with a light source and utilize a viewing telescope with a rigid or flexible telescopic lens or by direct vision. Some endoscopes utilize eyepiece couplers that attach to a camera video system that displays the surgical site on a high resolution monitor. This allows all members of the team to observe the procedure.

An external electrical light source supplies illumination through a fiberoptic cable attached to the telescope or through a metal light pipe inserted through the side of a rigid hollow scope. Fiberoptic cables have a series of glass tubes that deliver light to the field. Care is taken not to tightly flex the tubing because the fibers will break, preventing the transfer of light to the scope. The cable can be tested under sterile conditions during the sterile set-up procedure by holding one end of the cable up in the direction of the room light and simultaneously looking at the glow from the opposite end. The glowing end will look peppered with black spots if glass fibers are broken within the cable. Excessive black spots indicate that the cable may not deliver enough light to perform the procedure adequately.

The illuminated fiberoptic cable can radiate enough heat during the procedure to cause the drapes to smolder or burn if permitted to lay unattended. The cable should be attached to the telescope at all times when the power is on. Some light sources are considered "cooler" and pose less of a fire hazard.

MANIPULATION AND PROCEDURAL TASKS

Assorted clamps, graspers, dissectors, and other tissue manipulators can be introduced into the patient through additional trocars or working channels in the main trocar. The specimen can be extracted through the trocar.

ENDOSCOPY THROUGH THE SKIN

Laparoscopy

Laparoscopy refers to the percutaneous entry into the abdominal or pelvic cavity. The procedural steps are performed within the peritoneal sac. Percutaneous procedures of the trunk involving the extraperitoneal or retroperitoneal spaces or thorax utilize different instrumentation and are described later in this chapter.

Endoscopic Percutaneous Access – SPECIALTY SPECIFIC INSTRUMENTS

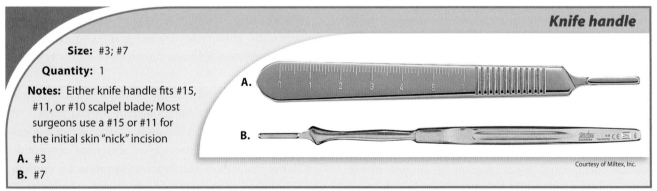

Knife handle

Size: #3; #7

Quantity: 1

Notes: Either knife handle fits #15, #11, or #10 scalpel blade; Most surgeons use a #15 or #11 for the initial skin "nick" incision

A. #3
B. #7

A.

B.

Courtesy of Miltex, Inc.

FIGURE 15-1

Endoscopic Percutaneous Access – SPECIALTY SPECIFIC INSTRUMENTS *continued*

Trocar with sleeve

Size: 5–13 mm diameter

Notes: Obturator can be blunt for open laparoscopy or sharp for puncture laparoscopy

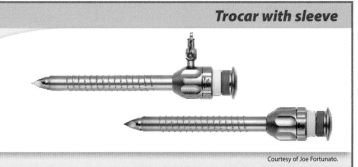

Courtesy of Joe Fortunato.

FIGURE 15-2

Reduction sleeve and reducer caps

Size: 6 to 13 mm

Quantity: Several as needed

Notes: A smaller sleeve can be seated inside a larger sheath after the access portal is inserted into the patient; The small sleeve accommodates a narrow instrument in a larger opening without permitting loss of gas

A. Reducer sleeve
B. Reducer cap

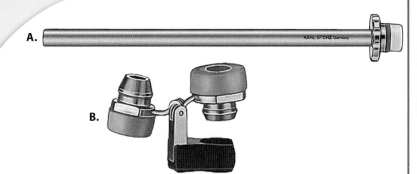

© Karl Storz Endoscopy America, Inc.

FIGURE 15-3

Thread sleeve

Size: 6 to 13 mm

Quantity: 1 for each access portal

Notes: A threaded outer cannula placed over the trocar and sleeve assembly before placement into the patient's abdomen secures and anchors the sleeve

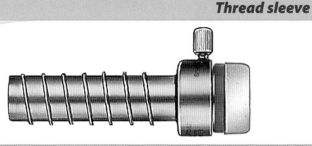

© Karl Storz Endoscopy America, Inc.

FIGURE 15-4

continues

Endoscopic Percutaneous Access – SPECIALTY SPECIFIC INSTRUMENTS *continued*

Blunt trocar with sleeve

Size: 7 mm; 11 mm

Quantity: 1

Notes: Initial pneumoperitoneum is created with this trocar and sleeve assembly; The procedure is referred to as "open laparoscopy;" No Veress needle is used; Carbon dioxide gas is insufflated after the trocar assembly is inserted through the patient's abdomen; Device can be sutured into place. Conical stopper prevents gas leakage; It is sometimes known as Hasson trocar; Reusable styles are completely disassembled for cleaning and steam sterilization; Disposable styles are commercially available

© Karl Storz Endoscopy America, Inc.

FIGURE 15-5

Tissue retractors "S" shape

Size: 1 size

Quantity: 2

Notes: Used to facilitate insertion of blunt insufflation trocar and sleeve assembly

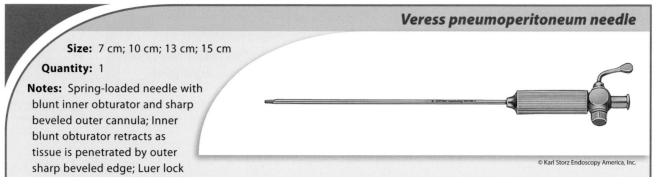

© Karl Storz Endoscopy America, Inc.

FIGURE 15-6

Creation of the Working Space – SPECIALTY SPECIFIC INSTRUMENTS

Veress pneumoperitoneum needle

Size: 7 cm; 10 cm; 13 cm; 15 cm

Quantity: 1

Notes: Spring-loaded needle with blunt inner obturator and sharp beveled outer cannula; Inner blunt obturator retracts as tissue is penetrated by outer sharp beveled edge; Luer lock end with stopcock for connection and control of carbon dioxide gas insufflation tubing; Reusable styles are steam sterilized and disassembled; Disposable styles are commercially available

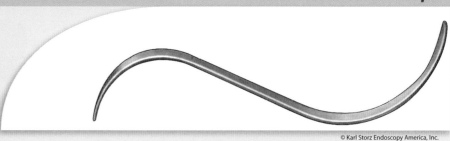

© Karl Storz Endoscopy America, Inc.

FIGURE 15-7

Illumination and Visualization – SPECIALTY SPECIFIC INSTRUMENTS

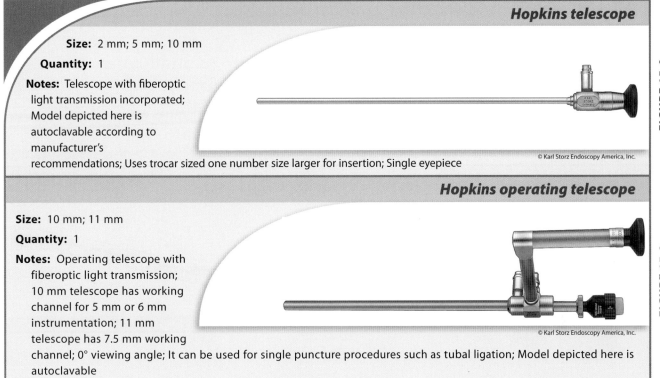

Hopkins telescope

Size: 2 mm; 5 mm; 10 mm

Quantity: 1

Notes: Telescope with fiberoptic light transmission incorporated; Model depicted here is autoclavable according to manufacturer's recommendations; Uses trocar sized one number size larger for insertion; Single eyepiece

© Karl Storz Endoscopy America, Inc.

FIGURE 15-8

Hopkins operating telescope

Size: 10 mm; 11 mm

Quantity: 1

Notes: Operating telescope with fiberoptic light transmission; 10 mm telescope has working channel for 5 mm or 6 mm instrumentation; 11 mm telescope has 7.5 mm working channel; 0° viewing angle; It can be used for single puncture procedures such as tubal ligation; Model depicted here is autoclavable

© Karl Storz Endoscopy America, Inc.

FIGURE 15-9

CLAMPS

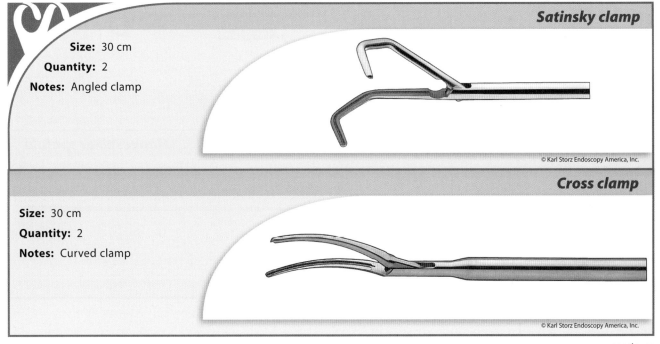

Satinsky clamp

Size: 30 cm

Quantity: 2

Notes: Angled clamp

© Karl Storz Endoscopy America, Inc.

FIGURE 15-10

Cross clamp

Size: 30 cm

Quantity: 2

Notes: Curved clamp

© Karl Storz Endoscopy America, Inc.

FIGURE 15-11

continues

CLAMPS *continued*

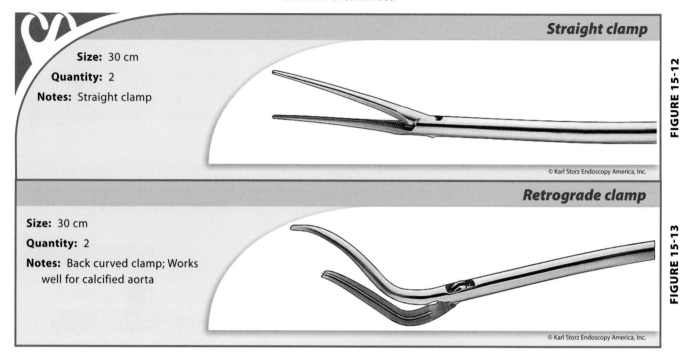

Straight clamp

Size: 30 cm

Quantity: 2

Notes: Straight clamp

© Karl Storz Endoscopy America, Inc.

FIGURE 15-12

Retrograde clamp

Size: 30 cm

Quantity: 2

Notes: Back curved clamp; Works well for calcified aorta

© Karl Storz Endoscopy America, Inc.

FIGURE 15-13

DISSECTION INSTRUMENTS

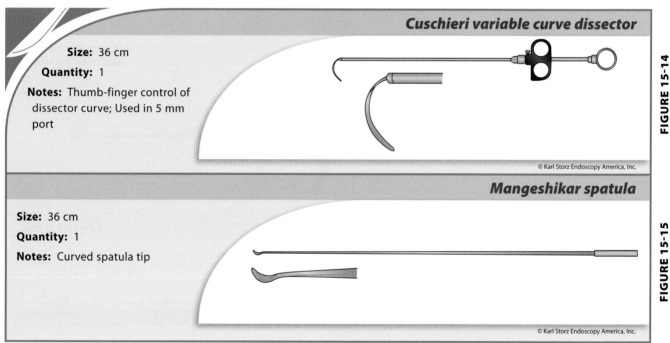

Cuschieri variable curve dissector

Size: 36 cm

Quantity: 1

Notes: Thumb-finger control of dissector curve; Used in 5 mm port

© Karl Storz Endoscopy America, Inc.

FIGURE 15-14

Mangeshikar spatula

Size: 36 cm

Quantity: 1

Notes: Curved spatula tip

© Karl Storz Endoscopy America, Inc.

FIGURE 15-15

PROBES AND DILATORS

Probe

Size: 43 cm

Quantity: 1

Notes: Graduated solid probe for manipulating tissues

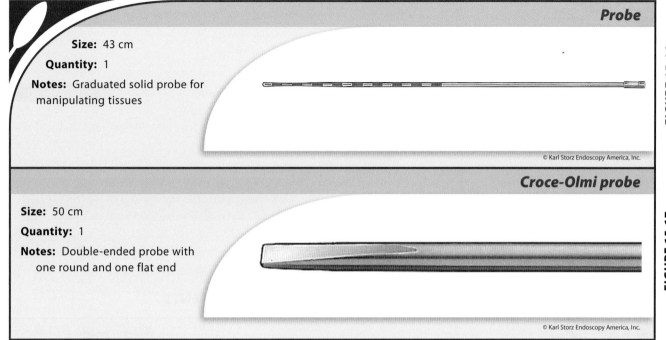

© Karl Storz Endoscopy America, Inc.

FIGURE 15-16

Croce-Olmi probe

Size: 50 cm

Quantity: 1

Notes: Double-ended probe with one round and one flat end

© Karl Storz Endoscopy America, Inc.

FIGURE 15-17

RETRACTION AND EXPOSURE INSTRUMENTS

Fan retractor

Size: 36 cm

Quantity: 1

Notes: Retractor with finger-like blades that spread wide to retract delicate tissues

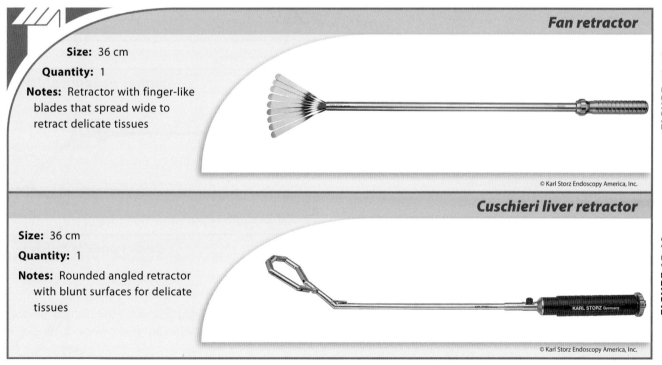

© Karl Storz Endoscopy America, Inc.

FIGURE 15-18

Cuschieri liver retractor

Size: 36 cm

Quantity: 1

Notes: Rounded angled retractor with blunt surfaces for delicate tissues

© Karl Storz Endoscopy America, Inc.

FIGURE 15-19

continues

RETRACTION AND EXPOSURE INSTRUMENTS *continued*

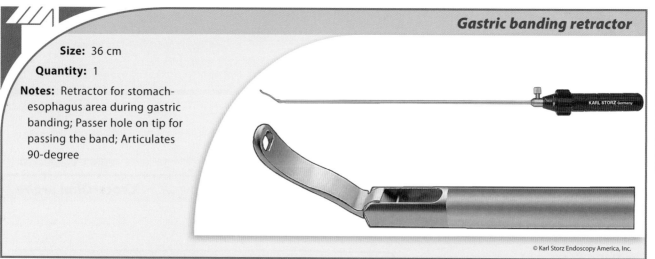

Gastric banding retractor

Size: 36 cm

Quantity: 1

Notes: Retractor for stomach-esophagus area during gastric banding; Passer hole on tip for passing the band; Articulates 90-degree

© Karl Storz Endoscopy America, Inc.

FIGURE 15-20

APPROXIMATION AND CLOSURE INSTRUMENTS

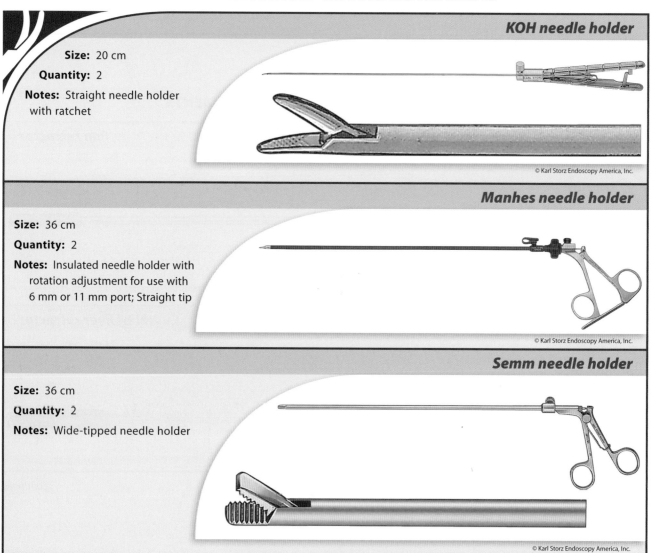

KOH needle holder

Size: 20 cm

Quantity: 2

Notes: Straight needle holder with ratchet

© Karl Storz Endoscopy America, Inc.

FIGURE 15-21

Manhes needle holder

Size: 36 cm

Quantity: 2

Notes: Insulated needle holder with rotation adjustment for use with 6 mm or 11 mm port; Straight tip

© Karl Storz Endoscopy America, Inc.

FIGURE 15-22

Semm needle holder

Size: 36 cm

Quantity: 2

Notes: Wide-tipped needle holder

© Karl Storz Endoscopy America, Inc.

FIGURE 15-23

APPROXIMATION AND CLOSURE INSTRUMENTS *continued*

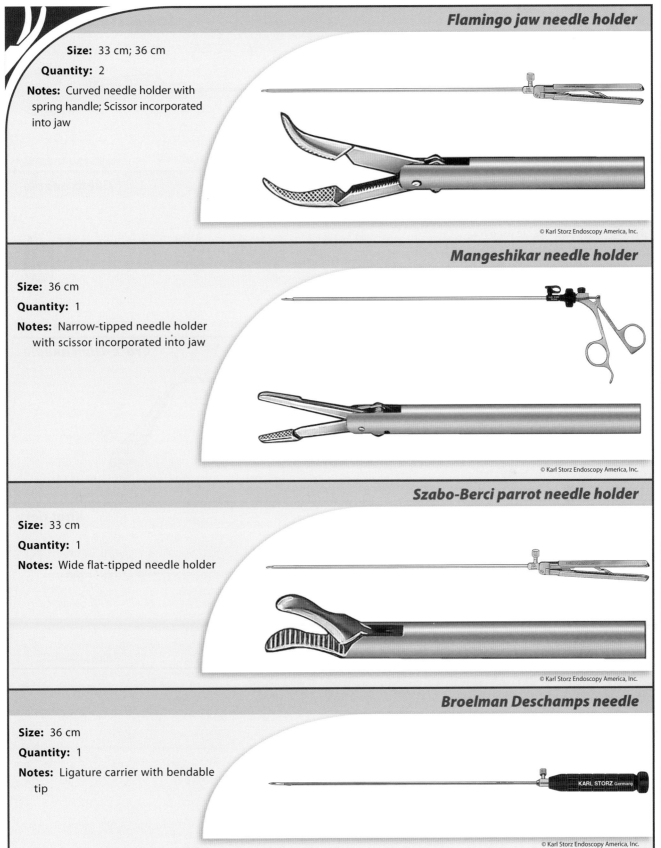

Flamingo jaw needle holder

Size: 33 cm; 36 cm

Quantity: 2

Notes: Curved needle holder with spring handle; Scissor incorporated into jaw

© Karl Storz Endoscopy America, Inc.

FIGURE 15-24

Mangeshikar needle holder

Size: 36 cm

Quantity: 1

Notes: Narrow-tipped needle holder with scissor incorporated into jaw

© Karl Storz Endoscopy America, Inc.

FIGURE 15-25

Szabo-Berci parrot needle holder

Size: 33 cm

Quantity: 1

Notes: Wide flat-tipped needle holder

© Karl Storz Endoscopy America, Inc.

FIGURE 15-26

Broelman Deschamps needle

Size: 36 cm

Quantity: 1

Notes: Ligature carrier with bendable tip

© Karl Storz Endoscopy America, Inc.

FIGURE 15-27

continues

APPROXIMATION AND CLOSURE INSTRUMENTS *continued*

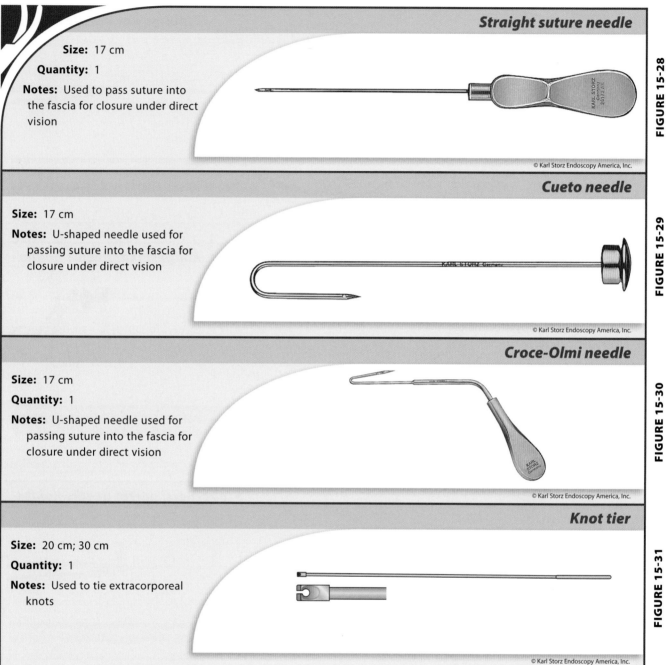

Straight suture needle

Size: 17 cm

Quantity: 1

Notes: Used to pass suture into the fascia for closure under direct vision

© Karl Storz Endoscopy America, Inc.

FIGURE 15-28

Cueto needle

Size: 17 cm

Notes: U-shaped needle used for passing suture into the fascia for closure under direct vision

© Karl Storz Endoscopy America, Inc.

FIGURE 15-29

Croce-Olmi needle

Size: 17 cm

Quantity: 1

Notes: U-shaped needle used for passing suture into the fascia for closure under direct vision

© Karl Storz Endoscopy America, Inc.

FIGURE 15-30

Knot tier

Size: 20 cm; 30 cm

Quantity: 1

Notes: Used to tie extracorporeal knots

© Karl Storz Endoscopy America, Inc.

FIGURE 15-31

SPECIALTY SPECIFIC INSTRUMENTS

Silastic ring applicator

Quantity: 1

Notes: Used to grasp the fallopian tube and apply a silastic band for tubal occlusion for sterilization

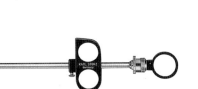

© Karl Storz Endoscopy America, Inc.

FIGURE 15-32

Tintara uterine manipulator

Size: 50 mm

Quantity: 1

Notes: Used during gynecologic procedures to manipulate the uterus for unobstructed view of the pelvis; Probe placed into the cervix for perturbation with contrast media or dye

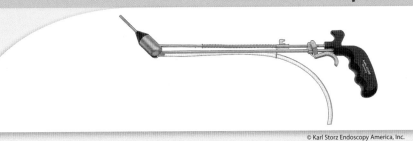

© Karl Storz Endoscopy America, Inc.

FIGURE 15-33

Koninck uterine rotator

Size: 37.5 cm

Quantity: 1

Notes: Used during gynecologic procedures to manipulate the uterus for unobstructed view of the pelvis; Probe placed into the cervix for uterine mobility

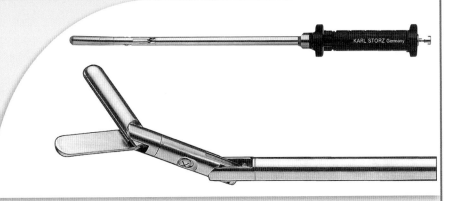

© Karl Storz Endoscopy America, Inc.

FIGURE 15-34

Endobag extractor

Notes: Three blades are used to dilate the access portal in the skin for removal of the specimen

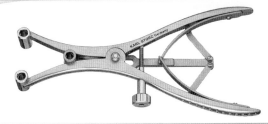

© Karl Storz Endoscopy America, Inc.

FIGURE 15-35

Arthroscopy

Arthroscopy is performed by percutaneously inserting trocars and working instrumentation into a joint space. Common sites for arthroscopy include the knee, wrist, shoulder, and hip. The surgeon creates the working space by instillation of sterile normal saline or lactated ringer's by gravity or by infusion pump. Infusion pump instillation allows more control of bleeding and measured administration of the fluid. Snug trocars prevent slippage of the sleeve and leakage of the fluid from the joint capsule into adjacent tissues.

Percutaneous Access, Illumination, and Viewing – SPECIALTY SPECIFIC INSTRUMENTS

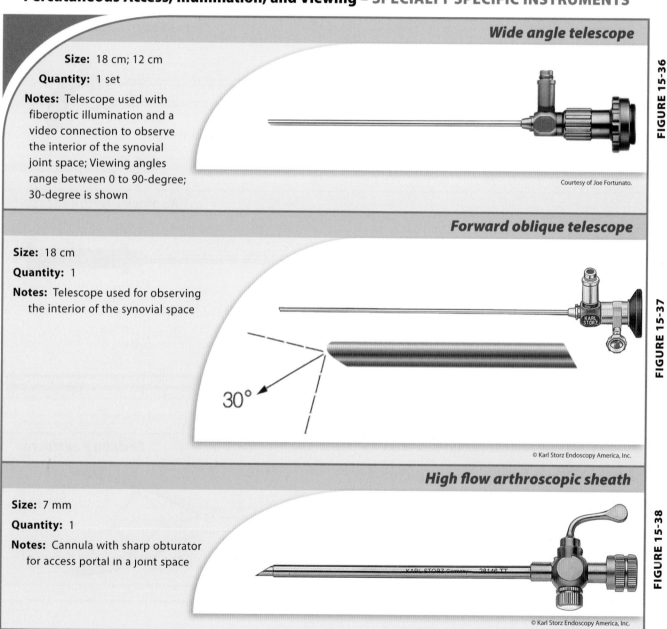

Wide angle telescope

Size: 18 cm; 12 cm

Quantity: 1 set

Notes: Telescope used with fiberoptic illumination and a video connection to observe the interior of the synovial joint space; Viewing angles range between 0 to 90-degree; 30-degree is shown

Courtesy of Joe Fortunato.

FIGURE 15-36

Forward oblique telescope

Size: 18 cm

Quantity: 1

Notes: Telescope used for observing the interior of the synovial space

30°

© Karl Storz Endoscopy America, Inc.

FIGURE 15-37

High flow arthroscopic sheath

Size: 7 mm

Quantity: 1

Notes: Cannula with sharp obturator for access portal in a joint space

KARL STORZ Germany   28146 TT

© Karl Storz Endoscopy America, Inc.

FIGURE 15-38

Percutaneous Access, Illumination, and Viewing – SPECIALTY SPECIFIC INSTRUMENTS *continued*

Anthroscope

Size: 12 cm

Quantity: 1

Notes: Autoclavable

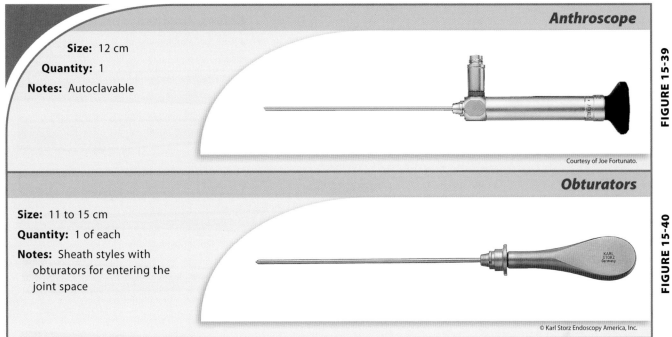

Courtesy of Joe Fortunato.

FIGURE 15-39

Obturators

Size: 11 to 15 cm

Quantity: 1 of each

Notes: Sheath styles with obturators for entering the joint space

© Karl Storz Endoscopy America, Inc.

FIGURE 15-40

Working Elements – SPECIALTY SPECIFIC INSTRUMENTS

Knives, curettes, and rasps

Size: 9.0 cm; 11.0 cm

Quantity: 1 set

Notes: Rigid instrumentation for manipulating tissues within the joint space

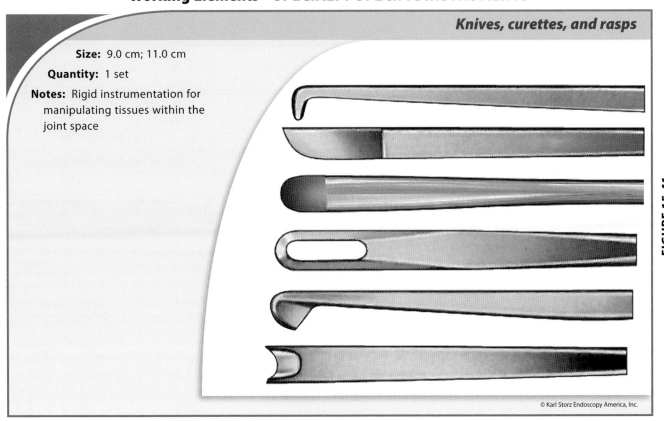

© Karl Storz Endoscopy America, Inc.

FIGURE 15-41

continues

Working Elements – **SPECIALTY SPECIFIC INSTRUMENTS** *continued*

Knives, curettes, and rasps, cont.

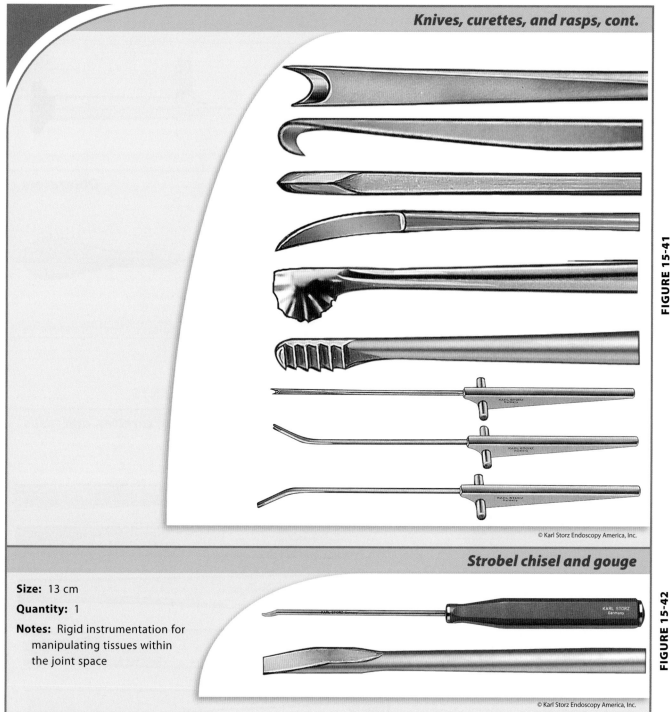

© Karl Storz Endoscopy America, Inc.

FIGURE 15-41

Strobel chisel and gouge

Size: 13 cm

Quantity: 1

Notes: Rigid instrumentation for manipulating tissues within the joint space

© Karl Storz Endoscopy America, Inc.

FIGURE 15-42

Working Elements – SPECIALTY SPECIFIC INSTRUMENTS *continued*

Anterior cruciate ligament repair

Size: 30 cm

Quantity: 1 set

Notes: Rigid instrumentation for manipulating ligaments within the joint space

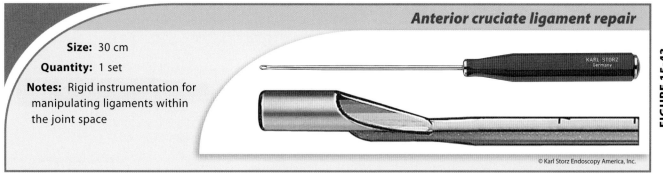

© Karl Storz Endoscopy America, Inc.

FIGURE 15-43

DEBULKING INSTRUMENTS

Strobel curettes

Size: 13 cm

Quantity: 1

Notes: Ring curettes used within the working channel of the arthroscope

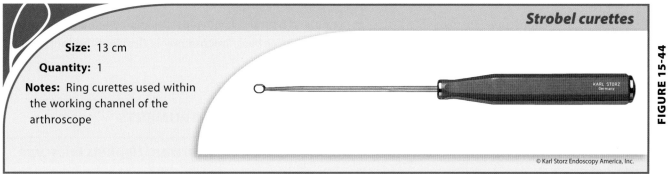

© Karl Storz Endoscopy America, Inc.

FIGURE 15-44

APPROXIMATION AND CLOSURE INSTRUMENTS

Intraarticular suture device

Size: 1 size

Quantity: 3

Notes: Three types of needle-suture passers for use in the joint space

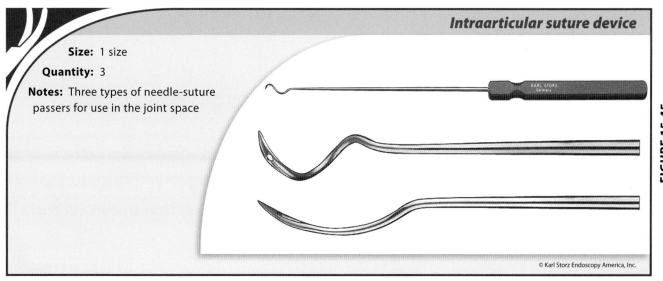

© Karl Storz Endoscopy America, Inc.

FIGURE 15-45

SPECIALTY SPECIFIC INSTRUMENTS

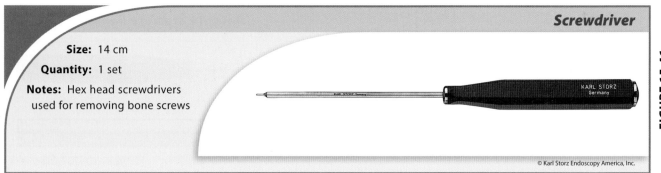

Screwdriver

Size: 14 cm

Quantity: 1 set

Notes: Hex head screwdrivers used for removing bone screws

FIGURE 15-46

© Karl Storz Endoscopy America, Inc.

Neuroendoscopy

Rigid and flexible endoscopes are used to visualize the brain and neural tissue. Ventricles can be unblocked, thereby avoiding the use of a shunt. One advantage of neuroendoscopy over basic microscopy is the ability to look around corners and in retrograde mode for greater field of vision.

Percutaneous Access – SPECIALTY SPECIFIC INSTRUMENTS

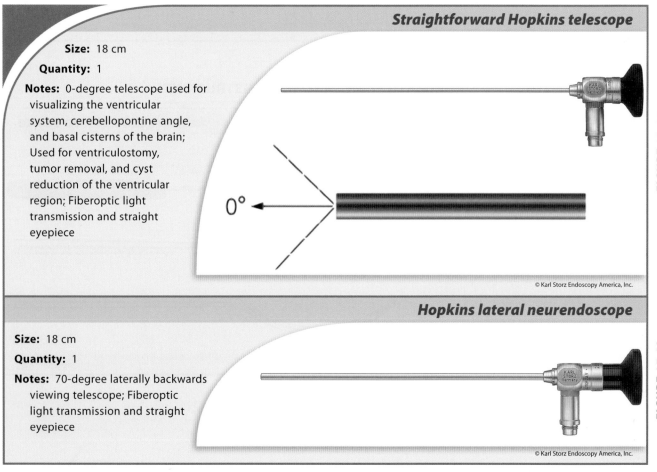

Straightforward Hopkins telescope

Size: 18 cm

Quantity: 1

Notes: 0-degree telescope used for visualizing the ventricular system, cerebellopontine angle, and basal cisterns of the brain; Used for ventriculostomy, tumor removal, and cyst reduction of the ventricular region; Fiberoptic light transmission and straight eyepiece

0°

FIGURE 15-47

© Karl Storz Endoscopy America, Inc.

Hopkins lateral neurendoscope

Size: 18 cm

Quantity: 1

Notes: 70-degree laterally backwards viewing telescope; Fiberoptic light transmission and straight eyepiece

FIGURE 15-48

© Karl Storz Endoscopy America, Inc.

Percutaneous Access – SPECIALTY SPECIFIC INSTRUMENTS *continued*

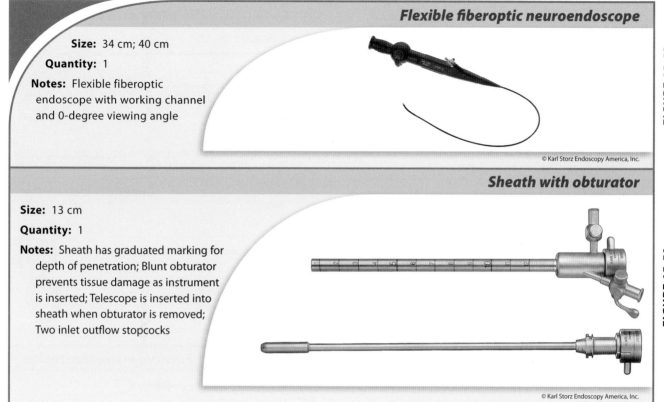

Flexible fiberoptic neuroendoscope

Size: 34 cm; 40 cm

Quantity: 1

Notes: Flexible fiberoptic endoscope with working channel and 0-degree viewing angle

© Karl Storz Endoscopy America, Inc.

FIGURE 15-49

Sheath with obturator

Size: 13 cm

Quantity: 1

Notes: Sheath has graduated marking for depth of penetration; Blunt obturator prevents tissue damage as instrument is inserted; Telescope is inserted into sheath when obturator is removed; Two inlet outflow stopcocks

© Karl Storz Endoscopy America, Inc.

FIGURE 15-50

Working Elements – SPECIALTY SPECIFIC INSTRUMENTS

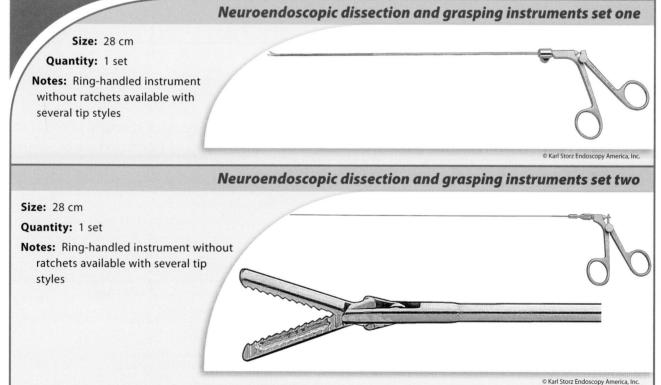

Neuroendoscopic dissection and grasping instruments set one

Size: 28 cm

Quantity: 1 set

Notes: Ring-handled instrument without ratchets available with several tip styles

© Karl Storz Endoscopy America, Inc.

FIGURE 15-51

Neuroendoscopic dissection and grasping instruments set two

Size: 28 cm

Quantity: 1 set

Notes: Ring-handled instrument without ratchets available with several tip styles

© Karl Storz Endoscopy America, Inc.

FIGURE 15-52

continues

Working Elements – SPECIALTY SPECIFIC INSTRUMENTS *continued*

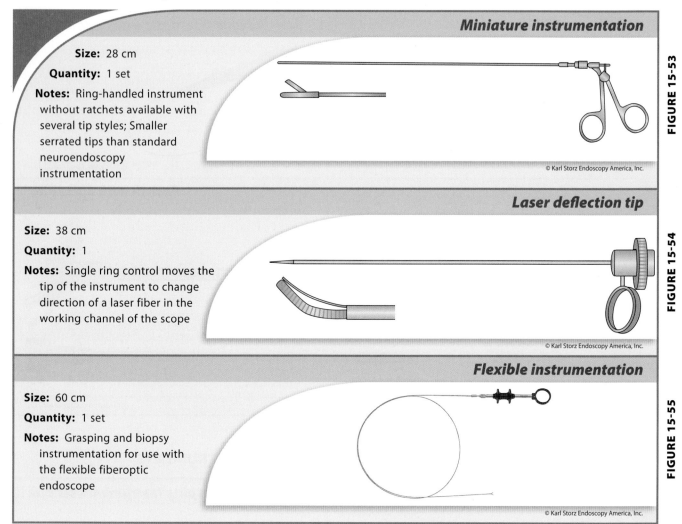

Miniature instrumentation

FIGURE 15-53

Size: 28 cm

Quantity: 1 set

Notes: Ring-handled instrument without ratchets available with several tip styles; Smaller serrated tips than standard neuroendoscopy instrumentation

© Karl Storz Endoscopy America, Inc.

Laser deflection tip

FIGURE 15-54

Size: 38 cm

Quantity: 1

Notes: Single ring control moves the tip of the instrument to change direction of a laser fiber in the working channel of the scope

© Karl Storz Endoscopy America, Inc.

Flexible instrumentation

FIGURE 15-55

Size: 60 cm

Quantity: 1 set

Notes: Grasping and biopsy instrumentation for use with the flexible fiberoptic endoscope

© Karl Storz Endoscopy America, Inc.

Thoracoscopy

Percutaneous access through the chest wall is performed for procedures involving the lungs, structural aspects of the upper airway, and surface access to great vessels and nodes. Standard laparoscopes and videoscopes can be inserted through the trocars for video-assisted endoscopy (VATS).

Percutaneous Access – SPECIALTY SPECIFIC INSTRUMENTS

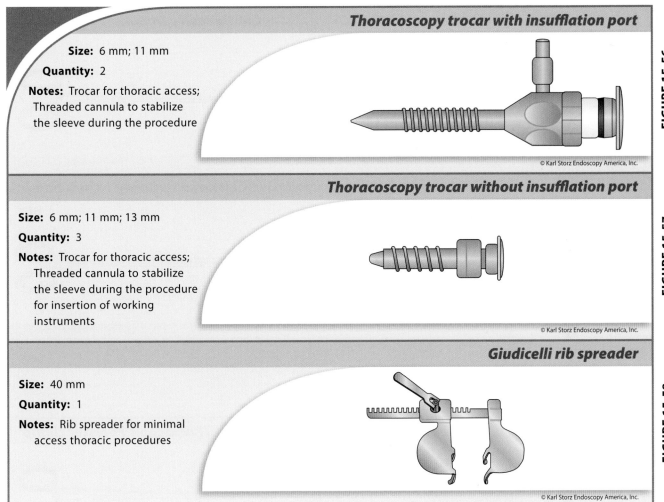

Thoracoscopy trocar with insufflation port

Size: 6 mm; 11 mm

Quantity: 2

Notes: Trocar for thoracic access; Threaded cannula to stabilize the sleeve during the procedure

© Karl Storz Endoscopy America, Inc.

FIGURE 15-56

Thoracoscopy trocar without insufflation port

Size: 6 mm; 11 mm; 13 mm

Quantity: 3

Notes: Trocar for thoracic access; Threaded cannula to stabilize the sleeve during the procedure for insertion of working instruments

© Karl Storz Endoscopy America, Inc.

FIGURE 15-57

Giudicelli rib spreader

Size: 40 mm

Quantity: 1

Notes: Rib spreader for minimal access thoracic procedures

© Karl Storz Endoscopy America, Inc.

FIGURE 15-58

Illumination and Viewing – SPECIALTY SPECIFIC INSTRUMENTS

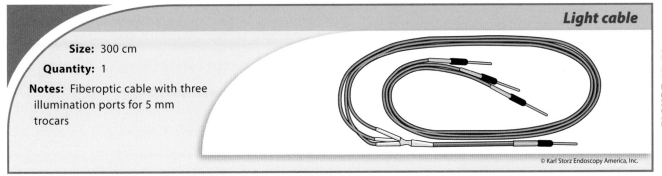

Light cable

Size: 300 cm

Quantity: 1

Notes: Fiberoptic cable with three illumination ports for 5 mm trocars

© Karl Storz Endoscopy America, Inc.

FIGURE 15-59

CLAMPS

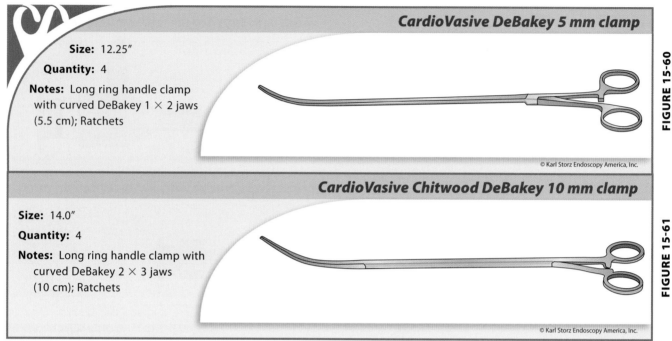

CardioVasive DeBakey 5 mm clamp

Size: 12.25"

Quantity: 4

Notes: Long ring handle clamp with curved DeBakey 1 × 2 jaws (5.5 cm); Ratchets

© Karl Storz Endoscopy America, Inc.

FIGURE 15-60

CardioVasive Chitwood DeBakey 10 mm clamp

Size: 14.0"

Quantity: 4

Notes: Long ring handle clamp with curved DeBakey 2 × 3 jaws (10 cm); Ratchets

© Karl Storz Endoscopy America, Inc.

FIGURE 15-61

GRASPING FORCEPS

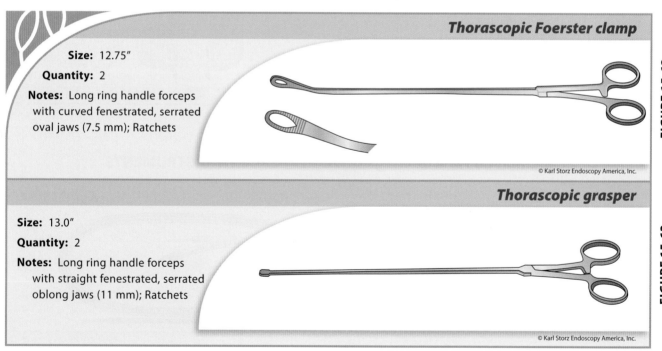

Thorascopic Foerster clamp

Size: 12.75"

Quantity: 2

Notes: Long ring handle forceps with curved fenestrated, serrated oval jaws (7.5 mm); Ratchets

© Karl Storz Endoscopy America, Inc.

FIGURE 15-62

Thorascopic grasper

Size: 13.0"

Quantity: 2

Notes: Long ring handle forceps with straight fenestrated, serrated oblong jaws (11 mm); Ratchets

© Karl Storz Endoscopy America, Inc.

FIGURE 15-63

GRASPING FORCEPS *continued*

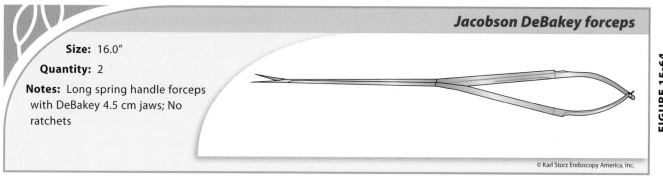

Jacobson DeBakey forceps

Size: 16.0"

Quantity: 2

Notes: Long spring handle forceps with DeBakey 4.5 cm jaws; No ratchets

© Karl Storz Endoscopy America, Inc.

FIGURE 15-64

DISSECTION INSTRUMENTS

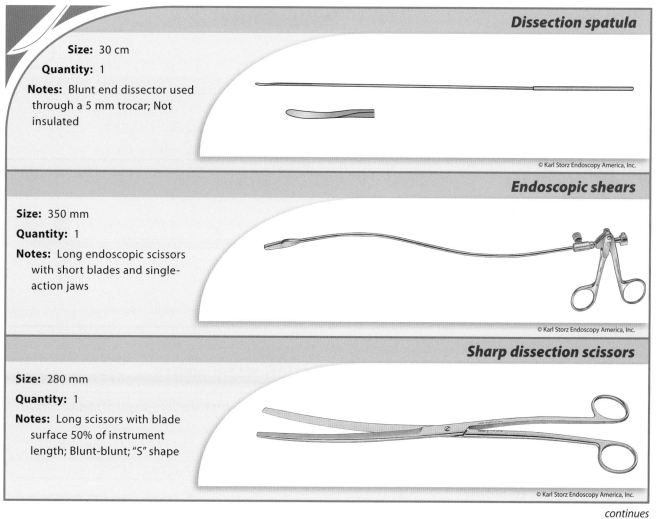

Dissection spatula

Size: 30 cm

Quantity: 1

Notes: Blunt end dissector used through a 5 mm trocar; Not insulated

© Karl Storz Endoscopy America, Inc.

FIGURE 15-65

Endoscopic shears

Size: 350 mm

Quantity: 1

Notes: Long endoscopic scissors with short blades and single-action jaws

© Karl Storz Endoscopy America, Inc.

FIGURE 15-66

Sharp dissection scissors

Size: 280 mm

Quantity: 1

Notes: Long scissors with blade surface 50% of instrument length; Blunt-blunt; "S" shape

© Karl Storz Endoscopy America, Inc.

FIGURE 15-67

continues

DISSECTION INSTRUMENTS *continued*

Sharp dissection scissors extra-long

Size: 330 mm

Quantity: 1

Notes: Long scissors with short blade surface 10% of instrument length; Blunt-blunt "S" shape

© Karl Storz Endoscopy America, Inc.

FIGURE 15-68

Sharp dissection scissors angled

Size: 260 mm

Quantity: 1

Notes: Long scissors with angled tip and "S" shanks; Blunt-blunt

© Karl Storz Endoscopy America, Inc.

FIGURE 15-69

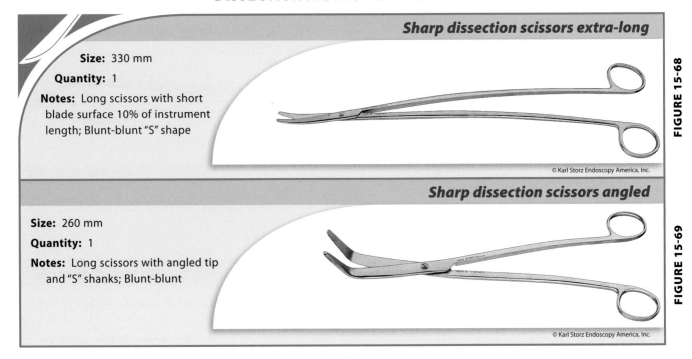

PROBES AND DILATORS

Suction tip

Size: 36 cm

Quantity: 1

Notes: Negative pressure controlled by pressing trumpet valve

Courtesy of Joe Fortunato.

FIGURE 15-70

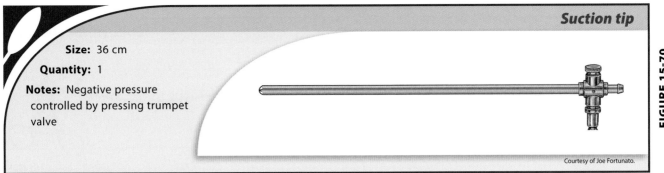

EVACUATION AND INSTILLATION INSTRUMENTS

Instillation-aspiration cannula

Size: 36 cm

Quantity: 1

Notes: Long hollow tube with a beveled needle tip for aspiration or instillation; Luer lock connector

© Karl Storz Endoscopy America, Inc.

FIGURE 15-71

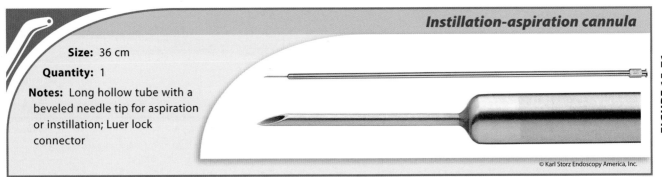

EVACUATION AND INSTILLATION INSTRUMENTS *continued*

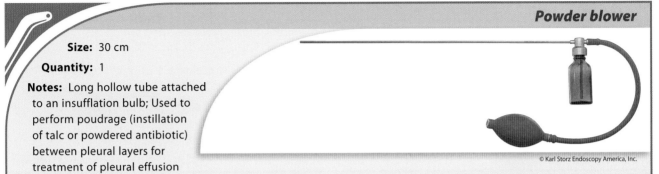

Powder blower

Size: 30 cm

Quantity: 1

Notes: Long hollow tube attached to an insufflation bulb; Used to perform poudrage (instillation of talc or powdered antibiotic) between pleural layers for treatment of pleural effusion

© Karl Storz Endoscopy America, Inc.

FIGURE 15-72

RETRACTION AND EXPOSURE INSTRUMENTS

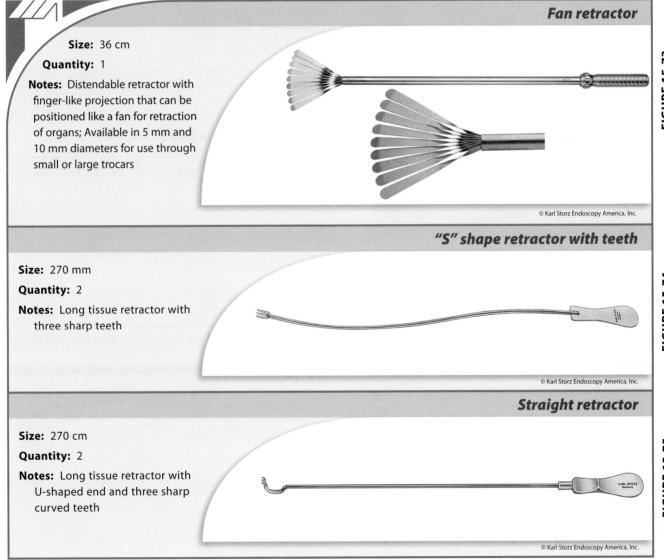

Fan retractor

Size: 36 cm

Quantity: 1

Notes: Distendable retractor with finger-like projection that can be positioned like a fan for retraction of organs; Available in 5 mm and 10 mm diameters for use through small or large trocars

© Karl Storz Endoscopy America, Inc.

FIGURE 15-73

"S" shape retractor with teeth

Size: 270 mm

Quantity: 2

Notes: Long tissue retractor with three sharp teeth

© Karl Storz Endoscopy America, Inc.

FIGURE 15-74

Straight retractor

Size: 270 cm

Quantity: 2

Notes: Long tissue retractor with U-shaped end and three sharp curved teeth

© Karl Storz Endoscopy America, Inc.

FIGURE 15-75

continues

RETRACTION AND EXPOSURE INSTRUMENTS *continued*

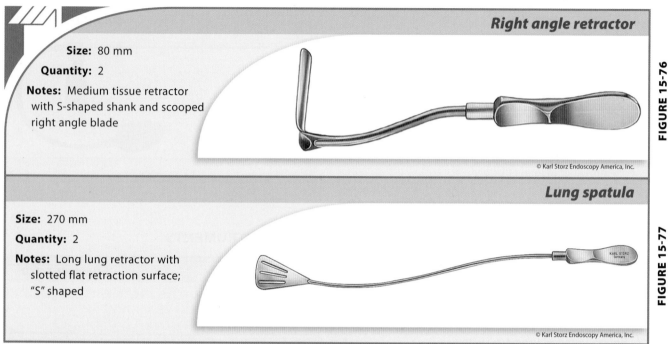

Right angle retractor

Size: 80 mm

Quantity: 2

Notes: Medium tissue retractor with S-shaped shank and scooped right angle blade

© Karl Storz Endoscopy America, Inc.

FIGURE 15-76

Lung spatula

Size: 270 mm

Quantity: 2

Notes: Long lung retractor with slotted flat retraction surface; "S" shaped

© Karl Storz Endoscopy America, Inc.

FIGURE 15-77

APPROXIMATION AND CLOSURE INSTRUMENTS

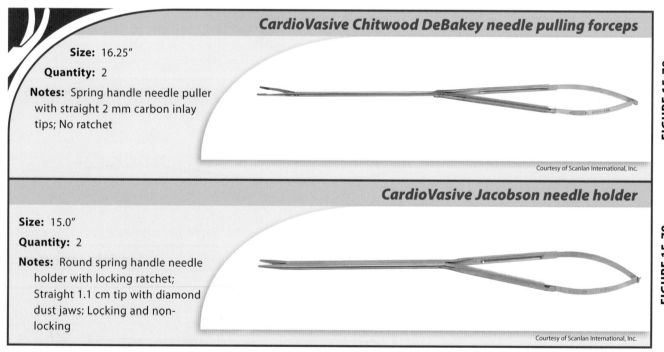

CardioVasive Chitwood DeBakey needle pulling forceps

Size: 16.25"

Quantity: 2

Notes: Spring handle needle puller with straight 2 mm carbon inlay tips; No ratchet

Courtesy of Scanlan International, Inc.

FIGURE 15-78

CardioVasive Jacobson needle holder

Size: 15.0"

Quantity: 2

Notes: Round spring handle needle holder with locking ratchet; Straight 1.1 cm tip with diamond dust jaws; Locking and non-locking

Courtesy of Scanlan International, Inc.

FIGURE 15-79

APPROXIMATION AND CLOSURE INSTRUMENTS *continued*

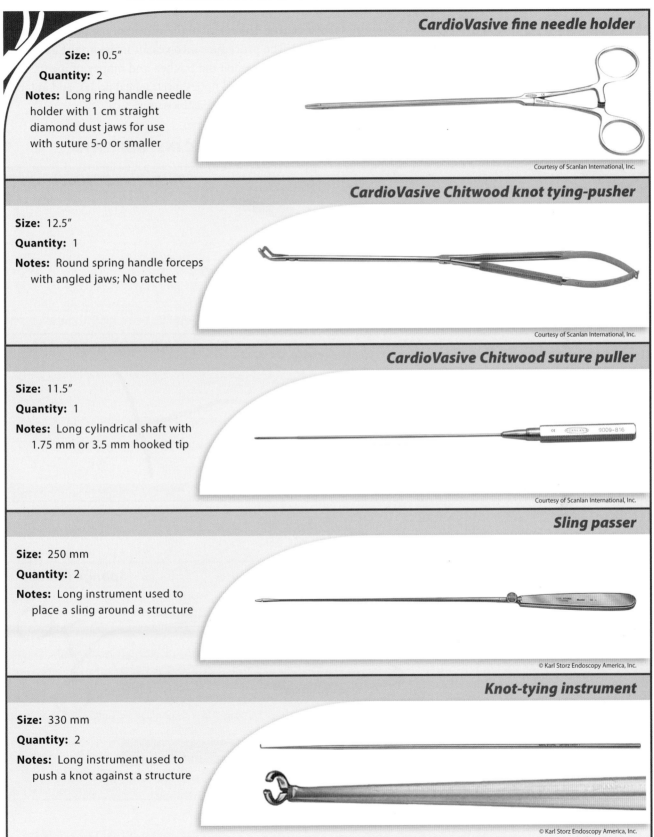

CardioVasive fine needle holder

Size: 10.5"

Quantity: 2

Notes: Long ring handle needle holder with 1 cm straight diamond dust jaws for use with suture 5-0 or smaller

Courtesy of Scanlan International, Inc.

FIGURE 15-80

CardioVasive Chitwood knot tying-pusher

Size: 12.5"

Quantity: 1

Notes: Round spring handle forceps with angled jaws; No ratchet

Courtesy of Scanlan International, Inc.

FIGURE 15-81

CardioVasive Chitwood suture puller

Size: 11.5"

Quantity: 1

Notes: Long cylindrical shaft with 1.75 mm or 3.5 mm hooked tip

Courtesy of Scanlan International, Inc.

FIGURE 15-82

Sling passer

Size: 250 mm

Quantity: 2

Notes: Long instrument used to place a sling around a structure

© Karl Storz Endoscopy America, Inc.

FIGURE 15-83

Knot-tying instrument

Size: 330 mm

Quantity: 2

Notes: Long instrument used to push a knot against a structure

© Karl Storz Endoscopy America, Inc.

FIGURE 15-84

Mediastinoscopy

Mediastinoscopy is performed to stage a disease entity such as cancer. The extent of the spread of the nodal advancement of disease is predictive of the patient's chances of survival. The procedure involves an incision just above the suprasternal notch followed by the insertion of a mediastinoscope alongside the trachea and biopsy of mediastinal nodes. Nodes accessible through this route are the left and right paratracheal nodes, pretracheal nodes, and anterior subcarinal nodes. Fine needle aspiration biopsy can be performed through mediastinoscopy.

Access, Illumination, and Viewing – SPECIALTY SPECIFIC INSTRUMENTS

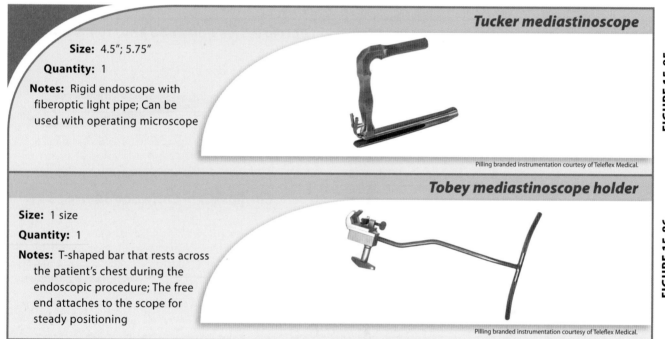

Tucker mediastinoscope

Size: 4.5"; 5.75"

Quantity: 1

Notes: Rigid endoscope with fiberoptic light pipe; Can be used with operating microscope

Pilling branded instrumentation courtesy of Teleflex Medical.

FIGURE 15-85

Tobey mediastinoscope holder

Size: 1 size

Quantity: 1

Notes: T-shaped bar that rests across the patient's chest during the endoscopic procedure; The free end attaches to the scope for steady positioning

Pilling branded instrumentation courtesy of Teleflex Medical.

FIGURE 15-86

GRASPING FORCEPS

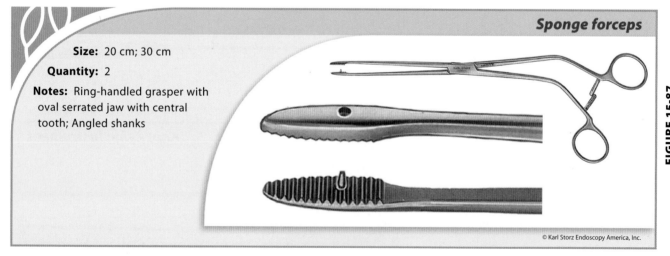

Sponge forceps

Size: 20 cm; 30 cm

Quantity: 2

Notes: Ring-handled grasper with oval serrated jaw with central tooth; Angled shanks

© Karl Storz Endoscopy America, Inc.

FIGURE 15-87

DISSECTION INSTRUMENTS

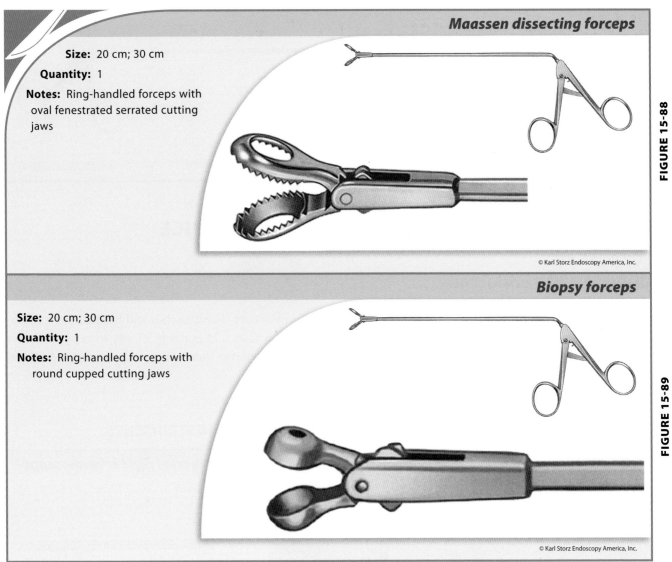

Maassen dissecting forceps

Size: 20 cm; 30 cm

Quantity: 1

Notes: Ring-handled forceps with oval fenestrated serrated cutting jaws

© Karl Storz Endoscopy America, Inc.

FIGURE 15-88

Biopsy forceps

Size: 20 cm; 30 cm

Quantity: 1

Notes: Ring-handled forceps with round cupped cutting jaws

© Karl Storz Endoscopy America, Inc.

FIGURE 15-89

EVACUATION AND INSTILLATION INSTRUMENTS

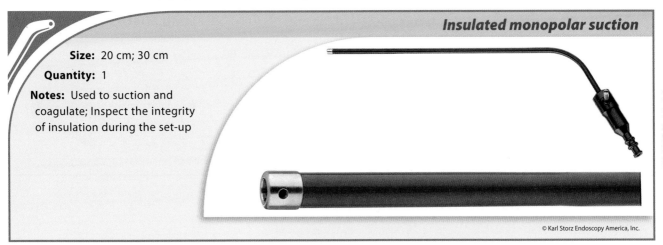

Insulated monopolar suction

Size: 20 cm; 30 cm

Quantity: 1

Notes: Used to suction and coagulate; Inspect the integrity of insulation during the set-up

© Karl Storz Endoscopy America, Inc.

FIGURE 15-90

APPROXIMATION AND CLOSURE INSTRUMENTS

Clip applier

Size: 22 cm; 30 cm

Quantity: 2

Notes: Endoscopic reusable clip applier

© Karl Storz Endoscopy America, Inc.

FIGURE 15-91

ENDOSCOPY THROUGH A NATURAL BODY ORIFICE

Upper Airway Endoscopy

Bronchoscopy is performed through the mouth or through a tracheostomy. The bronchus and bronchioles are visualized using a rigid or flexible fiberoptic endoscope. Working elements, such as graspers, biopsy forceps, and other devices, can be passed through the endoscope to perform surgical procedures. There is no need to use any additional instrumentation for access to the surgical site.

Illumination and Viewing – SPECIALTY SPECIFIC INSTRUMENTS

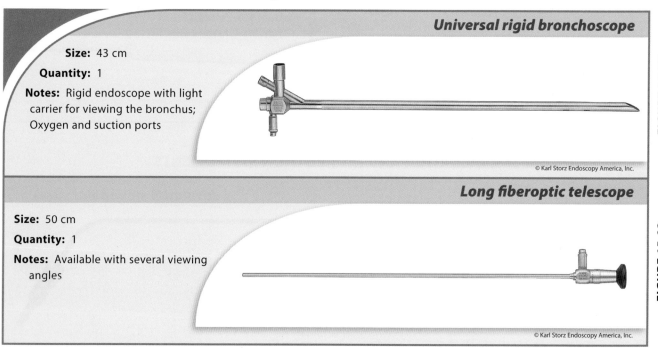

Universal rigid bronchoscope

Size: 43 cm

Quantity: 1

Notes: Rigid endoscope with light carrier for viewing the bronchus; Oxygen and suction ports

© Karl Storz Endoscopy America, Inc.

FIGURE 15-92

Long fiberoptic telescope

Size: 50 cm

Quantity: 1

Notes: Available with several viewing angles

© Karl Storz Endoscopy America, Inc.

FIGURE 15-93

Illumination and Viewing – SPECIALTY SPECIFIC INSTRUMENTS continued

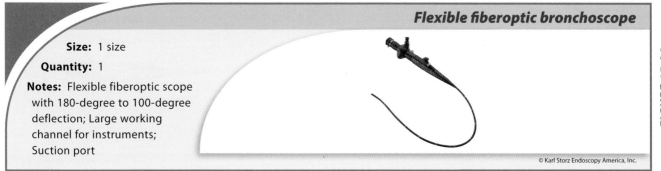

Flexible fiberoptic bronchoscope

Size: 1 size

Quantity: 1

Notes: Flexible fiberoptic scope with 180-degree to 100-degree deflection; Large working channel for instruments; Suction port

© Karl Storz Endoscopy America, Inc.

FIGURE 15-94

Working Elements – SPECIALTY SPECIFIC INSTRUMENTS

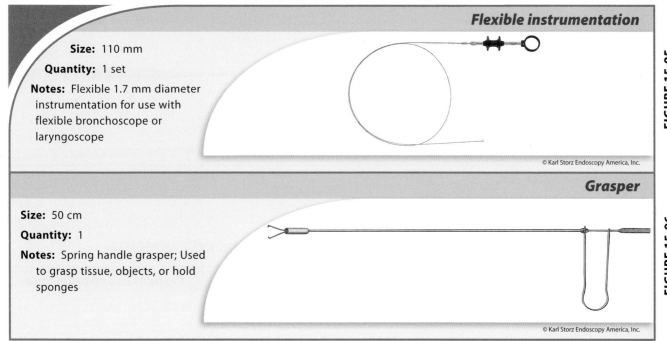

Flexible instrumentation

Size: 110 mm

Quantity: 1 set

Notes: Flexible 1.7 mm diameter instrumentation for use with flexible bronchoscope or laryngoscope

© Karl Storz Endoscopy America, Inc.

FIGURE 15-95

Grasper

Size: 50 cm

Quantity: 1

Notes: Spring handle grasper; Used to grasp tissue, objects, or hold sponges

© Karl Storz Endoscopy America, Inc.

FIGURE 15-96

EVACUATION AND INSTILLATION INSTRUMENTS

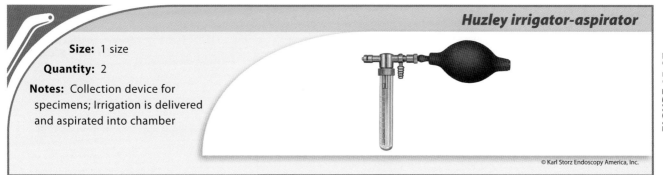

Huzley irrigator-aspirator

Size: 1 size

Quantity: 2

Notes: Collection device for specimens; Irrigation is delivered and aspirated into chamber

© Karl Storz Endoscopy America, Inc.

FIGURE 15-97

continues

EVACUATION AND INSTILLATION INSTRUMENTS *continued*

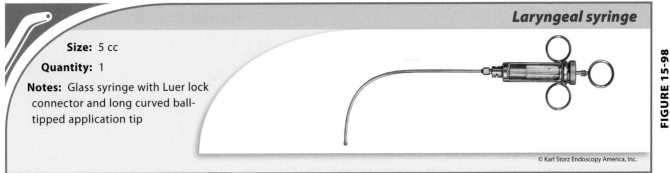

Laryngeal syringe

Size: 5 cc

Quantity: 1

Notes: Glass syringe with Luer lock connector and long curved ball-tipped application tip

© Karl Storz Endoscopy America, Inc.

FIGURE 15-98

SPECIALTY SPECIFIC INSTRUMENTS

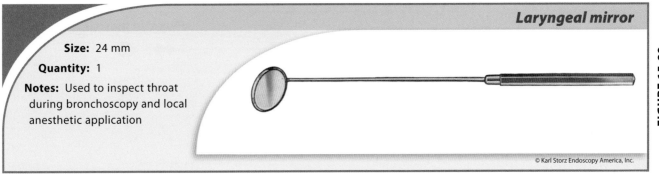

Laryngeal mirror

Size: 24 mm

Quantity: 1

Notes: Used to inspect throat during bronchoscopy and local anesthetic application

© Karl Storz Endoscopy America, Inc.

FIGURE 15-99

Upper Digestive Endoscopy

Illumination and Viewing – SPECIALTY SPECIFIC INSTRUMENTS

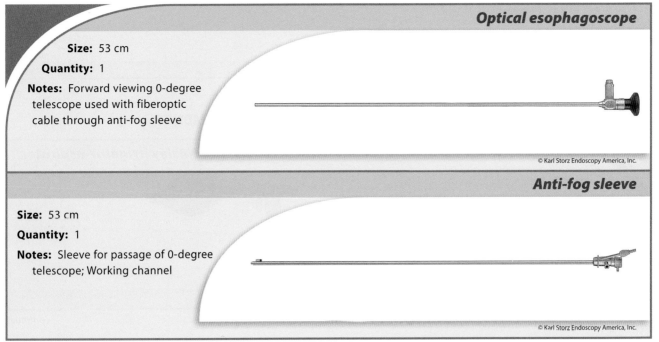

Optical esophagoscope

Size: 53 cm

Quantity: 1

Notes: Forward viewing 0-degree telescope used with fiberoptic cable through anti-fog sleeve

© Karl Storz Endoscopy America, Inc.

FIGURE 15-100

Anti-fog sleeve

Size: 53 cm

Quantity: 1

Notes: Sleeve for passage of 0-degree telescope; Working channel

© Karl Storz Endoscopy America, Inc.

FIGURE 15-101

Illumination and Viewing – SPECIALTY SPECIFIC INSTRUMENTS *continued*

Esophagoscope tube

Size: 53 cm

Quantity: 1

Notes: Rigid metal tube with working channels for air insufflation, suction, and fiberoptic light carrier; Glass eyepiece

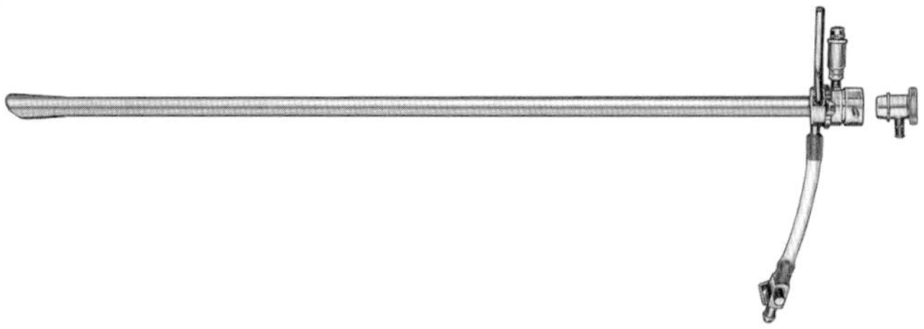

© Karl Storz Endoscopy America, Inc.

FIGURE 15-102

Insufflation bulb

Size: 1 size

Quantity: 1

Notes: Used to create a working space with insufflated room air

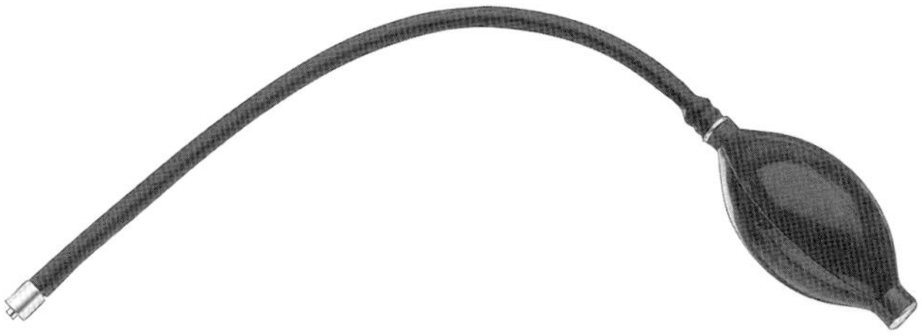

© Karl Storz Endoscopy America, Inc.

FIGURE 15-103

Light carrier

Size: Sized according to scope

Quantity: 1

Notes: Metallic rod with glass light fibers that fits inside a rigid scope for distal illumination; Attaches to fiberoptic light cable

© Karl Storz Endoscopy America, Inc.

FIGURE 15-104

GRASPING FORCEPS

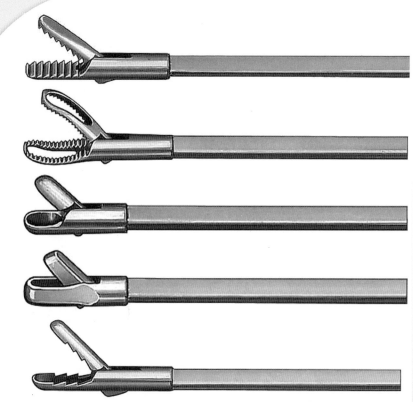

Single-action grasping forceps

Size: 55 cm

Quantity: 1 set

Notes: Grasper with serrated jaws; Used in rigid bronchoscope or esophagoscope

© Karl Storz Endoscopy America, Inc.

FIGURE 15-105

Snare basket grasper

Size: 35 cm; 55 cm

Quantity: 1

Notes: Thumb and finger action snare wire used for foreign body extraction

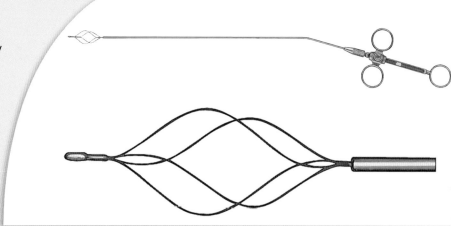

© Karl Storz Endoscopy America, Inc.

FIGURE 15-106

DISSECTION INSTRUMENTS

Single-action biopsy forceps

Size: 55 cm

Quantity: 1 set

Notes: Biopsy forceps with cupped, through cutting, or scissors dissection

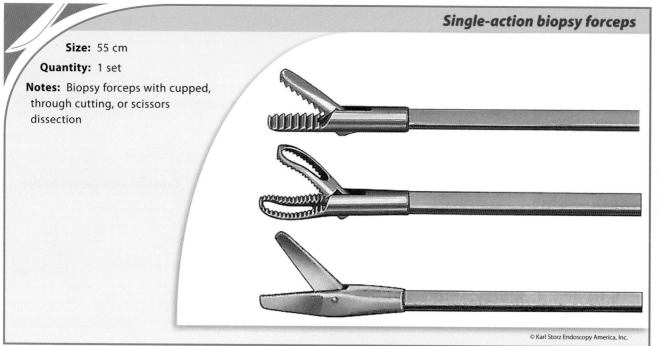

© Karl Storz Endoscopy America, Inc.

FIGURE 15-107

PROBES AND DILATORS

Jackson bougie

Size: 57 cm

Quantity: 1 set

Notes: Single-end dilators for the esophagus with diameters ranging between 10 mm and 40 mm

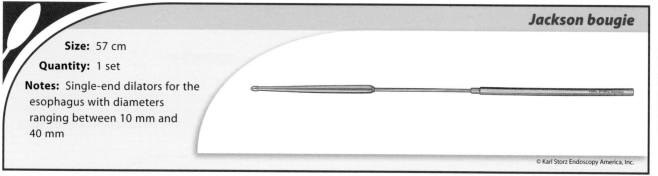

© Karl Storz Endoscopy America, Inc.

FIGURE 15-108

Gynecologic Transcervical Endoscopy

Access, Illumination, and Viewing – SPECIALTY SPECIFIC INSTRUMENTS

Hamou operating and contact hysteroscope

Size: 30 cm

Quantity: 1

Notes: Rigid forward oblique 30-degree view telescope for inspecting the interior of the uterus; Uses standard fiberoptic light cable

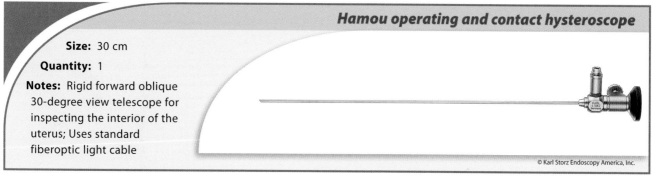

© Karl Storz Endoscopy America, Inc.

FIGURE 15-109

continues

Access, Illumination, and Viewing – SPECIALTY SPECIFIC INSTRUMENTS *continued*

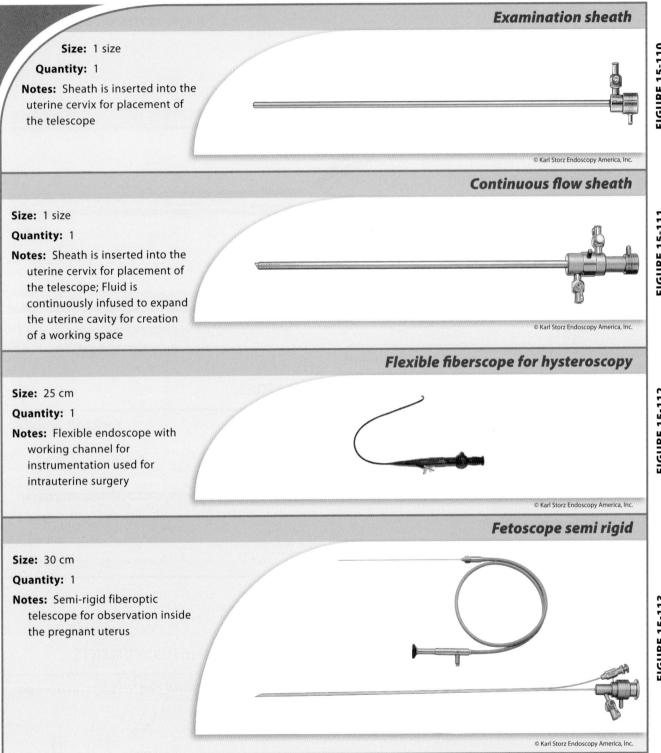

Examination sheath

Size: 1 size

Quantity: 1

Notes: Sheath is inserted into the uterine cervix for placement of the telescope

© Karl Storz Endoscopy America, Inc.

FIGURE 15-110

Continuous flow sheath

Size: 1 size

Quantity: 1

Notes: Sheath is inserted into the uterine cervix for placement of the telescope; Fluid is continuously infused to expand the uterine cavity for creation of a working space

© Karl Storz Endoscopy America, Inc.

FIGURE 15-111

Flexible fiberscope for hysteroscopy

Size: 25 cm

Quantity: 1

Notes: Flexible endoscope with working channel for instrumentation used for intrauterine surgery

© Karl Storz Endoscopy America, Inc.

FIGURE 15-112

Fetoscope semi rigid

Size: 30 cm

Quantity: 1

Notes: Semi-rigid fiberoptic telescope for observation inside the pregnant uterus

© Karl Storz Endoscopy America, Inc.

FIGURE 15-113

Access, Illumination, and Viewing – SPECIALTY SPECIFIC INSTRUMENTS *continued*

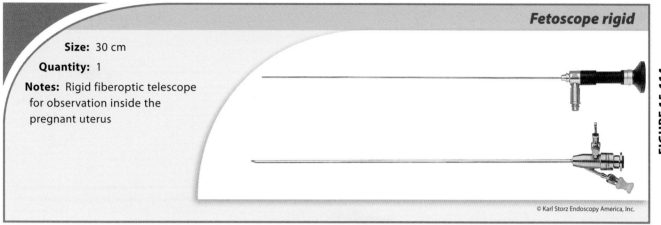

Fetoscope rigid

Size: 30 cm

Quantity: 1

Notes: Rigid fiberoptic telescope for observation inside the pregnant uterus

© Karl Storz Endoscopy America, Inc.

FIGURE 15-114

Working Elements – SPECIALTY SPECIFIC INSTRUMENTS

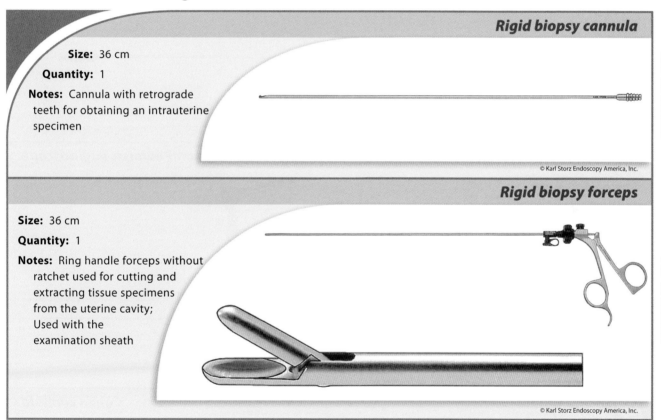

Rigid biopsy cannula

Size: 36 cm

Quantity: 1

Notes: Cannula with retrograde teeth for obtaining an intrauterine specimen

© Karl Storz Endoscopy America, Inc.

FIGURE 15-115

Rigid biopsy forceps

Size: 36 cm

Quantity: 1

Notes: Ring handle forceps without ratchet used for cutting and extracting tissue specimens from the uterine cavity; Used with the examination sheath

© Karl Storz Endoscopy America, Inc.

FIGURE 15-116

continues

Working Elements – SPECIALTY SPECIFIC INSTRUMENTS *continued*

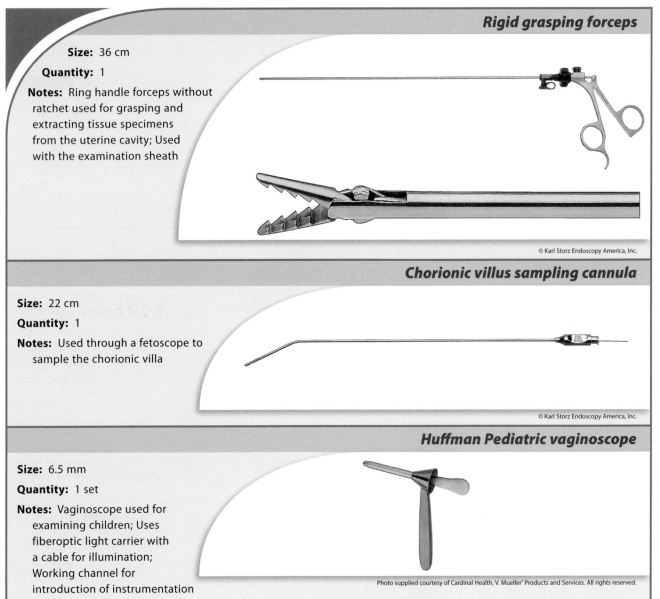

Rigid grasping forceps

Size: 36 cm

Quantity: 1

Notes: Ring handle forceps without ratchet used for grasping and extracting tissue specimens from the uterine cavity; Used with the examination sheath

FIGURE 15-117

Chorionic villus sampling cannula

Size: 22 cm

Quantity: 1

Notes: Used through a fetoscope to sample the chorionic villa

FIGURE 15-118

Huffman Pediatric vaginoscope

Size: 6.5 mm

Quantity: 1 set

Notes: Vaginoscope used for examining children; Uses fiberoptic light carrier with a cable for illumination; Working channel for introduction of instrumentation

FIGURE 15-119

PROBES AND DILATORS

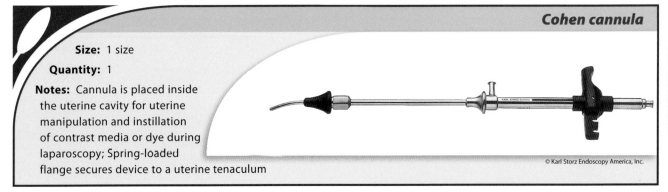

Cohen cannula

Size: 1 size

Quantity: 1

Notes: Cannula is placed inside the uterine cavity for uterine manipulation and instillation of contrast media or dye during laparoscopy; Spring-loaded flange secures device to a uterine tenaculum

FIGURE 15-120

PROBES AND DILATORS *continued*

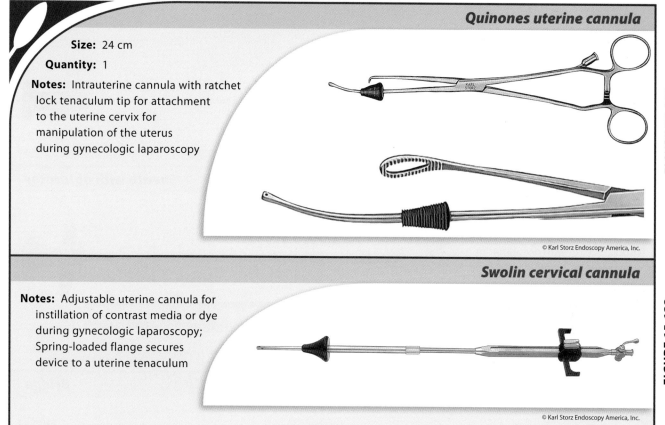

Quinones uterine cannula

Size: 24 cm

Quantity: 1

Notes: Intrauterine cannula with ratchet lock tenaculum tip for attachment to the uterine cervix for manipulation of the uterus during gynecologic laparoscopy

© Karl Storz Endoscopy America, Inc.

FIGURE 15-121

Swolin cervical cannula

Notes: Adjustable uterine cannula for instillation of contrast media or dye during gynecologic laparoscopy; Spring-loaded flange secures device to a uterine tenaculum

© Karl Storz Endoscopy America, Inc.

FIGURE 15-122

Urologic Endoscopy

Most urologic endoscopic instrumentation is used through the urethral orifice of either the male or the female during cystoscopic surgery. A sheath with an obturator is introduced through the urethra and the working space is created with sterile water instillation. The obturator is removed and a telescope is inserted. The sheath has a working channel for instrumentation. The surgeon controls the instillation and evacuation of the fluid expansion medium. Electrosurgical procedures can safely be performed inside the bladder and prostate through the cystoscope.

Cystoscopy can be performed with the patient under general or local anesthesia. If a gel-type local anesthetic is placed in the male urethra a gentle spring-loaded clamp is placed across the penis to prevent oozing of the gel before it can take effect.

An exception to the procedures performed through the urethra is nephroscopy. The scopes used to view the outside of the kidney via a percutaneous access portal are introduced through the patient's skin at the level of the organ. The process is not the same as laparoscopy because the peritoneal cavity is not entered.

Access, Illumination, and Viewing – SPECIALTY SPECIFIC INSTRUMENTS

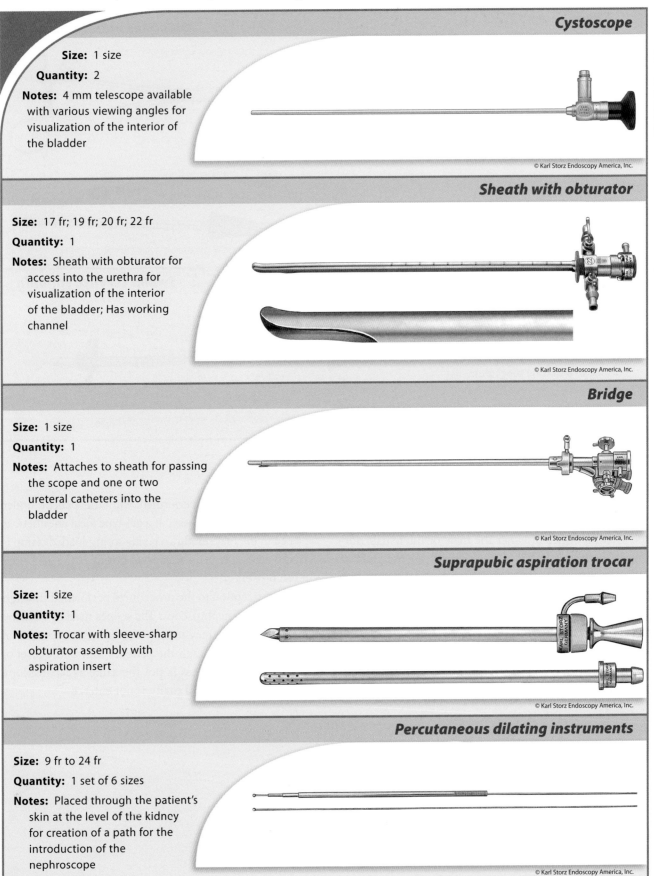

Cystoscope

Size: 1 size

Quantity: 2

Notes: 4 mm telescope available with various viewing angles for visualization of the interior of the bladder

© Karl Storz Endoscopy America, Inc.

FIGURE 15-123

Sheath with obturator

Size: 17 fr; 19 fr; 20 fr; 22 fr

Quantity: 1

Notes: Sheath with obturator for access into the urethra for visualization of the interior of the bladder; Has working channel

© Karl Storz Endoscopy America, Inc.

FIGURE 15-124

Bridge

Size: 1 size

Quantity: 1

Notes: Attaches to sheath for passing the scope and one or two ureteral catheters into the bladder

© Karl Storz Endoscopy America, Inc.

FIGURE 15-125

Suprapubic aspiration trocar

Size: 1 size

Quantity: 1

Notes: Trocar with sleeve-sharp obturator assembly with aspiration insert

© Karl Storz Endoscopy America, Inc.

FIGURE 15-126

Percutaneous dilating instruments

Size: 9 fr to 24 fr

Quantity: 1 set of 6 sizes

Notes: Placed through the patient's skin at the level of the kidney for creation of a path for the introduction of the nephroscope

© Karl Storz Endoscopy America, Inc.

FIGURE 15-127

Access, Illumination, and Viewing – SPECIALTY SPECIFIC INSTRUMENTS continued

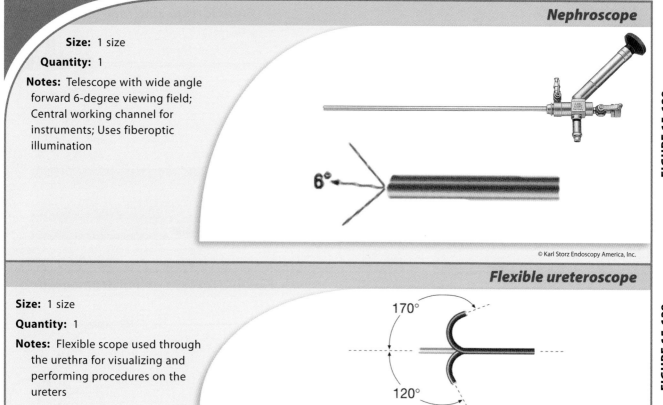

Nephroscope

Size: 1 size

Quantity: 1

Notes: Telescope with wide angle forward 6-degree viewing field; Central working channel for instruments; Uses fiberoptic illumination

© Karl Storz Endoscopy America, Inc.

FIGURE 15-128

Flexible ureteroscope

Size: 1 size

Quantity: 1

Notes: Flexible scope used through the urethra for visualizing and performing procedures on the ureters

© Karl Storz Endoscopy America, Inc.

FIGURE 15-129

CLAMPS

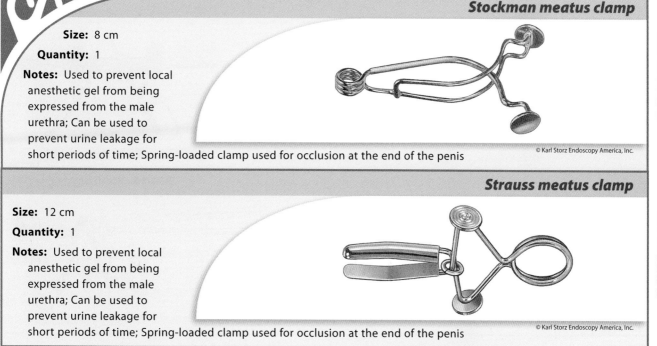

Stockman meatus clamp

Size: 8 cm

Quantity: 1

Notes: Used to prevent local anesthetic gel from being expressed from the male urethra; Can be used to prevent urine leakage for short periods of time; Spring-loaded clamp used for occlusion at the end of the penis

© Karl Storz Endoscopy America, Inc.

FIGURE 15-130

Strauss meatus clamp

Size: 12 cm

Quantity: 1

Notes: Used to prevent local anesthetic gel from being expressed from the male urethra; Can be used to prevent urine leakage for short periods of time; Spring-loaded clamp used for occlusion at the end of the penis

© Karl Storz Endoscopy America, Inc.

FIGURE 15-131

Working Elements – SPECIALTY SPECIFIC INSTRUMENTS

Rigid forceps and instrumentation

Size: 1 size

Quantity: 1 set

Notes: Rigid ring handle instruments that fit into the working channel of the cystoscope sheath

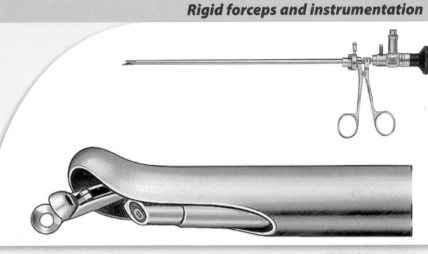

© Karl Storz Endoscopy America, Inc.

FIGURE 15-132

Flexible forceps and instrumentation

Size: 1 size

Quantity: 1

Notes: Flexible ring handle instruments that fit into the working channel of the cystoscope sheath

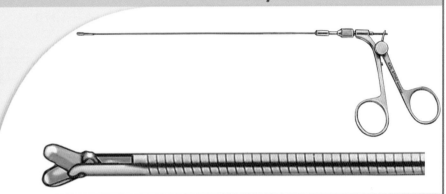

© Karl Storz Endoscopy America, Inc.

FIGURE 15-133

Lithotrite

Size: 1 size

Quantity: 1

Notes: Manual pistol grip 24 fr instrument for crushing bladder stones for passage through the urethra; Used with forward oblique telescopes

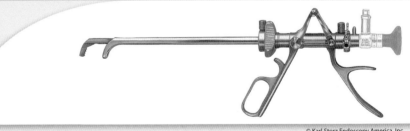

© Karl Storz Endoscopy America, Inc.

FIGURE 15-134

Stone crushing forceps

Size: 1 size

Quantity: 1

Notes: Manual ring-handled instrument for crushing bladder stones through the resectoscope sheath

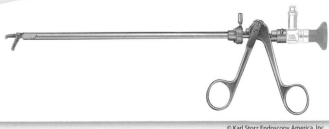

© Karl Storz Endoscopy America, Inc.

FIGURE 15-135

Working Elements – SPECIALTY SPECIFIC INSTRUMENTS *continued*

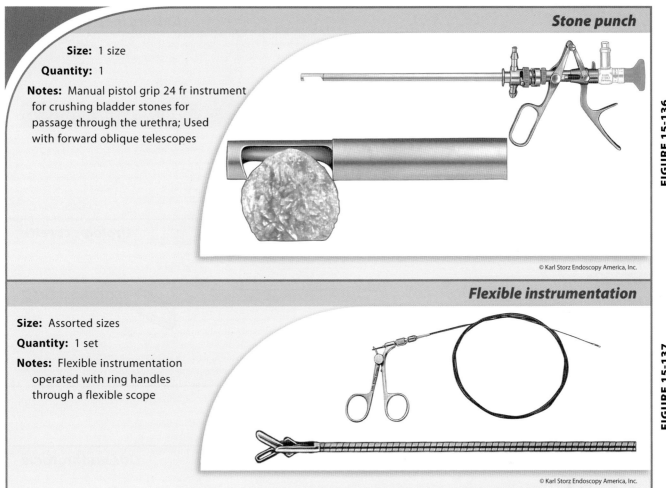

Stone punch

Size: 1 size

Quantity: 1

Notes: Manual pistol grip 24 fr instrument for crushing bladder stones for passage through the urethra; Used with forward oblique telescopes

© Karl Storz Endoscopy America, Inc.

FIGURE 15-136

Flexible instrumentation

Size: Assorted sizes

Quantity: 1 set

Notes: Flexible instrumentation operated with ring handles through a flexible scope

© Karl Storz Endoscopy America, Inc.

FIGURE 15-137

DEBULKING INSTRUMENTS

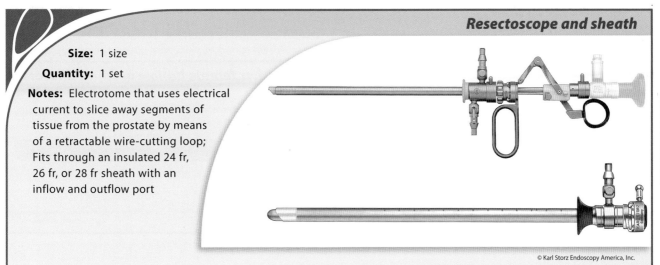

Resectoscope and sheath

Size: 1 size

Quantity: 1 set

Notes: Electrotome that uses electrical current to slice away segments of tissue from the prostate by means of a retractable wire-cutting loop; Fits through an insulated 24 fr, 26 fr, or 28 fr sheath with an inflow and outflow port

© Karl Storz Endoscopy America, Inc.

FIGURE 15-138

continues

DEBULKING INSTRUMENTS *continued*

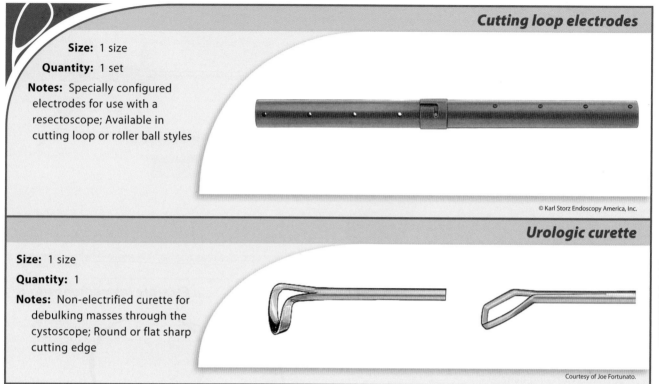

Cutting loop electrodes

Size: 1 size

Quantity: 1 set

Notes: Specially configured electrodes for use with a resectoscope; Available in cutting loop or roller ball styles

FIGURE 15-139

© Karl Storz Endoscopy America, Inc.

Urologic curette

Size: 1 size

Quantity: 1

Notes: Non-electrified curette for debulking masses through the cystoscope; Round or flat sharp cutting edge

FIGURE 15-140

Courtesy of Joe Fortunato.

PROBES AND DILATORS

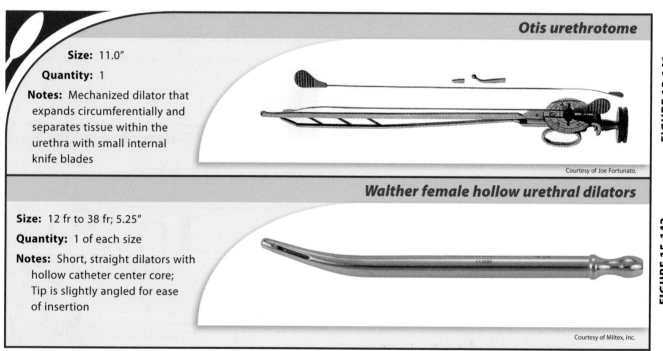

Otis urethrotome

Size: 11.0″

Quantity: 1

Notes: Mechanized dilator that expands circumferentially and separates tissue within the urethra with small internal knife blades

FIGURE 15-141

Courtesy of Joe Fortunato.

Walther female hollow urethral dilators

Size: 12 fr to 38 fr; 5.25″

Quantity: 1 of each size

Notes: Short, straight dilators with hollow catheter center core; Tip is slightly angled for ease of insertion

FIGURE 15-142

Courtesy of Miltex, Inc.

PROBES AND DILATORS *continued*

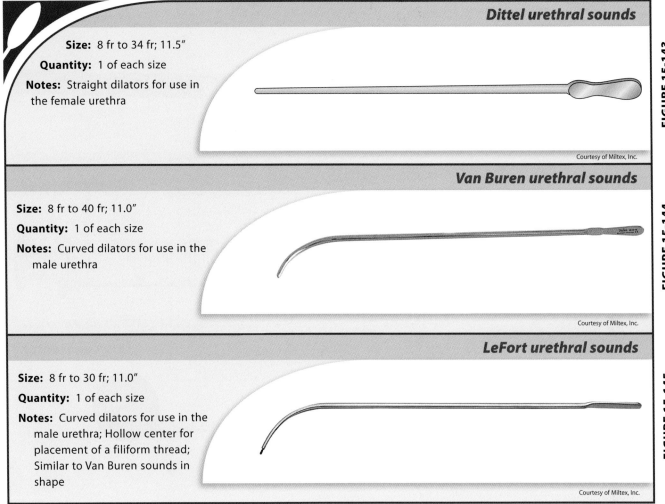

Dittel urethral sounds

Size: 8 fr to 34 fr; 11.5″

Quantity: 1 of each size

Notes: Straight dilators for use in the female urethra

Courtesy of Miltex, Inc.

FIGURE 15-143

Van Buren urethral sounds

Size: 8 fr to 40 fr; 11.0″

Quantity: 1 of each size

Notes: Curved dilators for use in the male urethra

Courtesy of Miltex, Inc.

FIGURE 15-144

LeFort urethral sounds

Size: 8 fr to 30 fr; 11.0″

Quantity: 1 of each size

Notes: Curved dilators for use in the male urethra; Hollow center for placement of a filiform thread; Similar to Van Buren sounds in shape

Courtesy of Miltex, Inc.

FIGURE 15-145

EVACUATION AND INSTILLATION INSTRUMENTS

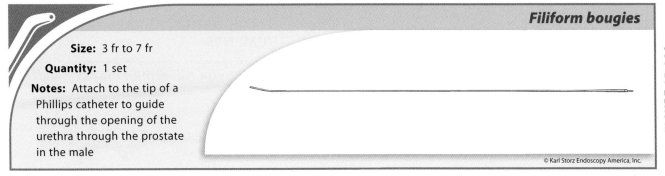

Filiform bougies

Size: 3 fr to 7 fr

Quantity: 1 set

Notes: Attach to the tip of a Phillips catheter to guide through the opening of the urethra through the prostate in the male

© Karl Storz Endoscopy America, Inc.

FIGURE 15-146

continues

EVACUATION AND INSTILLATION INSTRUMENTS *continued*

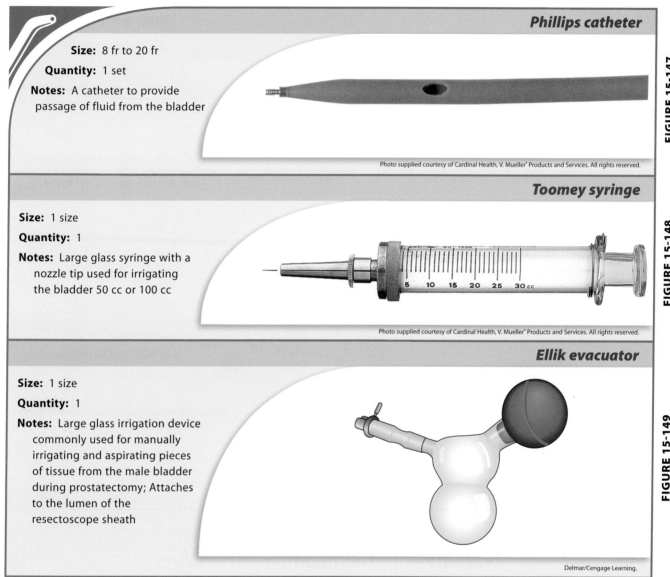

Phillips catheter

Size: 8 fr to 20 fr

Quantity: 1 set

Notes: A catheter to provide passage of fluid from the bladder

FIGURE 15-147

Toomey syringe

Size: 1 size

Quantity: 1

Notes: Large glass syringe with a nozzle tip used for irrigating the bladder 50 cc or 100 cc

FIGURE 15-148

Ellik evacuator

Size: 1 size

Quantity: 1

Notes: Large glass irrigation device commonly used for manually irrigating and aspirating pieces of tissue from the male bladder during prostatectomy; Attaches to the lumen of the resectoscope sheath

FIGURE 15-149

SPECIALTY SPECIFIC INSTRUMENTS

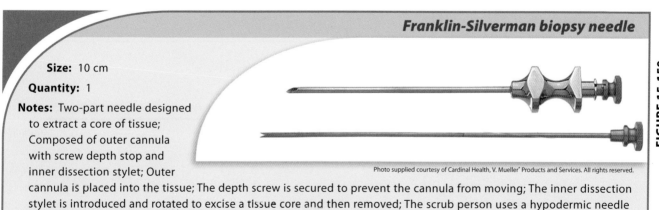

Franklin-Silverman biopsy needle

Size: 10 cm

Quantity: 1

Notes: Two-part needle designed to extract a core of tissue; Composed of outer cannula with screw depth stop and inner dissection stylet; Outer

FIGURE 15-150

cannula is placed into the tissue; The depth screw is secured to prevent the cannula from moving; The inner dissection stylet is introduced and rotated to excise a tissue core and then removed; The scrub person uses a hypodermic needle to tease the "worm-like" specimen onto gauze for transport to pathology

SUMMARY

Endoscopic surgery can be combined with robotics for procedural finesse unmatched by human capabilities. Some robotic components are merely hinged arms that attach to the rails of the operating bed. These flexible-locking arms can be positioned by the surgeon to facilitate the procedure. The robotic-steady position of the camera or grasper replaces a fatigable first assistant that could cause the field to shift, making the image on the video monitor difficult to visualize.

Other robotic devices have a remote control computerized component that permits the surgeon to use a voice-imprinted card to recognize verbal commands. In addition to voice cards, some robotic models have articulated "hands and arms" that respond to motions made on a console by a surgeon-operated joystick. Some of these endoscopic robotic units can perform maneuvers too small for human hands to perform with precision. The application of robotics to endoscopy has advanced the concept of minimally invasive surgery to new levels for the 21st century and beyond.

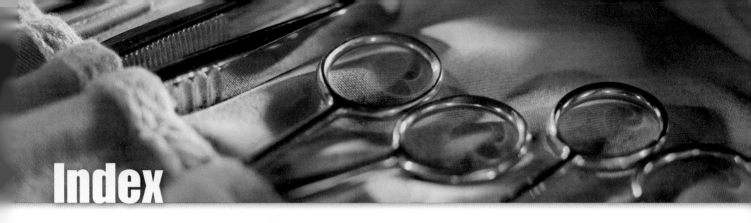

Index